W9-BFG-196

The Life Extension Foundation's

Disease
Prevention and Treatment
Protocols

The Life Extension Foundation's

Disease
Prevention and Treatment
Protocols

1998
Expanded Second Edition

❖ Offshore Medical Therapies
❖ Natural Alternatives to Toxic Drugs
❖ Therapies for "Untreatable" Diseases
❖ Based on Thousands of Research Studies

Visit The Life Extension Foundation website:
lef.org

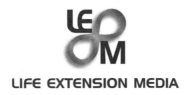

LIFE EXTENSION MEDIA

THE LIFE EXTENSION FOUNDATION DISEASE PREVENTION AND TREATMENT PROTOCOLS 1998. Copyright © 1997, 1998 William Faloon. All rights reserved. Printed in the United States. No part of this publication may be reproduced, stored in a retrieval system, or transmitted in any form by any means, electronic, mechancial, photo-copying, recording, or otherwise, without prior written permission of the Author.

Life Extension Foundation books may be purchased for personal, educational, business or sales promotional use. For information, please write: The Life Extension Foundation, P.O. Box 229120, Hollywood, Florida 33022-9120. Website: www.lef.org

SECOND EDITION

Cover design by Roy Rauschenberg/Jato Design

Set in Korinna

ISBN 0-9658777-1-X

Dedicated to those who needlessly suffered and died.

CONTENTS

Contents

Contents

Contents

Advanced Therapies for Diseases and Aging

In 1928, Dr. Alexander Fleming discovered penicillin. His work was published the very next year in the *British Journal of Experimental Pathology*. Nevertheless, the medical profession did not begin treating humans with this lifesaving therapy until 1941, and the general population did not gain access to penicillin until 1946.

Millions of people suffered and died from bacterial/infectious diseases when a cure had already been discovered and been published in a respected medical journal. For 18 years, millions of people could only watch helplessly as their loved ones suffered and died from a host of bacterial diseases that penicillin could have cured.

The leading cause of death and disability today is ignorance of therapies to prevent and treat the degenerative diseases of aging. This book is dedicated to eradicating the ignorance that is causing humans to suffer and die from diseases that may already have cures, or at least palliative therapies. Almost every therapy discussed in this book has been documented extensively by peer-reviewed, published studies from the most prestigious medical journals in the world. Despite this scientific evidence, these therapies are being largely ignored by the medical establishment.

The protocols in this book also are available on the Life Extension Foundation's web site (http://**www.lef.org**), enabling the user to access thousands of scientific abstracts that support the use of the therapies in these protocols in preventing and treating diseases.

The information in this book is not intended to replace the attention or advice of a physician or other health care professional. Anyone who wishes to embark on any dietary, drug, exercise, or other lifestyle change intended to prevent or treat a specific disease or condition should consult with, and seek clearance and guidance from, a qualified health care professional. The book offers general suggestions based upon scientific evidence, not specific advice or recommendations. Patients need to be treated in an individual manner by their own personal physician, and the information in this book must not be considered a substitute for the individual attention of a personal physician.

In some cases, we repeat scientific findings and recommendations verbatim in related protocols for which these findings and recommendations are valid.

For additional information on the therapies discussed in these protocols, and to examine the thousands of scientific abstracts that document their value, please pay a visit to the Life Extension Foundation website at **http://www.lef.org**. Just click on ***Disease Therapies*** on our home page. Protocols are updated regularly on the Foundation's website.

The Life Extension Foundation

Before you consider making use of the disease prevention and treatment protocols in this book, you should know something about the organization that developed them.

The Life Extension Foundation is the world's largest organization dedicated to the investigation of every possible method of preventing and treating diseases, aging and death. The Foundation funds scientific research aimed at achieving an indefinitely extended lifespan. Foundation members benefit now by having access to lifesaving information and therapies that will not be available to the general public for years.

Life Extension Foundation members are people who believe in taking advantage of documented scientific therapies to prevent diseases and slow aging. The medical literature contains thousands of papers on the use of antioxidant supplements, hormone therapies, and other medications that have been shown to improve the quality and length of life. Life extensionists attempt to use this scientific information, in conjunction with their physicians, to improve their chances of living longer in good health.

The Life Extension Foundation was incorporated in 1980, but its founders have been writing about and funding anti-aging research since the 1960s.

Research supported by the Life Extension Foundation has documented the value of antioxidants and other types of compounds in preventing diseases, and in protecting cells against ischemia (reduced blood flow). Ischemia can be caused by the blockage of a coronary artery, leading to a heart attack, or the blockage of a cerebral artery, which can lead to a stroke.

The Life Extension Foundation supports a research facility in Southern California that conducts path-breaking ischemia research. The Foundation also supports another Southern California facility that conducts research to stop death cold in its tracks by achieving suspended animation. Additional Foundation funds have been committed to evaluating the effects of nutrients and hormones on aging and lifespan in laboratory mice—nutrients and hormones commonly used by life extensionists. These experiments are being carried out by eminent scientists at institutions such as the University of Wisconsin at Madison and the University of California at Riverside.

The Life Extension Foundation maintains the highest quality-control standards by offering products that contain pharmaceutical-grade nutrients. The purity of your supplements is critical if you plan to take them for the rest of your life. For example, many discount products include low-grade vitamin C imported from China that contains traces of toxic arsenic, lead and iron. Since the Food and Drug Administration (FDA) does not believe anyone should take more than 100 mg a day of vitamin C, the agency permits the importation of this contaminated vitamin C. However, life extensionists take 3,000 to 20,000 mg a day of vitamin C, so it is crucial that they use pharmaceutical-grade vitamin C that has gone through 18 purification steps to remove contaminants.

Since the FDA does not properly regulate dietary supplement manufacturing, the Foundation employs an independent quality-control expert to verify that only pharmaceutical-grade nutrients are used in its products. The Life Extension Foundation also has access to a state-of-the art laboratory, where trained chemists conduct assays of the nutrients in its products, and develop new assays to guarantee quality control in even the most advanced formulas. The reason you take nutrients is because of published research indicating specific health benefits. In these studies, only pharmaceutical-grade nutrients are used. If you expect to obtain the same health benefits, you need to take the exact same nutrients used in these studies.

Members of the Life Extension Foundation receive large discounts that enable them to purchase premium-grade nutrient supplements at up to 60% below the prices charged at health-food stores for similar products.

The Foundation monitors thousands of scientific studies every week to make sure its disease-preventing formulas include the most effective life-extending nutrients in the world, and its protocols are up to date. The Foundation interacts with the foremost medical and anti-aging researchers in the world in order to obtain inside information about the latest life extension breakthroughs. Foundation members often gain access to their disease-preventing, anti-aging findings even before they are published in science and medical journals.

✔ In 1980, the Foundation recommended antioxidants to prevent the diseases of aging.
✔ In 1981, the Foundation introduced DHEA as a disease-preventing therapy.
✔ In 1983, the Foundation recommended aspirin to prevent heart attacks.
✔ In 1983, the Foundation introduced coenzyme Q10 to prevent and treat heart disease.
✔ In 1983, the Foundation warned that excessive iron causes cancer and heart disease.
✔ In 1985, the Foundation made lycopene available to help prevent cancer.
✔ In 1986, the Foundation recommended deprenyl as an anti-aging drug.
✔ In 1988, the Foundation made phosphatidylserine available to slow brain aging.
✔ In 1991, the Foundation sued the FDA for quicker approval of lifesaving drugs.
✔ In 1992, the Foundation introduced melatonin for sleep and the prevention of disease.
✔ In 1995, the Foundation introduced the first anti-aging drug formula in the world.
✔ In 1996, the Foundation published 110 disease prevention and treatment protocols based upon published medical research.

✔ In 1997, the Foundation introduced Americans to SAMe (S-adenosylmethionine), a safe-
and effective natural anti-depressant that also is effective for liver diseases, osteoarthritis
and other conditions.

✔ In 1998, the Foundation introduced Americans to the urtica dioca extract used in
Germany to treat benign prostate enlargement.

New medical information is expanding at an exponential rate. The first edition of *Disease Prevention and Treatment Protocols,* which was published less than a year ago, contained 327 pages and was based on about 2,500 scientific abstracts. Here, in the second edition, the Life Extension Foundation's protocols have been expanded and improved, based upon 1,500 additional scientific abstracts.

The Life Extension Foundation can assist you in finding offshore pharmacies that will sell to you advanced European and Asian medications that are usually five or more years ahead of FDA-approved drugs. The Foundation is the foremost organization in the fight for the rights of Americans to import lifesaving medications for their own personal use.

Call the Life Extension Foundation today for membership information: 1-800-841-5433. Or visit the Foundation's web site at **http://www.lef.org**.

Medical Advisory Board

Andrew M. Baer, M.D., focuses on anti-aging and mind/body medicine, consciousness technology, degenerative diseases, and the treatment of age-associated memory impairment. Dr. Baer has conducted numerous lectures, and hosts *Health Talk*, a radio program from Youngstown, Ohio.

Gustavo Tovar Baez, M.D., operates the Life Extension Clinic in Caracas, Venezuela. He is the first physician in Caracas to specialize in anti-aging medicine.

Sam Baxas, M.D., head of the Baxamed Medical Center for Youth Restoration, in Basel, Switzerland, has developed innovative cell therapy and growth hormone therapies used in the treatment of chronic fatigue syndrome, muscle-wasting disease, Parkinson's disease, arthritis and lupus.

Ricardo Bernales, M.D., is a general practitioner in Chicago, Ill., focusing on allergies, bronchial asthma and immunodeficiency. He is on the medical staff of St. Elizabeth Hospital in Chicago, and is a board-certified pediatrician and allergist/immunologist.

Michael Boone, M.D., is a clinician who devotes his entire practice to nutritional medicine. He participates in research conducted at Tufts University, in Medford, Mass., aimed at substantiating the role that nutrition plays in the prevention of disease. Dr. Boone is actively involved in developing non-invasive tests to measure oxidative stress, toxicities and nutritional deficiencies.

Thomas F. Crais, M.D., F.A.C.S., is a board-certified plastic surgeon, and is medical director of the microsurgical research and training laboratory, Southern Baptist Hospital, in New Orleans, La. He also has served as clinical instructor in surgery at Louisiana State University Medical Center, and is widely published in scientific and medical journals.

Martin Dayton, M.D., D.O., practices holistic, alternative and mainstream conventional medicine at the Sunny Isles Medical Center in North Miami Beach, Fla. His major therapeutic areas of concentration include nutrition, aging, chelation therapy, holistic medicine and oxidative medicine. Dr. Dayton also utilizes electroacupuncture, cellular therapy, and hormone therapies.

Arnold Fox, M.D., is an internist, cardiologist and practicing physician in Beverly Hills, Calif., specializing in anti-aging medicine using nutritional and hormone therapies, as well as more traditional medicine. He is the author of a number of books for the general public, including *The Fat Blocker Diet*.

Carmen Fusco, R.N., who has served on the advisory board of the Life Extension Foundation since its inception, is a research scientist and clinical nutritionist in New York City. Ms. Fusco has lectured about and written numerous articles on the biochemical approach to the prevention of aging and degenerative diseases, is a member of the New York Academy of Sciences, and is formulator of the Rejuvenex skin care line.

Miguelangelo Gonzalez, M.D., is a certified plastic and reconstructive surgeon at the Plastic and Reconstructive Surgery Institute of Jalisco, Guadalajara, Mexico. In private practice in Nogales, Mexico, Dr. Gonzalez is the founder of a non-profit organization called "New Face" ("Nueva Cara") that provides charity plastic and reconstructive surgery to children with cleft lip and palate deformities.

Garry F. Gordon, M.D., D.O., who lives and works in Payson, Ariz., conducts in-depth research into alternative medical approaches that may have applications for effective treatment of complex medical problems that are unresponsive to traditional therapies. Dr. Gordon also formulates and markets specialized vitamin, mineral and herbal products for the professional and lay markets.

Farhad Hakimi, D.M.D., is affiliated with St. Luke's-Roosevelt Hospital Center, New York City, and had been professor of dentistry for 15 years at New York University. He specializes in maxillofacial prosthodontics, with a practice in New York City. He invented the Snore/Stress Relieving Device, a non-invasive treatment for snoring and obstructive sleep apnea.

Richard Heifetz, M.D., is a board-certified anesthesiologist, specializing in the delivery of anesthesia for office-based plastic/cosmetic surgery, chelation therapy, pain management, and nutritional and longevity medicine. He is affiliated with The Surgery Center, Santa Rosa, Calif.

Maurice D. Marholin, D.O., D.C., was graduated from Cleveland Chiropractic College as well as Nova Southeastern University, and is currently serving his residency in family practice at the University of Alabama, in Birmingham. His expertise also encompasses osteoarthritis, and the effects of exercise in the elderly.

Herbert Pardell, D.O., operates an anti-aging clinical practice in North Miami, Fla., that specializes in hyperbaric oxygen, chelation and alternative medicine. He is the medical director of the Life Extension Foundation.

Lambert Titus K. Parker, M.D., practices internal medicine at the Schuyler Hospital Primary Care Clinic, in Montour Falls, N.Y. He is the director of the clinic's intensive care unit, is medical director of Schuyler Hospital Inc., and is a hospital board trustee. He has also been an associate professor of medicine with the State University of New York.

Joseph P. Pepping, Pharm.D., is assistant director of pharmacy services at St. Francis Medical Center in Honolulu, Hawaii, where he oversees all clinical pharmacy activities, with emphases on drug usage evaluation studies, adverse drug reaction reporting, and pain management consultation for oncology and hospice patients.

Patrick Quillan, Ph.D., R.D., C.N.S., is director of the Rational Healing Institute in Tulsa, Okla., where he develops programs and products to promote rational healing principles in world health care. He has served as vice president of nutrition for Cancer Treatment Centers of America, and is an internationally respected author and nutritional consultant.

Marc R. Rose, M.D., practices ophthalmology with his brother, Michael Rose in Los Angeles, Calif., and is president of the Rose Eye Medical Group. He is on the hospital staffs of Pacific Alliance Medical Center, Los Angeles; St. Joseph Medical Center, Burbank, Calif.; and North Hollywood Medical Center, North Hollywood, Calif.

Michael R. Rose, M.D., is a board-certified ophthalmologist with the Rose Eye Medical Group in Los Angeles, Calif., and is active on the hospital staffs at the University of Southern California Doheny Laser Vision Medical Center, and the UCLA Jules Stein Eye Institute.

Roman Rozencwaig, M.D., is a pioneer in research on melatonin and aging, and was the first to postulate the theory that aging is a syndrome of melatonin deficiency resulting from the gradual failure of the pineal gland. Dr. Rozencwaig practices in Montreal, Canada, and is on the staff at Reddy Memorial Hospital and Bishop Medical Centre, in Montreal.

Carol Ann Ryser, M.D., F.A.A.P., is medical director of Health Centers of America, in Kansas City, Mo. Dr. Ryser is on the advisory board of the University of Missouri for Family Studies and the Coalition for Positive Family Relationships, and focuses on pediatrics and mental health.

E.K. Schandl, Ph.D., is a clinical biochemist and oncobiologist with the Center for Metabolic Disorders, and director of American Metabolic Laboratories, in Hollywood, Fla. Dr. Schandl, Scientific Director of the Life Extension Foundation, is the developer of the Cancer Profile, a specialized battery of tests designed to predict the risk of developing cancer long before symptoms occur.

Ramon Scruggs, M.D., has established a national reputation as a clinical expert in the use of natural human hormones for the treatment of a variety of metabolic diseases, and is a leading practitioner in the field of anti-aging medicine. The Costa Mesa, Calif., physician has successfully treated such chronic illnesses as diabetes, asthma, hypertension, arthritis, allergies, heart disease, carpal tunnel syndromes, chronic fatigue and other ills, often with the reduction or elimination of drugs and surgery.

Herbert R. Slavin, M.D., is medical director of The Institute of Advanced Medicine, in Lauderhill, Fla., specializing in internal medicine, cardiovascular disease, anti-aging medicine, disease prevention, chelation therapy, natural hormone replacement therapy, detoxification programs and nutritional supplementation. He is a staff physician at Florida Medical Center, Fort Lauderdale.

R. Arnold Smith, M.D., is a clinical radiation oncologist who specializes in using immunotherapy to enhance the safety and efficacy of conventional cancer therapies. Dr. Smith operates an independent oncology practice where he integrates conventional and innovative therapies.

Stephen L. Smith, M.D., owns and operates Physicians Immediate Care Center, an ambulatory care center in Richland, Wash. A graduate of the University of Washington School of Medicine, Dr. Smith has conducted post-graduate training and certification in treating allergies, and is a member of the American Society for Lasers in Medicine and Surgery.

Stephen Strum, M.D., is a practicing clinical oncologist who specializes in integrating conventional and nutritional therapies for the treatment of prostate cancer. He practices in Playa del Rey, Calif.

Javier Torres, M.D., is a member of the American Academy of Physical Medicine and Rehabilitation, and is on the medical staffs of Sunrise Hospital, Desert Springs Hospital, Valley Hospital and Mountain View Hospital, all in Las Vegas, Nev.

Jonathan V. Wright, M.D., is a family practitioner at the Tahoma Clinic, in Kent, Wash. Dr. Wright emphasizes preventive medicine, nutritional biochemistry, allergy, anti-aging and natural hormone replacement therapy. Dr. Wright also is a board member of the Vitamin C Foundation and the American Preventive Medical Association, among many other groups.

PROTOCOLS

Acetaminophen (Tylenol) Poisoning: Acute and Chronic

Most over-the-counter (OTC) pain remedies can cause potentially lethal side effects. People in chronic pain often abuse OTC pain medications such as acetaminophen, which is sold under many brand names, the most popular being Tylenol. One result of acetaminophen injury is the generation of toxic free radicals in the liver.

If a person attempts to commit suicide by taking an entire bottle of acetaminophen, the emergency room doctor will administer an antioxidant drug called Mucosil (Mucomyst). If administered in time, Mucosil can save the patient's life by inhibiting free radical damage to the liver caused by acetaminophen-induced depletion of hepatic glutathione.

The active ingredient in Mucosil is the nutrient N-acetylcysteine (NAC). N-acetylcysteine suppresses the toxic free radicals generated by ingested acetaminophen. If you have to take acetaminophen, we suggest you take the amino acid N-acetylcysteine or L-cysteine along with at least one gram of vitamin C with each dose of acetaminophen.

One of the body's own antioxidants, glutathione, protects the liver against acetaminophen-induced free radical injury. Another approach to protecting against acetaminophen-induced free radical liver damage is to take one capsule of a multi-nutrient formula that contains glutathione, vitamin C and cysteine with each dose of acetaminophen. This antioxidant formula will provide significant protection to the liver.

Acetaminophen also can cause permanent kidney damage when taken over extended periods of time. This damage can be lethal to those with underlying kidney disease. There are no nutrient supplements known to protect against acetaminophen-induced kidney damage, although the amino acid taurine (1,000 mg two to three times a day) and high doses of vitamin E succinate (800 to 1,200 IU a day) might be helpful.

The Food and Drug Administration does not require the manufacturers of Tylenol and other brands of acetaminophen to warn people with kidney disease to avoid this pain medication. However, for those in chronic pain who cannot find relief from natural pain relief therapies (see protocols for Pain and Arthritis), it is suggested that Tylenol and other brands of acetaminophen be used sparingly.

Some people alternate other types of OTC pain-relieving drugs, such as Advil, aspirin and Naprosyn, to avoid using acetaminophen on a daily basis. Although these drugs also have dangerous side effects, alternating their use may help to reduce their toxicity.

To illustrate how dangerous acetaminophen can be, one study showed that people who used acetaminophen with other pain relievers on a regular basis had a three- to eightfold increase in their risk of kidney cancer. Kidney cancer is very difficult to treat. The liver/kidney/heart muscle toxicities and the cancer risks of analgesic drugs have not been reported by most media, which reap tremendous profits from the advertising of pain-relief products.

When using the drug Mucosil (N-acetylcysteine) to treat acute liver failure from aceta-minophen overdose, it is crucial that the drug be administered immediately, and that it be continued for at least 36 hours in all cases. Optimal results occur when N-acetylcysteine is administered within 10 hours of acetaminophen overdose. N-acetylcysteine also is effective when given after 15 hours of acetaminophen poisoning. Treatment with N-acetylcysteine should not be discontinued until all clinical signs of toxicity have subsided. Permanent liver injury can occur if N-acetylcysteine therapy is discontinued too soon. Patients who develop chronic liver failure should be treated with a prolonged course of N-acetylcysteine.

Product availability: Glutathione, vitamin C and cysteine capsules, NAC (N-acetylcysteine) caps, taurine, vitamin E succinate caps and vitamin C caps are available from the Life Extension Foundation. To order, phone 1-800-544-4440.

Adrenal Disease

Aging and the diseases of aging can cause a decline in critical hormones produced by the adrenal glands. The most important hormone produced primarily in the adrenal glands is pregnenolone. Pregnenolone is converted into crucial anti-aging hormones such as DHEA (dehydroepiandrosterone), estrogen, progesterone and testosterone.

Pregnenolone supplementation may help to rectify hormone imbalances caused by aging-induced adrenal insufficiency, which can cause life-threatening conditions. One of these imbalances involves over-production of the hormone cortisol, which has been called a "death hormone" because it is a cause of immune suppression, atherosclerosis, brain cell injury and accelerated aging. Pregnenolone or DHEA supplementation may protect against the over-production of cortisol from the adrenal glands. Vitamin C and aspirin may block excessive cortisol production.

A protocol to treat adrenal disease includes one 50-mg pregnenolone capsule once a day for one week. Increase to two capsules a day the second week and then three capsules a day the third week. Prior to starting the protocol and during week four, have DHEA sulfate and cortisol blood tests to help determine your state of adrenal function. If your cortisol levels remain elevated, one-quarter tablet a day of aspirin taken with a heavy meal and 3,000 mg of vitamin C a day could suppress your cortisol levels. The European drug KH3 (the active ingre-dient is procaine) can block some of the cell-damaging effects of cortisol. To help protect against cortisol toxicity, take one to two KH3 capsules in the morning on an empty stomach and one to two KH3 capsules in mid-afternoon on an empty stomach.

CAUTION: Some adrenal diseases, such as Addison's disease, involve under-production of cortisol. This is an acute, potentially life-threatening condition that requires expert physician intervention. Glucocorticoid and mineralocorticoid drugs are prescribed for Addison's dis-ease. Once cortisol levels are stabilized, serum levels of DHEA should be evaluated to deter-mine if DHEA-replacement therapy is warranted. In 80 percent of cases, Addison's disease is caused by an autoimmune attack on the adrenal glands. Before taking DHEA or pregnenolone, refer to the Foundation's DHEA-Pregnenolone Precautions in this book. Also refer to the Autoimmune Disease protocol for additional suggestions.

Product availability: Pregnenolone capsules, DHEA, vitamin C powder and capsules, and ¼ aspirin tablets (Healthprin) can be ordered by phoning 1-800-544-4440. KH3 is not available from the Life Extension Foundation. Call for a list of companies abroad that sell KH3 to Americans for personal use.

Age-Associated Mental Impairment (Brain Aging, Stroke, Head Trauma, Memory Loss)

Aging precipitates a progressive decline in overall cognitive function. Aging causes us to lose our ability to store and retrieve short-term memories and to learn new information. Many neurological diseases are directly related to aging.

The Life Extension Foundation has evaluated thousands of published studies showing that brain aging can at least be partially controlled. Some of these studies demonstrate a preventive effect, while others show a benefit in reversing cognitive impairment caused by normal aging or by a specific disease of aging, such as stroke.

There are several classes of agents that enhance cognitive function and protect against neurological aging. The most commonly used memory-enhancing nutrients are choline, lecithin and phosphatidylcholine, which are precursors to the chemical neurotransmitter acetylcholine in the brain. Acetylcholine helps brain cells communicate with each other, and plays an important role in learning and memory. Acetylcholine deficiency can predispose a person to a wide range of neurological diseases, including Alzheimer's disease and stroke. Suggested dosage ranges are:

- ❖ 2,500 to 10,000 mg a day of choline
- ❖ 10,000 to 15,000 mg a day of lecithin
- ❖ 1,200 to 6,000 mg of phosphatidylcholine

Take choline, lecithin and phosphatidylcholine early in the day for maximum improvements in brain productivity throughout the day.

Another mechanism of memory enhancement involves boosting the energy output of brain cells. Aging causes a decline in the ability of neurons to take up glucose and to produce mitochondrial energy. This decline in energy production causes memory and cognitive deficits and results in the accumulation of cellular debris that eventually kills brain cells. When enough brain cells have died from accumulated cellular debris, senility is usually diagnosed. Stroke and head trauma victims are especially in need of brain cell energy-enhancing agents, though everyone who undergoes normal aging will suffer from cerebral circulatory deficits and reduced brain cell energy output. Therapies that fit into the category of brain cell energy enhancers include:

- ❖ 1,000 to 2,000 mg a day of acetyl-L-carnitine
- ❖ 120 mg a day of ginkgo biloba extract
- ❖ 100 to 200 mg a day of coenzyme Q10
- ❖ 2,400 to 4,800 mg a day of piracetam
- ❖ 250 to 1,000 mg a day of centrophenoxine
- ❖ 4 to 10 mg of Hydergine (ergoloid mesylates)
- ❖ 5 to 10 mg a day of NADH (nicotinamide adenine dinucleotide)
- ❖ 100 to 300 mg a day of phosphatidylserine
- ❖ 50 to 100 mg three times a day of Picamilon
- ❖ 200 mg three times a day of pyritinol
- ❖ 30 mg three times a day of nimodipine

The most important of the above to take on a daily basis are ginkgo biloba extract, coenzyme Q10 (CoQ10) and acetyl-L-carnitine. Thousands of published studies show that ginkgo, coQ10 and acetyl-L-carnitine play a critical role in brain cell energy metabolism both in healthy people and in those suffering from neurological diseases.

For healthy people seeking to improve cognitive function, the other cerebral metabolic enhancers can be tried individually or in combination to assess their ability to boost memory and intelligence. The combination of centrophenoxine and piracetam is one of the more popular therapies in Europe to improve memory and enhance mental energy. The Russian drug Picamilon improves blood flow to cerebral vessels and enhances energy levels. Pyritinol has been used in Europe to enhance neuronal metabolism in order to help restore youthful cognitive function.

Stroke and head trauma victims should consider multiple brain cell energy-enhancing therapies to help restore circulation and energy levels of cells damaged by transient ischemic attack. It is especially recommended that stroke and head trauma victims consider taking 30 mg of the prescription drug Nimotop (nimodipine) three times a day in addition to the nutrients, hormones and drugs recommended in this protocol. Nimotop is a calcium-channel blocking drug specific to the central nervous system. It dramatically improves cerebral blood flow and blocks excess calcium infiltration into brain cells. Nimotop is an FDA-approved drug that has been ignored by most neurologists treating victims of stroke and other age-related neurological diseases.

Phosphatidylserine plays an important role in maintaining the integrity of brain cell membranes. The breakdown of brain cell membranes prevents glucose and other nutrients from entering the cell. By protecting the integrity of brain cell membranes, phosphatidylserine facilitates the efficient transport of energy-producing nutrients into cells, thus enhancing brain cell energy metabolism,

In order to take advantage of increases in brain cell energy, elevated levels of acetylcholine, and enhanced brain cell membrane function, it is important to take hormones to help restore the synchronization of youthful activity within the aging brain. Two hormones that are well documented to improve brain cell activity are DHEA and pregnenolone.

Pregnenolone and DHEA have been shown to be memory-enhancing hormones. Pregnenolone is converted into DHEA within the body. DHEA helps to preserve youthful neurological function. Together, pregnenolone and DHEA help to maintain the "program" brain cells need to store and retrieve short-term memories. Pregnenolone initiates the memory-storage process by stimulating adenylate cyclase activity, which is needed to activate and regulate other critical enzymes required for cellular energy production. Pregnenolone then regulates the sequential flow of calcium ions through the cell membrane. The pattern of calcium ion exchange has great informational content and may determine how memories are encoded by neurons. Pregnenolone also modulates chemical reactions, calcium-protein binding, gene activation, protein turnover, and enzymatic reactions involved in the storage and retrieval of memory. Aging results in a severe deficiency of pregnenolone and DHEA. Without adequate pregnenolone and DHEA, we gradually lose the neuronal synchronization required for optimal cognitive function.

DHEA is naturally synthesized in abundance in young people from pregnenolone in brain and adrenal cells. It is known to affect the excitability of hippocampal neurons. Current findings suggest that DHEA enhances memory by facilitating the induction of neural plasticity. Refer to the DHEA-Pregnenolone Precautions in this book before using DHEA or pregnenolone.

The dosage range for pregnenolone is 50 to 150 mg in three divided doses. The recommended dosage for DHEA is 25 mg three times a day for men, and 15 mg three times a day for women. Anyone who is planning to take pregnenolone or DHEA should have a DHEA-S blood test six weeks after initiating therapy, in order to help evaluate the correctness of the dosage.

A convenient way of taking pregnenolone (which may convert to DHEA), along with phosphatidylserine and choline, is to take five capsules a day of the nutrient formula Cognitex. Five capsules of Cognitex contain the suggested daily doses of pregnenolone, choline, vitamin B5 and phosphatidylserine.

Another hormone that may help prevent age-associated mental impairment is melatonin, which is secreted by the pineal gland. Melatonin is a powerful antioxidant that also plays a role in brain cell synchronization. The suggested dose of melatonin for neurological function for people over age 35 is 500 micrograms to 3 milligrams (mg) a night. For people already afflicted with an aging-related degenerative brain disease, 3 to 10 mg a night of melatonin is suggested.

Vitamins can protect and enhance cognitive function. A six-year study was done to determine nutritional status and cognitive performance in 137 elderly people. Several significant associations were observed between cognition and vitamin status. Intake of the B vitamins thiamine, riboflavin, niacin and folate resulted in better abstraction performance. Higher plasma vitamin C levels were associated with better visuospatial performance. Higher past intake of vitamin A, vitamin E, vitmain B6 and vitamin B12 was related to better performance on visuospatial recall and/or abstraction tests. The use of vitamin supplements was associated with better performance on a difficult visuospatial test and an abstraction test.

In a study of 70 male subjects, aged 54 to 81 years, elevated homocysteine levels were associated with poorer cognitive function. Elevated homocysteine was an independent factor in cognitive deficit, as were low levels of vitamin B12, folate and vitamin B6. Another study showed that less-than optimal levels of vitamin B6, B12 and folic acid were shown to create a deficiency of S-adenosylmethionine (SAMe). A deficiency of SAMe could be a cause of depression, dementia or demyelinating myelopathy. The neurotoxic effects of homocysteine may be a cause of psychiatric disturbances that are correctable by proper vitamin supplementation.

Free radicals have been implicated as an initiator of DNA damage that results in the breakdown of brain cell metabolism. Scientists suggest that the consumption of antioxidants, especially vitamin E, can reduce the risk of senility. The daily dose of Life Extension Mix provides broad-spectrum antioxidant protection for brain cells. The standard dose of Life Extension Mix (three tablets, three times a day) provides high doses of specific nutrients that may provide significant improvement in mental function based on several studies in well-nourished human populations. Vitamin B12 deficiency in particular is a major cause of neurological impairment in the elderly. Sublingual vitamin B12 tablets taste good and are a popular method for people to add an additional 1,000 to 2,000 micrograms a day of B12 to their diet.

Product availability: Cognitex, pregnenolone, DHEA, acetyl-L-carnitine, ginkgo biloba, DMAE, lecithin, NADH, coenzyme Q10, Life Extension Mix, and melatonin are available from the Life Extension Buyers Club by calling 1-800-544-4440. Piracetam and centrophenoxine are available from overseas companies for personal use only. A list of these companies can be obtained by phoning 1-800-544-4440.

Alcohol-Induced Hangover: Prevention

The consumption of alcohol results in the formation of two very toxic compounds: acetaldehyde and malondialdehyde. These compounds generate massive free radical damage to cells throughout the body. The free radical damage generated by these alcohol metabolites creates an effect in the body similar to radiation poisoning. That is why people feel so sick the day after consuming too much alcohol. If the proper combination of antioxidants are taken at the time the alcohol is consumed or before the inebriated individual goes to bed, the hangover and much of the cellular damage caused by alcohol may be prevented.

Aging makes us increasingly vulnerable to alcohol-induced hangover, liver injury and damage to the central nervous system. In the elderly, alcohol and drug-induced injury are more common, more serious, and recovery is more difficult.

Nutrients that neutralize alcohol by-products and protect cells against the damaging effects of alcohol include vitamin C, vitamin B1, the amino acids cysteine and glutathione, along with vitamin E and selenium. There are several commercial formulas that can be taken at the time the alcohol is consumed and/or before bedtime to help prevent a hangover. One of these formulas is called Anti-Alcohol Antioxidants. Six capsules of this formula contain the proper amounts of antioxidant nutrients to help prevent a hangover.

Another product drinkers use is Kyolic Garlic Formula 105. Garlic contains s-allyl-cysteine and this particular formula also contains vitamin C and vitamin E, beta-carotene and selenium. Since the heavy consumption of alcohol produces many deleterious effects within the body, including an increased risk of cancer, liver disease and neurological disease, it is suggested that hangover-prevention formulas such as Kyolic Garlic Formula 105 and Anti-Alcohol Antioxidants be taken any time alcohol is consumed.

Free radical damage is a major mechanism by which ethanol damages the liver. As has already been discussed, supplementing with the right antioxidants while consuming ethanol significantly reduces damage to cells throughout the body. Ethanol also damages the liver by depressing an enzyme required to convert methionine into S-adenosylmethionine (SAMe). A deficiency of SAMe can predispose an alcoholic to develop liver cirrhosis. An alcohol-induced depletion of SAMe can be bypassed by SAMe supplementation, which restores hepatic SAMe levels and attenuates parameters of ethanol-induced liver injury significantly.

Supplementation with 400 to 800 mg of SAMe twice a day may help to reverse alcoholic cirrhosis. For those alcoholics who cannot afford SAMe, supplementation with 500 mg of trimethylglycine (TMG, also known as glycine betaine), 800 micrograms of folic acid and 500 micrograms of vitamin B12, twice a day, could help the liver to synthesize S-adenosylmethionine. Phosphatidylcholine supplementation, at a dose of 2,000 mg a day, may protect against alcohol-induced septal fibrosis, cirrhosis and lipid peroxidation.

Chronic alcohol consumption can constrict arteries in the brain and lead to neurological deficit. Supplementation with 500 mg to 1,500 mg a day of magnesium could help keep cerebral blood vessels open by blocking excess infiltration of calcium into endothelial cells. European medications such as Picamilon (50 mg, three times a day) and pyritinol (200 mg, three times a day) could help prevent and restore neurological function lost because of chronic ethanol intake.

Product availability: The Anti-Alcohol Antioxidant formula, Kyolic Garlic Formula 105, magnesium and S-adenosylmethionine can be obtained from the Life Extension Buyers Club by calling 1-800-544-4440. You can also be referred you to suppliers of offshore medications such as Picamilon and pyritinol.

Allergies

Allergies are abnormal hypersensitive reactions to toxic substances (toxins). Allergic reactions occur when, in response to these allergens, our immune system turns against our body's own cells. These autoimmune reactions often involve the creation of damaging free radicals.

Toxins are normally handled within the body by detoxification systems. When the toxic load overwhelms these systems, the "gates" to our bodies (the skin, lungs and gastrointestinal tract) that interface with the environment close down. This stimulates the release of histamine and other inflammatory agents that generate the rashes, hives and other symptoms that plague allergy sufferers.

Allergic reactions can be suppressed by reprogramming immune cells not to react against the host. Allergic reactions can be mitigated, and sometimes eliminated, by maintaining high levels of antioxidants in the body to suppress the effects of an autoimmune attack. For allergy sufferers who are not taking high doses of vitamins, we suggest that three tablets, three times a day, of Life Extension Mix be taken for five weeks. If Life Extension Mix does not suppress the allergic reactions adequately, additional steps should be considered.

Gamma linolenic acid (GLA) is the active fatty acid in primrose, black current seed and borage oils that has been shown to suppress some autoimmune reactions. Studies on people suffering from autoimmune diseases indicate that the daily consumption of five capsules a day of borage oil (providing 1,500 mg of GLA) may be of help. In addition to borage oil, three to six capsules of a concentrated fish oil (Mega EPA) should be taken for long-term essential fatty acid balance and additional protection against allergic attacks.

DHEA can modulate immune system cytokines that cause autoimmune allergic reactions. The dose of DHEA required to suppress autoimmune cytokines varies, but 25 mg three times a day for men, and 15 mg three times a day for women, is suggested. Refer to DHEA-Pregnenolone Precautions before using DHEA.

Vitamin C can act as a natural antihistamine in doses of 2,500 to 12,000 mg a day. Bioflavonoids such as the proanthocyanidins found in grape seed-skin extract can work with vitamin C to further suppress allergic reactions. The recommended dose of proanthocyanidins to combat allergies is 100 to 300 mg a day.

Nutritionist Carmen Fusco recommends 300 to 500 mg twice a day of pantothenic acid in the form of calcium pantothenate or pantothine to help both the adrenals and the thymus gland in the fight against allergies. She also suggests that Drenamin helps in most allergies, while Antronex, which contains an antihistamine produced by the liver, helps in many nasal allergies. The stinging nettle (urtica dioica), especially when taken with vitamin C and bioflavinoids, is effective in reducing symptoms of allergies.

Product availability: Life Extension Mix, Mega GLA Mega EPA, DHEA, vitamin C and grape seed-skin extract can be obtained by calling 1-800-544-4440.

Alzheimer's Disease

Approximately 10 percent of Americans over age 65 show signs of dementia. For those over age 75 the incidence of dementia increases about 2 percent per year. About 70 percent of dementia cases are due to Alzheimer's disease, with blood vessel disease (including stroke) being the second most common cause. The memory loss, cognitive decline and personality disorders of Alzheimer's disease are undoubtedly due to the massive loss of neurons and synapses in those portions of the brain most concerned with intellectual function.

For more than 100 years, neuroscientists have debated whether the accumulation of lipofuscin (age pigments) in neurons is a cause of dementia. It has been argued that lipofuscin is formed by lipid peroxidation, but this seems unlikely insofar as these pigments are primarily composed of protein and carbohydrate. Recent evidence has shown that glycation (protein cross-linking by sugar) is probably a greater cause of lipofuscin formation than lipid peroxidation. Glycation is partially caused by free radicals. Although a role for lipofuscin cannot definitely be ruled out, few neurologists today believe that it is a central factor in Alzheimer's disease.

In the 1970s, many neurologists became convinced that Alzheimer's disease is due to the degeneration of the basal forebrain neurons that send the neurotransmitter acetylcholine to the cerebral cortex. Acetylcholine plays a key role in memory formation, but there are other neurotransmitters that may play a more important role in the development of Alzheimer's disease. Most neurologists now believe that degeneration of cholinergic neurons in Alzheimer's disease is only one manifestation of widespread degeneration of cognitively important neurons in the cerebral cortex and associated areas of the brain.

Recently, the most contentious issue among scientists studying Alzheimer's disease has been whether senile plaques of beta-amyloid peptide or neurofibrillary tangles containing tau protein are more critically associated with Alzheimer's. Neurofibrillary tangles are found inside neurons, whereas amyloid plaques are found outside neurons and on the walls of brain blood vessels. This dispute has whimsically been described as a "religious war" between the "Baptists" and the "Taoists." Despite a strong correlation of both amyloid plaques and neurofibrillary tangles with Alzheimer's disease, the cause of the disease is still unknown. It is possible that both amyloid plaques and neurofibrillary tangles are key factors. Or it is possible that both are merely symptoms of a more important underlying process.

Neurons, and in particular the axons of neurons, use microtubules to transport substances between the center of the neuron and its outer portions. The assembly and structural integrity of microtubules depend upon several proteins, the most important of which is probably the protein tau. When tau is abnormally phosphorylated, it forms the paired helical filaments known as neurofibrillary tangles. Why this abnormal phosphorylation occurs is unknown, but the loss of microtubule transport is particularly damaging in neurons that produce and release large amounts of neurotransmitters. The large pyramidal neurons of the cortex and the basal nucleus acetylcholine neurons (among others) are important for cognition. These large neurons have more microtubules than other neurons, and have the most neurofibrillary tangles in Alzheimer's disease. It is neurofibrillary tangle distribution (rather than amyloid plaque distribution) that correlates most closely with the severity of Alzheimer's dementia.

The role of beta-amyloid peptide in Alzheimer's disease seems most evident in the small percentage of cases caused by known genetic factors. Beta-amyloid is normally produced in the brain in a soluble form from amyloid precursor protein (APP), but certain genetic diseases result in large amounts of insoluble beta-amyloid production from APP. One genetic disease results in abnormal forms of apolipoprotein E (apo E), a substance that binds to cholesterol and helps to carry it outside of cells. Apo E also binds to beta-amyloid. People with two genes for the apo E-IV form of apolipoprotein E are eight times more likely to develop Alzheimer's than people with two genes for apo E-III.

Most cases of Alzheimer's disease do not involve genetic abnormalities, however, and amyloid plaques are commonly seen in both demented and non-demented elderly persons. No one knows why production of abnormal amyloid would increase in normal people. Beta-amyloid plaques are toxic to neurons and may "strangle" them by binding to neuronal surfaces. Beta-amyloid also damages brain blood vessels, and may thereby undermine the integrity of the blood-brain barrier, which normally protects the brain.

An ultimate cure for Alzheimer's disease will probably require some form of molecular engineering based on an understanding of how the disease actually works. No known chemical intervention can currently do more than slow the progression of the disease or provide temporary relief. For some people, this may seem futile. For others—family and friends—making the most of the remaining years of an Alzheimer's patient is both painful and precious.

Aging causes deficits in short-term memory and other cognitive functions, deterioration of brain cell structure, the degradation and death of brain neurons, and sporadic pathological lesions such as senile plaques and neurofibrillary tangles. Alzheimer's disease is an accelerated form of aging characterized by the widespread distribution of senile plaques and neurofibrillary tangles, the progressive loss of short-term memory and other cognitive functions, major brain cell structural deterioration, major behavioral disorders, and the eventual loss of one's identity . . . all of which lead eventually to death.

Among the proposed causes of the destruction of cholinergic neurons in Alzheimer's disease are the intracellular accumulation of beta-amyloid protein, aluminum, lipofuscin (cellular debris), and the generation of excessive free radical activity. One of the biochemical effects of beta-amyloid protein deposition is the inhibition of mitochondrial succinate dehydrogenase enzyme activity, which leads to a marked decrease in ATP formation, and a resulting decline in energy production

The ultimate cause of Alzheimer's disease is unknown, and the disease is currently incurable. It might seem that little can be done against it, but this is not true. Surprisingly, there are a number of chemical interventions that can slow its progress or even prevent its occurrence. Moreover, the diagnosis of Alzheimer's disease is only about 85 percent accurate, and the diagnosis is generally only confirmed by brain biopsy after death. Alzheimer's-like symptoms can be manifested by brain cancer, meningitis, neuro-syphilis, hypothyroidism, hypoglycemia, congestive heart failure, AIDS, vascular disease, Parkinson's disease, Huntington's disease, multiple sclerosis, subdural hematoma, and liver or kidney dysfunction. *Many of these conditions are treatable.* Nutritional deficiencies of vitamin E, magnesium and the B-vitamins (B12, folic acid, niacin and thiamine) can also produce symptoms that might be mistaken for dementia.

People who have had head injuries have a higher incidence of Alzheimer's disease. People who have had higher education and who live intellectually challenging lives have a lower incidence of the disease (or don't develop it as early). People who take aspirin or other non-steroidal anti-inflammatory drugs are less likely to get Alzheimer's. Women who take postmenopausal estrogen are less likely to get Alzheimer's.

The brains of Alzheimer's patients are known to be high in iron and aluminum, but the role of these elements remains controversial. Antioxidants may be of value against the free-radicals generated by these metals. Mercury may contribute to the disease by binding to protein and altering microtubule assembly. Selenium protects cells from mercury damage. Because glycation and oxidation causes so many other disorders, there is reason to suspect that they may underlie the metabolic disturbances of Alzheimer's disease. A varied mixture of different types of compounds to inhibit glycation and free radical formation, therefore, seems prudent. The drug aminoguanidine, available only in Europe, is a specific anti-glycating agent.

A program involving intake of a wide range of nutrients, hormones and drugs may be of value to slow the progress of Alzheimer's disease once it has begun. Antioxidants such as coenzyme Q10 and deprenyl may be of value in this regard.

Beta-amyloid peptide is known to generate free radicals, and vitamin E has been shown to protect neurons against this toxicity. Tacrine and other acetylcholine-promoting substances have been shown to slow cognitive decline in some Alzheimer's patients. Phosphatidylserine appears to protect cell membranes. Acetyl-L-carnitine also may be of benefit, although both the mechanism of action and benefits of this substance are disputed. Since Alzheimer's disease often coexists with vascular dementia, substances that promote brain circulation, such as ginkgo biloba, may be helpful.

Although several therapies can produce minor improvements in Alzheimer's patients, none of them can produce major therapeutic benefits when used alone. As a result, the Life Extension Foundation suggests a multi-modal approach to the treatment of Alzheimer's disease. This approach is based upon numerous published studies on the synergistic ability of nutrients, hormones and drugs in helping to protect brain cells from the deficits of normal aging, including the deposition of cellular debris in neurons, as well as the improvement of cognitive function in subjects of various ages.

Our approach also is based upon clinical results with multi-modal therapies in Alzheimer's patients in medical centers in the U.S. and Europe, including a highly successful program at the Alzheimer's Prevention Foundation, in Tucson, Ariz.

The Foundation recommends that several or all of the protocols below be used together in Alzheimer's disease patients for the best possible results. It is imperative that regular biochemical and functional tests be administered to the patient under the supervision of a knowledgeable physician to assess the effects of the treatment program selected, and to determine changes that may be required in the program for optimal results.

- ❖ **Protocol Number One**: To boost acetylcholine levels in the brain, enhance brain cell uptake of glucose, preserve the integrity of brain cell membranes, and synchronize neuronal activity:

  1. The nutrient-hormone formula Cognitex. The suggested dose is five capsules of Cognitex in the morning and five Cognitex capsules in the afternoon. Cognitex provides potent doses of two forms of the acetylcholine precursor choline and vitamin B5 to convert choline into acetylcholine; phosphatidylserine to maintain the integrity of brain cell membranes and boost brain cell energy metabolism; and pregnenolone, a hormone that improves memory by synchronizing neuronal activity in the brain.

  2. One capsule containing 120 mg of ginkgo biloba extract in the morning.

- ❖ **Protocol Number Two**: To combat excessive free radical activity with a potent combinations of antioxidants:

  Life Extension Mix, three tablets, three times a day, with meals.

- ❖ **Protocol Number Three**: To boost brain cell energy levels necessary for healthy metabolic activity:

  1. Acetyl-L-carnitine — 1,000 mg in the morning and 1,000 mg in the afternoon.

  2. Piracetam — 1,600 mg in the morning and 1,600 mg in the afternoon.

  3. Hydergine — 5 mg in the morning and 5 mg in the afternoon.

  4. NADH — 5 to 20 mg daily in the morning on an empty stomach.

  5. Coenzyme Q10 — 200 to 400 mg daily with or after meals.

- ❖ **Protocol Number Four**: To elevate dopamine levels, improve cellular communication, and enhance neurological function:

  1. Deprenyl — 5 mg, twice a week.

  2. NADH — 5 to 20 mg a day

  3. Vitamin B12, which is often deficient in elderly people suffering from neurological diseases. Take 2,000 micrograms a day in sublingual (under the

tongue) form.

❖ **Protocol Number Five**: To remove cellular debris, such as lipofuscin (aging pigment) caused by the breakdown by-products of cellular metabolism, and to strengthen neuronal membrane structure: *Enzymes.*

1. Centrophenoxine — one tablet in the morning and one in the afternoon.

2. Phosphatidylserine capsules — 100 to 300 mg daily with a meal. Note that phosphatidylserine is already included the Cognitex formula (Protocol Number One).

❖ **Protocol Number Six**: To replace critically important hormones that are severely depleted and/or inactive in Alzheimer's disease patients:

1. Human growth hormone — 1 to 2 units a day injected subcutaneously six days a week, or follow physician's prescribed dose based upon blood levels of somatomedin-C (IGF-1).

2. DHEA — 25 mg three times a day in men, or 15 mg three times a day in women, or follow physician's prescribed dose based upon blood levels of DHEA sulfate.

3. Pregnenolone — 50 to 150 mg a day. Pregnenolone is included in the Cognitex formula in Protocol Number One. Your physician may recommend additional pregnenolone based upon your blood levels of DHEA.

4. Melatonin — 3 to 10 mg nightly.

   Important Note: Pregnenolone and DHEA can cascade down into estrogen and testosterone. Estrogen has been shown to improve memory and reduce the risk of Alzheimer's disease in women, and is being used in some clinics as a treatment for Alzheimer's disease. The above hormone replacement protocol may provide enough estrogen (converted from pregnenolone and DHEA) to have a therapeutic effect. Some female patients may require additional estrogen and some males may require supplemental testosterone. The drug Premarin is often prescribed for women because this contains the most potent estrogens. Estrogen replacement therapy does not work for men because they do not have enough estrogen receptor sites on brain cells.

❖ **Protocol Number Seven**: To inhibit the enzyme acetylcholinesterase, which excessively degrades the neurotransmitter acetylcholine in Alzheimer's patients:

1. THA, also known as Cognex (tacrine) — 160 to 200 mg daily. Physician supervision is mandatory to test liver enzymes to make sure THA is not causing liver damage. One tablespoon of lecithin will reduce THA-induced liver toxicity and provide phosphatidylcholine, from which the brain can produce the neurotransmitter acetylcholine.

2. A drug called Aricept works via similar mechanisms as THA, but may be less toxic. Aricept should be used in place of THA in some people.

❖ **Protocol Number Eight**: To inhibit protein cross linking-induced lipofuscin deposits in brain cells caused by glycation. Glycation occurs when a protein molecule binds with a glucose molecule to form a non-functioning structure within the cell.   *Enzymes.*

1. Aminoguanidine, available only in Europe. Initial dose should be 300 mg a day. Toxicity can occur when doses higher than 300 mg a day are administered, but some people tolerate up to 600 mg a day.

2. The nutrients recommended in Protocol Number Two also may provide some protection against excessive glycation.

Product availability: Cognitex, ginkgo caps, Life Extension Mix, acetyl-L-carnitine, NADH, coenzyme Q10, vitamin B12, phosphatidylserine, DHEA, pregnenolone, lecithin and melatonin can be obtained by calling 1-800-544-4440. THA and Aricept are FDA-approved prescription drugs that must be prescribed by a physician. Piracetam, Hydergine, deprenyl, aminoguanidine and centrophenoxine are available from overseas companies for personal use only. For a list of companies offering these products, call 1-800-544-4440.

Amnesia

European doctors use the drugs piracetam and vasopressin to help people suffering from amnesia recover their memories. Published studies show that the recovery of memory in amnesia patients can take from several hours to a few days when vasopressin and/or piracetam are used.

The recommended dosage of vasopressin is at least 16 international units (IU) a day, usually in the form of a nasal spray, though physicians may prescribe higher amounts to treat acute amnesia. The recommended dose of piracetam is 4,800 mg a day until memory is restored.

Product availability: Vasopressin is a prescription drug produced by the Sandoz pharmaceutical company. You must see a physician and get a prescription for this medication. Piracetam is an unapproved drug that has to be ordered from offshore pharmacies. For a list of such pharmacies, call 1-800-544-4440.

Amyotrophic Lateral Sclerosis (Lou Gehrig's Disease)

Amyotrophic lateral sclerosis (ALS) is a disabling disease involving the breakdown of the neurons leading from the brain and spinal cord to the muscles. The result is the progressive wasting of the muscles that leads to death from respiratory complications in two to five years.

There is no established therapy to treat ALS, but understanding some of the mechanisms of neuron destruction involved in ALS can enable a person to follow a protocol that, in theory, could slow the progression of the disease.

Acetyl-L-carnitine has produced dramatic results in protecting neurons in a wide range of disease states. We therefore suggest that ALS patients take 3,000 mg a day of acetyl-L-carnitine.

— B_6 + B_{12}

Neuron damage can be caused by degeneration of the myelin sheath, a fatty layer that wraps the signal-moving neuronal fibers. Taking two tablespoons a day of Udo's Choice Essential Fatty Acids will provide omega-3 and omega-6 fatty acids, which may help to repair the myelin sheath required for proper neuron conduction.

Since pregnenolone and DHEA are involved in the regulation of neurologic function, supplementation with 50 mg three times a day of pregnenolone, and/or 25 mg three times a day of DHEA should be considered.

Innovative drug therapies for ALS also might include 10 to 20 mg a day of Hydergine, 40 mg a day of vinpocetin, and human growth hormone replacement therapy.

To protect against respiratory dysfunction, 600 mg of N-acetylcysteine (NAC) and 1,000 mg of vitamin C, three times a day, are suggested.

Free radicals have been implicated in the ALS disease process, so the standard dose of Life Extension Mix, which is three tablets three times a day, might be helpful. While Life Extension Mix contains a considerable amount of magnesium, 500 mg a day of additional magnesium also is suggested.

Alpha-lipoic acid is a potent antioxidant that is especially effective in preventing diabetic neuropathy. Therefore, we suggest a dose of 1,000 mg a day of alpha-lipoic acid to protect the neurons affected by ALS.

Nutritionist Carmen Fusco reports that, while under her care for ALS, Senator Jacob Javits seemed to improve enough to reduce his hospital admissions with the following nutrients: octocosonol as it occurs in raw wheat germ oil; mega doses of pantothenic acid (viamin B5, the "stress vitamin"); and DMG sublingual. Fusco also has used the branch chain amino acids and sublingual vitamin B12. Dr. Benjamin Frank recommended the coenzyme form of the B vitamins which were administred intramuscularly by injection.

Product availability: For a listing of physicians in your area who might be knowledgeable in these innovative approaches, call 1-800-544-4440. To order acetyl-L-carnitine, alpha-lipoic acid, N-acetylcysteine, pregnenolone, DHEA, Life Extension Mix and magnesium, phone 1-800-544-4440. Hydergine is available by prescription in the U.S. or from overseas pharmacies. Vinpocetin is available from overseas pharmacies. For a list of such pharmacies, call 1-800-544-4440.

Anemia-Thrombocytopenia-Leukopenia

Aging, viral infections, blood diseases, cancer chemotherapy and radiation therapy can cause deficits in red blood cell, white blood cell and blood platelet production.

Studies have shown that supplemental melatonin in doses of 10 to 40 mg a night can protect and restore normal blood-cell production caused by the toxicity of chemotherapy. A recent study was performed in 80 patients with metastatic solid tumors to evaluate the benefits of melatonin. Patients either received chemotherapy alone or chemotherapy plus 20 mg each night of melatonin. Thrombocytopenia was significantly less frequent in patients receiving melatonin.

Other common side effects of cancer chemotherapy, such as malaise, asthenia, stomatitis and neuropathy, occurred less frequently in patients receiving melatonin. This corroborated previous studies showing that the administration of melatonin during chemotherapy can prevent some side effects, especially myelosuppression (blood cell production suppression) and neuropathy.

Infection by the human immunodeficiency virus (HIV) is commonly associated with hematologic abnormalities (anemia, leukopenia and thrombocytopenia). Several causes have been identified, including direct HIV injury on bone marrow, anti-HIV drugs such as AZT, opportunistic infections in bone marrow, vitamin B12 and folate deficiency, radiation therapy, and hemophagocytic syndrome. Patients have an increased risk of infection, since the neutrophils play an important role in the defense against bacterial and certain fungal infections.

Treatment strategies may include reducing or eliminating anti-HIV drugs and other conventional therapies that suppress bone-marrow production of blood cells. Supplementation with 2,000 micrograms of vitamin B12 sublingual tablets and 1,600 micrograms of folic acid is strongly suggested, because deficiencies of these vitamins can cause numerous AIDS-related complications.

If these therapies are not successful, then the FDA-approved drug Neupogen, which is a granulocyte colony-stimulating factor (G-CSF), can be used to stimulate bone-marrow granulopoiesis. A modified version of this drug, known as a granulocyte macrophage-colony stimulating factor (GM-CSF), also may be considered by your immunologist or hematologist.

Another therapy to restore healthy blood platelet production is five capsules a day of standardized shark liver oil capsules containing 200 mg of alkylglycerols per capsule. Studies have shown that shark liver oil can boost the production of blood platelets. Shark liver oil capsules should only be taken in high doses for a maximum period of 30 days, because too many blood platelets might be produced.

Anemia can be caused by deficiencies in vitamin B1, vitamin B2, vitamin B6, vitamin B12, folic acid and iron. Supplementation of these nutrients should be considered when there are deficiencies. Regular blood testing should be done to monitor the effectiveness of these blood cell-boosting therapies.

Product availability: Standardized shark liver oil capsules, vitamin B1, vitamin B2, vitamin B6, vitamin B12, folic acid and pharmaceutical grade melatonin can be obtained by phoning 1-800-544-4440.

Anesthesia and Surgery Precautions

Anesthesia and surgery can cause temporary or permanent brain damage. Surgical complications can be caused by the free radicals that occur during anesthesia or during the surgical process.

Some of the mechanisms of neurologic injury caused by anesthesia and surgical procedures have been identified in the scientific literature. There are specific nutrients and drugs that can be taken ahead of time to help protect against the most common forms of neurologic injury caused by anesthesia and surgery.

During open-heart surgery, free radicals have been identified as a primary culprit in preventing the reestablishment of a regular heart rhythm, and in causing the common complication of pancreatitis.

A study was conducted on 30 patients undergoing vascular surgery for abdominal aortic aneurysm or obstructive aorto-iliac disease. Patients in group one were treated with coenzyme Q10 (150 mg a day) for seven days before the operation. Those in group two received a placebo. The results showed that markers of free radical activity and tissue damage (i.e. malondialdehyde, conjugated dienes, creatine kinase and lactate dehydrogenase) were significantly lower in patients who received coenzyme Q10 than in the placebo group. A decrease of plasma malondialdehyde correlated positively with a decrease in both creatine kinase and lactate dehydrogenase. The doctors concluded that pre-treatment with coenzyme Q10 may play a protective role during routine vascular procedures by attenuating the degree of peroxidative free radical damage.

Some forms of anesthesia administered during surgical procedures that can cause temporary reduced blood flow may lead to significant free radical damage to cells. A study was performed to assess the administration of vitamin E during severe anesthesia. The administration of vitamin E produced a statistically significant decrease in the content of peroxidation products in the blood.

A growing body of evidence supports the role of free radicals in delayed functional and metabolic myocardial recovery following cardiopulmonary bypass in humans. A clinical study was designed to evaluate the extent that ginkgo extract could inhibit reperfusion-induced lipid peroxidation, ascorbate depletion, tissue necrosis and cardiac dysfunction. Patients received either ginkgo extract (320 mg a day) or a matching placebo before surgical intervention. Plasma samples were obtained up to eight days post-operatively, from the peripheral circulation and the coronary sinus, at crucial stages of the operation (i.e., before incision, during ischemia, and within the first 30 minutes after unclamping). Upon aortic unclamping, ginkgo extract inhibited the formation of free radicals, significantly reduced the delayed leakage of myoglobin, preserved the ascorbic acid pool, and had an almost significant effect on ventricular myosin leakage. The surgeons concluded that these results demonstrate the usefulness of adjuvant (assisting) ginkgo extract therapy in limiting oxidative stress in cardiovascular surgery. They discussed the possible role of highly bioavailable terpene constituents of the drug.

The most convenient way of obtaining high-potency antioxidants to protect against free radicals induced by anesthesia and surgery is to take—at least one week prior to surgery—three tablets, three times a day, of Life Extension Mix, along with 200 mg a day of coenzyme Q10, 2,000 mg a day of acetyl-L-carnitine, and 120 mg a day of ginkgo extract.

Also, at least 3 to 10 mg of melatonin should be taken every night for one week before the surgery, and 10 mg of melatonin may be taken just before anesthesia is administered to provide further protection against anesthesia and surgery-induced complications. Research funded by the Life Extension Foundation has shown that melatonin given prior to anesthesia protects cells throughout an animal's body (but especially in the brain) against ischemic injury caused by lack of blood flow.

In addition to these antioxidants, at least 5 mg a day of the drug Hydergine and 2,400 mg a day of piracetam should be taken one week before surgery to protect brain cells against the effects of erratic blood flow that may occur during the procedure.

Some surgeons ask their pre-surgical patients to avoid aspirin and nutrients that may promote excessive bleeding during surgery. Ginkgo biloba and some of the nutrients in Life Extension Mix, such as vitamin E, can inhibit abnormal blood clotting and may cause excessive bleeding during and after surgery. For some surgical procedures, excessive bleeding can be a problem, but experienced surgeons should be able to deal with this.

On the other hand, a significant risk factor during and after surgical procedures and long hospital stays is the development of abnormal blood clots inside blood vessels that can cause a stroke, heart attack or a lethal pulmonary embolism. The platelet aggregation-inhibiting effect of vitamin E, ginkgo and other nutrients in Life Extension Mix could prevent surgically induced blood clots from forming.

Published studies have shown that when open-heart surgery patients take antioxidants before surgery, fewer complications develop. There are contradictions in the scientific literature as to whether or not vitamin E and other antioxidants cause enough excessive bleeding to create a problem. But when you consider the neurologic benefits, the protection against free radicals, the protection against abnormal blood-clot formation, and the overall health benefits these nutrients provide, you (and your physician) may choose to include the nutrients that have been suggested as part of your pre-surgery medication protocol.

Product availability: Life Extension Mix, ginkgo biloba, acetyl-L-carnitine, coenzyme Q10 and melatonin can be ordered by calling 1-800-544-4440. Hydergine can be obtained with a physician's prescription. Piracetam can be ordered from offshore pharmacies. For a list of these pharmacies, call 1-800-544-4440.

Anxiety and Stress

In today's high-pressure world, it's not surprising that many people suffer from chronic stress and fatigue, along with such associated conditions as anxiety, phobias and depression. Vast numbers of Americans use FDA-approved drugs to mitigate chronic stress and fatigue. These drugs have adverse side effects and often fail to address the underlying anxiety, irritability, depression and learning dysfunction associated with stress and fatigue.

Europeans and Japanese are increasingly turning to a natural alternative to drugs to alleviate chronic stress and fatigue. One of these products, Adapton, is now being used by innovative medical doctors in the United States in place of such FDA-approved drugs as Xanax, Prozac and Buspar. Adapton comes from a species of deep sea fish called garum whose only known habitat is off the coast of England.

Adapton is being used throughout Europe and Japan for the treatment of a wide range of stress-induced disorders.

1. In a recent crossover clinical trial, 20 patients who had been ill with various forms of chronic fatigue were studied. The patients' anxiety, depression, muscle fatigue, mental fatigue, sleep disorders and headache were measured. Placebo capsules were given to these patients during the first two weeks of the study. This study showed that, after two weeks on placebo, fatigue symptoms were reduced by an average of 14 percent and overall symptoms of anxiety, depression and insomnia were reduced by 4 percent (the "placebo effect."). However, when Adapton was given for the next two weeks of the study, fatigue symptoms were reduced by 51 percent and overall symptoms by 65 percent. These results showed broad-spectrum benefits in taking Adapton for people suffering from chronic stress and fatigue.

2. Another study involved 40 patients who had been suffering from various forms of chronic fatigue syndrome. Four capsules of Adapton per day were prescribed for two weeks. The results, based upon the Fatigue Study Group criteria, showed benefit in 50 percent of the subjects for the 10 functions that most accurately measure fatigue and depression. No serious side effects were reported. The researchers concluded that Adapton is extremely

well-tolerated and is without contraindications.

3. In a study of 60 patients on Adapton, only three mild reactions were noted: one case of nervous irritation, one case of heartburn and one of diarrhea. It was concluded that Adapton is extremely well-tolerated and is without contraindications. Other studies are showing that when Adapton reduces anxiety it also improves learning and enhances electroencephalogram (EEG) brain-wave activity.

4. Adapton benefits 90 percent of patients with chronic stress and fatigue, compared with only 30 percent of patients on placebo. An analysis of the human clinical studies of Adapton shows overall positive results for the symptoms of chrionic stress, including fatigue, anxiety and depression.

Adapton is comprised of a standardized dose of polypeptides that exerts a regulatory effect on the nervous system, enabling people to better adapt to stressful conditions. These unique polypeptides act as precursors to endorphins and other neurotransmitters that improve our ability to adapt to mental and physical stress. Adapton also contains an omega-3 essential fatty acid complex that enhances prostaglandins and prostacyclins, the chemical mediators that regulate major biological functions in the body. Omega-3 extract is thought to contribute to the stress-reducing effects of this European therapy.

If you suffer from chronic stress-induced anxiety, fatigue or depression, Adapton could provide you with substantial relief. Hyperactive children in Europe with such learning disabilities as attention deficit disorder are being treated successfully with Adapton in place of drugs like Ritalin.

The recommended dosage is four capsules of Adapton on an empty stomach in the morning for 15 consecutive days. After two weeks, the dose should be reduced to two capsules every morning. If complete relief is obtained, Adapton can be discontinued until symptoms return. Some people take two to three Adapton capsules every other day. There is no toxicity risk in taking Adapton every day, although it doesn't have to be taken every day for it to work.

For those who suffer from anxiety attacks, 10 mg of the prescription drug propranolol can provide immediate relief. Propranolol works by blocking beta-adrenergic sites on cell membranes so that cells do not overreact to the increased amount of adrenaline secreted in response to anxiety-provoking situations. Propranolol is a cardiovascular drug, and those with very low blood pressure, asthma or congestive heart failure may not be able to use it. The low dose of propranolol required to prevent or treat anxiety attacks is tolerable by the vast majority of people.

Anxiety and stress can result in excessive production of the adrenal hormone cortisol. Cortisol damages the immune system, the arterial system and brain cells, and causes premature aging. While some people never gain complete control over stress and anxiety, the effects of excessive cortisol production can be mitigated by taking one to two tablets of the

European medication KH3 in the morning on an empty stomach, and one to two tablets of KH3 in mid-afternoon on an empty stomach.

Important: People allergic to procaine (the active ingredient in KH3) or who are on sulfa drugs should not take KH3.

The regulatory hormones melatonin and DHEA also may protect against the effects of stress-induced excessive cortisol production. Suggested dosage for melatonin is 500 micrograms to 10 mg each night. Men should take 25 mg three times a day of DHEA, while women should take 15 mg three times a day of DHEA. Refer to the DHEA-Pregnenolone Precautions protocol before taking DHEA.

Conventional doctors often prescribe selective serotonin reuptake inhibitor (SSRI) drugs, such as Prozac, Zoloft or Paxil, for the treatment of anxiety, phobias and obsessive-compulsive symptoms. It is argued that serotonergic dysfunction may underlie such non-psychotic disorders as anxiety, as well as affective and compulsive-obsessive disorders. While the SSRIs are safer than such tranquilizers as Xanax and Valium, there are concerns in the life extension community about such long-term side effects as serotonin overload. When looking at the safety profile of the natural therapies available to treat anxiety and stress, it makes sense to try natural therapies that have potential side *benefits*, rather than drugs that many believe produce dangerous long-term side effects.

Among Carmen Fusco's treatments for stress and anxiety are 500 mg of magnesium aspartate, 50 to 100 mg of vitamin B6, 300 to 500 mg of pantothenic acid, kava kava and taurine.

Product availability: Adapton, melatonin and DHEA are available by calling 1-800-544-4440. Ask for a listing of offshore companies that sell KH3 to Americans by mail for personal use. Propranolol can be prescribed by a doctor.

Arrhythmia (Cardiac)

Heart arrhythmia is caused by a variety of medical conditions that have to be identified by a cardiologist before appropriate therapies can be suggested. Once the underlying cause of the cardiac arrhythmia has been established, there are a number of natural therapies that may be of help in reestablishing normal heart rhythms. *These therapies should be used with a great deal of caution.*

Anti-arrhythmia nutrients include the minerals magnesium at 500 to 2,000 mg a day, potassium at 200 to 500 mg a day, and selenium at 300 to 600 micrograms a day. Coenzyme Q10 is used in Japan as a treatment for cardiac arrhythmia at 100 to 300 mg a day. Acetyl-L-carnitine is used in Europe to treat cardiac arrhythmia at 1,000 to 2,000 mg a day. Also in Japan, taurine is used at 1,000 to 2,000 mg a day with carnitine and coenzyme Q10 as a treatment for congestive heart failure.

Forskolin is an Indian herbal extract that improves contractile strength in the heart muscle when taken at 10 to 60 mg a day. Forskolin may alleviate cardiac arrhythmia or, over an extended period of time, exacerbate it. Forskolin is most appropriately used when arrhythmia is accompanied by severe congestive heart failure.

CAUTION: Do not use forskolin if you have prostate cancer.

Vitamin D3 enhances calcium metabolism in the sinoatrial node of the heart when given at 1,000 IU a day. Vitamin E at 400 to 800 IU a day is used to treat coronary artery disease, but also helps establish normal heart rhythms. Five to eight capsules a day of fish oil concentrates have been shown in several published studies to regulate cardiac arrhythmias.

A novel anti-arrhythmia agent may be vitamin A. One study showed that retinoic acid, a vitamin A derivative of vitamin A, produced marked anti-arrhythmia effects in rats. Those who want to avoid vitamin A drugs that can produce adverse side effects should use 100,000 IU a day of water-soluble vitamin A liquid drops as a potential therapy to restore normal heart rhythms.

Important: Refer to the Symptoms of Vitamin A Toxicity, in Appendix A, for safety information about long-term use of high doses of vitamin A.

The use of any of these natural therapies should be done with the full cooperation of a trained cardiologist, as any errors could result in sudden death from a heart attack. Those with cardiac arrhythmias should avoid caffeine, heavy alcohol intake and saturated fats.

Product availability: Magnesium, potassium, acetyl-L-carnitine, coenzyme Q10, taurine, Mega EPA, selenium, vitamin D3, forskolin and vitamin A liquid drops can be obtained by calling 1-800-544-4440.

Arthritis

Arthritis is epidemic throughout the world. There are two basic forms of arthritis: osteoarthritis and rheumatoid arthritis.

Osteoarthritis is characterized by the inability of the cartilage in joints to maintain and repair itself. The results of osteoarthritis are cartilage degradation, erosion of joint lining and eventual loss of mechanical function in the joint, all of which involve chronic pain. The initial symptoms of osteoarthritis are joint pain, stiffness and decreased joint movement. In severe cases, the cartilage in the joint disintegrates entirely, causing the joint bones to rub against each other, which causes severe pain and rapid loss of joint function.

Rheumatoid arthritis is characterized by autoimmune attack on the linings of the joints, resulting in severe inflammation, joint disfigurement, loss of joint function and chronic pain. The initial symptom of rheumatoid arthritis is enlargement of the joints, often in the fingers, with increasing pain and loss of function as the disease flares up.

The Life Extension Foundation recommends natural therapies for arthritis and other inflammatory disorders. Newly published scientific research studies confirm the benefits of natural therapies in suppressing inflammation and pain without adverse side effects.

Mainstream medicine treats arthritis patients with corticosteroids and nonsteroidal anti-inflammatory drugs. While these drugs may work in the short term, they can produce such serious adverse side effects as gastric ulceration, and liver and kidney damage when taken chronically (over long periods). *Estimates are that conventional arthritis drugs kill more than 7,000 Americans a year, and are responsible for 70,000 hospitalizations yearly.*

Also, long-term use of many of these drugs can result in complete joint immobilization because they fail to treat the underlying cause of most forms of arthritis. FDA-approved drugs can exacerbate catabolic cartilage breakdown and prevent the expression of natural anabolic-repair mechanisms.

European doctors have been using non-toxic natural therapies to treat arthritis with great success for many years. These natural therapies work because they treat the underlying degenerative process affecting the linings of the joints in osteoarthritis, and/or improve the autoimmune disorder that destroys the joint linings in rheumatoid arthritis.

The cartilage in our joints is vulnerable to a wide range of insults that can result in cartilage degeneration. When a joint becomes inflamed, the blood supply is reduced, thereby reducing the ability to repair the cartilage in the joint. The attack on the cartilage in our joints intensifies as we grow older. First, our vascular system becomes blocked, which prevents normal cartilage repair and maintenance. Then, our natural antioxidant enzyme systems break down and free radicals attack joint cartilage. Finally, our immune system becomes disoriented and starts attacking the linings of our own joints.

The initial result of joint injury is the formation of free radicals that attack the cartilage and the lubricating synovial fluid within the joint. This free radical activity can trigger a cascade of autoimmune events to cause chronic loss of cartilage structure and function. Conventional doctors usually accept these events as the normal, irreversible progression of arthritis.

Research indicates that a deficiency of antioxidants often is a factor in the development of arthritis. While antioxidants can be of help in some early stage arthritis patients, more direct anti-arthritic therapies are required for those whose joint degeneration has progressed significantly.

In order for osteoarthritis to be treated effectively, the cartilage and synovial fluid in the joint must be protected against further destruction. At the same time, it is desirable to stimulate anabolic restoration of joint cartilage and synovial fluid. Chondroprotective agents are compounds the body manufactures naturally to regenerate cartilage and healthy joint function. Aging and trauma disrupt the body's ability to use its own chondroprotective agents. Here are therapies that have been shown to be helpful for osteoarthritis patients:

❖ **Therapy Number One:** Glucosamine, which has been used extensively in Europe to treat osteoarthritis. Studies document glucosamine's ability to function as a chondroprotective agent. Glucosamine provides the raw material needed for chondrocytes to regenerate cartilage. A glucosamine deficiency caused by aging and/or trauma leads to osteoarthritis.

In nine European studies, the oral administration of glucosamine produced major reductions in joint pain, joint tenderness and joint swelling. Improvements in joint function and overall physical performance were noted in these studies, compared with placebo and/or the drug ibuprofen. While ibuprofen worked faster than glucosamine in relieving pain, glucosamine improved overall condition better, without any of the toxic side effects associated with ibuprofen.

The research and clinical results with glucosamine have been so impressive that it has become a first-line therapy against osteoarthritis in Europe. It is only when glucosamine doesn't work that European doctors resort to toxic nonsteroidal anti-inflammatory drugs. Glucosamine salts exhibit no toxicity at doses far higher than patients need to treat their arthritis successfully. Glucosamine salts are easily absorbed and distributed in the joint cartilage matrix.

Studies show that glucosamine takes four to 10 weeks to produce noticeable results. A new arthritis formula that contains glucosamine has been producing noticeable reductions in inflammation and pain in most arthritis patients in less than four weeks! This formula, which will be described later in this protocol, contains two forms of glucosamine, chondroitin sulfates and the essential fatty acids that have been shown to suppress inflammation.

❖ **Therapy Number Two:** The chondroitin sulfates, which provide the structural components of the cartilage found in the joint. Chondroitin sulfate is a constituent of shark cartilage, which helps to explain the beneficial effects that shark cartilage produces in some arthritis patients. The chondroitin sulfates have been tested extensively in humans with outstanding success. The FDA has ruled, however, that, because each chondroitin sulfate molecule is different from all other chondroitin sulfate molecules, it cannot be approved because it is impossible to produce a precisely standardized product. Nevertheless, research studies have provided much useful data on the safety and effectiveness of chondroitin sulfates in arthritis patients. Chondroitin sulfates inhibit enzymes that degrade joint cartilage and collagen.

❖ **Therapy Number Three:** The anti-inflammatory essential fatty acids. The most potent fatty acid is GLA (gamma linolenic acid), which is found in evening primrose oil, borage oil and black currant seed oil. Fish oils rich in EPA and DHA also have been shown to suppress chronic inflammation. Here are findings from some of the studies documenting the benefits of essential fatty acids in treating arthritis:

> In the *Annals of Internal Medicine* (1993, 119/9), the findings of a 24-week, double-blind, placebo-controlled trial with GLA derived from borage oil was reported. The patients receiving the borage oil experienced a 36-percent reduction in the number of tender joints, a 45-percent reduction in the tender joint score, a 41-percent reduction in the swollen joint score, and a 28-percent reduction in the swollen joint count. The placebo group showed no benefits.

A paper in the *British Journal of Rheumatology* (1994, 33/9) reports the findings of a 24-week, double-blind, placebo-controlled trial in rheumatoid arthritis patients treated with black currant seed oil rich in gamma linolenic acid (GLA) and alpha linolenic acid. Patients receiving black currant seed oil showed reductions in the signs and symptoms of the disease. The placebo group showed no change in disease status. According to the researchers, the study showed that black currant seed oil is a potentially effective treatment for active rheumatoid arthritis. No adverse reactions were observed, although some people dropped out of the trial because of the size and number of capsules they were required to take.

In *Seminars in Arthritis and Rheumatism* (1995, 25/2), there was a review of all the published literature on the use of GLA for the treatment of rheumatoid arthritis. GLA reduced the effects of autoimmune disease on joint linings, though more research was said to be needed to determine the ideal dose of GLA for arthritis.

A study in the *Journal of Clinical Epidemiology* (1995, 48/11) reviewed all the published studies on the use of fish oil to treat rheumatoid arthritis. It revealed that, in general, after three months of use there was a significant reduction in tender-joint count and morning stiffness in patients receiving fish oils. The placebo groups experienced no relief from pain.

In a study in *Arthritis and Rheumatism* (1995, 38/8), rheumatoid arthritis patients stopped taking non-steroidal anti-inflammatory drugs and switched to fish oil. This placebo-controlled, double-blind study showed that the group receiving the fish oil experienced significant decreases in the number of tender joints and the duration of morning stiffness, improvements in the physicians' and patients' evaluation of global arthritis activity, and improvements in the physicians' evaluation of pain. Patients receiving fish oil exhibited improvement in clinical functions compared with patients receiving placebo. Some patients were able to stop taking conventional arthritis drugs altogether.

A unique formula called Natural Pain Relief For Arthritis has been developed for the treatment of such chronic inflammatory diseases as osteoarthritis, rheumatoid arthritis and bursitis. This formula combines the most effective anti-inflammatory agents European doctors are prescribing as first-line therapies against arthritis and other chronic inflammatory diseases. Natural Pain Relief For Arthritis also may be effective for conditions such as tendinitis, sprained ankles and knees, lupus, rheumatism, cancer and ulcers.

The ingredients in Natural Pain Relief For Arthritis have been shown to:

✔ Relieve the inflammation, stiffness and pain associated with osteoarthritis and rheumatoid arthritis.

✔ Contribute to the regeneration of joint cartilage and joint-lubricating synovial fluid.

✔ Contribute to the suppression of autoimmune components that attack joint linings.

✔ Be almost totally free of adverse side effects, especially those associated with nonsteroidal anti-inflammatory drugs.

In addition to relieving chronic joint inflammation and pain, the natural ingredients in Natural Pain Relief For Arthritis have been shown to:

❖ Reduce the risk of abnormal blood clot formation that can lead to a sudden heart attack or stroke.

❖ Contribute to the alleviation of autoimmune disorders not associated with chronic inflammatory diseases.

❖ Help maintain the health of the endothelial linings of the arterial system.

❖ Contribute to the suppression of such common inflammatory skin disorders as eczema.

❖ Reduce serum triglyceride levels.

❖ Reduce blood pressure in some hypertensive patients.

The recommended dose of this new natural formula is based upon weight. For those weighing less than 150 pounds, take one capsule three times a day. For those weighing 150 to 200 pounds, take two capsules, three times day. Those weighing more than 200 pounds should take three capsules, three times a day.

If reductions in inflammation and pain do not begin to occur within a week after starting Natural Pain Relief For Arthritis, increase your dosage by taking one additional capsule with each dose. Instead of taking one capsule three times a day, increase it to two capsules three times a day.

Natural Pain Relief For Arthritis comes in oil-filled, soft gel capsules. Three capsules contain the following:

✔ 400 mg EPA (from fish oil)
✔ 300 mg DHA (from fish oil)
✔ 300 mg GLA (from black currant seed or borage oil)
✔ 500 mg n-acetyl-glucosamine
✔ 500 mg glucosamine sulfate
✔ 200 mg chondroitin sulfate
✔ 1 mg magnesium aspartate
✔ 5 mg ascorbyl palmitate
✔ 10 IU vitamin E

This formula has a patent pending with the U.S. Patent Office. The owner of the patent is INHOLTRA Inc.

A study investigated patients with rheumatoid arthritis to determine if dietary factors might play a role in their disease. Rheumatoid arthritis patients were shown to ingest too much total fat, too little polyunsaturated fatty acids and too little fiber, compared with healthy controls. Their diets were deficient in vitamin B6, zinc, magnesium, copper and folate. The researchers noted that these findings, also documented in previous studies, suggest that routine dietary supplementation with multivitamins and trace elements is appropriate for rheumatoid arthritis patients.

Because oxidative damage has been implicated in such autoimmune diseases as rheumatoid arthritis and lupus, a study was designed to assess serum concentrations of vitamin E, beta-carotene and vitamin A. This study examined cases of rheumatoid arthritis and systemic lupus erythematosus that developed two to 15 years after people donated blood to a serum bank in 1974. Stored serum samples were assayed for vitamin E, beta-carotene and vitamin A. People who later developed rheumatoid arthritis or lupus were shown to have had lower serum concentrations of vitamin E, beta-carotene and vitamin A in 1974 than did matched controls. For rheumatoid arthritis, the difference for beta-carotene (minus 29 percent) was statistically significant. These findings supported those of a previous study showing that low-antioxidant status is a risk factor for rheumatoid arthritis and systemic lupus erythematosus.

With regard to juvenile rheumatoid arthritis, a study examined the markers of free radical activity, vitamin E and superoxide dismutase in the blood of 74 young patients with juvenile rheumatoid arthritis, as well as in 138 healthy children aged 3 to 15. The results showed a statistically significant increase of free radical markers in the blood plasma of the children with juvenile arthritis, compared with those in the healthy control group. The vitamin E concentration was significantly lower in the blood plasma of the experimental subjects than in the subjects in the control group. Superoxide dismutase activity in the red blood cells also was significantly lower in children who had suffered from juvenile arthritis.

Based upon these results showing low antioxidant levels in children with rheumatoid arthritis, high potency antioxidant supplementation may be advisable. Some parents use Life Extension Mix powder in their child's juice to provide high doses of antioxidant and SOD-boosting nutrients.

Nutritionist Carmen Fusco offers the following recommendations for rheumatoid arthritis: two soft eggs (organic) daily to provide the antiinflammatory sulfur amino acids, and raw fresh vegetable juices on an empty stomach for nutritional treatment of rheumatoid arthritis. Also helpful is GH3 and fever few.

Product availability: You can order glucosamine-chondroitin sulfate formulas or essential fatty acid concentrates as single products. However, we recommend the Natural Pain Relief For Arthritis formula that combines all the natural pain and inflammation-suppressing therapies. To order any of these products, call 1-800-544-4440.

Asthma

Asthma is characterized by recurrent airway obstructions that may resolve by themselves or may require treatment. Asthma may be a response to inhaled allergens, infectious agents, irritants (such as dust, chemical vapors or cold air) or may come from emotional stress. Symptoms may range from wheezing, mild coughing and slight breathlessness, to severe attacks that can lead to total airway obstruction and death. The lungs become over-inflated because of impaired emptying and respiratory gas-exchange deterioration.

The immune system components histamine and leukotrienes generate free radicals, involved in the inflammatory process, that results in lung irritation and airway obstruction. The same mechanisms that cause allergies also can cause asthma. When Life Extension Mix was introduced in 1983, many asthmatics called the Foundation to report that their asthma unexpectedly went away.

Studies document that asthmatics who take high-potency vitamin supplements have a significant reduction in the incidence and severity of asthmatic attacks. They also show that high dietary magnesium intake is associated with improvement in lung function, less wheezing and fewer asthma attacks. Life Extension Mix contains high levels of magnesium, which may partially explain why so many asthmatics no longer have asthma attacks after taking Life Extension Mix.

Asthmatics should consider taking an additional 500 mg a day of elemental magnesium. Histamine is a major factor in asthmatic attacks, and vitamin C is involved in the natural destruction of excess histamine. Asthmatics should take at least two 600-mg capsules of N-acetylcysteine (NAC) a day, along with two grams or more of vitamin C, to break up mucus that could worsen an asthmatic attack.

Asthmatics also should consider taking either the drug Hydergine or the herbal extract forskolin to safely boost intracellular levels of the messenger molecule cyclic adenosine monophosphate (cAMP). Higher levels of cAMP often reduce bronchial constriction. Forskolin has been shown to relax smooth muscles in the airways of guinea pigs, both in vitro and in vivo, by raising tissue cAMP levels. The recommended dose of Hydergine is 5 mg to 10 mg a day with food. Forskolin can be taken in the dosage range of 10 mg to 60 mg a day. The FDA-approved drug theophylline is used to treat asthma because it boosts cAMP levels.

Important: Forskolin may lower blood pressure, so avoid it if you are hypotensive. Do not take forskolin if you have prostate cancer.

Buffered vitamin C, 500 to 1,000 mg, taken at bedtime seems to lessen or prevent the asthmatic attacks that occur around 4 a.m., according to Carmen Fusco. Sublingual DMG before vigorous activity, vitamins B6 and B12, and cirtrus bioflavonoids prove helpful, she adds.

Product availability: Life Extension Mix, forskolin, N-acetylcysteine (NAC), magnesium and vitamin C are available by calling 1-800-544-4440. You also can ask for a listing of offshore pharmacies that sell high potency generic Hydergine to Americans for personal use.

Atherosclerosis

Atherosclerosis is the leading cause of death and disability in the Western world. Atherosclerosis can be defined as the progressive narrowing of the arteries. A heart attack or stroke can occur as a result of a blood clot that forms in an atherosclerotic artery, and/or when the artery narrows to the point of severely restricting blood flow. Restricted blood flow results in cell injury and cell death in the heart, brain, kidneys and other organs.

Specific diseases caused by atherosclerosis include coronary artery disease, angina pectoris, cerebral vascular disease, thrombotic stroke, transient ischemic attacks and diabetic vascular complications.

The mechanisms that have been identified as the most probable causative factors in the development of atherosclerosis and reduced blood flow include:

- ❖ LDL cholesterol oxidation. LDL stands for low-density lipoprotein and is often referred to as "bad cholesterol." Oxidation of LDL renders it "sticky," which enables it to be readily deposited on the internal lining of blood vessel walls. The oxidation of LDL cholesterol and other blood fats can initiate and significantly contribute to the development of atherosclerosis.

- ❖ Homocysteine. Homocysteine is a by-product of methionine metabolism. Homocysteine often causes the initial lesions on arterial walls that enable LDL cholesterol and fibrinogen to accumulate and eventually to occlude blood flow. Homocysteine also contributes to the oxidation of LDL cholesterol and the accumulation of arterial plaque. Homocysteine also can cause abnormal arterial blood clots (thrombosis) that can completely block an artery. Homocysteine alone promotes atherosclerosis and thrombosis, even if cholesterol and triglyceride levels are not significantly elevated.

- ❖ Abnormal platelet aggregation. Fibrinogen, platelets and other clotting factors aggregate with LDL cholesterol, triglycerides and calcium on the arterial wall to further promote the development of atherosclerotic plaques. Abnormal platelet aggregation can lead to the development of a blood clot on the arterial walls inside the heart, brain or any other organ, resulting in ischemia (reduced blood flow) and/or infarction (cell death). Abnormal platelet aggregation can cause an acute arterial blood clot that can lead to a suddenly fatal heart attack or stoke.

To prevent the known atherogenic factors from causing a heart attack, stroke or other arterial occlusive disease, the following protocols should be followed:

1. To inhibit the oxidation of serum cholesterol we suggest:

    a) Life Extension Mix — Three tablets, three times a day, preferably with meals. Life Extension Mix contains a potent spectrum of such antioxidants as vitamin E, which have been shown to inhibit the oxidation of cholesterol.

b) Coenzyme Q10 — 100 mg to 200 mg a day. CoQ10 works synergistically with vitamin E to prevent LDL cholesterol oxidation. CoQ10 also enhances heart cell energy function. CoQ10 in a base of rice bran oil should be used, based on studies showing superior assimilation and cardiac benefits.

c) Life Extension Herbal Mix — One tablespoon early in the day. This formula contains plant extracts that have been documented to maintain the health of the vascular system and reduce the incidence of cardiovascular disease. Life Extension Herbal Mix contains pharmaceutical doses of such premium grade herbal extracts as green tea, ginkgo biloba, ginseng, bilberry and grape seed-skin extract. The suggested dose is one tablespoon mixed with water or juice early in the day.

2. To inhibit the formation of atherogenic homocysteine, we suggest:

a) Folic Acid — 800 micrograms with every meal. Folic acid has been shown to significantly lower blood levels of artery-clogging homocysteine. Folic acid stays in the body only for four to five hours after oral ingestion, so it is crucial to take 800 micrograms of folic acid with every meal. Use a folic acid supplement that also contains at least 300 micrograms of vitamin B12. Folic acid works synergistically with vitamin B12 to lower homocysteine levels.

b) Vitamin B6 — 100 to 200 mg a day. Vitamin B6 reduces homocysteine via a different mechanism than folic acid. There is enough vitamin B6 in Life Extension Mix to keep homocysteine levels under control in most people. In the case of the disease called familial homocysteinemia, however, folate will not reduce homocysteine levels adequately, but doses of vitamin B6 in excess of 500 mg daily can do so. Since high doses of vitamin B6 can cause peripheral nerve toxicity, high doses (500 mg a day and higher) should only be used when a blood test documents the failure of folic acid to lower homocysteine levels.

c) Trimethylglycine (TMG) —500 to 1,500 mg a day with meals. TMG is the most effective homocysteine-lowering substance known.

3. To inhibit the formation of blood clots inside arteries, we suggest:

a) Low-dose aspirin — Take ¼ of an aspirin tablet every day with the heaviest meal of the day.

b) Fish Oils — Take four to eight capsules daily of a concentrated EPA/DHA fish oil supplement. Flax oil may work as well as fish oils.

c) Garlic — Take 800 to 4,000 mg a day.

4. To lower cholesterol levels, we suggest:

a) Herbal Cardiovascular Formula — Take one capsule in the morning and one in the evening. If your cholesterol levels are not significantly lower in 30 days, double or triple this dose.

b) Soy protein concentrate — Take one heaping tablespoon (10 to 20 grams) of soy protein powder containing a standardized amount of soy isoflavones such as genistein and daidzein. A product called Mega Soy Extract provides, in two small capsules, the amount of genistein and other isoflavones found in 10 to 20 grams of soy protein powder. It is not yet known if these two capsules of genistein extract will lower cholesterol levels. The Mega Soy Extract supplement is used primarily for cancer and osteoporosis risk reduction.

c) Fiber — Take 10 to 30 grams of soluble fibers, including pectins, guar and psyllium. You can take fiber powder along with soy protein powder.

It should be noted that there is an overlapping beneficial effect in the above recommendations. For example, the homocysteine-reducing effect of folic acid can inhibit the progression of atherosclerosis and also reduce the risk of abnormal blood clots forming inside arteries. Folic acid, therefore, protects against heart attack and stroke via two well-documented mechanisms of action.

Also, fish oil has been shown in published studies to reduce triglyceride levels by about 35 percent on average. Thus, fish oil may prevent abnormal arterial clotting and reduce triglyceride-induced arterial clogging.

In addition to lowering cholesterol levels, soy protein has been shown to induce a significant improvement in insulin sensitivity, glucose effectiveness, fasting insulin levels, and insulin-to-glucose ratios. In female monkeys, soy genistein has been shown to enhance the dilator response to acetylcholine in atherosclerotic arteries. This means that the daily ingestion of soy could prevent sudden heart attack or stroke by mechanisms other than its known cholesterol-lowering effect.

Linus Pauling recommended that 500 mg of the amino acid lysine be taken three times a day as a therapy for reversing atherosclerosis. Dr. Pauling showed that the combination of lysine and vitamin C inhibits lipoprotein(a) and (b) from accumulating on the arterial wall. Thus, individuals with coronary atherosclerosis or aortic valve stenosis may want to add vitamin C and lysine to their regimens.

Herbal Cardiovascular Formula contains potent extracts of ginger and curcumin. These extracts produce anti-inflammatory effects that may slow the progression of aortic stenosis. Ginger also inhibits abnormal platelet aggregation. For further information on aortic valve stenosis, refer to the Valvular Insufficiency/Heart Valve Defects protocol.

These protocols are designed to prevent the development of atherosclerosis and arterial blockage by :

1. Lowering and inhibiting the oxidation of LDL cholesterol;
2. Elevating beneficial HDL cholesterol;
3. Lowering serum triglycerides, fibrinogen, glucose, homocysteine and iron levels; and
4. Inhibiting the propensity of the blood to clot within blood vessels.

Following these protocols involves a lot of pill-taking, but it must be understood that there are many factors that can cause atherosclerosis and abnormal blood clots that can lead to a heart attack or stroke. If you fail to use all the known therapies for preventing atherosclerosis and abnormal blood clotting, one missing link could cause a life-threatening cardiovascular event. Many Foundation members already are following our atherosclerosis protocols because the same antioxidant nutrients used to prevent cardiovascular disease may also help to prevent cancer, cataract, Alzheimer's disease and a host of other aging-related illnesses.

Product availability: You can obtain Life Extension Mix, coenzyme Q10, Life Extension Herbal Mix, folic acid, vitamin B6, fish oils, Herbal Cardiovascular Formula, garlic, Fiberfood, Healthprin (aspirin), Mega EPA, TMG and Super Soy Extract powder by calling 1-800-544-4440.

Attention Deficit Disorder (ADD)

Children with learning difficulties often have attention deficit disorder. ADD can be a symptom of vitamin deficiency. Studies document improvement in cognitive function when children and young adults take vitamin supplements. The most difficult aspect of treating ADD in children is compliance. Chewable vitamin supplements do not taste good, and it is sometimes hard to get children to swallow pills.

Many parents have their children drink a glass of juice spiked with Life Extension Mix powder every morning before school. Life Extension Mix is the most concentrated vitamin supplement in the world. Children should take a proportionally smaller dose than an adult, based upon their weight. If the child will not drink Life Extension Mix with juice, then other forms of high-potency vitamin supplementation should be tried to correct learning disorders and behavior problems.

Elevating acetylcholine levels in the brain can improve cognitive function and concentration. A convenient supplement for children to take is the acetylcholine precursor product called Choline Cooler. This product was designed by life extension scientists Durk Pearson and Sandy Shaw and is a good tasting powder that can be mixed in water or juice. Choline Cooler contains a synergistic blend of acetylcholine precursors that are ideal to help boost memory and concentration.

Cognitex contains a broad array of brain-boosting nutrients. If a child is able to swallow capsules, four to six capsules in the morning are suggested.

Udo's Choice Oil Blend also can be helpful for maintaining proper growth and helping to make prostaglandins that are essential for brain function. Essential fatty acids are a structural component of all brain cells, the blood-brain barrier, the myelin sheath that wraps around nerves, and cellular walls. Essential fatty acids comprise more than 50 percent of the brain itself, and help with nerve transmission.

If desired results do not occur with supplements of vitamins, choline and essential fatty acids, then the European drug piracetam should be added. Piracetam dosing for adults is 1,600 to 4,800 mg a day. Children should take slightly less piracetam, though piracetam does not appear to be toxic even when children take adult doses. All these nutrients and drugs should be taken in the morning.

Product availability: Cognitex, Udo's Choice Oil Blend, Choline Cooler and Life Extension Mix can be ordered by calling 1-800-544-4440. Call to receive a list of offshore pharmacies that sell piracetam to Americans for personal use.

Autoimmune Diseases

A wide range of degenerative diseases are caused by the immune system attacking a person's own cells. Our immune system becomes increasingly defective as we age, though some people suffer from autoimmune diseases very early in life. Immune dysfunction can cause immune responsive cells to manufacture antibodies that attack the linings of the joints, resulting in arthritis. It could also prompt defectively functioning immune cells to attack the insulin-producing islet cells of the pancreas, resulting in insulin-dependent diabetes. Lupus is thought to be primarily an autoimmune disease.

As noted in a previous protocol (but which bears repeating in this context), because oxidative damage has been implicated in such autoimmune diseases as rheumatoid arthritis and lupus, a study was designed to assess serum concentrations of vitamin E, beta-carotene and vitamin A in patients. The study examined cases of rheumatoid arthritis and systemic lupus erythematosus that developed two to 15 years after people donated blood to a serum bank in 1974. Stored serum samples were assayed for vitamin E, beta-carotene and vitamin A.

People who later developed rheumatoid arthritis or lupus showed lower serum concentrations of vitamin E, beta-carotene and vitamin A in 1974 than did matched controls. For rheumatoid arthritis, the difference for beta-carotene (minus 29 percent) was statistically significant. These findings support those of a previous study showing that low antioxidant status is a risk factor for rheumatoid arthritis and systemic lupus erythematosus.

A host of diseases have been linked to a defective immune system. Many people find that taking three tablets three times a day of Life Extension Mix can help correct a defective immune system.

People with existing autoimmune diseases may need more help than just Life Extension Mix. The hormone DHEA can help suppress certain unwanted immune system reactions in autoimmune-disease patients. A recent clinical study showed that DHEA reduced symptoms in patients with lupus, a common autoimmune disease.

CAUTION: Refer to the DHEA-Pregnenolone Precautions for safety and proper dosing information before beginning DHEA therapy.

Fish oils that provide concentrated amounts of the essential fatty acids EPA and DHA, and borage oil that contains gamma linolenic acid (GLA), can be effective in alleviating the symptoms of autoimmune diseases. Suggested doses are four capsules a day of the fish oil concentrate Mega EPA, and five capsules a day of Mega GLA, along with the standard daily dose of Life Extension Mix.

Product availability: Mega EPA, Mega GLA, DHEA and Life Extension Mix can be obtained by calling 1-800-544-4440.

Bacterial Infections

Acute bacterial infections require immediate conventional medical care. If FDA-approved antibiotics fail to work, European antibiotics, which are several years more advanced than American antibiotics, may be effective.

The following natural therapies are suggested:

* Herbal extracts from goldenseal and echinacea may be effective natural antibiotics. Raw garlic has potent antibacterial effects. Kyolic, an aged garlic product, does not kill bacteria directly, but does boost immune function, thus enabling the body to fight off some chronic bacterial infections.

* Shark liver oil capsules containing a minimum of 200 mg of alkylglycerols per capsule, at the dose of five capsules a day, can have a direct antibiotic effect. Do not take shark liver oil for more than 30 days because it may cause the overproduction of blood platelets.

* Bromelain can potentiate the effects of conventional antibiotics, making them more effective in killing bacteria. Suggested dose is 2,000 mg of

bromelain per day.

❖ Arginine in doses ranging from 6 to 20 grams a day can stimulate antibacterial components of the immune system. Arginine promotes nitric oxide synthesis, which may protect against bacterial infections. The role of nitric oxide was studied in host defense against Klebsiella pneumoniae infection of the lung. The results suggested that nitric oxide plays a critical role in antibacterial host defense against Klebsiella pneumoniae, in part by regulating macrophage phagocytic and microbicidal activity.

❖ Recent electron microscope studies show that bee propolis has a potent anti-bacterial effect by preventing cell division and inhibiting protein synthesis.

CAUTION: Bee products should not be administered to children under the age of three.

For more information about treating bacterial infections, refer to the Foundation's Immune Enhancement protocols.

Product availability: For information on European antibiotics, call 1-800-544-4440. Kyolic garlic, Norwegian shark liver oil, bromelain, echinacea, arginine and bee propolis can be obtained by calling 1-800-544-4440.

Balding

Although hair loss is an integral part of the aging process, its impact is most pronounced in young people who suffer from a condition called androgenetic alopecia (AGA), which causes accelerated hair loss. AGA is commonly called male pattern baldness but, in fact, occurs in both men and women.

The pattern of hair loss varies by gender. With men, it usually begins with a receding hair line, with further loss at the vertex of the scalp. In women, the pattern is more diffuse, typically sparing the anterior hairline and predominately affecting the crown.

The current model of how accelerated hair loss occurs involves a combination of genetic, hormonal and immunologic factors.

Despite what some doctors (and TV infomercials) would have you believe, AGA has nothing to do with clogged hair follicles, which has been the basis for many "hair growth" products. Good scalp hygiene will improve hair's appearance, and can add volume to existing hair, but it will do nothing to prevent AGA or actually increase hair counts. There are at least 20 different products on the market today which claim, either directly or indirectly, that they will grow hair or prevent baldness by "unclogging" your hair follicles. The effectiveness of virtually all these products can be summed up in three simple words—they don't work!

The only exceptions to this are the compounds polysorbate 60 and polysorbate 80, both of which are in Life Extension Shampoo sold by the Life Extension Buyers Club. Polysorbate 60 and 80 appear to be useful in slowing down hair loss when applied topically because of their ability to emulsify androgen-rich sebum deposits from the scalp. They are rarely able to generate any degree of hair regrowth, however, but may be useful in conjunction with other agents.

There's little doubt that some people are genetically susceptible to accelerated hair loss caused by AGA. Generations of young men with bald fathers have traditionally dreaded the first signs of hair loss, which to them signified the beginning of a process that would inevitably end in baldness at an earlier-than-normal age.

The latest scientific model to explain baldness involves the action of dihydrotestosterone (DHT), the major metabolite of the male hormone testosterone. Scientists have found that excessive secretion of DHT stimulates a localized immune reaction, which in turn generates an inflammatory response that damages hair follicles. This results in their miniaturization and eventual loss.

What appears to happen is that DHT (and perhaps other androgenic hormones) causes the immune system to react to the hair follicles in the affected areas as foreign bodies. This is suggested by the presence of hair-follicle antibodies, as well as by the infiltration of immune system cells around the hair follicles of balding men and women.

Successful prevention and treatment of accelerated hair loss necessitates dealing with some, if not all, of these factors involved in the process, except for the genetic component of baldness that is still in the research phase.

Since the male hormone dihydrotestosterone is involved in premature hair loss, scientists have experimented with a wide variety of anti-androgens in an attempt to prevent or reverse the process. Among the anti-androgens that have been used to treat hair loss are progesterone, spironolactone (Aldactone), flutamide (Eulexin), finasteride (Proscar), cimetidine (Tagamet), serenoa repens (Permixon) and cyproterone acetate (Androcur/Diane). Of these anti-androgens, the most effective have proven to be oral finasteride (Proscar) and topical spironolactone, both of which have been able to grow hair to some degree with minimal side effects.

In the hair-loss process, it is the immune reaction caused by male hormones such as DHT that plays, perhaps, the most significant role. Stimulated by androgens, the immune system targets hair follicles in genetically susceptible areas to cause the premature loss of hair that is characteristic of male pattern baldness.

Among the most potent hair growth stimulators are topical oxygen radical scavengers such as the superoxide dismutases (SODs), enzymes that play a critically important role in countering excessive free radical activity throughout the body.

SODs not only inhibit oxygen radicals, but also may inhibit the localized immune response responsible for so much hair loss, and may offset some of the damage and inflammation already incurred. Unless the immunologic factors involved in the hair loss process are dealt with effectively, the potential for significant hair regrowth may be very limited.

A Multi-Modal Approach To Hair Treatment

There are many agents available (such as Rogaine) that can stimulate some degree of hair growth in some people, but cannot by themselves produce the kind of health and cosmetic benefits that balding people desire. What's needed is a multi-modal approach that combines anti-androgens with autoimmune protective agents, oxygen free radical inhibitors, and other hair-growth stimulators to halt hair loss and generate hair regrowth to a degree well beyond the abilities of single compounds.

Dr. Peter Proctor is the only hair treatment practitioner in the world who has developed unique, patented multi-ingredient hair formulas that address all the known factors in the balding process. He is the author of more than 30 scientific articles and book chapters, and holds several broad patents for hair-loss treatment.

Dr. Proctor offers both prescription and non-prescription hair treatment formulas which vary both in potency and cost. However, even the least-potent of Dr. Proctor's formulas has proven to be superior to Rogaine, the only FDA-approved hair treatment product on the market.

The least expensive of Dr. Proctor's hair growth formulas is sold under the name Dr. Proctor's Hair Regrowth Shampoo. This formula includes an abundant supply of the most potent natural hair growth stimulator available—NANO (3-carboxylic acid pyridine-N-oxide), which is known as "natural" minoxidil.

Dr. Proctor's Hair Regrowth Shampoo has been shown to work effectively in many people who did not respond to Rogaine. It may be all you need if you have experienced only small to moderate hair loss, or if your primary need is for a prophylactic program that will prevent hair loss in the future. Dr. Proctor's Hair Regrowth Shampoo should be used whenever you shower or wash your hair (at least three times a week). It should be used just like any other shampoo.

The second formula developed by Dr. Proctor, which is sold under the name Dr. Proctor's Advanced Hair Regrowth Formula, includes a potent dose of "natural" minoxidil (NANO) combined with the following natural hair protection and hair growth agents: EDRF enhancers, SODs and various free radical scavengers.

This multi-agent natural formula is the most potent natural hair growth formula you can buy. It includes every type of natural hair-treatment agent available to counter the DHT, autoimmune and inflammatory effects that are at the root of hair loss and baldness. Dr. Proctor's Advanced Hair Regrowth Formula is a liquid that is applied to the scalp.

Dr. Proctor's Advanced Hair Regrowth Formula should be used in the following manner: eight to 10 drops applied once or twice a day to the thinning areas. Its side effects include contact dermatitis, an itchy, scaly rash at the site of application.

If you have a really serious hair-loss problem, you may need to try Dr. Proctor's most potent hair-growth formula—Dr. Proctor's European Prescription Hair Regrowth Formula—which uses an array of natural hair growth protectors combined with several drugs compounded into a cream base. The natural agents in Dr. Proctor's European Prescription Hair Regrowth Formula include topical anti-androgens, which increase EDRF levels and oxygen free radical scavengers. These agents are combined with the following drugs: minoxidil, phenytoin (Dilantin), tretinoin (Retin-A) and spironolactone.

The protocol for using Dr. Proctor's European Prescription Hair Regrowth Formula is as follows: Apply 1/10 of a teaspoon (a dab on the end of your finger) once a day for eight to 12 months, then every other day for maintenance. Its side effects include contact dermatitis.

Product availability: You can order Dr. Proctor's Hair Regrowth Shampoo and Advanced Hair Regrowth Formula by calling 1-800-544-4440. European Prescription Hair Regrowth Formula is available by prescription from his office. For further information, call 1-800-544-4440.

Bladder Conditions

Bladder conditions, benign and malignant, often are treated successfully by innovative doctors with the FDA-approved biological, non-toxic solvent dimethyl sulfoxide (DMSO).

For bladder infections, refer to the Foundation's Urinary Tract Infections protocol in this book.

For bladder cancer, refer to the Foundation's Cancer protocols.

For use of DMSO in interstitial cystitis, have your doctor contact Research Industries Corporation at 1-801-972-5500. This company offers a DMSO product called Rimso-50.

Blood Testing

Please refer to the Medical Testing protocol.

Breast Cancer

In 1971, when President Richard Nixon declared "war on cancer," the chance of a woman getting breast cancer was one in 20. Today, after billions of dollars of government research money has been spent fighting the disease, the odds are a shocking one out of eight women who will develop breast cancer.

According to the American Cancer Society, more than 180,000 women will be diagnosed with breast cancer in the coming year, and about 46,000 women will die from it. Breast cancer has become the second largest cause of cancer death in women, after lung cancer, and the leading cause of death for women between 35 and 54. Ever since the "war on cancer" was declared, more women have died of breast cancer than the total number of Americans who lost their lives in World Wars I and II, the Korean War, and the Vietnam War combined!

Clearly, we are in the midst of a breast cancer epidemic. By the time the tell-tale lump is detected in the breast, there already are an average of 45 billion cancer cells present, and some of these malignant cells have been metastasized to other parts of the body. Conventional medicine recommends radiation and chemotherapy after the cancerous lump has been removed in an attempt to kill escaped, metastasized cancer cells. The net effect of radiation and chemotherapy is the weakening of the immune system and the rendering of the cancer patient more vulnerable to the development of metastatic lesions in critical organs of the body.

There are alternative therapies that are crucial to the successful treatment of breast cancer. Breast cancer cells differ from other cancer cells, thus mandating the incorporation of immune- and hormone-modulating therapies that interfere with breast cancer cell proliferation.

One of the most important supplements for the breast cancer patient is high doses of the hormone melatonin at bedtime. Melatonin blocks estrogen receptors somewhat similarly to the drug tamoxifen without the long-term side effects of tamoxifen. Further, when melatonin and tamoxifen are combined, synergistic benefits occur. Melatonin can be safely taken for an indefinite period of time. The suggested dose of melatonin for breast cancer patients is 10 to 50 mg at bedtime.

Melatonin not only blocks estrogen receptor sites on breast cancer cells, but directly inhibits breast cancer cell proliferation and boosts the production of immune components that kill metastasized cancer cells.

It should be noted that new studies on tamoxifen indicate that after two years, it can cause a significant increase of estrogens in the blood. This may be a mechanism by which cancer cells become resistant to tamoxifen therapy. Since serious side effects of tamoxifen also begin at two years, it may be prudent not to use tamoxifen for more than two years.

CAUTION: Although melatonin is strongly recommended for breast cancer patients, inter-leukin-2 (IL-2), which often is combined with melatonin, should be avoided by breast cancer patients. IL-2 may promote breast cancer cell division.

Vitamin A and vitamin D3 inhibit breast cancer cell division and can induce cancer cells to differentiate into mature, non-cancer cells. Vitamin D3 works synergistically with tamoxifen to inhibit breast cancer cell proliferation. Breast cancer patients should take 4,000 to 6,000 IU of vitamin D3 every day on an empty stomach. Water-soluble vitamin A can be taken in doses of 100,000 IU to 300,000 IU every day. Monthly blood tests are needed to make sure toxicity does not occur in response to these relatively high daily doses of vitamin A and vitamin D3. After six months, the doses of vitamin D3 and vitamin A can be reduced.

Vitamin E and vitamin E succinate negatively regulate tumor cells in vitro and in vivo. In a recently published study, vitamin E succinate, a derivative of fat soluble vitamin E, inhibited growth and induced apoptic cell death in estrogen receptor-negative human breast cancer cell lines. The study concluded that vitamin E succinate may be of clinical use in the treatment of aggressive human breast cancers, particularly those that are resistant to anti-estrogen therapy.

Estrogen receptor-negative breast cancer patients should consider taking 1,200 IU of vitamin E succinate a day.

Important: Refer to the Symptoms of Vitamin A Toxicity, in Appendix A.

Soy extracts have become very popular in the last few years as an adjuvant (assisting) cancer therapy. However, there are some cancer patients who should not use soy, or who are less likely to benefit from soy.

Cancer patients (and their doctors) may find the following information complicated, but it is crucial that it be understood if the cancer patient is to use high concentrations of soy properly.

Cancer patients undergoing radiation therapy should not take soy supplements one week before, during, and one week after being treated. Soy inhibits protein kinase C activity in cancer cells. Since cancer cells use protein kinase C for energy production, inhibiting this enzyme is usually desirable. Radiation therapy, on the other hand, depends on protein kinase C to help generate free radicals that kill cancer cells. It's possible, therefore, that large amounts of genistein in cancer cells could protect them against radiation-induced free-radical-mediated destruction.

In studies, genistein has shown anti-angiogenesis effects. Angiogenesis (new blood vessel growth) is a key step in tumor growth, invasion and metastasis. To date, a number of anti-angiogenic agents have been identified. In animal models, treatment with angiogenesis inhibitors has proven anti-tumor effects. Early clinical experience with angiogenic inhibitors indicates that optimal anti-angiogenic therapy will likely be based on the long-term administration of genistein to cancer patients as an adjunct to surgery and conventional chemotherapy. Genistein is one of the more potent nutritional anti-angiogenesis agents.

Genistein also has been shown to have cancer cell adhesion inhibition properties, and apoptosis-inducing (programmed cancer cell death inducing) effects.

An investigation into the effects of soy genistein on the growth and differentiation of human melanoma cells showed that genistein significantly inhibited cell growth. Some studies suggest that genistein may enhance the benefits of certain chemotherapy regimens.

One study showed that genistein inhibited the proliferation and expression of the invasive capacity of prostate cancer cells in vitro. Genistein proved to be cytotoxic to a line of prostate cancer cells. The more aggressively the prostate cancer cells grew, the more genistein was effective in inhibiting both growth factors and the rate of cellular proliferation. Prostate cancers often have similarities to breast cancers.

Curcumin and genistein both have been shown to inhibit the growth of estrogen-positive human breast cancer cells induced by pesticides. When curcumin and genistein were added to breast cancer cells, a synergistic effect resulted in a total inhibition of cancer cell growth caused by pesticide-induced estrogenic activity. This study suggested that the combination of curcumin and genistein in the diet has the potential to reduce the proliferation of estrogen-positive cells induced by mixtures of pesticides or estrogen. Since it is difficult to remove pesticides completely from the diet and since both curcumin and soy genistein is not toxic to humans, their inclusion in the diet in order to prevent hormone related cancers deserves consideration.

A study was conducted to determine if genistein can induce human breast adenocarcinoma cell maturation and differentiation. Treating these cells with genistein resulted in growth inhibition accompanied by increased cell maturation. These maturation markers were optimally expressed after nine days of treatment with genistein. Both estrogen receptor-positive and estrogen receptor-negative cells became differentiated in response to genistein, which is a crucial step in inducing cancer cell apoptosis (programmed cell death).

Naturally occurring flavonoids were tested for their effects on the proliferation of an estrogen receptor-positive human breast cancer cell line. Genistein inhibited cell proliferation, but was reversed with the addition of excess competing estrogen. The flavonoids hesperidin, naringenin and quercetin inhibited breast cancer cell proliferation, even in the presence of high levels of estrogen. These flavonoids apparently exert their anti-proliferative activity via a mechanism different from that of genistein.

A study was conducted to determine if genistein can induce human breast adenocarcinoma cell maturation and differentiation. Treating these cells with genistein resulted in growth inhibition accompanied by increased cell maturation. Optimal maturation was achieved after nine days of treatment with genistein. Both cancer cells with positive estrogen-receptors and negative estrogen-receptor cells differentiated in response to genistein, a crucial step in the induction of cancer cell apoptosis.

Despite these studies, we do not recommend that women with estrogen receptor-positive breast cancer use soy genistein. The Foundation has made a preliminary determination that women with estrogen receptor-positive breast cancer should not take soy supplements based on evidence that an estrogenic growth effect could occur in some forms of estrogen receptor-positive breast cancer. Until more is known about the effects of soy phytoestrogens in this type of cancer, compounds such as genistein should be avoided in those with estrogen receptor-positive breast cancer.

The most potent soy extract on the market is called Mega Soy Extract. It contains almost 40 percent pure soy isoflavones . . . much higher than previous soy products. The suggested dose for non-estrogen receptor-positive breast cancer patients is five 700-mg capsules of Mega Soy Extract four times a day. This provides the optimal daily dose of approximately 2,800 mg of standardized genistein. Genistein is rapidly metabolized within the body, which makes it necessary for cancer patients to take Mega Soy Extract in four divided doses spaced evenly throughout the day.

Soy genistein may inhibit an enzyme that normally recycles cyclooxygenases in the colon. This may lead to excess levels of Cox-2 (cyclooxygenase 2) in the colon. Cox-2 causes excess production of prostaglandin E2, which in turn can promote cancer growth, stimulate angiogenesis and induce immunosuppression. Colon cancer patients taking soy supplements should consider taking an aspirin with their heavy meal every day to inhibit Cox-2. Other Cox-2 inhibitors include a daily dose of fish oil concentrate containing 2,400 mg of EPA and 1,800 mg of DHA, 2,000 mg of ginger extract and 6,000 mg a day of garlic. For some cancers, inhibition of Cox-2 can be an effective adjuvant therapy in and of itself.

Women with any type of breast cancer should test their serum estrogen levels to make sure that too much estrogen is not present if they are taking high doses of soy. Estrogen can combine with the genistein to cause some breast cancer cells to grow faster. Other studies show that genistein blocks certain types of estrogen-receptor sites, thus inhibiting the proliferation of these types of breast cancer cells.

Breast cancer patients whose tumor cells have a mutant p53 oncogene are far more likely to benefit from soy extract supplementation. Only a pathology examination of the actual cancer cells can determine p53 status. An immuno-histochemistry test can help to determine the p53 status of tumor cells. The following laboratory can perform this new test:

IMPATH Laboratories
1010 Third Avenue, Suite 203
New York, N.Y. 10021
Phone: 1-800-447-5816

IMPATH Labortories measures mutant p53. If the test is positive, you have mutant p53 and are *more* likely to benefit from soy extracts. If the test is negative, this indicates that you have functional p53 and are *less* likely to benefit from soy extracts. The Foundation realizes that many cancer patients seeking to use soy supplements may find it difficult to have an immuno-histochemistry test performed to ascertain p53 status.

Monthly blood testing for breast cancer patients is mandatory. Every patient responds differently to both conventional and alternative cancer therapies. The results of blood tests provide critically important data to evaluate the effectiveness of whatever therapies are being used. The blood tests commonly used by doctors to evaluate progression or regression of breast cancer are CA 27.29, CEA, prolactin, GGTP and alkaline phosphatase. If, for instance, the CA 27.29 tumor marker were to continue to elevate 30 to 60 days after initiating soy extract supplementation, discontinue its use and seek another therapy immediately.

Breast cancer patients often have elevated levels of the pituitary hormone prolactin. Abnormally high levels of prolactin can interfere with successful breast cancer therapy. If a blood test reveals elevated prolactin levels, the oncologist should be encouraged to prescribe 1.25 to 2.5 mg of the drug Parlodel, also known as bromocriptine. Parlodel must be taken after meals because severe nausea can occur when it is taken on an empty stomach. A better way to suppress prolactin is with Dostinex. Just twice a week dosing of 0.25 mg to 0.50

mg is needed, and side effects are rare.

There are phytochemicals in cabbage and broccoli that interfere with breast cancer cell growth. Studies show that the phytochemical 3-indole carbinol can inhibit activation of the estrogen receptor, thus lowering estrogenic stimulation in estrogen-dependent breast cancer cells.

The daily juicing of fresh organic cabbage and/or broccoli is suggested for breast cancer patients. For those who find it too inconvenient to juice cabbage and broccoli every day, there is a product called Phyto-Food powder that is composed of potent concentrations of broccoli, cabbage and other cruciferous vegetables that contain phytochemicals that help fight cancer. Breast cancer patients should take two heaping tablespoons of Phyto-Food powder every day.

Preliminary research from Europe indicates extremely encouraging results when breast cancer patients take 300 to 400 mg a day of coenzyme Q10. Breast cancer patients should thus consider taking 300 to 400 mg a day of coenzyme Q10 in oil-filled capsules for maximum absorption.

The most current research shows that some of the ingredients in green tea may have a beneficial effect in treating cancer. While drinking green tea is a well-documented method of preventing cancer, it is difficult for the cancer patient to obtain a sufficient quantity of anti-cancer components in that form. We suggest that a person with breast cancer take four to 10 decaffeinated green tea extract capsules every day. These capsules contain a standardized extract of epigallocatechin gallate, which is the component of green tea that makes it an effective adjunct therapy in the treatment of breast cancer.

Radiation exposure as a result of the Chernobyl nuclear power plant accident in the Soviet Union in April 1986 increased the cancer risk of the nearby population and emergency workers. A long-term experiment in 400 rats exposed to radiation following the Chernobyl pattern showed that a selenium-enriched diet started after exposure caused a longer average lifespan and a 1.5 to 3.5-fold decrease of leukemias and other malignancies including breast cancer. Selenium has been shown to directly induce growth arrest and death of mammary cancer cells in mice, though it cannot be inferred that selenium by itself can result in breast cancer remission in humans. Breast cancer patients should consider 200 micrograms of organic selenium (selenomethionine), two to three times a day.

One of the most exciting new therapies in the prevention and treatment of breast cancer is conjugated linoleic acid (CLA). CLA is the component of beef that has direct breast cancer cell inhibitory effects. CLA has been shown both in vitro and in animal models to have strong anti-tumor activity. Particular effects were observed on the growth and metastatic spread of transplantable mammary tumors. One study examined the effect of dietary CLA on the growth of human breast adenocarcinoma cells in mice. Dietary CLA inhibited local tumor growth by 73 percent and 30 percent at nine and 14 weeks post-inoculation, respectively. Moreover, CLA completely abrogated the spread of breast cancer cells to lungs, peripheral blood, and bone marrow. This indicates the ability of dietary CLA to block the local growth and systemic spread of human breast cancer. For breast cancer prevention and treatment, it is suggested that six to 10 500-mg capsules of CLA a day be taken. Estrogen receptor negative breast cancer patients should take at least 800 mg of soy genistein when taking CLA.

Lignans are an important class of phytochemicals found in flax seed. When rats are fed a diet containing ground flax seed, it becomes very difficult to develop a breast tumor, even when breast cancer cells have been injected directly into the animal. Rats not given flax seed readily develop breast cancers in response to injections with live cancer cells.

When rats with large breast tumors were fed flax seed, the breast tumors shrunk. In laboratory monkeys who eat lignans in their lab chow, it is very difficult to induce breast tumors. Ground flax seed (but not flax oil) provides a healthy dose of lignans. The most efficient way of consuming fresh flax seed with other cancer fighting phytochemicals is to consume two to five tablespoons a day of The Missing Link for Humans, a specially designed flax seed based meal replacement food.

Garlic is a well-established cancer-preventing nutrient. A study investigated aged garlic extract in an effort to determine whether it could inhibit proliferation of cancer cells. The proliferation and viability of erythroleukemia, hormone-responsive breast and prostate cancer cell lines were evaluated. The eyrtholeukemia cells were not significantly affected by the garlic extract, but the breast and prostate cancer cell lines clearly were susceptible to the growth-inhibitory influence of aged garlic extract. The anti-proliferative effect of aged garlic extract was limited to actively growing cells. This study provided evidence that garlic can exert a direct effect on established cancer cells.

Aberrant hyper proliferation is a late-occurring event that precedes mammary tumorigenesis in vivo. A study conducted on pre-cancer cells showed that eicosapentaenoic acid (EPA), indole-3-carbinol (broccoli-cabbage extract) , and green tea extract resulted in a 70 to 99 percent inhibition of aberrant hyperprolifertion.

Whey appears to inhibit the growth of breast cancer cells at low concentrations. One clinical study with cancer patients showed a regression in some patient's tumors when fed whey protein concentrate at 30 grams per day.

Research using whey protein concentrate has led researchers to a discovery regarding the relationship between cancerous cells, whey protein concentrate and glutathione, an antioxidant that protects the body against harmful compounds. It was found that whey protein concentrate selectively depletes cancer cells of their glutathione, thus making them more susceptible to cancer treatments such as radiation and chemotherapy.

It has been found that cancer cells and normal cells will respond differently to nutrients and drugs that affect glutathione status. What is most interesting to note is the fact that the concentration of glutathione in tumor cells is higher than that of the normal cells that surround them. This difference in glutathione status between normal cells and cancer cells is believed to be an important factor in cancer cells' resistance to chemotherapy.

As the researchers put it, "Tumor cell glutathione concentration may be among the determinants of the cytotoxicity of many chemotherapeutic agents and of radiation, and an increase in glutathione concentration in cancer cells appears to be at least one of the mechanisms of acquired drug resistance to chemotherapy." They further state, "It is well-known that rapid glutathione synthesis in tumor cells is associated with high rates of cellular proliferation. Depletion of cancer cell glutathione in vivo decreases the rate of cellular proliferation and inhibits cancer growth."

The problem is, it's difficult to reduce glutathione sufficiently in tumor cells without placing healthy tissue at risk and putting the cancer patient in a worse condition. What is needed is a compound that can selectively deplete the cancer cells of their glutathione, while increasing, or at least maintaining, the levels of glutathione in healthy cells. This is exactly what whey protein appears to do.

In this new research, it was found that cancer cells subjected to whey proteins were depleted of their glutathione, and their growth was inhibited, while normal cells had an increase in glutathione and increased cellular growth. These effects were not seen with other proteins. Not surprisingly, the researchers concluded, "Selective depletion of tumor cell glutathione may in fact render cancer cells more vulnerable to the action of chemotherapy and eventually protect normal tissue against the deleterious effects of chemotherapy." The exact mechanism by which whey protein achieves this is not fully understood, but it appears that it interferes with the normal feedback mechanism and regulation of glutathione in cancer cells. It is known that glutathione production is negatively inhibited by its own synthesis. Since baseline glutathione levels in cancer cells are higher than that of normal cells, it is probably easier to reach the level of negative-feedback inhibition in the cancer cells' glutathione levels than in the normal cells' glutathione levels.

Monthly blood tests should include a complete blood chemistry with tests for liver function and serum calcium levels, prolactin levels, parathyroid hormone levels and the tumor marker CA 27.29, and Cancer Profile tests (CA Profile) that includes the CEA and GGTP tests. These tests monitor the progress or failure of whatever therapies are being used, and also are able to detect toxicity from high doses of vitamin A and vitamin D3. The patient should insist on obtaining a copy of their blood workups every month.

Please refer to the Cancer Treatment Protocol for additional suggestions.

Product availability: Melatonin, Phyto-Food, Mega Soy Extract, coenzyme Q10, green tea, Water-soluble vitamin A, vitamin D3 caps, conjugated linoleic acid and The Missing Link For Humans, can be ordered by calling 1-800-544-4440. Ask for a listing of innovative physicians in your area who may be able to help you implement an alternative therapy cancer program.

Bursitis

The same therapies used to treat arthritis may also be used for the treatment of bursitis and other inflammatory disorders. Refer to the Foundation's Arthritis protocol.

Cancer Chemotherapy

There are nutrient and hormone therapies that can mitigate the toxicity brought about by cancer chemotherapy. In peer-reviewed scientific papers, nutrients such as coenzyme Q10 and vitamin E have been shown to protect against chemotherapy-induced cardiomyopathies, and melatonin has been shown to protect against chemotherapy-induced immune depression.

One study suggested that cancer patients treated with adriamycin should supplement with vitamin A, vitamin E and selenium to reduce the side effects of this toxic chemotherapy drug.

Another study showed that the antioxidants vitamin C, vitamin E and N-acetylcysteine could protect against heart muscle toxicity when cancer patients are receiving high doses of chemotherapy and/or radiation therapy. This study documented that in the antioxidant group, no chemotherapy patient showed a fall in the left ventricular ejection fraction, while 46 percent of patients in the chemotherapy group not receiving antioxidants did experience a fall in left ventricular function. No patient showed a significant fall in overall ejection fraction in the antioxidant group, whereas 29 percent in the group not getting the antioxidants showed a reduction. In the radiation therapy group, left ventricular ejection fraction did not change in patients treated with antioxidants, but 66 percent of patients in the group not receiving the antioxidants showed a fall in ejection fraction.

Experimental data have suggested that the pineal hormone melatonin may counteract chemotherapy-induced myelosuppression and immunosuppression. In addition, melatonin has been shown to inhibit the production of free radicals, thus playing a part in mediating the toxicity of chemotherapy. A study was performed in an attempt to evaluate the influence of melatonin on chemotherapy toxicity. Patients were randomized to receive chemotherapy alone or chemotherapy plus melatonin (20 mg per day in the evening). Thrombocytopenia was significantly less frequent in patients treated with melatonin. Malaise and asthenia also were significantly less frequent in patients receiving melatonin. Finally, stomatitis and neuropathy were less frequent in the melatonin group. Alopecia and vomiting were not influenced by melatonin.

This pilot study seems to suggest that administration of melatonin during chemotherapy may prevent some chemotherapy-induced side effects, particularly myelosuppression and neuropathy.

Expensive drugs such as Leukine (granulocyte macrophage-colony stimulating factor, or GM-CSF) and intron A alpha interferon (an immune modulating cytokine) can restore immune function debilitated by toxic cancer chemotherapy drugs. In a recent published study, patients with refractory (resistant to treatment) solid tumors treated with standard chemotherapy and GM-CSF had a 33.3 percent objective response rate, versus 15 percent with chemotherapy alone.

If you are on chemotherapy, and your blood tests show immune suppression, you should demand that your oncologist use the appropriate immune restoration drug(s).

Melatonin also has been seen to amplify interleukin-2 anticancer action and to reduce its toxicity. Melatonin use in association with IL-2 cancer immunotherapy has been shown to have the following actions:

1. amplification of IL-2 biological activity by enhancing lymphocyte response and by antagonizing macrophage-mediated suppressive events;

2. inhibition of production of tumor growth factors, which stimulate cancer cell proliferation by counteracting lymphocyte-mediated tumor cell destruction;

3. maintenance of a circadian rhythm of melatonin, which is often altered in human neoplasms and influenced by cytokine exogenous injection.

The subcutaneous administration of 3 million IU a day of interleukin-2 (IL-2) and high doses of melatonin (40 mg a day orally) in the evening has appeared to be effective in tumors resistant either to IL-2 alone or to chemotherapy. The dose of 3 million IU a day of interleukin-2 is a low dose, while serious toxicity normally begins at 15 million IU a day. At present, 230 patients with advanced solid tumors and life expectancy less than six months have been treated with this melatonin/IL-2 combination. Objective tumor regressions were experienced in 44 patients (18 percent), mainly in patients with lung cancer, hepatocarcinoma, cancer of the pancreas, gastric cancer and colon cancer. A survival longer than one year was achieved in 41 percent of the patients. The preliminary data show that melatonin synergizes with tumor necrosis factor (TNF) and alpha interferon by reducing their toxicity.

Drugs to mitigate chemotherapy-induced nausea include Megace and Zofran. The high cost of Zofran has kept many cancer patients not covered by insurance from obtaining this potentially beneficial drug. If you are receiving chemotherapy and are suffering from nausea, you should be able to demand that any HMO, PPO or insurance carrier pay for this drug. Zofran can enable a cancer patient to tolerate chemotherapy long enough for it to be possibly effective.

One study evaluated glutathione, vitamin C and vitamin E for their anti-vomiting activity against cisplatin-induced vomiting in dogs. Cisplatin-induced vomiting was significantly reduced by glutathione, vitamin C and vitamin E. The anti-vomiting activity of antioxidants was attributed to their ability to react with free radicals generated by cisplatin. This study provides further evidence that free radicals play a role in cancer chemotherapy-induced vomiting.

Research using whey protein concentrate has led researchers to a discovery regarding the relationship among cancerous cells, whey protein concentrate and glutathione. Glutathione is an antioxidant that protects cells against harmful compounds. It was found that whey protein concentrate selectively depletes cancer cells of their glutathione, thus making them more susceptible to cancer treatments such as radiation and chemotherapy.

It has been found that cancer cells and normal cells will respond differently to nutrients and drugs that affect glutathione status. What is most interesting to note is that the concentration of glutathione in tumor cells is higher than that of the normal cells that surround them. This difference is believed to be an important factor in cancer cells' resistance to chemotherapy. As the researchers put it, "Tumor cell glutathione concentration may be among the determinants of the cytotoxicity of many chemotherapeutic agents and of radiation, and an increase in glutathione concentration in cancer cells appears to be at least one of the mechanisms of acquired drug resistance to chemotherapy."

They further state, "It is well-known that rapid glutathione synthesis in tumor cells is associated with high rates of cellular proliferation. Depletion of cancer cell glutathione in vivo decreases the rate of cellular proliferation and inhibits cancer growth." The problem is, it's difficult to reduce glutathione sufficiently in tumor cells without placing healthy tissue at risk and putting the cancer patient in a worse condition. What is needed is a compound that can selectively deplete the cancer cells of their glutathione while increasing, or at least maintaining, levels of glutathione in healthy cells. This is exactly what whey protein appears to do.

In this new research, it was found that cancer cells subjected to whey proteins were depleted of their glutathione and their growth was inhibited, while normal cells had an increase in glutathione and increased cellular growth. These effects were not seen with other proteins. Not surprisingly, the researchers concluded, "Selective depletion of tumor cell glutathione may, in fact, render cancer cells more vulnerable to the action of chemotherapy and eventually protect normal tissue against the deleterious effects of chemotherapy."

The exact mechanism by which whey protein achieves this is not fully understood, but it appears that it interferes with the normal feedback mechanism and regulation of glutathione in cancer cells. It is known that glutathione production is negatively inhibited by its own synthesis. Since baseline glutathione levels in cancer cells are higher than those of normal cells, it is probably easier to reach the level of negative-feedback inhibition in the cancer cells' glutathione levels than in the normal cells' glutathione levels.

Cancer chemotherapy patients may consider taking 30 grams a day of whey protein concentrate 10 days before, during and at least 10 days after chemotherapy is discontinued.

NOTE: Refer to the Cancer Treatment protocol for additional information about cancer chemotherapy.

Product availability: Coenzyme Q10, whey protein concentrate, vitamin C, vitamin E, selenium and melatonin can be obtained by calling 1-800-544-4440.

Cancer Radiation Therapy

Cancer radiation therapy inflicts tremendous damage to healthy cells in the body. However, there are specific nutrients that have been shown to protect the body against cancer radiation therapy.

The amino acid taurine is severely depleted when people undergo radiation therapy. Supplementation with 2,000 mg a day of taurine is, therefore, recommended to people undergoing cancer radiation therapy. Also, when ginseng was administered along with radiation therapy in animal studies, a far greater percentage of the animals survived in the ginseng-supplemented group, compared with the group administered radiation without ginseng. Cancer patients should consider taking two to four capsules daily of Sports Ginseng by Nature's Herbs, which combines Korean and Siberian ginseng.

Shark liver oil containing standardized alkylglycerols can prevent immune impairment and irradiation injury to healthy tissues. Cancer patients should take six 200-mg of standardized shark liver oil capsules a day for 30 days. Shark liver oil can cause an overproduction of blood platelets, so high doses of shark liver oil should not be taken for more than 30 days.

Antioxidant supplements can reduce the amount of free radical damage to healthy cells caused by cancer radiation therapy.

Radiation pneumonitis is thought to occur as the result of excess free radical generation following cancer radiation therapy. In vitro studies have shown that large doses of radiation can cause membrane lipid peroxidation and the oxidation of protein groups. In a study of radiation-induced pneumonitis, blood samples were taken over a three-month period in 25 patients with inoperable non-small cell lung cancer treated with radiation therapy. Ten patients developed radiation pneumonitis. The patients who developed pneumonitis showed a tendency toward significantly higher levels of free radical markers and iron in the blood, compared with the non-pneumonitis group.

The doctors concluded that patients who have an increased susceptibility to develop radiation pneumonitis could benefit from intervention therapies with antioxidants.

Radiation fibrosis represents a severe complication of radiation therapy, and standardized treatment protocols are lacking so far. Surgical excision of radiation-induced fibrosis rarely results in complete healing. A physician reported on a 58-year-old woman who developed, 17 years ago, a squamous cell carcinoma within the fibrotic area of the irradiation field on the right chest caused by radiotherapy following mastectomy for breast cancer. After surgical excision of the carcinoma a combined treatment with three 400-mg pentoxifylline tablets a day and one 400-mg vitamin E capsule a day was initiated. The patient noted an increasing improvement of the condition of the affected skin starting from four months. A continuing decrease of skin thickness could be demonstrated from the sixth month on. The treatment was tolerated well, and no side effects were observed.

The data indicate a beneficial therapeutic effect of pentoxifylline and vitamin E on radiation-induced fibrosis.

The prognosis of brain glioblastoma is still very poor and the median survival time is generally less than six months. However, when 20 mg a night of melatonin was administered in patients with glioblastoma treated with radical or adjuvant (assisting) radiotherapy, both the survival curve and the percentage of survival at one year were significantly higher in patients treated with radiation therapy plus melatonin, than in those receiving radiotherapy alone. Moreover, radiotherapy or steroid therapy-related toxicities were lower in patients concomitantly treated with melatonin.

This preliminary study suggested that radiation therapy plus melatonin may prolong the survival time and improve the quality of life of patients affected by glioblastoma.

While soy extracts are strongly recommended as an adjuvant cancer therapy, do not take soy or genistein extracts one week before and during radiation therapy because soy may prevent radiation from killing cancer cells.

Whey protein concentrate selectively depletes cancer cells of their glutathione, thus making them more susceptible to cancer treatments such as radiation and chemotherapy.

It has been found that cancer cells and normal cells will respond differently to nutrients and drugs that affect glutathione status. As has been noted in related protocols, the concentration of glutathione in tumor cells is higher than those of the normal cells that surround them. This difference in glutathione status between normal cells and cancer cells is believed to be an important factor in cancer cells' resistance to chemotherapy.

As the researchers put it, "Tumor cell glutathione concentration may be among the determinants of the cytotoxicity of many chemotherapeutic agents and of radiation, and an increase in glutathione concentration in cancer cells appears to be at least one of the mechanisms of acquired drug resistance to chemotherapy." They further state, "It is well-known that rapid glutathione synthesis in tumor cells is associated with high rates of cellular proliferation. Depletion of cancer cell glutathione in vivo decreases the rate of cellular proliferation and inhibits cancer growth."

Again, as cited in a related protocol, it's difficult to reduce glutathione sufficiently in tumor cells without placing healthy tissue at risk and putting the cancer patient in a worse condition. What is needed is a compound that can selectively deplete the cancer cells of their glutathione, while increasing or at least maintaining the levels of glutathione in healthy cells. This is exactly what whey protein appears to do.

It was found that cancer cells subjected to whey proteins were depleted of their glutathione, and their growth was inhibited, while normal cells had an increase in glutathione and increased cellular growth. These effects were not seen with other proteins. Not surprisingly, the researchers concluded, "Selective depletion of tumor cell glutathione may in fact render cancer cells more vulnerable to the action of chemotherapy and eventually protect normal tissue against the deleterious effects of chemotherapy."

The exact mechanism by which whey protein achieves this is not fully understood, but it appears that it interferes with the normal feedback mechanism and regulation of glutathione in cancer cells. It is known that glutathione production is negatively inhibited by its own synthesis. Being that baseline glutathione levels in cancer cells are higher than that of normal cells, it is probably easier to reach the level of negative-feedback inhibition in the cancer cells' glutathione levels than in the normal cells' glutathione levels.

Cancer patients undergoing radiation therapy may consider taking 30 grams a day of whey protein concentrate at least 10 days before beginning therapy and during therapy, and then continuing with the whey protein for at least 10 days after completion of the therapy.

It is well established that solid tumors contain oxygen deficient hypoxic (oxygen tension) areas and that cells in such areas will cause tumors to be resistant to ionizing radiation. Irresectable cervical cancer is normally treated with radiotherapy. Several previous in vivo and in vitro trials suggest an improvement of radiosensitivity by adding retinoids and alpha interferon in squamous cell cervical cancer.

In a recently reported pilot trial, 33 women with squamous cell cervical cancer were treated with 6 million units of alpha interferon per day and 1 mg per kilogram of body weight of the retinoid drug Accutane per day for 12 days prior to radiotherapy. During radiotherapy all dosages were reduced to prevent toxic side effects: 3 million units of alpha interferon three times a week and 0.5 milligrams per kilogram of Accutane daily were administered until the maximum dosage of radiation was reached. Twenty-nine patients were totally evaluated and four patients were still under treatment.

Complete response occurred in 26 patients, partial response in three patients, and almost all patients tolerated treatment well while toxicity was mild. World Health Organization grade IV side effects were not observed. Treatment with alpha interferon and Accutane improves oxygenation of squamous cell cancers and may enhance the efficacy of radiotherapy.

Product availability: Shark liver oil capsules, whey protein concentrate, taurine, ginseng and melatonin can be obtained by calling 1-800-544-4440.

Cancer Surgery

Most people don't realize that surgery places tremendous stress on the body that causes significant immune depression. This is particularly dangerous to the cancer patient who undergoes surgery to remove a primary tumor. Billions of cancer cells often remain in the body after the surgery and a strong immune system is required to eradicate these remaining cancer cells.

A study conducted several years ago in Germany showed that for most forms of cancer, surgical removal of the primary tumor did not result in prolonged survival, compared with cancer patients who refused surgery. For many forms of cancer, however, the surgical removal of the primary tumor is crucial if long-term remission is to occur. The nutrients and hormones in the Cancer Treatment protocol can help protect against surgically induced immune depression, thus improving the odds of long-term survival.

Cancer Treatment

The Life Extension Foundation's cancer treatment protocol incorporates a wide range of therapies designed to boost immune function, inhibit cancer cell division, induce cancer cells to differentiate into mature cells, inhibit the ability of cancer cells to metastasize, prevent angiogenesis, and modulate the effects of hormones on cancer cell growth. The studies substantiating the Foundation's protocol are impressive, but more aggressive therapies still need to be utilized to achieve a long-term remission.

Every cancer is different, and there are new tests (immuno-histochemistry) available that look for specific mutations in the individual cancer cell in order to help determine the best conventional and alternative therapies to use.

Whole-body cytotoxic chemotherapy drugs are widely used in an attempt to kill the metastasized tumor cells. However, conventional oncologists are failing to incorporate newly published findings into their chemotherapy regimens that could make chemotherapy more effective. Chemotherapy destroys immune function, thereby condemning the cancer patient to the likelihood of a recurrence of tumor metastasis, along with life-threatening infections. If the immune system is unable to recognize and destroy metastasized cancer cells, then the chances of achieving a permanent remission are remote.

In the 30 years that cancer chemotherapy has been used, it has proved effective for relatively few cancers. The cancers that chemotherapy has been shown to benefit include testicular cancer, choriocarcinoma, Hodgkin's disease, leukemia and lymphoma. For the majority of cancers, however, chemotherapy has been a failure. The Life Extension Foundation has identified methods of making chemotherapy more toxic to cancer cells and less toxic to healthy cells. Please refer to the Cancer Chemotherapy protocol for suggestions about making chemotherapy more effective and how to protect healthy cells against injury and death from highly toxic chemotherapy drugs.

When cancer is first diagnosed, the primary tumor often is too large for the Foundation's Cancer Treatment Protocols to be effective by themselves. In these cases, conventional cancer therapy (surgery and/or radiation) often is necessary to eradicate the primary tumor. However, surgery and radiation place tremendous stress on the body that severely weakens immune function and can put the body into a catabolic (wasting) state that leads to noticeable weight loss. The Foundation's Cancer Treatment Protocol provides nutritional and hormonal therapies that are needed to mitigate the damaging effects of surgery/radiation therapy. Conventional cancer doctors seldom include any of the nutritional support that is so desperately needed by the cancer patient.

At this time, the Life Extension Foundation does not have a good alternative for conventional therapies when it comes to large primary tumors. Even the advanced therapies used at offshore cancer clinics are usually not potent enough to shrink large, primary tumors.

It is crucial for cancer patients to monitor the effectiveness of any cancer therapy they are using under the care of a physician, preferably an oncologist. Blood tests should be done monthly that measure tumor markers in the blood and measure the effects of immune-boosting therapies on specific immune components of the blood.

We cannot overemphasize the importance of monthly blood testing for all cancer patients. Every patient responds differently to both conventional and alternative cancer therapies. The results of blood tests provide critically important data to evaluate the effectiveness of these therapies.

Some of the blood tests commonly used by doctors to evaluate different types of cancers are:

Type of Cancer	Blood Test
Ovarian cancer	CA 125
Prostate cancer	PSA and prolactin
Breast cancer	CA 27.29, CEA, alkaline, phosphatase and prolactin
Colon, rectum, liver, stomach and other organ cancers	CEA, GGTP
Pancreatic	CA 19.9, CEA, GGTP
Leukemia, lymphoma, and Hodgkin's disease	CBC with differential, immune cell differentiation and leukemia profile
Lung cancer	CEA, CA 125, alkaline phosphatase PT, PTT and D-Dimer of fibrin

Dr. Emil Schandl's Cancer Profile, which has had an excellent track record for more than 10 years, is strongly recommended for all cancers (refer to the Medical Testing Protocols for in-depth information). For cancers that do not have an established blood tumor marker test, one should use MRI, CAT scans, and other imaging diagnostics every 30 to 60 days to determine whether tumor shrinking is actually occurring. This will provid some evaluation about the benefits of whatever therapy is being used.

While you may have to rely on conventional cancer therapy to treat a primary tumor, the nutrients and hormones in the Cancer Treatment protocol improve the chances of bringing metastasized cancer cells under control.

Melatonin may be the single most effective alternative cancer therapy because it boosts immune function, suppresses free radicals, inhibits cell proliferation, and helps to change cancer cells into normal cells.

Nutrients that have an inhibitory effect on cancer-cell proliferation include vitamin A (and synthetic vitamin A analogs) and such phytochemicals found in cruciferous vegetables as sulforaphane, 3-indole-carbinol and isothiocyanate. Soy contains numerous anti-cancer agents such as genistein and other isoflavones. Vitamin D3 inhibits cancer cell growth and induces cancer cells to differentiate into normal cells.

The best example of the effectiveness of vitamin A and beta-carotene in inhibiting cell proliferation is in patients with cancer of the mouth. Vitamin A or beta-carotene supplementation puts most forms of early stage mouth cancer in remission as long as these nutrients continue to be consumed.

The Foundation's Cancer Treatment Protocol is for most forms of cancer, including metastasized prostate cancer.

This protocol assumes that the patient's primary tumor has been eradicated, at least partially, by surgery or some other treatment. However, it may be followed even if the primary tumor has not yet been eradicated.

Here is the Life Extension Foundation's Cancer Treatment Protocol:

❖ **Step One: Arrange for monthly blood tests, to include:**

1. Tumor marker test—The type of cancer dictates the type of test used. Some cancers do not have a specific tumor marker test available. The CA Profile is not organ specific and has been shown to be effective in monitoring the progression and regression of cancer.

2. Immune cell subset test (This is an expensive test.)

3. Complete blood chemistry—to include all standard liver, thyroid, heart and kidney function tests. This is a low-cost test.

   These blood tests must be taken on a regular basis under the supervision of a physician in order to follow scientifically the Foundation's Cancer Treatment Protocol. It's the best way of knowing whether what you are taking is working, and/or whether significant toxicity is developing. This is no time to guess!

   Since you will be having these tests performed monthly, you should price-shop for the best deal. The Life Extension Foundation now offers these tests at discount prices.

❖ **Step Two: Total nutritional support**

1. Life Extension Mix—The standard daily dose involves three tablets, three

times a day. Also available in powder or capsule form to be taken in three divided doses.

2. Life Extension Herbal Mix—powder only. One tablespoon early in the day.

3. Super selenium complex. One tablet, two times a day.

4. Green tea capsules (decaffeinated) —Four to 10 capsules a day in divided doses.

5. Coenzyme Q10—oil filled capsules, 200 to 400 mg early in the morning.

6. Garlic—Kyolic Galic Formula 105, four capsules a day; and PureGar (high allicin garlic), four 900-mg capsules a day with meals.

7. Essential fatty acids—Mega EPA fish oil or Udo's Choice Ultimate Oil. Highest tolerable doses. Suggested dose is 12 Mega EPA caps or two table-spoons of Udo's Choice Ultimate Oil daily. Some studies suggest not taking these oils if you have prostate cancer.

8. Vitamin C—Capsules or powder. Highest tolerable dose of pharmaceutical grade vitamin C to be taken throughout the day.

9. Phyto-Food powder. One to two tablespoons daily. Juicing organic vegeta-bles is an alternative to Phyto-Food powder.

10. L-carnitine capsules (600 mg)—Four capsules early in the day. Use acetyl-L-carnitine if affordable.

11. Curcumin—four 500-mg capsules daily.

12. Conjugated linoleic acid (CLA)—10 500-mg capsules in two divided doses

❖ Step Three: Boosting immune function

1. If the immune system is weakened enough, cancer cells can survive and multiply. The most critical part of the immune system is the thymus gland, a small organ just below the breast bone that governs the entire system. There are two products that promote healthy thymic activity:

   a) Thymic Protein A has been shown in laboratory and animal experiments to cause the T-4 lymphocyte to mature, there-by initiating a specific cell-mediated immune response.

   Thymic Protein A is a protein that has been shown to be a stimulant in animal models for the production of inter-leukin-2. Interleukin-2 production by T-4 cells is the bench-mark measurement for T-cell maturity and initiation of immune response.

   A daily dose of four micrograms of Thymic Protein A may strengthen the immune system through its T-cell "programming" role. The more T-cells that are properly functioning, the more immune response may be mounted against metastasized cancer cells.

Initial reports from those undergoing chemotherapy indicate that Thymic Protein A has maintained their total white blood count at acceptable levels during the therapy. (It is well known among oncologists that chemotherapy and radiation often will induce a drop in white blood count to dangerous levels, which may dictate cessation of therapy.) Healthy people can take one packet every day or every other day. Those with disease whose treatment is dependent on a strong immune system may need three packets a day for several months.

b) Another product, Thymex, provides extracts of fresh, healthy tissue from the thymus and other glands that produce the disease-fighting cells of our immune system.

The primary ingredient in Thymex is immunologic tissue from the thymus gland. Also included in Thymex is tissue from the lymph nodes and spleen that produces the white blood cells that engage in life or death combat with invading organisms in our bloodstream under the "instruction" of the thymus gland.

Thymex is a synergistic formula that contains herbal activators and a full complement of natural homeopathic nutrients, in addition to fresh, healthy thymus, lymph and spleen tissues. Thymex is a professional formula normally dispensed through doctor's offices. Thymex has been extensively used to amplify the immune potentiating effect of DHEA replacement therapy. According to a physician most familiar with DHEA, thymus extract is required to obtain the immune system-boosting benefit of DHEA.

2. Cancer patients usually have elevated cortisol levels that can suppress immune function. Take one to two tablets of KH3 daily on an empty stomach first thing in the morning, and one or two KH3 tablets in the mid-afternoon on an empty stomach to suppress the damaging effects of cortisol.

3. DHEA can also suppress dangerously high cortisol levels while boosting immune function via other mechanisms. Doctors usually prescribe at least 25 mg per day of DHEA for their male cancer patients and a minimum of 15 mg a day of DHEA for females. Your monthly or bimonthly DHEA-S and

immune cell subset tests and tumor marker tests will determine if DHEA is producing a beneficial effect.

Do not use DHEA if you have prostate cancer or estrogen-sensitive breast cancer.

4. Melatonin boosts immune function via several mechanisms of action. It also exerts an inhibitory effect on cancer cell proliferation and induces the differentiation of cancer cells into normal cells. Melatonin should be taken every night in doses ranging from 3 to 40 mg.

   CAUTION: Some doctors are under the impression that leukemia, Hodgkin's disease, and lymphoma patients should avoid melatonin until more is known about its effects on these forms of cancer. If melatonin is tried in these types of cancer, tumor blood markers should be watched closely for any sign that melatonin is promoting tumor growth.

5. Show your oncologist the information in this book regarding the use of the FDA-approved drugs interleukin-2 or interferon and melatonin. Studies document that low doses of interleukin-2 or alpha interferon combined with high doses of melatonin (10 to 50 mg nightly) are effective against advanced, normally untreatable cancers. Ask your doctor to prescribe these agents:

   a) Interleukin-2 at a dose of 3 million units injected subcutaneously six out of every seven days for six weeks.

   And one month later:

   b) Alpha interferon at a dose of 100,000 to 300,000 units injected subcutaneously six out of seven days for six weeks. Subcutaneous injections can be self-administered at home.

CAUTION: Breast cancer patients should *not* use interleukin-2. While low-dose IL-2 and high-dose melatonin have been shown to be effective against many forms of cancer, interleukin-2 could promote breast cancer cell division. Breast cancer patients are encouraged to take 10 to 50 mg of melatonin nightly (See the Breast Cancer protocol).

This immune-boosting program should be adjusted if the immune cell subset test or the CA Profile fails to show marked improvement in the patient's immune function. For example, if there are too many T-suppressor cells, 800 mg a day of the drug Tagamet (now available over the counter) can lower the T-suppressor cell activity. T-suppressor cells often are elevated in cancer patients, which prevents them from mounting a strong immune response to the cancer.

❖ Step Four: Inhibiting cancer cell proliferation

1. Water-soluble vitamin A liquid in doses of 100,000 to 300,000 IU a day should be used for several months.

   CAUTION: Monthly blood tests can help ascertain if toxicity is occurring in response to these high doses of vitamin A. Do *not* take vitamin A if you have thyroid cancer or suffer severe thyroid deficiency. Refer to the Vitamin A Precautions appendix before taking vitamin A.

2. Melatonin taken to boost immune function also inhibits cancer cell proliferation.

3. Mega Soy Extract. Five 700-mg capsules four times a day. Soy may be effective in treating certain cancers. Genistein is the most substantiated soy isoflavone that produces multiple cancer-inhibiting effects. Genistein has been shown to work especially well against certain leukemias and cancers of the skin, prostate and brain.

   CAUTION: For most cancers, the determining factor of whether soy may work is if your cancer cells carry a mutated p53 tumor suppressor gene, or carry functional p53. If functional p53 is present, then soy genistein will probably *not* work. In small-cell lung cancer, however, it was recently determined that genistein's growth inhibitory effects were independent of p53 function. Only specialized tumor cell tests (immuno-histochemistry) can determine the p53 status of your particiular cancer.

   Estrogen-receptor positive breast cancer patients should avoid high doses of genistein.

4. Whey protein concentrate powder. 30 to 60 grams a day (one to two scoops). Whey protein concentrate inhibits cancer cell glutathione levels, making cancer cells more vulnerable to free radical destruction than normal cells.

❖ Step Five: Inducing cancer cell differentiation

Cancer cells are aberrant, transformed cells that proliferate (divide) more rapidly than normal cells until they kill the patient. Inducing cancer cells to "differentiate" back into normal cells is a primary objective of cancer researchers.

1. The Total Nutritional Support protocol supplies nutrients like beta-carotene and the phytochemicals found in fresh fruits and vegetables that induce cancer cell differentiation into normal cells and inhibit cancer cell proliferation.

2. Melatonin, which boosts immune function and inhibits cancer cell proliferation, also induces cancer cell differentiation.

3. Vitamin D3 and its analogs may be the most effective therapies to induce cancer cell differentiation. Vitamin D3 can cause too much calcium to be absorbed into the bloodstream, so the monthly blood chemistry test, which includes serum calcium levels and kidney and liver function tests, is crucial to guard against vitamin D3 overdose. A daily dose of 2,000 to 3,000 IU of vitamin D3 is suggested. Increase vitamin D3 if blood tests show blood calcium levels are not being affected and parathyroid hormone (PTH) levels are not suppressed. Decrease or eliminate vitamin D3 supplementation if hypercalcemia occurs. Underlying kidney disease precludes high-dose vitamin D3 supplementation.

Note the importance of competent, professional guidance by a physician. **Monthly blood testing is mandatory when taking high doses of vitamin A or vitamin D3.**

❖ Step Six: Preventing cancer cell metastasis

Modified citrus pectin interferes with cancer cell communication, enhances killer cell activity, and inhibits cancer cell metastasis. Suggested dose of this powder is 15 grams a day.

❖ Step Seven: Call the Life Extension Foundation

If following the above protocols does not result in significant immune enhancement, improvements in blood tumor markers, tumor shrinkage, weight stabilization, and an overall improvement in well being within two months, please call the Life Extension Foundation at 1-800-544-4440 for other, more aggressive options.

It is impossible to fit a description about the mechanisms of action of all the nutrients and hormones in this Cancer Treatment protocol. That would require a separate book. What follows are some recent reports that substantiate some components of the Cancer Treatment protocol. The inclusion of certain nutrients in the following descriptions does not mean that they are more important than nutrients like vitamin C and selenium, whch are not discussed because of lack of space.

Conjugated linoleic acid (CLA) has been shown both in vitro and in animal models to have strong anti-tumor activity. Particular effects have been observed on the growth and metastatic spread of mammary tumors. A study investigated the effect of dietary CLA on the growth of human breast adenocarcinoma cells in immuno-deficient mice. CLA inhibited the development and growth of mammary tumors. Moreover, CLA completely abrogated the spread of breast cancer cells to lungs, peripheral blood and bone marrow. These results indicate the ability of dietary CLA to block both the local growth and systemic spread of human breast cancer via mechanisms independent of the host immune system.

CLA has been shown to inhibit initiation and promotion stages of carcinogenesis in several experimental animal models. A study of mice with skin tumors showed that CLA inhibited tumor yield. This study confirmed previous studies showing that CLA inhibits tumor promotion in a manner that is independent of its cancer-prevention effects.

Genistein has shown significant cell-inhibiting effects in many different types of cancer. A study was conducted to examine the role genistein played in growth factors such as protein tyrosine kinase and thymidine incorporation into cancer cells. Genistein suppressed protein tyrosine kinase activity and the subsequent growth stimulatory incorporation of thymidine into cancer cells. The scientists speculated that genistein has potential value in the prevention and treatment of some tumors in vivo. In other studies, genistein has shown anti-angiogenesis properties, cancer cell adhesion-inhibition properties, estrogen-receptor blocking properties and apoptosis-inducing effects. An investigation into the effect of soy genistein on the growth and differentiation of human melanoma cells showed that genistein significantly inhibited cell growth. Some studies suggest that genistein may enhance the efficacy of certain chemotherapy regimens.

Curcumin and genistein both have been shown to inhibit the growth of estrogen-positive human breast cancer cells induced by pesticides. When curcumin and genistein were added to breast cancer cells, a synergistic effect resulted in a total inhibition of cancer cell growth caused by pesticide-induced estrogenic activity. This study suggested that the combination of curcumin and genistein in the diet has the potential to reduce the proliferation of estrogen-positive cells induced by mixtures of pesticides or estrogen. Since it is difficult to remove pesticides completely from the diet, and since both curcumin and soy genistein are not toxic to humans, their inclusion in the diet in order to prevent hormone-related cancers deserves consideration. Curcumin appears to function via several different mechanisms to inhibit cancer cell proliferation.

Genistein appears to be especially effective against prostate cancers. One study showed that genistein inhibited the proliferation and expression of the in vitro invasive capacity of tumoral prostatic cells. In a cell culture system, genistein appeared to be cytotoxic and inhibitory to PC-3 cells. The more aggressive the prostate cancer cell culture studies, the more genistein was effective, both with respect to proliferation rate and inhibition of growth factors.

Angiogenesis (new blood vessel growth) is a key step in tumor growth, invasion and metastasis. To date, a number of anti-angiogenic agents have been identified. In animal models, treatment with angiogenesis inhibitors has proven anti-tumor effects. Early clinical experience with angiogenic inhibitors indicates that optimal anti-angiogenic therapy in the future will likely be based on their long-term administration to cancer patients in adjunct to surgery, radiotherapy and conventional chemotherapy.

Differentiation-inducing agents such as genistein, retinoids and vitamin D analogs inhibited tumor cell induced angiogenesis in vitro and in vivo. Simultaneous administration of retinoids and 1,25-Dihydroxy vitamin D3 led to a synergistic inhibition of tumor associated angiogenesis in mice. Recently, these compounds have been shown to induce and act in concert with natural angiogenic inhibitors such as interferons.

A study was conducted to determine if genistein can induce human breast adenocarcinoma cell maturation and differentiation. Treating these cells with genistein resulted in growth inhibition accompanied by increased cell maturation. These maturation markers were optimally expressed after nine days of treatment with genistein. Both estrogen receptor-positive and estrogen receptor-negative cells became differentiated in response to genistein, which is a crucial step in inducing cancer cell apoptosis (programmed cell death).

Despite this study, we do not recommend that women with estrogen receptor-positive breast cancer use soy genistein because of the following evidence.

The Foundation has made a preliminary determination that women with estrogen-receptor positive breast cancer should not take soy supplements based on evidence that an estrogenic growth effect could occur in some forms of estrogen-receptor positive breast cancer. Until more is known about the effects of soy phytoestrogens in this type of cancer, compounds such as genistein should be avoided in those with estrogen-receptor positive breast cancer.

One study tested the effects of naturally occurring flavonoids on the proliferation of an estrogen receptor-positive human breast cancer cell line. Genistein inhibited cell proliferation, but this effect was reversed when estrogen was added. The flavonoids hesperidin, naringenin and quercetin inhibited breast cancer cell proliferation even in the presence of high levels of estrogen. These flavonoids apparently exert their anti-proliferative activity via a mechanism that is different from genistein.

Women with any type of breast cancer should test their serum estrogen levels to make sure that too much estrogen is not present if they are taking high doses of soy. Estrogen can combine with the phytoestrogen genistein to cause some breast cancer cells to grow faster. Other studies, however, show that genistein blocks certain types of estrogen-receptor sites, thus inhibiting the proliferation of these types of breast cancer cells.

Cancer patients whose tumor cells have a mutant p53 oncogene are far more likely to benefit from soy extract supplementation. Only a pathology examination of the actual cancer cells can determine p53 status. An immuno-histochemistry test can help to determine the p53 status of tumor cells. The following laboratory can perform this new test:

IMPATH Laboratories
1010 Third Avenue, Suite 203
New York, N.Y. 10021
Phone: 1-800-447-5816

IMPATH Laboratories measures mutant p53. If the test is positive, you have mutant p53 and are *more* likely to benefit from soy extracts. If the test is negative, this indicates that you have functional p53 and are *less* likely to benefit from soy extracts. The Foundation realizes that many cancer patients seeking to use soy supplements may find it difficult to have an immuno-histochemistry test performed to ascertain p53 status.

Because all cancer therapies produce individual responses, the Foundation reiterates its recommendation that all cancer patients have monthly blood tumor marker tests to determine whether the therapies they are using are working. If, for instance, tumor markers were to continue to elevate for 30 to 60 days after initiating soy extract supplementation, discontinue its use and seek another therapy immediately.

Fish oil may enhance the effectiveness of cancer chemotherapy drugs. A study compared different fatty acids on colon cancer cells to see if they could potentiate the effect of the chemotherapy drug mitomycin C. Eicosapentaenoic acid (EPA) from fish oil was shown to make colon cancer cells more vulnerable to mitomycin C without affecting normal cells. The scientists found that EPA induced alternations of the fatty-acid composition of cancer cells, which made them more vulnerable to chemotherapy destruction. Although preliminary, these findings imply that EPA specifically enhances the chemosensitivity of malignant cells. Fish oil has been shown to specifically induce apoptosis of pancreatic cancer cells and to inhibit metastasis of breast and lung cancer cells.

Garlic is a well-established cancer preventing nutrient. A study investigated aged garlic extract in an effort to determine whether it could inhibit proliferation of cancer cells. The proliferation and viability of erythroleukemia, hormone-responsive breast and prostate cancer cell lines were evaluated. The eyrtholeukemia cells were not significantly affected by the garlic extract, but the breast and prostate cancer cell lines clearly were susceptible to the growth-inhibitory influence of aged garlic extract. The anti-proliferative effect of aged garlic extract was limited to actively growing cells. This study provided evidence that garlic can exert a direct effect on established cancer cells.

Aberrant hyperproliferation is a late occurring event that precedes mammary tumorigenesis in vivo. A study conducted on pre-cancer cells showed that EPA, indole-3-carbinol (broccoli-cabbage extract) and green tea extract resulted in a 70 to 99 percent inhibition of aberrant hyperprolifertion.

Whey protein concentrate has been studied for cancer prevention and treatment. When different groups of rats were given a powerful carcinogen, those fed whey protein concentrate showed fewer tumors and a reduced pooled area of tumors. The researchers found that whey protein offered "considerable protection to the host" over that of other proteins, including soy.

Whey appears to inhibit the growth of breast cancer cells at low concentrations. One clinical study with cancer patients showed a regression in some patient's tumors when fed whey protein concentrate at 30 grams per day.

As noted in a related protocol, but worth repeating in this context, this led researchers to discover a relationship between cancerous cells, whey protein concentrate and glutathione. Glutathione is an antioxidant that protects the body against harmful compounds. It was found that whey protein concentrate selectively depletes cancer cells of their glutathione, thus making them more susceptible to cancer treatments such as radiation and chemotherapy.

It has been found that cancer cells and normal cells will respond differently to nutrients and drugs that affect glutathione status. What is most interesting is that the concentration of glutathione in tumor cells is higher than that of the normal cells that surround it. This difference in glutathione status between normal cells and cancer cells is believed to be an important factor in cancer cells' resistance to chemotherapy. As the researchers put it, "Tumor cell glutathione concentration may be among the determinants of the cytotoxicity of many chemotherapeutic agents and of radiation, and an increase in glutathione concentration in cancer cells appears to be at least one of the mechanisms of acquired drug resistance to chemotherapy."

They further state, "It is well-known that rapid glutathione synthesis in tumor cells is associated with high rates of cellular proliferation. Depletion of cancer cell glutathione in vivo decreases the rate of cellular proliferation and inhibits cancer growth." The problem is, it's difficult to reduce glutathione sufficiently in tumor cells without placing healthy tissue at risk and putting the cancer patient in a worse condition. What is needed is a compound that can selectively deplete the cancer cells of their glutathione, while increasing, or at least maintaining, the levels of glutathione in healthy cells. This is exactly what whey protein appears to do.

This research found that cancer cells subjected to whey proteins were depleted of their glutathione and their growth was inhibited, while normal cells had an increase in glutathione and increased cellular growth. These effects were not seen with other proteins. Not surprisingly, the researchers concluded, "Selective depletion of tumor cell glutathione may in fact render cancer cells more vulnerable to the action of chemotherapy and eventually protect normal tissue against the deleterious effects of chemotherapy." The exact mechanism by which whey protein achieves this is not fully understood, but it appears that it interferes with the normal feedback mechanism and regulation of glutathione in cancer cells. It is known that glutathione production is negatively inhibited by its own synthesis. Since baseline glutathione levels in cancer cells are higher than that of normal cells, it is probably easier to reach the level of negative-feedback inhibition in the cancer cells' glutathione levels than in the normal cells' glutathione levels.

Molecular Oncology

CAUTION: The following information is extremely technical. The cooperation of your oncologist is vital to most cancer patients who seek to use the following information in an attempt to save their lives:

❖ Determining RAS mutations.

The family of RAS proteins plays a central role in the regulation of cell growth and integration of regulatory signals that govern the cell cycle and proliferation. Mutant RAS genes were among the first oncogenes described for their ability to transform cells to a cancerous phenotype. Mutations in one of three genes (H, N and K-RAS) encoding RAS proteins have been intimately associated with unregulated cell proliferation, and are found in an estimated 30 percent of all human cancers. The frequency of RAS mutations appears to depend upon the specific tumor type analyzed. For example, 90 percent of pancreatic carcinomas contain a mutated oncogenic RAS protein while RAS mutations are rarely found in breast carcinomas.

Approximately one-third of liver cancers harbor a mutated RAS oncogene. Pravastatin, an inhibitor of the rate-limiting enzyme of cholesterol synthesis, inhibits growth of liver cancer cells. One of the possible mechanisms of pravastatin inhibition of cell growth is that pravastatin may inhibit the activity of RAS proteins. In a recently published study, patients with primary liver cancer were treated either with the chemotheraputic drug 5-FU or a combination of 5-FU and 40 mg per day of pravastatin. Median survival was 26 months in the combination therapy group, versus 10 months in the monotherapy (5-FU) group.

The highest incidences of RAS mutations are found in adeno-carcinomas of the pancreas (90 percent), the colon (50 percent) and the lung; in thyroid tumors (50 percent); in liver tumors (30 percent); and in myeloid leukemia (30 percent). If you have one of these cancers, you should consider requesting an immuno-histochemistry for the mutated RAS oncogene or a biopsied specimen in order to ascertain if the combination of chemotherapy and a statin drug may be effective.

❖ **Determining p53 status.**

Another of the most widely studied molecular changes in epithelial malignancies is mutation in the p53 tumor suppressor gene. A p53 mutation has been found in approximately 50 percent of solid tumors. The p53 gene product is regarded as a cell-cycle checkpoint, arresting progression through the G phase of the mitotic cycle in response to cellular injury and allowing time for repair of replication errors. Mutant p53 allows tumor cells to bypass the cell cycle constraints that facilitate repair or promote apoptosis (programmed cell death).

P53 dysfunction promotes the spontaneous emergence of mutant cells and encourages progression of cancer. Mutant p53 might restrict therapeutic efficacy since many cancer drugs and radiotherapy operate via the induction of DNA damage and p53 dependent apoptosis. Clinically, the presence of p53 mutations is indeed associated with intransigence to treatment, and both in vitro and in vivo studies with human cell lines and transplantable tumors have demonstrated enhanced survival of p53 mutant or null cells in the face of normally lethal concentrations of cytotoxic drugs and ionizing radiation. A determination of p53 status, by an immuno-histochemistry, can help to ascertain whether genotoxic chemotherapy and/or radiotherapy are likely to work, and can even help determine whether natural therapies such as soy genistein will be effective.

In a recently published study, genistein was shown to inhibit growth and induce differentiation in human melanoma cells in vitro. The effects of genistein were regulated by cellular p53. Functional p53-containing cells were not suppressed by genistein. However, mutant p53-containing cells were significantly more sensitive to genistein's inhibitory and cell-differentiating effects.

IMPATH Laboratories, cited earlier in this protocol, can ascertain immuno-histochemistries which will ascertain RAS and p53 status.

❖ **Determining thrombotic risk factors.**

In patients affected with different tumors, disorders concerning blood clotting are frequently observed. The biological processes leading to coagulation are probably involved in the mechanisms of metastasis. About 50 percent of all cancer patients, and up to 95 percent of those with metastatic disease, show some abnormalities—a pre-thrombic state—in the coagulation-fibrinolytic system. Thromboembolic complications are seen in up to 11 percent of cancer patients, and hemorrhage occurs in about 10 percent. Thromboembolism and hemorrhage, as a whole, are the second most common cause of death after infection.

In a recently published study, subclinical changes in the coagulation-fibrinolytic system were frequently detected in lung cancer patients. Five conventional and one new test of blood coagulation—that is, platelet count (P), prothrombin time (PT), partial thromboplastin time (PTT), fibrinogen (F) and D-Dimer of fibrin (DD)—were prospectively recorded in a series of 286 patients with new primary lung cancer. A pre-thrombotic state (depicted by a prolongation of PT, PTT and increase of D-Dimer of fibrin) was significantly associated with an adverse outcome.

Anticoagulant treatment of cancer patients, particularly those with lung cancer, has been reported to improve survival. These interesting though preliminary results of controlled trials lent some support to the argument that activation of blood coagulation plays a role in the natural history of tumor growth. Recently, two studies compared the effectiveness of standard heparin with low molecular weight heparin (LMWH) in the treatment of deep vein thrombosis (DVT). In both studies, mortality rates were lower in the patients randomized to LMWH. The analysis of these deaths reveals a striking difference in cancer-related mortality.

Cancer-related mortality of patients treated with standard heparin was 31 percent, versus only 11 percent among those treated with low molecular weight heparin. This difference cannot solely be attributed to thrombotic or bleeding events. Because large numbers of cancer patients were included in the studies, it seems unlikely that ones with more advanced tumors were present in the standard heparin group. Although it is also possible that standard heparin increases cancer mortality, such an adverse effect has not been reported. These considerations suggest that low molecular weight heparin might exert an inhibitory effect on tumor growth that is not apparent with standard heparin. The evidence of lowered cancer mortality in patients on LMWH has renewed interest in these agents as antineoplastic drugs. If your oncologist will not test for thrombotic risk factors, contact the Life Extension Foundation at 1-800-544-4440.

❖ **Assessing immune function.**

In order to assess the effectiveness of immune-boosting therapies, a complete immune cell subset test could be performed bimonthly in order to measure CD4 (T-helper) total count, CD4/CD8 (T-helper to T-suppressor) ratio, and NK (natural killer cell) activity.

CD4 T-cells have been shown to differentiate into TH1 or TH2 cells, with different cytokine profiles and functions. TH1 cells produce interleukin-2 and gamma interferon, activate macrophages, and cause delayed type hypersensitivity reactions, whereas TH2 cells produce interluken-4, interluken-5 and interluken-10, cause eosinophilia, and are more specialized in providing B cell (antibody) help for immunoglobin production. The differential development of these immune system subjects is a major determinant of the outcome of physiological as well as pathological immune responses to cancer.

One of the soluble factors secreted by monocytes, interleuken-12, is a major cause of differentiation of T cells towards the TH1 type, while suppressing TH2 cytokine development. The capacity of interleukin-12 to stimulate growth and gamma interferon production in T cells and NK cells is probably the main reason for its TH1-inducing capacity. Another product of activated monocytes, prostaglandin E2, has been shown to be an important regulatory factor in inducing TH2 responses. PGE2 affects T helper responses opposite to interleukin-12: the synthesis of TH1 cytokines (interleukin-2 and gamma interferon) is much more sensitive to inhibition by PGE2 than TH2 cytokine production (IL-4, IL-5, IL-10). Because TH1 and TH2 cytokines negatively cross-regulate each other's production, the selective inhibition of TH1 cytokines by PGE2 could result in dominant TH2 responses. These findings provide opportunities to treat patients with dominant TH2 responses by selectively inhibiting synthesis of PGE2 during therapy, as this would increase interleukin-12 production and cause a shift toward TH1 cytokine production.

Many human tumors, including gastric, colon, estrogen receptor-negative breast, prostate and lung produce more prostaglandin E2 than their associated normal tissues. The mechanisms and implications are not fully understood, but PGE2 may act as a tumor promotor in tumor angiogenesis, in cachexia (wasting syndrome) and in the suppression of immune function.

Prostaglandins are synthesized from arachidonic acid by the enzyme cyclooxygenase. There are two isoforms of cyclooxygenases: Cox-1 is expressed constitutively in most tissues and helps maintain gastric mucosal integrity; Cox-2 is inducible and is associated with cellular growth and differentiation. In a recently published study, PGE2 was shown, for the first time, to up-regulate the levels of its own synthesizing enzyme, Cox-2, in four human cells lines. In this regard, it is conceivable that cells continuously sustain their growth in part by using extra cellular PGE2 that they themselves produce and release to up-regulate the expressions of Cox-2 and possibly other growth related genes. Elevated Cox-2 expression may make cancer cells resistant to apoptosis. Inhibition of excess activity with Cox-2 specific nonsteroidal anti-inflammatory drugs might restore the cell's ability to die by apoptosis and so cause tumor regression.

Super aspirins that selectively inhibit Cox-2 are being developed by several drug companies to try and avoid the side effects of NSAIDS. The currently commercially available NSAIDS are nonselective Cox inhibitors and are associated with peptic ulceration in the stomach. Nimesulide is a novel NSAID that is one hundred times more selective for Cox-2 than for Cox-1. In a recently published study, patients received either nimesulide or aspirin for 14 days. PGE2 formation fell markedly in the nimesulide treated patients, whereas aspirin had no effect. In contrast, nimesulide had no significant effect on Thromboxane B2 which was suppressed by aspirin. Nimesulide suppressed Cox-2 in vivo with no detectable effect on platelet Cox-1.

Nimesulide has been commercially available throughout most of the rest of the world for more than 10 years. It has not been licensed by the FDA for use in the United States. The Life Extension Foundation has identified sources that will ship nimesulide to Americans for personal use.

There are several thousand studies that substantiate the anti-cancer potential of the nutrients listed in this Cancer Treatment protocol. There is not room in this book to describe each component in detail. Please refer to the References section for additional studies. Refer to the Foundation's Web Site—**www.lef.org**—to obtain actual abstracts that substantiate the benefits of all the nutrients and hormones the Life Extension Foundation recommends as adjuvant treatments of cancer.

Product availability: You can order Life Extension Mix, Life Extension Herbal Mix, selenium complex, Thymex, DHEA, melatonin, vitamin A emulsified drops, vitamin D3, Mega Soy Extract, green tea caps, coenzyme Q10, garlic, vitamin C, Phyto-Food, carnitine, acetyl-L-carnitine and modified citrus pectin by calling 1-800-544-4440. Ask for the names of companies that will ship nimesulide and other cancer drugs to Americans for personal use.

For some forms of cancer, you may be able to get in a free program utilizing experimental cancer therapies sponsored by the National Cancer Institute. For information about experimental cancer therapies, call 1-800-4-CANCER. Make sure you do not enroll in a study where you may be part of a placebo group or where the potential toxicity of the drug may kill you before the cancer does.

Cancer Vaccine Therapy

Ever since doctors noticed that at least some cases of spontaneous cancer remissions could be credited to the patients' immune mechanisms, they have dreamed of immune-based treatments for cancer. Such an approach should be far less toxic than conventional chemotherapy, yet able to track down dispersed tumor cells and metastases that elude the surgeon's scalpel.

As with all cancer therapeutics, developers of cancer vaccines have had to find targetable structures present on cancer cells, but not on the normal cells from which they evolve. And even when that's possible, there's an extra obstacle unique to the immunotherapeutic approach: getting the immune system to notice the structure and mount an effective attack. Although cancer vaccine development is now well into its second decade, no product has been licensed. But at least seven different products of various types are in late stage clinical trials. Encouraging results from trials have been reported for small-cell lung cancer and malignant melanoma. Cancer vaccines no longer seem to be a matter of "if," but of "when."

For more information, contact the Cancer Information Service at 1-800-4-CANCER.

Candida (Fungal, Yeast) Infections

Chronic fungal infections often are found in the gastrointestinal (GI) tract, due to the yeast-like fungi called Candida. Improving the bacterial flora and the overall health of the GI tract can help to prevent recurring Candida infections throughout the body.

The intake of bifido bacteria concentrate capsules every day can dramatically increase the quantity of beneficial bacteria in the gut to help fight Candida infections. Acidophilus bacteria also can help to fight Candida in the upper intestinal tract. Bifido bacteria feed on a special sugar trademarked under the name Nutraflora. One teaspoon a day of Nutraflora promotes the proliferation of friendly bifido bacteria in the gut.

Garlic (not Kyolic garlic), biotin and caprylic acid have a direct yeast-killing effect in the intestine. Fiber in the diet also can help remove yeast and fungus from the intestines. A product called Yeast Fighters Capsules contains an odorless garlic concentrate, caprylic acid, biotin, acidophilus and a fiber blend to control Candida overgrowth in the intestine before it spreads to other parts of the body.

Chronic Candida infections can be caused by a deficient immune system. If you suffer from an acute Candida infection, or one that has not responded to standard therapy, the most potent FDA-approved drug available is called Diflucan. One month's treatment with Diflucan can temporarily eradicate a systemic Candida infection so that anti-Candida nutritional supplements like Yeast Fighters, bifido bacteria and Nutraflora can prevent a new Candida infection from occurring.

Shark liver oil has demonstrated an antifungal effect in laboratory studies. Shark liver oil capsules, containing 200 mg of alkylglycerol, can be taken in doses of five capsules a day for up to 30 days. As for dietary modifications, you should avoid sucrose and fructose, since these types of sugars can cause yeast overgrowth.

Studies have shown that the daily ingestion of 150 mL of yogurt enriched with live Lacto acidophilus is associated with an increased colonization of friendly bacteria in the rectum and vagina. This results in reduced episodes of bacterial vaginitis. Yogurt often is used by women with chronic vaginal Candida infections.

Natural agents are frequently neglected for the treatment and prevention of selected intestinal and vaginal infections. To evaluate the potential of natural agents (microorganisms with therapeutic properties) for the prevention and/or treatment of selected intestinal and vaginal infections, the MEDLINE computer database was searched for all relevant articles. All placebo-controlled human studies on natural biotherapeutic agents were reviewed. Placebo-controlled studies showed that natural agents have been used successfully to prevent antibiotic-associated bacterial infections and Candida vaginitis. Few adverse effects have been reported. There is now significant evidence that administration of selected microorganisms is beneficial in the prevention and treatment of certain intestinal infections, and possibly in the treatment of vaginal infections.

Product availability: Yeast Fighters capsules, bifido bacteria, standardized shark liver oil capsules, and Nutraflora can be ordered by calling 1-800-544-4440. Diflucan is an expensive prescription drug that needs to be prescribed by your physician.

Catabolic Wasting

Cancer, HIV infection, congestive heart failure, aging, surgery and a host of degenerative diseases can result in the body shifting from a healthy anabolic cell-replacement metabolism into a catabolic wasting state. Catabolism, also known medically as cachexia, is characterized by severe weight loss and muscle breakdown. If untreated, catabolic wasting can result in death.

Depletion of muscle and adipose tissue in cancer cachexia appears to arise not only from decreased food intake but also from the production of catabolic factors secreted by certain tumors such as tumor necrosis factor and other autoimmune cytokines. Experiments with a cachexia-inducing tumor in mice showed that, when part of the carbohydrate calories in their diet was replaced by fish oil, host body weight loss was inhibited. The catabolic-inhibiting effect occurred without an alteration of either the total calorie consumption or nitrogen intake.

Fish oil that is high in EPA (the fatty acid eicosapentaenoic acid) was found to directly inhibit tumor-induced lipolysis. The effect of EPA-preventing catabolic fat loss arose from an inhibition of the elevation of cyclic AMP (adenosine monophosphate, a nucleotide involved in energy metabolism) in fat cells. The increased protein degradation in the skeletal muscle of catabolic animals also was inhibited by EPA. This effect was due to the inhibition of muscle prostaglandin E2 in response to a tumor-produced proteolytic factor by EPA. Thus, reversal of cachexia by EPA in this mouse model results from its capacity to interfere with tumor-produced catabolic factors. Similar factors have been detected in human cancer cachexia. Catabolic wasting patients should consider taking five capsules a day of the Mega EPA fish oil concentrate.

Glutamine has been one of the most intensively studied nutrients in the field of nutrition support in recent years. Animal studies show that glutamine is effective against catabolic stress. Glutamine supplementation was shown to improve organ function and/or survival in most published studies. These studies also have supported the concept that glutamine is a critical nutrient for the gut mucosa and immune cells.

Recent molecular and protein chemistry studies are beginning to define the basic mechanism involved in glutamine action in the gut, liver and other cells and organs. Double-blind prospective clinical investigations to date suggest that glutamine-enriched diets are generally safe and effective in catabolic patients. Intravenous glutamine has been shown to increase plasma glutamine levels, exert protein anabolic effects, improve gut structure and/or function, and reduce important indices of disease, including infection rates and length of hospital stay in selected patient subgroups.

Glutamine is the most abundant free amino acid in the human body. In catabolic stress situations—such as after surgical operations, trauma and during sepsis—glutamine is rapidly transported to organs and to blood cells. This results in an intracellular *depletion* of glutamine in the muscles, and the ensuing catabolic-wasting effect. Increasing evidence suggests that glutamine is a crucial substrate for immunocompetent cells. Glutamine depletion decreases the proliferation of lymphocytes, possibly by arresting a critical phase of the cells' growth cycle.

Glutamine is a precursor for the synthesis of glutathione and stimulates the formation of heat-shock proteins. Moreover, there are suggestions that glutamine plays a crucial role in the stimulation of intracellular protein synthesis. Experimental studies revealed that glutamine deficiency causes a necrotizing enterocolitis—an inflammation of the small intenstine and colon, leading to cell death—and increases the mortality of animals subjected to bacterial stress.

A clinical human study involving bone-marrow transplant patients demonstrated, after supplementation with glutamine, a decrease in the incidence of infections and a shortening of hospital stay. In critically ill patients, parenteral glutamine reduced nitrogen loss and caused a reduction of the mortality rate. In surgical patients, glutamine evoked an improvement of several immunological parameters. Moreover, glutamine exerted a nutritional (trophic) effect on the intestinal mucosa, decreased the intestinal permeability and thus may prevent the translocation of bacteria.

In conclusion, glutamine is an important metabolic substrate of rapidly proliferating cells. It influences the cellular hydration (combined with water) state and has multiple effects on the immune system, intestinal function and protein metabolism. In several disease states, glutamine may become an indispensable nutrient supplement. Catabolic wasting patients should consider supplementing with 2,000 mg of glutamine a day.

In addition, scientists have examined the impact of a designer whey protein concentrate on preventing or treating catabolic wasting, immune dysfunction and cancer. A study involving HIV-positive men fed whey protein concentrate found dramatic increases in glutathione levels, with most men reaching their ideal body weight. In another study, when different groups of rats were given a powerful carcinogen, those fed whey protein concentrate showed fewer tumors and reduced tumor masses. Whey appears to inhibit the growth of breast cancer cells at low concentrations. In one clinical study, when cancer patients were fed whey protein concentrate at 30 grams a day, some patients' tumors showed a regression.

The research using whey protein concentrate has led researchers to a discovery regarding the relationship between cancerous cells, whey protein concentrate and glutathione. Glutathione is an antioxidant that protects the body against harmful compounds. It was found that whey protein concentrate selectively depletes cancer cells of their glutathione, thus making them more susceptible to such cancer treatments as radiation and chemotherapy. It has been found that cancer cells and normal cells will respond differently to nutrients and drugs that affect glutathione status.

The concentration of glutathione in tumor cells is higher than that of the normal cells that surround it. This difference in glutathione status between normal cells and cancer cells is believed to be an important factor in cancer cells' resistance to chemotherapy. Research has shown that cancer cells subjected to whey proteins were depleted of their glutathione, and their growth was inhibited, while normal cells had an increase in glutathione, and increased cellular growth. These effects were not seen with other proteins.

Not surprisingly, the researchers concluded, "Selective depletion of tumor glutathione may, in fact, render cancer cells more vulnerable to the action of chemotherapy and eventually protect normal tissue against the deleterious effects of chemotherapy."

Whey protein also appears to play a direct role in bone growth. Researchers found that rats fed whey protein concentrate showed increased bone strength, as well as such bone protein as collagen. Whey protein was found to stimulate, dose dependently, total protein synthesis, DNA content and increased hydroxyproline contents of bone cells.

It should be noted that not all whey protein concentrates are created equal. Processing whey protein to remove the lactose and fats, but without losing its biological activity, takes special care by the manufacturer. The protein must be processed under low-temperature and low-acid conditions so as not to "denature" it. Maintaining the natural state of the protein is essential to its biological activity.

Whey protein has the highest biological value rating of any protein. When the biological value is high, that means protein is absorbed, used and retained better in the body. High biological values also are associated with tissue-sparing. Thus, whey protein concentrate can be beneficial for people suffering from wasting catabolic diseases.

The essential fatty acid conjugated linoleic acid (CLA) has anti-catabolic properties. The suggested dose of CLA for a person in a catabolic state is four 500-mg capsules taken twice a day. Cancer patients taking CLA also should take a soy supplement that provides at least 800 mg a day of genistein.

The amino acid arginine can help to generate anabolic cell replacement throughout the body, and can suppress excess levels of ammonia in the body, a common problem associated with catabolic breakdown. The suggested dose for arginine to counteract catabolism is 5 to 20 grams a day. Additional amino acid supplementation should include 2,400 mg of L-carnitine and four capsules a day of the branched chain amino acid complex that includes leucine, isoleucine and valine.

To summarize, catabolic wasting can be counteracted by proper nutrient supplementation. A daily dose of 2,000 mg of glutamine is suggested. Fish oil supplementation, in the dose of five Mega EPA fish oil capsules a day, should be considered. Four 500-mg CLA capsules should be taken twice a day to facilitate the transport of glucose into muscle cells. The intake of 30 grams a day of biologically active whey protein concentrate, 10 to 20 grams of arginine, 2,400 mg of L-carnitine and a branched chain amino acid complex may produce a dramatic anti-catabolic tissue-sparing effect, and regulate immune system cytokines that are thought to cause cachexia.

The standard dose of Life Extension Mix should be given to all people suffering from catabolic breakdown to provide the nutrient building blocks the body needs to start rebuilding.

WARNING: Some nutritionists are concerned about the use of high doses of glutamine and/or arginine in cancer patients. Glutamine and arginine promote cellular growth, and the concern is that these amino acids could cause cancer cells to grow faster. Scientific studies, however, show glutamine and arginine provide a beneficial effects to cancer patients. Only one study on breast cancer patients hinted at a risk for arginine supplementation.

Product availability: Glutamine, specially designed whey protein, arginine, Life Extension Mix, CLA, Mega EPA, L-carnitine, and the branched chain amino acid formula can be ordered by calling 1-800-544-4440.

Cataract

Cataract surgery costs Medicare more money than any other medical procedure. Cataract is epidemic among the aged. It is usually caused by the excessive production of free radicals throughout life.

It is difficult to treat cataract with oral antioxidants because there is only a minimal amount of blood circulation within the eye compared to other parts of the body. Yet, there is evidence that the progression of cataract disease can be slowed by taking nutrients that improve blood circulation to the eye.

Ginkgo biloba extract should be taken at a dose of 120 mg a day by anyone suffering from cataracts. Bilberry extract should be taken at a dose of 150 mg a day by cataract patients. These two flavonoid nutrients may help to restore micro-capillary circulation to the eye.

After taking ginkgo and bilberry for a month, add 600 micrograms of the mineral selenium, 500 mg of the amino acid glutathione and 1,000 mg of alpha-lipoic acid every day.

Melatonin is a potent antioxidant that may be especially effective in treating cataract. Melatonin production slows down in people over the age of 40, and by age 60 there is virtually no melatonin being naturally produced. It is over the age of 60 when most cataracts develop. The suggested dose for melatonin is 3 mg taken at bedtime.

Glycation (glycosylation) of proteins has been shown to play a prominent role in the development of diabetic cataract formation and retinopathy. This process also occurs as a result of general aging. Investigations have been conducted to explore the possibility of preventing glycation through the use of pyruvate and alpha-ketoglutarate. The results demonstrate that both these compounds are effective in preventing the initial glycation reaction, as well as the formation of eye disease.

Both pyruvate and alpha-keto glutarate also inhibit the generation of high molecular weight aggregates associated with cataract formation. The preventive effects appear to be due to competitive inhibition of glycation by the keto acids and the antioxidant properties of these compounds. These agents might be useful in preventing glycation related protein changes and consequent tissue pathological manifestations associated with cataract, diabetes and normal aging. Those with cataract disease should consider taking 650 mg of ornithine alpha-ketoglutarate three times a day.

The best form of pyruvate is calcium pyruvate. A 500-mg capsule of calcium pyruvate provides 405 mg of elemental pyruvic acid. One to three capsules a day of calcium pyruvate are suggested.

The European drug aminoguanidine in the dose of 300 mg a day has been shown to specifically inhibit glycation.

Arginine facilitates the natural synthesis of nitric oxide, and has been shown to enhance arterial elasticity in the diabetic patient. Nitric oxide enables arteries to easily expand and contract with each heart beat. One study also showed that supplementation with only two daily dosages of arginine free base (2 grams a day) produced a significant reduction in lipid peroxidation and free radical by-products after three months. The researchers concluded that arginine supplementation could reduce the long-term micro-capillary complications seen in diabetic patients.

Those suffering from cataract disease might benefit from the circulatory-enhancing effects of arginine. An arginine formula called Powermaker II provides a potent dose of arginine and related co-factors. The dose of Powermaker II Sugar Free (without fructose) should be one to two tablespoons a day.

It is crucial for cataract patients to wear protective eyeglasses to shield against free radical damage induced by ultraviolet (UV) sunlight. If UV-blocking sunglasses were to be worn throughout life, the risk of cataract would be reduced greatly. Exposure to sunlight is a major risk factor in the development and progression of cataract disease. Low-cost, wrap-around sunglasses called Sun-Shields are available; they fit over regular glasses to provide almost 100-percent protection against UV penetration to the eye.

Some cataract patients apply vitamin drops, called Viva Drops, to their eyes every day. While there is no published data on whether vitamin drops can slow the cataract disease process, these vitamin drops do provide antioxidant protection directly to the lens of the eye.

Carmen Fusco has written an article on the prevention of cataracts and the treatment of early cataract with riboflavin, chromium, SOD and catalase. She also recommends reducing sugars, including milk sugar.

Product availability: You can order ginkgo biloba and bilberry, high-potency glutathione capsules, a special selenium complex that contains three different forms of selenium, alpha-lipoic acid, calcium pyruvate, ornithine ketoglutarate, melatonin, Sun-Shields and Viva Drops by calling 1-800-544-4440. Ask how to contact a European supplier of aminoguanidine.

Cerebral Vascular Disease

For those suffering from hemorrhagic cerebral vascular disease, cerebral hemorrhage or cerebral aneurysm, it is suggested that nutrients that help build collagen and elastin be taken to help rebuild the endothelial lining of the arterial system.

Vitamin C at 5,000 mg a day is suggested, along with 300 mg a day of the flavonoid proanthocyanidin (grape seed-skin extract). Magnesium is crucial for arterial structure, and it is suggested that 1,500 mg a day of elemental magnesium be taken along with 1,000 mg a day of calcium and 500 mg a day of potassium.

Mechanisms that regulate cerebral circulation have been intensively investigated in recent years, and the effects of nitric oxide have been examined. Nitric oxide is an important regulator of cerebral vascular tone. Nitric oxide maintains the cerebral vasculature in a dilated state and appears to be an important vasodilator. Arginine specifically enhances nitric oxide synthesis. Those with cerebral vascular disease may consider taking 4 to 5 grams of arginine, three times a day,

Activation of potassium channels appears to be a major mechanism for dilatation of cerebral arteries. Agents that increase the intracellular concentration of cyclic adenosine monophosphate (cAMP) produce vasodilatation. Supplementation with 500 mg a day of potassium and 20 to 60 mg a day of forskolin might enhance vasodilatation in cerebral vascular disease. Do not take forskolin if you have prostate cancer or hypotension (low blood pressure).

Alcohol ingestion poses a risk for development of hypertension (high blood pressure), stroke and sudden death through the depletion from the body of magnesium. The dietary intake of magnesium modulates the hypertensive actions of alcohol. Experiments indicate that chronic ethanol ingestion results in the contraction of the cerebral arteries and capillaries, a contraction that causes increased cerebral vascular resistance. Chronic ethanol ingestion increases the reactivity of intact micro vessels to vasoconstrictors and results in decreased reactivity to vasodilators.

However, pretreatment of animals with magnesium prevents ethanol from inducing stroke, and prevents the adverse cerebral vascular changes from taking place. Magnesium influences the response of cerebral arteries to several other natural or synthetic stimulators (agonists), and has been shown to decrease cerebral vascular resistance. Contractility of cerebral arteries is dependent upon the actions and interactions of calcium and magnesium.

It is clear from published studies that magnesium can induce healthy vascular tone in all types of vascular smooth muscle. Magnesium appears to act on voltage-, receptor-, and leak-operated membrane channels in vascular smooth muscle. Standard channel blocker drugs do not have this uniform capability. Calcium channel-blocking drugs, however, can block calcium infiltration into brain cells, lower cerebral vascular resistance, relieve cerebral vasospasm, and lower arterial blood pressure.

Magnesium also can cause significant vasodilatation of intact cerebral arteries. Although magnesium is three to five orders of magnitude less potent than the standard calcium channel-blocking drugs, it possesses unique and potentially useful effects in maintaining healthy cerebral vascular circulation. Those with cerebral vascular disease, and especially those who consume alcohol, should take 1,500 mg a day of elemental magnesium.

Nimotop (nimodipine) is an FDA-approved calcium channel-blocking drug specific to cerebral circulation and brain-cell activity. It has been shown to work better in the restoration of cerebral circulation than any other calcium channel-blocking drug yet tested. The normal dose is 30 mg of Nimotop, taken three times a day.

Essential fatty acids in the form of fish oil concentrates also should be considered. Mega EPA enables a person to get pharmacologic doses of fish oils by taking only five capsules a day. Extreme caution should be exercised when taking these supplements because they inhibit blood-clotting. There is a chance that a cerebral hemorrhage could occur because of the blood-thinning effects these nutrients can produce. Blood tests that measure clotting time can be used to make sure these nutrients are not reducing the clotting factors in your blood too much.

Reducing hypertension is crucial when cerebral vascular disease is present.

Refer to the Age Associated Mental Impairment and Stroke protocols for additional suggestions about restoring cerebral circulation.

Product availability: Mega EPA, proanthocyanidins (grape seed-skin extract), vitamin C, magnesium, calcium, and potassium are available by calling 1-800-544-4440.

Cholesterol Reduction

Elevated LDL cholesterol is associated with a greater-than-normal risk of atherosclerosis and cardiovascular disease. The objective is to lower total cholesterol to 200 mg/dL or less, and to lower dangerous LDL cholesterol to under 120 mg/dL. The best way of lowering cholesterol is through dietary modification, yet for some people, no matter how little fat and cholesterol they consume, their livers produce too much cholesterol.

FDA-approved cholesterol-lowering drugs can produce serious long-term side effects. However, there are nutrients that lower cholesterol as well or better than FDA-approved drugs. By having regular blood tests to measure cholesterol levels, you can choose less-costly herbal supplements that produce beneficial side effects.

An herbal extract that can lower cholesterol levels is curcumin, the yellow pigment of turmeric. Curcumin is a potent antioxidant that helps to prevent several diseases. When rats were fed small doses of curcumin, their cholesterol levels fell to one-half those of rats not receiving curcumin (*Journal of Nutrition* 100:1307-16, 1970).

Curcumin's mechanisms of cholesterol reduction include interfering with intestinal cholesterol uptake, increasing the conversion of cholesterol into bile acids, and increasing the excretion of bile acids, according to the *International Journal of Vitamin Nutritional Research* (61:364-9, 1991).

Curcumin inhibits abnormal blood clot formation by blocking the formation of thromboxane A2, which is a promoter of platelet aggregation. Curcumin increases a prostacyclin that is a natural inhibitor of abnormal platelet aggregation (*Arzneim Forsh* 36:715-7,1986). When 500 mg a day of curcumin was administered to 10 human volunteers, there was a 29-percent increase in beneficial HDL cholesterol after only seven days. In this study, total cholesterol was reduced by 11.6 percent and lipid peroxidation was reduced by 33 percent (*Indian Journal of Physiology* 36(4):273-275, 1992).

If you are taking cholesterol-lowering drugs, you may be able to substitute curcumin and other nutrients in a product called Herbal Cardiovascular Formula. In order to document the effectiveness of nutritional cholesterol-reducing formulas, test your cholesterol first, then obtain another cholesterol test 45 days later. If curcumin and other nutrients work for you, you will save money, avoid potential side effects and obtain additional health benefits.

While FDA-approved cholesterol-lowering drugs can cause liver damage, curcumin has well-documented cancer- and viral-inhibiting effects. Curcumin also has anti-inflammatory effects. It neutralizes dietary carcinogens and inhibits cancer at the initiation, promotion and progression stages of development.

Curcumin is a potent antioxidant and an inhibitor of HIV replication. Unlike FDA-approved drugs, curcumin may protect against viral hepatitis-induced liver damage. Do not use curcumin if a biliary tract obstruction exists because curcumin increases the excretion of cholesterol bile acids. High doses of curcumin on an empty stomach can cause stomach ulceration.

Another cholesterol-lowering herbal extract is gugulipid, an extract from the mukjul tree. In a study in the *Journal of Associated Physicians-India*, 37(5):323-8, 1989, 125 patients receiving gugulipid experienced an average 11-percent decrease in total cholesterol, and a 16.8-percent decrease in triglycerides within three to four weeks. Patients with elevated cholesterol responded better than did normal patients. Beneficial HDL cholesterol levels increased in 60 percent of the patients receiving gugulipid.

In a placebo-controlled study, 205 patients received gugulipid at a dose of 25 mg three times a day. Of the gugulipid-treated patients, 70 to 80 percent experienced cholesterol reduction, compared with virtually none in the placebo group (*Journal of Associated Physicians-India* 37(5):328-8 1989). In another placebo-controlled trial in 40 patients with high blood-fat levels, serum cholesterol declined by 21.75 percent, and triglycerides by 27.1 percent after three weeks of gugulipid administration. After 16 weeks of gugulipid administration, HDL cholesterol increased by 35.8 percent.

Foundation members who have been following a life extension lifestyle normally have healthy vascular systems. Newly identified herbal extracts may provide further protection against cardiovascular disease risk factors. These herbs have been combined into the Herbal Cardiovascular Formula to provide the ideal potency of each pharmaceutical-grade herbal extract at a far lower price than these herbs cost separately.

Each capsule of the Herbal Cardiovascular Formula contains:

Curcumin (97 percent purity)	250 mg
Bromelain (2,000 gdu per gram)	250 mg
Ginger (gingerol standardized)	500 mg
Gugulipid	35 mg

Take one capsule in the morning and one in the evening. Cardiovascular patients should test their cholesterol/fibrinogen levels within 45 days to make sure the formula is providing sufficient cholesterol- and fibrinogen-lowering effects. Higher doses of Herbal Cardiovascular Formula can be taken to provide additional cholesterol-fibrinogen lowering effects.

Note: Fibrinogen appears to be a greater risk factor for developing vascular disease than cholesterol. For information about fibrinogen, refer to the Fibrinogen And Cardiovascular Disease protocol in this book.

While blood testing is not mandatory for healthy people seeking to reduce their risk of heart attack or stroke, it is recommended that everyone have an annual blood test to fine-tune and optimize their life-extension program.

Another cholesterol-lowering therapy is soy. Phyto extracts from soy can help prevent cancer, and may even be effective in the treatment of certain cancers. Evidence for the cholesterol-lowering effect of soy protein has been in the medical literature for 80 years. *The New England Journal of Medicine* (Aug. 3, 1995) published an analysis of all studies relating to the use of soy to lower blood fat levels. The results of their analysis of 38 controlled studies showed that soy protein produced a reduction of 9.3 percent in total cholesterol, 10.5 percent in triglycerides, and 12.9 percent in dangerous artery-clogging LDL cholesterol. A small increase of 2.4 percent in beneficial HDL was observed.

The primary mechanism by which soy protein lowers cholesterol appears to be related to the phytoestrogen genistein, and to other isoflavones in soy. It seems that soy boosted thyroxine levels, which caused enhanced metabolism of serum cholesterol. This means that people using FDA-approved cholesterol-lowering drugs might be able to substitute soy extracts to lower their cholesterol-triglyceride levels.

The side benefit of taking soy extracts is cancer prevention. In addition to lowering blood fat levels, soy may protect against the development of atherosclerosis and cerebrovascular disease via other mechanisms.

Anyone contemplating using nutrients to replace drugs should have their cholesterol-triglyceride levels checked regularly to make sure the desired blood-fat reducing effect is really occurring. It is advisable to do this under the supervision of a competent physician.

Super Soy Extract and Soy Power are soy concentrates that contain standardized levels of genistein and other isoflavones. These soy extracts contain high standardized potencies of the active phytoestrogens from soy. The minimum dose for cholesterol reduction is five 1,000-mg tablets a day, or one heaping teaspoon (5 to 6 grams) of powder a day. For those with elevated cholesterol levels, we suggest one to two heaping teaspoons of powder or 20 to 40 tablets a day. Soy powder is easily dispersed and has a light peanut butter taste.

A soy supplement called Mega Soy Extract contains in two capsules more genistein and other isoflavones than are contained in a heaping tablespoon of soy supplement powders. It has not been established whether the Mega Soy Extract supplement can lower cholesterol, but preliminary evidence in female primates indicates a protective cariovascular effect due to soy genistein.

Another cholesterol-lowering nutrient is niacin. The best form of niacin is inositol hexanicotinate, which is sold under such brand names as Flush-Free Niacin. This form of niacin is tolerable for most people in daily doses of 2,400 mg.

High intakes of fiber will facilitate serum cholesterol reduction.

Garlic is well-documented to lower serum LDL cholesterol levels. The published studies indicate that high doses of garlic are required to induce a significant cholesterol-lowering effect. The suggested dose is to take a 6,000 to 8,000 mg of a high allicin garlic extract with a heavy meal. This much garlic can cause stomach irritation if taken on an empty stomach.

Fish oil has been shown in published studies to reduce triglyceride levels by about 35 percent on average. Thus, fish oil may prevent abnormal arterial clotting and reduce triglyceride-induced arterial clogging. Fish oil does not appear to lower cholesterol levels as was originally thought.

Product availability: Herbal Cardiovascular Formula containing curcumin and gugulipid, Flush-Free Niacin and soy extracts are available by phoning 1-800-544-4440.

Chronic Fatigue Syndrome (Low Energy)

Chronic fatigue is sometimes an outward manifestation of multiple nutrient deficiencies. For many people, taking high-potency vitamin supplements alleviates chronic fatigue and restores youthful energy levels.

However, there are those who suffer from chronically low energy levels who need more than just vitamins. Victims of chronic fatigue syndrome often are helped by taking 100 mg of coenzyme Q10 three times a day. Another energy-boosting therapy involves taking 5 mg of NADH two times a day.

The amino acid L-carnitine has been approved by the FDA as an energy-boosting drug. People with low energy have been helped by taking 1,000 to 2,000 mg a day of acetyl-L-carnitine. Also, a potent antioxidant called alpha-lipoic acid has improved energy levels in some people on doses of 500 to 800 mg a day.

Some people's low energy levels are caused by deficiencies in brain hormones and neuro-transmitters. The amino acids phenylalanine or tyrosine, taken in daily doses of 1,500 mg, can boost epinephrine and norepinephrine levels. Refer to Phenylalanine And Tyrosine Precautions before taking phenylalanine or tyrosine products. Phenylalanine and tyrosine are available in capsule and powder forms.

The European anti-anxiety therapy Adapton has been shown to alleviate chronic fatigue symptoms when two to four capsules a day are used.

If none of these energy-boosting therapies work, there may be a chronic viral condition causing your chronic fatigue. You should have a medical test for herpes, Epstein-Barr virus and cytomegalovirus antibody activity. If you are infected with a chronic energy-depleting virus, there are conventional and alternative therapies that may be of help. It should be noted that most individuals have been exposed to pathogenic viruses that can be reactivated by adverse environmental conditions and cause chronic fatigue and other diseases. Studies indicate that the Epstein-Barr virus may be suppressed with bilberry extract (anthocyanins), cur-cumin, carotenoids and chlorophylls. The exact doses of these natural plant extracts that might be effective against Epstein-Barr have yet to be determined.

Thyroid deficiency can cause chronic fatigue syndrome. Refer to the Thyroid Deficiency protocol to find out how you can determine if you are deficient in thyroid hormone production.

DHEA has been reported to improve energy levels in chronic fatigue patients. One study showed the value of DHEA and vitamin C-infusion treatment in the control of chronic fatigue syndrome. Refer to DHEA-Pregnenolone Precautions in this book before embarking on this therapy.

For those with a viral-induced chronic fatigue syndrome, refer to the Foundation's protocol on Immune Enhancement.

Product availability: Alpha lipoic acid, acetyl-L-carnitine, NADH, coenzyme Q10, Adapton, DHEA, phenylalanine and tyrosine are available by phoning 1-800-544-4440.

Cirrhosis

Refer to the protocol on Liver (Cirrhosis) for diseases of the liver, and also the Hepatitis B and Hepatitis C protocols.

Cognitive Enhancement

Refer to Age-Associated Mental Impairment and Attention Deficit Disorder protocols.

Common Cold

There are more than 300 viruses that have been identified as causing the common cold. Most cold viruses replicate in the throat.

A randomized, double-blind, placebo-controlled clinical trial has shown that zinc gluconate lozenges produce a significant reduction in the duration of cold symptoms. In this study, patients received zinc lozenges or placebo lozenges every two hours for the duration of cold symptoms. The median time to complete resolution of cold symptoms was 4.4 days in the zinc group, compared with 7.6 days in the placebo group.

Another study to test the benefits of zinc gluconate lozenges showed that the time to complete resolution of symptoms was significantly shorter in the zinc group than in the placebo group. The zinc group had significantly fewer days with coughing, headache, hoarseness, nasal congestion, nasal drainage and sore throat. By dissolving two zinc lozenges in the mouth every few hours, the zinc will help inactivate cold viruses multiplying in the throat. Vitamin C in doses of 5,000 to 20,000 mg has been used by many people as a natural antihistamine and antiviral therapy to treat common colds.

In 1971, Linus Pauling carried out a meta-analysis of four placebo-controlled trials, concluding that it was highly unlikely that the decrease of common cold symptoms in vitamin C groups was caused by chance alone. Studies carried out since then have found that high doses of vitamin C alleviate common cold symptoms, indicating that the vitamin does indeed have physiologic effects on colds. However, despite the large number of placebo controlled studies showing that vitamin C supplementation alleviates the symptoms of the common cold, widespread skepticism about vitamin C persists.

In a review of six large studies on vitamin C supplementation of 1,000 mg a day or less, it was shown that common-cold incidence is not reduced in the low-dose vitamin C-supplemented groups. A further analysis of these studies, however, reveals that some groups do benefit from low-dose vitamin C supplementation. In four studies with British male schoolchildren and students, a statistically significant reduction in common-cold incidence was found in groups supplemented with low-dose vitamin C. One study showed that those who engaged in heavy exercise were 50 percent less likely to get a common cold if they took only 600 to 1,000 mg a day of vitamin C.

Also, echinacea standardized liquid herbal extract is effective at a dose of six full droppers followed by two full droppers every two waking hours until the 2-ounce bottle is empty. Astragalus herbal extract at 300 mg a day can boost immune function and produce direct antiviral effects.

The amino acid N-acetylcysteine (NAC) helps to break excessive mucous and can have a direct antiviral effect. If you get a cold, it is suggested that 600 mg of N-acetylcysteine be taken with at least 2,000 mg of vitamin C three times a day.

Ribavirin is a broad-spectrum antiviral approved in almost every country in the world except the United States. There is evidence that some cold virus strains can be stopped from replicating with ribavirin at a dose of 800 mg a day.

Carmen Fusco uses in her practice tea taken one hour before vitamin C and an immune-boosting formula containing thymus at the very first symptom of cold.

A well-documented but little-used therapy to treat the common cold involves a one-time injection of 500,000 to 3 million IU of interferon (alpha interferon-2a), combined with 40 mg of melatonin every night. Studies document the ability of interferon to kill many common-cold viruses. Interferon is a component of your immune system that kills viruses (and cancer cells). Since it is a prescription drug, you will have to convince your doctor to prescribe and inject the one-time dose of interferon to combat your cold. For additional suggestions, refer to the Immune Enhancement protocol in this book.

Product availability: Zinc lozenges, NAC, echinacea, astragalus, vitamin C and melatonin are available by calling 1-800-544-4440. Ask for a listing of offshore companies that sell ribavirin to Americans by mail. If you live close to the Mexican border, you can buy ribavirin in a Mexican pharmacy and bring it back into the United States under the FDA's personal-use importation policy.

Congestive Heart Failure and Cardiomyopathy

Energy deficiencies at the cellular level cause a gradual weakening of the heart muscle until a transplant becomes necessary. These energy deficits often are a cause of congestive heart failure and many forms of cardiomyopathy. Treatment of a weakened heart muscle involves the use of several different therapies known to boost cardiac energy levels and decrease vascular resistance.

We will discuss several different therapies being used to treat heart muscle energy deficits, and provide a step-by-step approach to the treatment of heart muscle energy deficiencies that are clinically diagnosed as congestive heart failure or cardiomyopathy.

Coenzyme Q10 is a naturally occurring substance that has antioxidant and membrane-stabilizing properties. Administration of coenzyme Q10 in conjunction with standard medical therapy has been reported to increase cardiac output and enhance functional capacity in patients with congestive heart failure. A study evaluated 17 congestive heart failure patients after four months of coenzyme Q10 therapy and found the following results:

❖ Functional class improved 20 percent, with the mean congestive heart failure score improving 27 percent;

❖ Left ventricular ejection fraction was improved by 34.8 percent;

❖ Cardiac output improved by 15.7 percent;

❖ Stroke volume index improved by 18.9 percent;

❖ End-diastolic volume area decreased by 8.4 percent; and

❖ Systolic blood pressure decreased by 4.4 percent.

Therapy with coenzyme Q10 was associated with a mean 25.4-percent increase in exercise duration and a 14.3-percent increase in workload. The doctors concluded by stating, "Coenzyme Q10 therapy is associated with significant functional, clinical, and hemodynamic improvements within the context of an extremely favorable benefit-to-risk ratio. Coenzyme Q10 enhances cardiac output by exerting a positive inotropic effect upon the myocardium, as well as mild vasodilatation."

Published clinical research, as well as various theoretical considerations, suggest that supplemental intakes of taurine, coenzyme Q10 and L-carnitine, as well as the minerals magnesium, potassium and chromium, may be of therapeutic benefit in congestive heart failure. High intakes of fish oil may likewise be beneficial. Fish oil may decrease vascular resistance, thus reducing the energy requirements of the weakened heart muscle. Fish oil also reduces blood viscosity, may reduce arrhythmic risk, and may reduce the risk of developing an arterial blood clot.

There appears to be little, if any toxic risk, to combining these nutritional therapies with conventional drugs.

Magnesium therapy has been shown to be beneficial in improving hemodynamics and in treating arrhythmias. Magnesium toxicity rarely occurs except in patients with kidney dysfunction. In patients with congestive heart failure, the presence of adequate total-body magnesium stores serves as an important prognostic indicator because of an amelioration of arrhythmias, digitalis toxicity and hemodynamic abnormalities. While magnesium appears important as part of an overall treatment program, some studies have shown that magnesium by itself is not effective in treating congestive heart failure.

In another study, seven patients with idiopathic dilated cardiomyopathy, and moderate to severe heart failure, were studied at base line after three months of therapy with human growth hormone, and three months after the discontinuation of growth hormone. Standard therapy for heart failure was continued throughout the study. When administered at a dose of 14 IU per week, growth hormone doubled the serum concentrations of insulin-like growth factor I. Growth hormone improved cardiac output, particularly during exercise, and enhanced ventricular function despite reductions in myocardial oxygen consumption and energy production. Ventricular mechanical efficiency more than doubled. Growth hormone also improved clinical symptoms, exercise capacity and the patients' quality of life.

After growth hormone was discontinued for three months, many of the positive improvements partially reversed. In this study, recombinant human growth hormone administered for three months to patients with idiopathic dilated cardiomyopathy resulted in improvement in hemodynamics, myocardial energy metabolism and clinical status.

Those who suffer from cardiac insufficiency diagnosed as cardiomyopathy or congestive heart failure may be substantially helped by taking the following energy-enhancing nutrients:

1. Coenzyme Q10 — 100 mg, three times a day.
2. Taurine — 2,000 mg a day.
3. Acetyl-L-carnitine — 2,000 mg daily.
4. Fish oil — five to eight capsules a day containing at least 400 mg of EPA and 300 mg DHA.
5. Magnesium — 1,000 mg a day.
6. Potassium — 500 mg a day (if needed).
7. NADH — 5 to 10 mg a day.
8. Life Extension Mix — three tablets, three times a day.
9. Human Growth Hormone — one to two international units (IU) a day, or as prescribed by your physician. Advise your physician about everything you are doing so he can adjust your treatment program. For additional suggestions, refer to the Foundation's Atherosclerosis protocol.

Angiotension-converting enzyme-inhibiting prescription drugs such as Capoten or Zestril relax the vascular system, thus reducing the workload of the heart. Fish oil also can relax the vascular system.

For those who cannot afford growth hormone, 6 to 10 grams a day of arginine is suggested. There are studies showing that arginine can boost cardiac output by itself.

One study reported on the conventional drugs doctors use to treat congestive heart failure. Here is the order and percentage of frequency: diuretics, 82 percent; angiotensin-converting enzyme inhibitors (such as Zestril or Capoten), 53 percent; nitrates, 49 percent; digoxin, 46 percent; potassium, 40 percent; aspirin, 36 percent; calcium antagonists, 20 percent; warfarin, 17 percent; beta-blockers, 15 percent; and magnesium, 10 percent.

Diuretic drugs deplete the body of the electrolyte minerals magnesium and potassium. Those taking diuretic drugs often are prescribed potassium and magnesium supplements by their physicians. If your doctor is not prescribing these two critical minerals, ask him why.

Digoxin (Lanoxin) improves the strength and efficiency of the heart. Coenzyme Q10, , taurine, acetyl-L-carnitine and other nutrients also improve cardiac energy output.

You should review the nutrients you plan to take with the doctor who is prescribing the medications used to treat your cardiomyopathy and/or congestive heart failure.

Carmen Fusco recommends that, since lasix often is given for congestive heart failure, it is extremely important to replace not only potassium but also magnesium and folic acid during lasix treatment.

Product availability: Coenzyme Q10, acetyl-L-carnitine, taurine, magnesium, potassium, NADH and high potency fish oil capsules are available by calling 1-800-544-4440. Growth hormone must be prescribed by a knowledgeable physician.

Constipation

Conventional and alternative doctors often recommend fiber supplements to prevent constipation. Yet, published studies show that a significant number of chronically constipated people do not find relief from fiber supplements. Many chronically constipated people become laxative addicts.

Dietary modifications can help some people, but many people's constipation is caused by insufficient peristalsis, which means there is not enough colon contractile activity to completely evacuate the bowel. There are specific nutrients that, if taken at the right time, can induce healthy colon peristaltic action without producing side effects. While pharmaceutical laxatives have been linked to the development of cancer, nutritional laxatives have many health benefits.

Nutrients that induce healthy colon peristalsis work best when taken on an empty stomach. One combination is 4 to 8 grams of vitamin C powder and 1,500 mg of magnesium oxide taken with the juice of a freshly squeezed grapefruit. If that's too tart for you, use vitamin C and magnesium capsules with fresh orange juice. This therapy has to be individually adjusted so it will not cause diarrhea.

Most Americans suffer from a deficiency of magnesium, and the use of a magnesium laxative several times a week could prove beneficial for cardiovascular health. However, chronic use of very high doses (over 3,000 mg every day) of magnesium could allow excessive magnesium into the bloodstream, and this could affect kidney function.

Vitamin B5 (pantothenic acid) in a dose of 3,000 mg on an empty stomach will produce a rapid evacuation of bowel contents. Durk Pearson and Sandy Shaw's Powermaker II Sugar Free formula contains vitamin B5, vitamin C, arginine and choline, all of which induce significant peristaltic action when one to two tablespoons of the product are taken on an empty stomach.

One study evaluated whether laxatives and fiber therapies improve symptoms and bowel movement frequency in adults with chronic constipation. Fiber and laxatives decreased abdominal pain and improved stool consistency, compared with placebo. The conclusions were that both fiber and laxatives modestly improved bowel movement frequency in adults with chronic constipation. There was inadequate evidence to establish whether fiber was superior to laxatives, or if one laxative class was superior to another.

A trial on functional constipation in children showed that most children with fecal incontinence benefit from a strict treatment plan that includes defecation trials, a fiber-rich diet and laxative medications. Surgery followed by medical treatment was required in patients with

Hirschsprung's disease (congenital colon defect) and in some patients with anal stenosis (narrowing).

Chronic constipation can be a disabling condition that may require removal of part or all of the colon (colectomy). However, one study showed fiber, cathartic laxatives or biofeedback therapy to be successful in 65 percent of patients. Among the remaining patients, two-thirds underwent surgery, of which 83 percent were successful.

Laxative use was significantly reduced in a long-term care facility when an interdisciplinary program based on a philosophy of prevention and health promotion was implemented. Specifically, increased fluid and fiber intake, timely toileting habits and regular activity or exercise led to a halving of the number of patients receiving laxatives as required, relative to pre-program levels and a control unit not receiving the program.

Constipation is a problem frequently encountered during pregnancy, as is excessive weight gain. Treatments commonly used to control constipation are endowed with some drawbacks, and often do not help control weight. However, a preparation of lactulose and glucomannan was shown to be effective and well-tolerated in patients affected by constipation and in controlling excessive food intake. Fifty pregnant females affected by constipation were treated with a preparation of glucomannan (3 to 6 grams) and lactulose (8 to 16 grams) twice a day for one to three months. This preparation resulted in a return to normal frequency of weekly number of evacuations, and a parallel control of weight gain.

An example of fiber *not* working was a trial that showed that 80 percent of patients with slow transit and 63 percent of patients with a disorder of defecation did not respond to dietary fiber treatment. In 85 percent of patients without these disorders, fiber was effective. This study showed that slow GI transit and/or a disorder of defecation may explain a poor outcome of dietary fiber therapy in some patients with chronic constipation.

Another example of fiber not working was a trial with 73 consecutive constipated children whose mean fiber intake was the same as in healthy controls, although energy and fluid intake was lower. The conclusion was that the amount of dietary fibers played no role in chronic constipation. Dietary advice did not change the mean fiber content of the diet. In addition, changes in fiber intake had no effect on colonic transit time or cure.

It is common for constipation to occur following severe spinal cord injury. One study suggested that increasing dietary fiber in spinal cord injury patients does not have the same effect on bowel function as has been previously demonstrated in individuals with "normally functioning" bowels. Indeed, the effect may be the opposite to that desired. As had been seen in previous studies, fiber will work only in certain people suffering from constipation.

Nutritional laxatives such as magnesium, ascorbic acid, arginine and pantothenic acid are becoming more popular in those afflicted with constipation that is resistant to fiber therapies.

Product availability: You can order pure ascorbic acid crystals, magnesium oxide powder, vitamin B5 powder, vitamin C caps, magnesium caps and Powermaker II Sugar Free by calling 1-800-544-4440.

Deafness

Refer to the Hearing Loss protocol.

Depression

Depression is now acknowledged to be an epidemic disease. The most widely sold prescription drug to treat depression in the United States is Prozac.

However, the safest and most effective antidepressant in the world is the European drug S-adenosylmethionine (SAMe). SAMe is a natural compound found in every cell within the body that plays an important role in critical biochemical processes. When compared with other antidepressants, SAMe works faster and more effectively, with virtually no adverse side effects. In fact, unlike FDA-approved antidepressants that have both lethal and non-lethal side effects, SAMe produces side *benefits*, such as improved cognitive function, protection of liver function, and a potential slowing of the aging process. Some people take SAMe for its anti-aging properties alone.

The major drawback of SAMe is that it is a difficult-to-produce natural substance with high manufacturing and packaging costs. At this time, the retail price of using SAMe to treat depression is more than the price of Prozac. The suggested dose of SAMe to treat depression ranges from 400 to 1,600 mg a day. In one study, as little as 25 mg a day was used to treat depression, while most have used 800 mg to 1,600 mg a day of SAMe.

A more affordable antidepressant being used in Europe and sold in some American health food stores is an extract from the herb St. John's wort called hypericum or hyperforat (St. John's wort extract). For treating depression we suggest 300 mg three times a day of hypericum (with a standardized concentration of 0.3 percent hypericin, the primary active ingredient in hypericum). Small children should be limited to 300 mg a day; larger children may take 600 mg a day; adolescents may take the full adult dose. One caution when using St. John's wort is to avoid prolonged sunlight exposure, since hypericin may make the skin more sensitive to UV light.

A meta-analysis and review of 23 randomized clinical trials involving 1,757 people with mild or moderately severe depressive disorders showed that St. John's wort was 2.67 times superior to placebo in relieving depressive symptoms and as effective as standard anti-depressant drugs. Side effects occurred in 19.8 percent of patients on St. John's wort, compared with 52.8 percent of those taking standard anti-depressant drugs. The conclusion of the researchers was that St. John's wort is more effective than placebo for the treatment of mild to moderately severe depressive disorders.

Another European antidepressant drug called adrafinil is being successfully used by Europeans and Americans who import it for personal use. The dose of adrafinil is two tablets twice a day.

Some people with depression benefit by the inhibition of the enzyme monoamine oxidase (MAO). While MAO-inhibiting drugs have many side effects, the use of the European drug KH3 can safely alleviate depression in some people without classic MAO-inhibiting drug side effects. KH3 is a mild inhibitor of MAO and is very inexpensive.

The amino acid acetyl-L-carnitine has been reported to safely alleviate depression in some people in doses of 1,000 mg twice a day. Acetyl-L-carnitine has cognitive-enhancing and anti-aging effects. Also, the brain cell energy-enhancing NADH (nicotinamide-adenine-dinucleotide) has alleviated depression in studies where 5 to 10 mg a day were used.

Nutrition plays a critical role in the treatment of depression. The supplementation of specific nutrients can correct an underlying deficiency that may be the cause of some depressive states. The most comprehensive nutrient supplement formula is Life Extension Mix, which contains high doses of 56 different ingredients. Depressed people who have not taken vitamin supplements before should try three tablets, three times a day, of Life Extension Mix for five weeks to see if it helps correct their depressive state. If vitamin supplements already have been tried and failed to correct a depressive state, nutritional anti-depressant therapy should begin immediately in conjunction with Life Extension Mix and any needed pharmacologic anti-depressant.

The amino acid dl-phenylalanine, when taken with the nutrients in Life Extension Mix, can boost endorphin levels in the brain to help lift a person out of a depressed state. The suggested dose is two 500-mg capsules of dl-phenylalanine in the morning on an empty stomach and one 500-mg capsule of dl-phenylalanine in midafternoon on an empty stomach.

Some people use the powder formula Rise & Shine, designed by Durk Pearson and Sandy Shaw, which provides phenylalanine and co-factors. The suggested dose is one tablespoon in the morning and one in midafternoon. If phenylalanine does not work after several weeks, then the amino acid tyrosine should be tried at the same dose. Some people find that 500 mg to 1,500 mg a day of the amino acid tyrosine works better than phenylalonine.

There are some people who are genetically sensitive to phenylalanine and cannot take it. Hypertensive people should use phenylalanine with caution because it can elevate blood pressure in people who already have high blood pressure. Cancer patients should avoid taking extra phenylalanine and tyrosine because these amino acids can contribute to cancer cell proliferation.

CAUTION: None of the above natural therapies may be effective in patients suffering from serious clinical depression or manic-depression. Such patients may require FDA-approved antidepressant drugs and/or lithium. Anyone suffering from clinical depression of any type should be under the care of a physician.

Product availability: SAMe, dl-phenylalanine, l-tyrosine, Life Extension Mix, St. John's wort extract, NADH, Rise & Shine and acetyl-L-carnitine are available by calling 1-800-544-4440. Ask for a listing of offshore companies that sell adrafinil and KH3 to Americans by mail.

DHEA-Pregnenolone Precautions

DHEA replacement is becoming a very popular anti-aging therapy. However, there are some precautions that should be exercised when taking DHEA. Since the hormone pregnenolone can cascade down into DHEA and estrogen, some of the precautions discussed for DHEA replacement therapy also may apply to pregnenolone replacement therapy.

A DHEA blood test should be taken three to six weeks after beginning DHEA and/or pregnenolone therapy to help determine optimal dosing. Some people take a DHEA blood test before beginning DHEA replacement therapy, but the Life Extension Foundation has found that every person evaluated who is over 39 years of age shows marked DHEA deficiency.

For the DHEA test, blood should be drawn between the second and third daily dose of DHEA (or pregnenolone). While this test can be costly, it can save you money in the long-run if it shows that you should take less of the hormone to produce youthful DHEA levels.

Take antioxidant supplements after every DHEA dose to protect your liver against free radicals that could be generated in response to DHEA's metabolic-enhancing effects.

CAUTION: Men with prostate cancer or severe benign prostatic hypertrophy should not take DHEA because it can be converted into the metabolites testosterone and dihydrotestosterone, which could promote prostate cell proliferation.

Men over 40 who take DHEA also should take an extract of saw palmetto (320 mg) and pygeum (100 mg) every day, or another 5-alpha reductase inhibitor, to reduce the conversion of testosterone to dihydrotestosterone. Men over 40 also should consider checking their PSA (prostate specific antigen) levels when they have their first DHEA blood tests, and every year thereafter. This test can reveal the presence of prostate cancer.

Do not take DHEA if you have prostate cancer.

DHEA can increase serum estrogen levels in women. It could reduce or eliminate the need for estrogen replacement therapy by naturally elevating estrogen levels in the body. To help protect cells (especially breast cells) from excessive proliferation in response to estrogen in the blood, women should consider taking 1 to 10 mg of melatonin every night, especially if they take DHEA. High doses of soy provides phytoestrogens that may also reduce breast cancer risk.

Note: Women taking DHEA or any form of estrogen therapy are strongly advised to take a soy supplement that provides at least 50 mg of elemental genistein for the specific purpose or reducing the overall risk of breast cancer.

Women with an estrogen-dependent cancer may want to avoid taking DHEA. However, some physicians find physiological DHEA replacement is beneficial for patients with such cancers. Women should consider estrogen testing when they take their DHEA blood test, in order to evaluate DHEA's effect on their blood levels of estrogen when a follow-up test is performed.

If you have liver disease, it is more important that you take DHEA sublingually (under your tongue) to reduce the amount of DHEA entering your liver. Check your liver enzyme levels to make sure DHEA is not making an existing liver disease worse. Some animal studies suggest the possibility of liver damage from large doses of DHEA. Antioxidants should be taken to protect against DHEA-induced free radical damage to the liver.

Pregnenolone can be taken in doses of 50 to 200 mg a day. If more than 50 mg of pregnenolone is taken, it should be taken in divided doses. Pregnenolone also can be converted into progesterone in the body, which may be beneficial for women.

Product availability: To obtain low-cost DHEA, pregnenolone and blood tests to measure these hormones by mail, phone 1-800-544-4440.

Diabetes Type I
(Juvenile Diabetes)

Type I diabetes is caused by the destruction of the insulin-producing cells in the pancreas. The resulting insulin deficiency requires the lifelong administration of insulin by injection several times a day in precise doses for proper glucose utilization. Juvenile diabetes is thought to be caused by an autoimmune or viral attack on the insulin-producing beta cells of the pancreatic islets.

The frequency and dose of insulin used by Type I diabetics is determined by the results of blood-sugar readings on a glucometer. Type I diabetics should use the glucometer at least three times a day to regulate their insulin dosing.

Juvenile diabetes may be prevented or mitigated by following the Autoimmune Disease protocol in this book. Once the insulin-producing cells are destroyed, the best alternative therapy involves protecting against the pathological effects caused by wide variations in blood sugar levels.

Diabetics are at risk of becoming disabled or dying from premature cardiovascular disease. Both insulin-dependent (Type I) and non insulin-dependent (Type II) diabetic patients have been shown to have significantly lower levels of antioxidant protection, compared with age-matched controls. Anyone with diabetes should follow the Atherosclerosis protocol that provides potent doses of antioxidants and other nutrients that have been shown to be especially beneficial in protecting against diabetic-induced cardiovascular disease.

To facilitate the cellular metabolism of glucose, diabetics should take 200 micrograms of chromium picolinate with every meal. Chromium may reduce the amount of injected insulin required, so using the glucometer can enable the diabetic patient to determine the proper amount of insulin to inject.

Diabetic retinopathy is a leading cause of blindness. Studies show that supplementation with vitamin B6 can help to prevent diabetic retinopathy. The appropriate amount of vitamin

B6 is included in the Atherosclerosis protocol. Diabetic neuropathy can cause severe pain throughout the body. It has been shown that the nutrients alpha-lipoic acid (in doses of 500 to 1,200 mg a day) and acetyl-L-carnitine (at 1,000 to 2,000 mg a day) have been effective for diabetic neuropathies.

The premature aging caused by diabetes is primarily the result of uncontrolled glucose that binds with protein in the blood to form nonfunctioning structures within the body. This devastating process is known as glycosylation. Everyone suffers from glycosylation as a normal consequence of aging. However, diabetics suffer from accelerated glycosylation that causes many of the health problems associated with juvenile diabetes. Vitamin C and chromium may inhibit glycosylation. Juvenile diabetics may want to take an additional 5 grams of vitamin C to further inhibit glycosylation.

DHEA is an adrenal hormone that may protect against some diabetic complications. Refer to DHEA-Pregnenolone Precautions protocol before using DHEA.

An interesting study on Swedish children showed that high levels of zinc in the drinking water dramatically reduced the incidence of developing juvenile diabetes. Previous studies have shown that a zinc deficiency increases the risk for diabetes in diabetes-prone experimental animals. This new study showed for the first time that long-term deficiency of zinc significantly increased the risk of a child developing juvenile diabetes. Children who may be genetically susceptible to developing diabetes should supplement with zinc.

Small children may need only 10 mg a day of zinc added to their food or drink. (An adult should not take more than 100 mg of zinc a day on a longterm basis.) There are good-tasting zinc lozenges available that contain 23 mg of zinc that could be given to older children.

Glycation (glycosylation) of proteins has been shown to play a prominent role in the development of many diseases related to diabetes, including atherosclerosis, cataract formation and retinopathy. This process also occurs as a result of general aging. Investigations have been conducted to explore the possibility of preventing glycation by the use of pyruvate and alpha-keto glutarate. The results demonstrate that both these compounds are effective in preventing the initial glycation reaction as well as the formation of eye disease.

Both pyruvate and alpha-keto glutarate also inhibit the generation of high molecular-weight aggregates associated with cataract formation. The preventive effects appear to be due to competitive inhibition of glycation by the keto acids and the antioxidant properties of these compounds. These agents might be useful in preventing glycation-related protein changes and consequent tissue pathological manifestations associated with cataract, diabetes and normal aging.

Diabetics should consider taking 650 mg of ornithine alpha-ketoglutarate three times a day. The best form of pyruvate is calcium pyruvate. A 500-mg capsule of calcium pyruvate provides 405 mg of elemental pyruvic acid. One to three capsules a day of calcium pyruvate are suggested.

The European drug aminoguanidine inhibits an enzyme required for glycosylation. The recommended dose of aminoguanidine is 300 to 600 mg a day. Some doctors believe that aminoguanidine could produce toxicities in doses over 300 mg a day.

Those with juvenile (Type I) diabetes should refer to the Type II Diabetes protocol for additional suggestions.

Product availability: Chromium picolinate, DHEA, alpha-lipoic acid, acetyl-L-carnitine, vitamin B6, zinc lozenges and capsules, calcium pyruvate, ornithine ketoglutarate and vitamin C are available by phoning 1-800-544-4440. Ask for the name of an offshore supplier of the anti-glycosylation drug aminoguanidine.

Diabetes Type II (Adult Onset Diabetes)

Type II diabetes is very different from Type I diabetes. Unlike Type I diabetes, which is characterized by a severe deficiency in pancreatic insulin production, Type II diabetes usually involves normal or overproduction of insulin by the pancreas. Type II diabetes occurs when the cells become resistant to insulin due to receptor malfunction. Insulin is the hormone that normally drives glucose into cells. Insulin resistance causes elevated blood sugar levels because sugar is not able to be absorbed and utilized by the cells. The pancreas may recognize the elevated blood sugar levels and secrete more insulin in a futile attempt to lower the elevated sugar levels.

Chronically elevated levels of serum glucose and insulin predispose a person to premature cardiovascular disease and other diabetic complications. In order to effectively treat Type II diabetes, insulin resistance needs to be alleviated so that glucose can freely enter cells for proper disposal.

Aging causes a breakdown in normal glucose metabolism, and dietary fat and obesity can contribute directly to Type II diabetes. A possible dietary cure for Type II diabetes involves eating a reduced-calorie diet comprised of 10 percent fat that is high in protein and low in carbohydrates. Since most people are unable to restrict their fat intake to only 10 percent, the Life Extension Foundation has specific nutrient, hormone and drug recommendations to help break down insulin resistance.

Both insulin-dependent (Type I) and non insulin-dependent (Type II) diabetic patients have been shown to have significantly lower levels of antioxidant protection, compared with age-matched controls. Anyone with Type II diabetes should follow the Atherosclerosis protocol in this book that recommends potent doses of antioxidants and other nutrients that have been shown to help protect against diabetic-induced cardiovascular diseases.

To help bring blood sugar levels under control, 200 micrograms of chromium picolinate and 7.5 mg of vanadyl sulfate should be taken with each meal. Aging people often suffer a chromium deficiency. Insufficient chromium levels also can be a manifestation of Type II diabetes because the cell membrane insulin receptors require chromium to properly take up insulin and metabolize glucose. Some Type II diabetics find that one to three 200-microgram capsules of chromium picolinate can reduce blood sugar levels.

Niacin helps the chromium work better, and the amount of niacin found in most multi-vitamin formulas is usually sufficient to facilitate the glucose-lowering effect of chromium.

Magnesium may be more important than chromium in controlling blood-sugar levels. Those with Type II diabetes should supplement with at least 500 mg a day of elemental magnesium. Magnesium supplementation should be used with caution in diabetics who also suffer from severe kidney impairment.

One of the factors involved in cellular-insulin resistance is a deficit of nitric oxide. Arginine induces the production of nitric oxide so that sugar molecules can more easily enter cells. Arginine's ability to facilitate the natural synthesis of the nitric oxide has been shown to enhance arterial elasticity in the diabetic patient. Nitric oxide enables arteries to easily expand and contract with each heart beat. One study also showed that supplementation with only two daily dosages of arginine free base (2 grams a day) produced a significant reduction in lipid peroxidation and free radical by-products after three months. The researchers concluded that arginine supplementation could reduce the long-term micro-capillary complications seen in diabetic patients.

An arginine formula called Powermaker II Sugar Free can be of significant benefit to most Type II diabetic patients, and possibly Type I diabetics. The dose of Powermaker II Sugar-Free should be one to two tablespoons a day.

CAUTION: For a minority of Type II diabetics, arginine can elevate their blood sugar by neutralizing insulin. Therefore, diabetics contemplating using arginine or Powermaker II Sugar Free should check their blood sugar with a glucometer every time they take an arginine supplement for the first three weeks.

The therapeutic benefits of biotin was evaluated on 43 Type II diabetic patients. The serum biotin levels were significantly lower than the 64 healthy control subjects. The lower the biotin levels, the greater the serum glucose level. The oral administration of 9,000 micrograms a day of biotin corrected the hyperglycemia in Type II diabetics. This finding suggests that biotin administration ameliorates abnormal glucose metabolism in the diabetic patient by enhancing the activity of the biotin-dependent enzyme required for the promotion of proper glucose utilization. The administration of biotin also enhanced the effectiveness of the anti-diabetic drug glibenclamide in patients who had been resistant to the drug. Neither a relapse of clinical symptoms nor an occurrence of undesirable side effects was observed in patients taking these relatively high doses of biotin.

DHEA hormone replacement therapy also can be beneficial in restoring youthful carbohydrate metabolism. See the DHEA Precaution protocol, for proper DHEA dosing and safety precautions. The combination of chromium, DHEA and thyroid hormone therapy can slowly produce weight loss, further reducing the risk factors for Type II diabetes. Since being overweight is usually a contributing factor in Type II diabetes, please check the Weight Management protocols in this book for further suggestions.

A common complication of diabetes is painful peripheral-nerve disease. Two nutrients that have been shown to be beneficial in preventing and treating diabetic neuropathy are alpha-lipoic acid and acetyl-L-carnitine. Suggested dosing is 500 mg to 1,200 mg a day of alpha-lipoic acid and/or 1,000 mg to 2,000 mg a day of acetyl-L-carnitine. In Europe, these nutrients are used as "drugs" to treat neuropathies.

Acetyl-L-carnitine has been shown to accelerate nerve regeneration after experimental surgical injury in rats. In diabetic rats, acetyl-L-carnitine has been shown to preserve and improve nerve conduction velocity. In one study, just one month of acetyl-L-carnitine treatment produced near-normalization of nerve conduction velocity in diabetic rats with no adverse effects. A human study showed that 1,500 mg a day of acetyl-L-carnitine could improve sensory nerve conduction in Type II diabetics suffering from neurogenic impotence. Another study showed that acetyl-L-carnitine treatment promoted nerve-fiber regeneration.

Free radicals can cause neuropathy. Supplementation with such antioxidants as vitamin E and alpha-lipoic acid has been shown to reduce the severity of diabetic neuropathies. Alpha-lipoic acid also improves glucose metabolism.

A study in Germany on 12 patients with severe Type II diabetes showed that a single infusion of 600 mg of alpha-lipoic acid improved insulin sensitivity. Longer-term studies show that 800 to 1,200 mg a day of alpha-lipoic acid produce a significant reduction in all the major symptoms of diabetic neuropathy. Alpha lipoic acid may lower blood sugar levels by correcting muscle glucose metabolic disorders.

Numerous studies show that diabetic patients have significant defects of antioxidant protection, and that many diabetic complications are caused by free radicals. Type II diabetics should consider taking three tablets, three times a day, of the Life Extension Mix nutritional formula that provides high potencies of a wide range of antioxidants, as well as minerals such as magnesium.

One study showed that vitamin-B6 supplementation combined with insulin produced a lower blood-glucose response, compared with insulin treatment without vitamin B6. Vitamin B6 also was able to lower thrombotic (clotting inside blood vessel) risk factors in diabetics taking insulin.

There is an increased requirement for nutrients in normal pregnancy, not only due to increased demand for those nutrients, but because of increased loss of them as well. In addition, there is an increased insulin-resistant state during pregnancy. A review of the published literature showed that vitamin/mineral supplementation may be useful to prevent or ameliorate pregnancy-related diabetic conditions.

Soy protein has been shown to induce a significant improvement in insulin sensitivity, glucose effectiveness, fasting insulin levels and insulin-to-glucose ratios. Type II diabetics are encouraged to consume one to two tablespoons (20 to 40 grams) a day of a concentrated soy protein extract powder, or take one capsule twice a day of Mega Soy Extract.

If, in following the Atherosclerosis protocol and taking arginine, chromium, magnesium, vanadyl sulfate, etc., blood sugar levels are not brought under control, then Glucophage, also known as metformin, should be prescribed by your doctor. Glucophage was used in Europe for 40 years before it was approved by the FDA for use in the United States. Glucophage can break down insulin resistance so cells are better able to absorb and utilize glucose. Lower glucose levels in the blood will result in reduced insulin output by the pancreas. Glucophage also may lower blood pressure. The dose of Glucophage most commonly prescribed is 500 mg twice a day. Glucophage has been shown to work synergistically with the amino acid arginine to enhance arterial elasticity.

In addition to Glucophage, thyroid-hormone replacement therapy can further help to drive glucose into your cells. Your doctor should prescribe the proper dose of thyroid hormone if this is required. Blood tests may not always reveal a thyroid-hormone deficiency, even though most people over the age of 40 have altered thyroid hormone metabolism. Refer to the Thyroid protocol for specific information about thyroid-hormone replacement. Soy may boost tyroid hormone output.

One of the newest drugs approved by the FDA to treat Type II diabetes is called Rezulin. In about 15 percent of those who tested the drug, insulin shots were no longer needed because the cells became more sensitive to insulin. Most diabetics studied still needed insulin but required fewer injections each day. Rezulin's side effects are rare and relatively mild, the FDA has said. These side effects include some infections, pain, liver degeneration, and headache. It also can cause an increase in cholesterol levels, but the FDA said the rise is not alarming. Nevertheless, any side-effects are good reasons for first trying diet, exercise and supplementation with safe nutrients that may lower elevated blood glucose levels. Your doctor then can determine whether to try Glucophage or Rezulin if drug therapy is needed.

Glycation (glycosylation) of proteins has been shown to play a prominent role in the development of many diseases related to diabetes, including atherosclerosis, cataract formation and retinopathy. Glycation also occurs as a result of general aging. Investigations have been conducted to explore the possibility of preventing glycation by use of pyruvate and alpha-keto glutarate. The results demonstrate that both these compounds are effective in preventing the initial glycation reaction as well as the formation of eye disease.

Both pyruvate and alpha-ketoglutarate also inhibit the generation of high molecular-weight aggregates associated with cataract formation. The preventive effects appear to be due to competitive inhibition of glycation by the keto acids and the antioxidant properties of these compounds. These agents might be useful in preventing glycation-related protein changes and consequent tissue-pathological manifestations associated with cataract, diabetes and normal aging.

Diabetics should consider taking 650 mg of ornithine alpha-ketoglutarate three times a day. The best form of pyruvate is calcium pyruvate. A 500-mg capsule of calcium pyruvate provides 405 mg of elemental pyruvic acid. One to three capsules a day of calcium pyruvate are suggested.

The European drug aminoguanidine inhibits an enzyme required for glycosylation. The recommended dose of aminoguanidine is 300 to 600 mg a day. Some doctors believe that aminoguanidine could produce toxicities in doses over 300 mg a day.

Refer also to the Neuropathy and Retinopathy protocols.

Product availability: Chromium, DHEA, vanadyl sulfate, Powermaker II, Mega Soy Extract, alpha-lipoic acid, calcium pyruvate, ornithine ketoglutarate, acetyl-L-carnitine, and arginine can be ordered by calling 1-800-544-4440. Your doctor can prescribe Glucophage and thyroid hormone replacement therapy.

Digestive Disorders

Aging causes a decline in the natural production of digestive enzymes, thereby making the efficient processing of food more difficult. Digestive enzyme deficiencies can cause the liver and pancreas to be overworked and become pathologically enlarged. There are specific enzymes and acids that are needed to break down proteins, carbohydrates and fats.

Many people over the age of 40 begin using digestive enzymes when eating a heavy meal. The enzymes quicken the digestive process so that the feeling of being bloated, heavy and tired after eating does not occur. There are many enzyme products available, but most people choose a multi-enzyme formula called Super Enzyme Caps that contains a concentrated standardized pancreatin enzyme, along with enzymes to break down every food group. Super Enzyme Caps also contain hydrochloric acid and ox bile. For people seeking a vegetable derived multi-enzyme supplement without pancreatin, hydrochloric acid and ox bile, a product called N-Zymes is often used.

The benefits of enzyme supplementation were validated in a study showing pancreatin could maintain post-operative digestion and nutrition in patients who had surgery for chronic pancreatitis. The effects of post-operative pancreatic enzyme supplementation was studied by measurements of intestinal absorption and nutritional status in a randomization trial in which the patients received the enzyme pancreatin or placebo.

All patients demonstrated abnormal digestion of fat, protein and total energy at baseline and three weeks after surgery. Pancreatin supplementation significantly improved the coefficients of absorption of dietary fat and total energy over the next four weeks. Between four and eight weeks, pancreatin significantly improved protein absorption and nitrogen balance, whereas placebo substitution worsened the absorption of dietary fat and total energy. Nutritional status was not significantly altered over the eight-week study period, although four patients receiving pancreatin gained an average of more than 3.6 kilograms (7.9 pounds) of body weight apiece. The data suggest that long-term post-operative pancreatic enzyme supplementation is both efficacious and necessary in chronic pancreatitis patients after surgery.

For those who do not benefit from digestive enzymes, an FDA-approved prescription drug called Propulsid can be taken 20 minutes before a meal in order to initiate a quicker peristaltic movement of food out of the stomach. The dose of Propulsid is 10 mg, ideally taken before every meal and at bedtime. This drug can induce diarrhea.

Conventional medicine has finally recognized that most stomach ulcers are caused by the Helicobacter pylori (H. pylori) bacteria. If you suffer from stomach ulcers, ask your doctor to prescribe the new antibiotic H. pylori-eradication therapies in combination. The determination of whether you suffer from an H. pylori infection in your stomach can be made by having your blood tested for an antibody to the H. pylori bacteria.

For heartburn problems, refer to the Esophageal Reflux protocol.

Product availability: You can order Super Enzyme Caps and N-Zymes by calling 1-800-544-4440.

Down Syndrome

Until recently, the birth defect that causes severe mental retardation, known as Down syndrome, was thought to be untreatable. A search of the scientific literature, however, indicates that high potency vitamin supplements, along with the European drug piracetam, can be effective in treating children with Down syndrome.

One study showed that Down-syndrome patients who progressed to Alzheimer's disease had low levels of serum vitamin E. The doctors suggested that vitamin E might protect against Down syndrome-induced premature Alzheimer's dementia.

Another study found a causal relationship between cognitive decline in Down syndrome that could be related to undetected folate vitamin deficiency.

Yet another study found a value from thyroid replacement therapy, vitamin-mineral therapy and 5-hydroxytryptophan in treating Down patients.

It has been suggested that malabsorption plays a role in a number of the vitamin and mineral deficiencies found in people with Down syndrome. A review of the published studies demonstrates that patients with Down syndrome are prone to suffer multiple deficiencies of vitamins and lifelong shortages of some trace metals. A significant reason for these deficiencies is malabsorption from the intestine. Treatment of vitamin deficiencies has shown success in some studies. The brain in Down syndrome does not develop adequately. The hippocampus region of the brain, which is concerned with memory, is especially poorly developed. The deficiency of nutrients in Down syndrome may play a significant role in relation to the failure of the brain to develop.

One study showed that Down syndrome patients had higher-than-normal levels of vitamin A and beta-carotene. These high levels of vitamin A may be caused by a thyroid deficiency. The correction of a thyroid deficiency may reverse this impairment in the utilization of vitamin

A at its site of action. Thyroid hormone is needed to produce transthyretin, which is required for the formation of retinol-binding protein. Retinol-binding protein stores about 99 percent of vitamin A in the blood until it is needed somewhere in the body.

Autopsy studies reveal significant reductions in noradrenaline, serotonin and choline acetyl transferase in the brains of Down-syndrome patients. These autopsy results indicate profound neurotransmitter deficits and neuropathological abnormalities in adult patients with Down syndrome that closely resemble those of Alzheimer's disease.

One study suggested that phosphatidylcholine therapy may be useful for improving neuro-physiological and intellectual functioning of some Down-syndrome children. A definitive increase in speech and language skills, as well as general motor-skills improvement, were seen in response to phosphatidylcholine supplementation.

Desperate parents have been using high-potency vitamin supplements and piracetam to treat Down syndrome with astonishing results. News reports have documented the before-and-after effects when Down syndrome children followed this protocol.

The Life Extension Foundation suggests that children with Down syndrome be given Life Extension Mix powder in doses slightly below the adult dose. We suggest that a teaspoon of choline bitartrate powder be added to the Life Extension Mix powder to potentiate the neuro-logic-enhancing effect of this vitamin formula.

Adding 50 mg a day of 5-hydroxytryptophan and 250 mg of tyrosine to this daily powder regimen could boost serotonin and noradrenaline levels in the brain.

Piracetam should be administered in doses beginning at 800 mg a day, and then working up to as high as 4,800 mg a day for short periods of time. Small children should be given lower doses of all the above. Daily compliance is the most difficult aspect of the protocol, because children often do not like the taste of vitamins. Life Extension Mix powder, choline bitartrate powder, and crushed piracetam and phosphatidylcholine caplets all can be administered together in juice to help improve the palatability of the mixture.

If a thyroid deficiency is present, then the vitamin A and beta-carotene in Life Extension Mix could become toxic, because there would be a lack of retinol-binding protein to store serum vitamin A. Contact the Life Extension Foundation at 1-800-841-5433 to enquire about the availability of a multi-nutrient powder without vitamin A or beta-carotene.

Product availability: Life Extension Mix powder and choline are available by phoning 1-800-544-4440. When calling the Foundation, ask for a listing of offshore suppliers of piracetam.

Emphysema and Chronic Obstructive Pulmonary Disease

Emphysema is a pulmonary deficiency usually caused by years of free radical damage that results in degenerative changes in the air sacs of the lung. Emphysema patients suffer shortness of breath, congestive heart failure, cough and increasingly troubled breathing. Pulmonary emphysema results in the destruction of the lung's gas-exchange structures, called alveoli.

Chronic obstructive pulmonary disease (COPD) is a disease of the bronchi in the lungs, characterized by the production of large amounts of thick mucus that cause difficulties in breathing.

A potential therapy for emphysema involves the FDA-approved drug all-trans-retinoic acid. Previous studies showed that treatment of normal rats with all-trans-retinoic acid increases the number of alveoli. Further animal studies showed that treatment with all-trans-retinoic acid reversed changes associated with emphysema, thus providing nonsurgical remediation of emphysema, and suggesting the possibility of a similar effect in humans. All-trans-retinoic acid also was shown to improve lung elasticity recoil and to enhance alveolar surface area.

All-trans-retinoic acid is a drug that should be prescribed by your doctor. If the high cost of this drug makes it cost-prohibitive, consider taking four drops of emulsified liquid vitamin A (100,000 IU) a day. Refer to the Vitamin A Precautions in Appendix A.

Free radicals and changes of antioxidant enzymes are thought to play a role in chronic obstructive pulmonary disease. Pulmonary oxygen radical injury, and the protective role of antioxidant enzymes in COPD, were measured in one study. The results suggest that the increased free-radical toxicity and decreased glutathione peroxidase and catalase activities in red blood cells are involved in chronic obstructive pulmonary disease.

An imbalance between oxidants and antioxidants in smokers and in patients with airway diseases such as asthma has been proposed as a factor here. Antioxidants were measured in a group of chronic obstructive pulmonary disease patients. The results showed that smoking, acute COPD attacks and asthma are associated with a marked oxidant/antioxidant imbalance in the blood, associated with evidence of increased oxidative stress.

The suggested daily dose of high-potency vitamins for patients with these lung diseases is three tablets three times a day of Life Extension Mix and one capsule a day of Life Extension Booster. In order to help break up the thick mucus, 600 mg of N-acetylcysteine should be taken three times a day, along with two grams of vitamin C.

If the combination of these nutrients does not sufficiently break up the mucus, Pulmozyme, a drug used to treat cystic fibrosis, can be prescribed by your doctor. Pulmozyme is the most effective mucous-eradicating drug available. However, it is approved only for cystic fibrosis and, as a result, physicians often fail to prescribe it for acute mucus problems. To restore energy production to damaged cells in the lungs, the following nutrients are suggested:

1. Coenzyme Q10 — 100 mg three times a day
2. Forskolin — 10 to 60 mg a day
3. Acetyl-L-carnitine — 1,000 mg twice a day
4. NADH — 5 mg twice a day
5. Taurine — 1,000 mg twice a day
6. Magnesium — 500 mg of elemental magnesium once a day
7. Potassium — if needed

CAUTION: Do not use forskolin if you have prostate cancer. Forskolin may lower blood pressure.

Carmen Fusco reports that, in her practice she gives all patients with breathing problems DMG, and increases their consumption of fatty fish for the omega-3 fatty acids.

Product availability: Life Extension Mix, Life Extension Booster, N-acetylcysteine, vitamin C, coenzyme Q10, forskolin, acetyl-L-carnitine, NADH, taurine, magnesium and potassium can be obtained by phoning 1-800-544-4440.

Esophageal Reflux (Heartburn)

About 40 percent of Americans suffer from heartburn to one degree or another. Heartburn is caused by an incomplete closure of the sphincter muscle at the end of the esophagus, causing stomach acids to wash up against the relatively delicate esophageal lining, resulting in the pain and discomfort of heartburn. This is technically known as esophageal reflux.

Conventional management of symptoms in patients with mild to moderate esophageal reflux without erosive esophagitis requires a systematic approach beginning with lifestyle modification, plus over-the-counter H2 antagonists (Tagamet, Pepcid, Zantac, Axid) and/or antacids (Tums, Maalox, etc). If these measures do not suppress heartburn, then prescription pharmacologic management with H2 antagonists may be attempted.

Some lifestyle changes involve sleeping with two pillows to keep stomach acid out of the esophagus at night, taking antacids after each meal, avoiding certain foods, and not eating before bedtime.

Proton pump-inhibiting drugs such as Prevacid and Prilosec completely suppress hydrochloric acid production, and normally provide relief after one week. The benefits, safety and costs of the available therapeutic alternatives must be considered in choosing acute and long-term therapy. Appropriate use of endoscopy and other diagnostic tests is important in ruling out erosive esophagitis, Barrett's syndrome, esophageal cancer, stomach ulcers or stomach cancer.

Gastroesophageal reflux disease requires long-term therapy in most patients. The appropriate medical therapy should be individualized according to the severity of symptoms, the degree of esophagitis, and the presence of other acid-reflux complications. In most patients, maintenance therapy is vital.

The constant irritation of stomach acids on the lining of the esophagus can result in an increased risk of esophageal cancer and esophagitis. Antioxidant nutrients can protect against esophageal inflammation and, according to published studies, they may lower the risk of esophageal cancer. If you suffer from heartburn, you should consider taking three tablets of Life Extension Mix with each meal to help reduce your risk of esophageal cancer and esophagitis.

It is important to remind the patient to limit or avoid orange and tomato juice, mint and peppermint, chocolate and excess caffeine and alcohol. The best time for taking an antacid is 40 minutes to 1 hour after eating when HCL is no longer needed for the digestion of food in the stomach. Decaffeinated green tea is protective against esophageal cancer.

Product availability: Life Extension Mix can be ordered by phoning 1-800-544-4440. Zantac, Tagamet, Pepcid and Axid are now sold over-the-counter.

Estrogen Replacement Therapy

Few gynecologists are using estrogen replacement therapy safely to help prevent osteoporosis, heart disease and premature aging. A recent study in *The New England Journal of Medicine* showed that women taking estrogen and a synthetic progestin had a 32- to 46-percent increase in their risk of breast cancer.

The most popular estrogen drug in the United States is Premarin, which contains estrogens derived from the urine of pregnant mares. Provera is the name of a popular synthetic progestin that, when taken with Premarin, helps to prevent estrogen-induced uterine cancer, but does not prevent estrogen-induced breast or ovarian cancer.

The mechanisms by which estrogen causes cancer are well-documented in the scientific literature, and new studies continue to show that conventional estrogen-replacement therapy significantly increases the risk of breast cancer.

Although estrogen increases the risk of some types of cancer, it also has critical anti-aging benefits, including the prevention of osteoporosis and heart disease, and the reversal of some aspects of neurologic decline. Many doctors don't believe that estrogen causes cancer at all, while others believe that combining estrogen with a synthetic progestin neutralizes the cancer-causing potential of estrogen. The scientific facts are obscured by studies that appear to contradict each other about estrogen's carcinogenic potential. Some studies show that estrogen may not cause cancer in the short term. However, in women taking estrogen and/or a synthetic progestin for more than 10 years, there appears to be a significantly elevated risk of breast, ovarian and uterine cancer.

The Life Extension Foundation bases its warning about the carcinogenic risk of estrogen-progestin replacement therapy on these longer term studies. *The New England Journal of*

Medicine's report, showing an increased risk of breast cancer, was based upon data from the famous Nurses' Health Study conducted at Harvard Medical School. The nurses participating in this study represented 725,550 person-years of followup. Because of the sheer size of this study, its findings are persuasive. They showed that women who took estrogen plus a synthetic progestin actually had a higher rate of breast cancer than women who took estrogen alone.

The authors of the study concluded, "The addition of progestins to estrogen therapy does not reduce the risk of breast cancer among post-menopausal women. The substantial increase in the risk of breast cancer among older women who take hormones suggests that the trade-offs between risks and benefits should be carefully assessed."

Another report in the *American Journal of Epidemiology* showed that long-term estrogen-replacement therapy increased the risk of fatal ovarian cancer. This seven-year study included 240,073 pre- and post-menopausal women. After adjusting for other risk factors, women who used estrogen for six to eight years had a 40 percent higher risk of fatal ovarian cancer, and women who used estrogen for 11 or more years had a shocking 70 percent higher risk of fatal ovarian cancer!

The increased ovarian cancer risk from estrogen is a serious concern. Cancers of the breast, uterus and ovary account for 41 percent of cancer incidence among women in the U.S. Breast cancer is running at epidemic levels, striking one in eight women, up from one in 30 women in 1960 (coinciding with the use since that time of conventional hormone replacement therapy and oral contraceptives). Clearly, an alternative is needed to provide the anti-aging benefits of these youth hormones, while protecting against their potential cancer-causing effects.

In addition to increased cancer risks, some of the risks of estrogen/progestin therapy include:

- ✔ weight gain
- ✔ abnormal blood clot formation
- ✔ increased risk of gallstones, fibroid tumors, headaches
- ✔ premenstrual-type symptoms , such as irritability and fluid retention

Some of these side effects may be attributable to the synthetic progestins prescribed with estrogen, and not necessarily to estrogen itself.

It is important to note that dangerous forms of estrogen can be produced naturally within the body, so avoiding FDA-approved drugs like Premarin does not always protect against estrogen-induced cancer. As noted, while estrogen may increase the risk of cancer, it is an important anti-aging hormone that provides us with many health benefits. This creates a dilemma that conventional medicine admits it has yet to resolve.

Estrogens are steroid hormones that promote youthful cell division in target organs of the body. The benefits of maintaining this youthful cellular division with the proper estrogen replacement therapy include:

- enhanced skin smoothness, firmness, and elasticity
- enhanced moistness of skin and mucus membranes
- enhanced muscle tone
- reduced genital atrophy and enhanced sex drive in women
- reduced menopausal miseries
- reduced risk of heart disease and osteoporosis
- reduced risk of colon cancer
- improved memory and overall neurologic function
- protection against Alzheimer's disease
- enhanced immune function
- a greater feeling of well-being

Given all this, it is no wonder that Premarin is the number-one prescription drug in the United States.

Despite conventional medicine's enthusiastic endorsement, Premarin is not for everyone. According to a 1987 survey, more than 50 percent of women quit estrogen therapy after a year because they didn't feel right, or were concerned about the long-term cancer risks. On the other hand, many women feel wonderful on estrogen-replacement therapy and plan to take it for the rest of their lives.

The Life Extension Foundation has suggested alternative approaches for women who are afraid of the cancer risks or side effects of long-term therapy with FDA-approved estrogen drugs such as Premarin.

The primary forms of estrogen are estrone, estradiol and estriol. Estrone sulphate is the form of estrogen found in Premarin, and estradiol-17B is the form found in Estrace and Estraderm. Estrone is the oxidized form of estradiol. Estrone and estradiol are the estrogens that significantly increase the risk of breast and ovarian cancer when taken for more than 10 years. According to the Merck Manual, conjugated estrogens (Premarin) are substances that "have been listed as known carcinogens."

Estriol, on the other hand, is a weak estrogen that provides the anti-aging benefits of estro-gen-replacement therapy without the apparent increased risk of cancer. During pregnancy, huge amounts of estriol are secreted by the placenta to protect the fetus. Urinary assay of estriol is used to assess the viability of the fetus. Estriol is used extensively in Europe for estro-gen-replacement therapy in menopausal and post-menopausal women, but is rarely used for that purpose in the United States.

Since estriol is a weak estrogen, larger amounts must be used for estrogen replacement therapy. Estriol is used in doses of 2 to 8 mg per day. A dose of 2 to 4 mg of estriol is equiv-alent to, and as effective as, 0.6 to 1.25 mg of conjugated estrogens (Premarin).

One of the most common side effects of standard estrogen therapy such as Premarin when used without a progestin is endometrial hyperplasia, or hyper-proliferation of the cells of the uterine lining, a condition that often turns into uterine cancer. Most investigators have found that estriol therapy, even at the high dose of 8 mg per day, does not cause endometrial hyperplasia.

In one study by scientists at the Medical College of Georgia, in Augusta, 52 women with severe menopausal symptoms were given estriol succinate continuously for six months in doses of 2 to 8 mg a day. Significant improvements in symptoms were noted within one month of the start of the study, and they persisted as long as estriol therapy was continued. The degree of symptom improvement was directly related to the dose. Symptom relief was moderate at 2 mg a day, but marked at 8 mg a day.

Estriol therapy also reversed vaginal atrophy and improved the quality of cervical mucus. No breakthrough bleeding occurred in any of the subjects and endometrial biopsies failed to show endometrial hyperplasia in any case, regardless of the dose of estriol used.

The scientists concluded, "Estriol therapy may be employed in dosages up to 8 mg/day continuously, especially in those patients in whom other estrogens induce undesired side effects such as nausea, breakthrough bleeding or endometrial hyperplasia, and the recurrence of hot flushes during cyclic therapy of more potent estrogens. Because of these features, estriol deserves a place in our therapeutic resources. Being a weak estrogen, it does not induce endometrial proliferation or breakthrough bleeding of any consequence, while modifying menopausal symptoms."

A longer-term and larger prospective study of estriol therapy for the symptoms of menopause was conducted by C. Lauritzen at the University of Ulm in Germany, who concluded, "Estriol therapy was successful in 92 percent of all cases. In 71 percent, hot flushes and sweating were completely eliminated, in 21 percent they were ameliorated, becoming weaker and occurring more seldom. Depressive moods were abolished in 24 percent of the cases and in 33 percent they were ameliorated, so that an overall improvement occurred in 57 percent.

"Also," Lauritzen continued, "forgetfulness, loss of concentration, irritability and heart palpitations were remarkably improved towards normal. The number of patients suffering from migraine headaches decreased from 33 to 12. Atrophic changes of the vulva were completely eliminated in 44 of 61 cases and improved in 12 cases. . . . Remarkably the quality of the skin improved according to the subjective impression of patients and physicians in a high percentage of cases. In no case did a deterioration of symptoms occur."

One of the major benefits of estrogen therapy is prevention of the bone loss associated with osteoporosis. Postmenopausal women taking estrogen experience 50-percent fewer bone fractures than women of comparable age who have not taken estrogen. Although no studies have yet been conducted in the U.S. to determine if estriol therapy can prevent osteoporosis, a prospective, double-blind study was conducted in 136 postmenopausal women at the Chinese Great Wall Hospital in Beijing, using nylestriol (CEE), a long-acting estriol derivative. The doctors found significantly greater loss of bone mass and higher low-density lipoprotein levels in the placebo group, compared with the estriol-derivative group.

The researchers concluded, "CEE is an effective estrogen for preventing bone loss and lipid disorders in post-menopausal women just as the most popular conjugated estrogen (Premarin), but is more convenient. Long-term CEE medication, its effects on endometrium and the regimen of progestin combination await further study."

There also is direct evidence from animal studies and indirect evidence from human studies that estriol can prevent breast cancer. Much of this work has been done by Dr. H.M. Lemon and associates of the department of internal medicine at the University of Nebraska Medical Center, in Omaha. In one study, the researchers induced mammary tumors by whole-body gamma radiation in female Sprague-Dawley rats. Subcutaneous treatment with estriol for 331 to 449 days reduced the incidence of mammary tumors, from the high of 75 percent in controls down to 48 percent in the animals receiving the estriol.

In another study by Lemon and his colleagues, estriol was shown to have "the most significant anti-mammary carcinogenic activity of 22 tested compounds (because) . . . estriol is less likely to induce proliferative changes in the target organs of cancer-prone women than estrone or estradiol."

Because of these anti-cancer effects of estriol in animals, Lemon looked at the question of whether estriol is related in any way to breast cancer in humans. He found that women with breast cancer have low levels of estriol relative to other forms of estrogen.

Doctors have found that many women can benefit by using estriol alone or in combination with low doses of more potent estrogens (estradiol and estrone). For women who do not benefit from 8 mg a day of estriol, the ideal therapy may be a combination of 80 percent estriol, 10 percent estrone and 10 percent estradiol. The name of this triple estrogen product is TriEst.

Another reason for taking TriEst is that its 10 percent of estradiol is the form of estrogen involved in improving learning, memory and other mental functions that decline with advancing age.

Estriol or TriEst can be obtained in capsule form from European companies. You should pursue estrogen replacement therapy only under the care of a physician, preferably a gynecologist.

As far as estriol alone is concerned, each capsule normally contains 2 mg. Dosage ranges are from 2 mg to 8 mg a day. Do not take more than 8 mg a day of estriol since nausea can occur. If estriol alone does not sufficiently alleviate menopausal symptoms, then the combination preparation TriEst normally does.

To treat mild-to-moderate hot flashes, 1.25 mg of TriEst should be taken twice a day. For moderate to severe estrogen deficiency symptoms, 2.5 mg of TriEst capsules should be taken twice a day. Some women may need 5 mg a day of TriEst.

Blood tests can measure the relative levels of the different forms of estrogen within your body. Each woman is different, which means that for some women Premarin may produce high levels of safe estriol, while other women may find that Premarin elevates their estradiol and estrone levels. The same may be true for DHEA-replacement therapy. In some women, DHEA may cascade down to safe estriol, or it could convert into the more potent estradiol and estrone.

DHEA replacement therapy may be a more natural way than FDA-approved estrogen drugs of replacing estrogen levels diminished by the aging process. Most women take 15 mg of DHEA three times a day. DHEA is naturally converted to estrogen compounds within the body. Refer to DHEA-Pregnenolone Precautions for proper DHEA dosing and safety precautions.

It is important for women taking DHEA also to take melatonin and high potency soy extracts to reduce breast cancer risk associated with any therapy that could boost estrogen levels.

Eating soy products such as miso is another natural way of boosting estrogen levels. There are soy extracts available in tablet and powder form that contain standardized phytoestrogens. Phytoestrogens are weak estrogens that protect against cancer and provide some anti-aging benefits of estrogen replacement.

Oriental women who consume high soy diets appear to gain the same protection against post-menopausal diseases. Also, Oriental women taking high levels of phytoestrogens from soy have very low levels of breast cancer and vascular disease. The companies that extract phytoestrogens from soy are well aware of the huge market potential, and are constantly increasing the amounts of phytoestrogens they are extracting from soy. There is a new phytoestrogen soy extract that may safely provide the estrogen replacement therapy that menopausal and post-menopausal women need.

Based upon records of dietary soy consumption in Japan, where breast and prostate cancer rates are very low, the typical daily isoflavone intake has been estimated at 50 mg per person. By contrast, the typical Western diet has been estimated to provide only two to three mg a day of genistein.

Two capsules of a new supplement called Mega Soy Extract provide 110 mg of soy phytoestrogens, more than twice the amount in the typical Japanese diet. Since the phytoestrogen genistein is water-soluble, it is suggested that one capsule of Mega Soy Extract be taken in the morning and one in the evening. Some women seeking to use Mega Soy Extract as an estrogen-replacement therapy may take two to three capsules twice a day.

Not only are certain cancer levels lower in those who consume soy, but menopausal symptoms and the incidence of osteoporosis also are reduced. One study shows that soy isoflavones promote an anabolic effect on bone density in post-menopausal women by binding to an estrogen receptor in bone.

Cruciferous vegetables protect against estrogen-induced cancers. Many women take a tablespoon of Phyto-Food powder every day to obtain the vegetable concentrates of broccoli and cabbage that naturally contain breast cancer-preventing phytochemicals. Flax seed and fish oils may lower production of toxic estrogens and may block some of their tumor-initiating effects.

Vitamin E supplementation may boost estriol levels in the body, while the B-complex vitamins may protect against some of the toxic effects of estrogen. Estrogen may produce some of its toxicity by binding to vitamin B6 in the body, thus causing a vitami n B6 deficiency.

If pregnenolone, DHEA and/or soy extracts fail to provide you with enough estrogen, estriol should be considered as the ideal form of estrogen for supplementation. While it may not be available at your corner drug store, doctors are free to prescribe it, and there are European pharmacies that sell it.

Blood tests may not accurately reflect a women's individual need for hormone replacement. Some clinicians believe that hot flashes, dry skin and vaginal dryness during and after menopause may be better indicators of the need for estrogen replacement therapy than blood tests. However, blood tests can be important indicators for dosage determination.

Other symptoms, these for progesterone deficiency, may manifest themselves as depression, irritability, mood swings and insomnia.

Women using estriol therapy should do so in conjunction with the regular application of topical natural progesterone cream (not Provera) and the nightly intake of 1 to 10 mg of melatonin.

One protocol to treat vaginal dryness is to use 1 gram of low potency estriol cream for seven continuous days, and then drop back to two to three applications a week. If low-potency estriol cream does not work, then order a more potent concentration. The objective is to provide the minimum estrogen replacement therapy your body needs for optimal, overall anti-aging benefits.

Calcium and vitamin D augment estrogen's ability to prevent osteoporosis. The suggested daily doses are 1,500 to 2,000 mg of calcium and 400 IU of vitamin D, along with high doses of soy protein extract and a progesterone cream.

To reiterate, the objective is to use the *minimum* amount of estrogen replacement to achieve anti-aging benefits, without increasing the risk of cancer. That is why it is imperative that women using any form of estrogen-replacement therapy use a topical natural progesterone cream and take melatonin to protect against the side effects of estrogen.

Women should try soy-derived phytoestrogens first to see if these safe forms of natural estrogen will provide the desired anti-aging benefits of estrogen.

A complete blood hormone profile that includes estrogen, progesterone, testosterone and DHEA should be considered.

Members of the Life Extension Foundation can have total estrogen, progesterone, testosterone and DHEA-S tests performed by mail. To enquire about these tests, call the Foundation at 1-800-544-4440.

Product availability: Soy extracts, pregnenolone, DHEA, vitamin E, melatonin, Phyto-Food and progesterone cream are available by calling 1-800-544-4440. When calling the Foundation, ask for a listing of offshore companies that sell estriol and TriEst.

Fibrinogen and Cardiovascular Disease

Blood clots that form inside arteries are the leading cause of death in the Western world. Most heart attacks and strokes are caused by a blood clot that obstructs the flow of blood to a portion of the heart or the brain. No blood flow, and thus no oxygen, means no life to the heart or brain cells. Blood clots kill more than 600,000 Americans every year, yet conventional medicine has largely ignored well-documented methods of reducing abnormal blood-clot formation.

Low-dose aspirin and certain nutrients provide partial protection against abnormal blood clots, but a newly identified clotting factor—fibrinogen—mandates that additional measures be taken to prevent heart attack and stoke. High levels of fibrinogen predispose a person to coronary and cerebral artery disease, even when other known risk factors such as cholesterol are low.

Fibrinogen elevation in cigarette smokers, for example, has been identified as a primary mechanism causing heart disease and stroke. Cigarette smoking increases cardiovascular disease risk, and it also raises fibrinogen levels in the blood. Published studies documenting the dangers of cigarette smoking show that cigarette smokers who suffer from cardiovascular disease also have high fibrinogen levels. In fact, *high fibrinogen levels may be a more powerful predictor of cardiovascular mortality than cigarette smoking itself.*

The role of fibrinogen in the development of cardiovascular disease has been fully confirmed by the results of all relevant studies conducted during the past 10 years. High fibrinogen levels have at least as great a predictive value as any other known risk factor, such as elevated LDL cholesterol, elevated triglycerides, obesity and diabetes.

In persons with a family history of heart disease, fibrinogen levels are high. Fibrinogen levels are primarily genetically inherited, meaning that fibrinogen may be the genetic factor causing familial premature heart disease. Also, exposure to cold increases fibrinogen levels by 23 percent, and mortality from heart attack and stroke are higher in winter than in summer.

Fibrinogen hinders blood flow and oxygen delivery by deforming red blood cells, causing red-cell aggregation and a thickening of the blood, all of which lead to diminished circulation. Fibrinogen binds blood platelets together, thus initiating abnormal arterial blood clots. Fibrinogen is then converted to fibrin, which is the final step in the blood-clotting cascade.

Fibrinogen contributes to the development of atherosclerosis by incorporating itself into the arterial plaque. Further, fibrinogen and LDL cholesterol work together to generate atherosclerotic plaques. Fibrinogen initiates the atherosclerotic plaque, then converts to fibrin and serves as a scaffold for LDL cholesterol in the atherosclerotic plaque that slowly occludes an artery.

Fibrinogen and its derivatives trigger a variety of other mechanisms thought to be involved in the atherosclerotic process. Fibrinogen and LDL cholesterol have a synergistic effect in promoting atherosclerosis, though fibrinogen may play a more important role in the development of atherosclerotic lesions.

Most heart attacks occur because a blood clot forms inside a coronary artery and chokes off the blood supply to the heart. Most strokes, on the other hand, occur because a blood clot forms inside a cerebral artery and blocks the blood supply to the brain. In either case, it is crucial to take steps to reduce the risk of fibrinogen causing an abnormal arterial clot.

Platelet-aggregation inhibitors reduce the risk that fibrinogen will cause an abnormal blood clot. Platelet-aggregation inhibitors include aspirin, green tea, ginkgo biloba and vitamin E. For optimal protection against the formation of arterial blood clots, it makes sense to utilize therapies that lower elevated fibrinogen levels.

High vitamin A and beta-carotene serum levels have been associated with reduced fibrinogen levels in humans. For example, animals fed a vitamin A-deficient diet have an impaired ability to break down fibrinogen, but when they are injected with vitamin A, they produce tissue plasminogen activator that breaks down fibrinogen. In addition, both fish and olive oil have been shown to lower fibrinogen in women with elevated fibrinogen levels. The daily amount of fish oil required to produce a fibrinogen-lowering effect is 6 grams, which equals about five capsules of Mega EPA fish oil concentrate capsules.

Elevated homocysteine levels have been shown to block the natural breakdown of fibrinogen by inhibiting the production of tissue plasminogen activator. Folic acid and vitamin B6 help to reduce elevated homocysteine levels.

One of the more interesting studies involved the use of vitamin C to break down excess fibrinogen. The FDA has stated that Americans need only 60 to 100 mg of vitamin C a day, while a government report published in early 1996 says that Americans need only 200 mg of vitamin C a day. This report received widespread media support. The media used this government report to ridicule the use of vitamin C supplements in excess of 200 mg.

However, in an earlier report published in the journal *Atherosclerosis*, heart-disease patients were given either 1,000 or 2,000 mg a day of vitamin C to assess its effect on the breakdown of fibrinogen. At 1,000 mg a day, there was no detectable change in fibrinolytic activity (fibrinogen breakdown) or cholesterol. At 2,000 mg a day of vitamin C, however, there was a 27-percent decrease in the platelet-aggregation index, a 12-percent reduction in total cholesterol, and a 45-percent increase in fibrinolytic activity.

Even in the face of this and other studies, the U.S. government and the medical establishment have tried to convince Americans they do not need vitamin supplements. Those Americans who believe the government are dying of artery disease.

For maximum fibrinogen-lowering effect, the proteolytic enzyme bromelain may be the most effective nutrient supplement. For those seeking to lower elevated fibrinogen levels, two to six capsules a day of Herbal Cardiovascular Formula containing a standardized bromelain concentrate should be considered.

Some non-pharmacologic ways of lowering fibrinogen include stopping smoking, avoiding obesity, lowering LDL cholesterol and avoiding exposure to cold.

Don't depend on FDA-approved drugs to lower fibrinogen levels. The popular cholesterol lowering drug Lopid (gemfibrozil) *increases* fibrinogen levels by 9 to 21 percent. Other FDA-approved heart medications have shown little effect on fibrinogen levels.

However, a European drug called Bezafibrate has been shown to lower fibrinogen levels by 25 percent in patients with fibrinogen levels between 300 and 415 mg/dL. In patients whose fibrinogen levels were over 600, Bezafibrate lowered fibrinogen levels by 45 percent. Bezafibrate has been used extensively in Europe since 1978 to lower LDL cholesterol by 20 to 30 percent, and increase beneficial HDL cholesterol. It has more than 9 million patient-years of safety documentation. The fact that Bezafibrate still is not approved by the FDA reflects a serious lack of care by our government about the health care of its citizens.

For those with vascular disease, please refer to the Atherosclerosis protocol for additional suggestions.

Nutritionist Carmen Fusco suggests the use of niacin as well as red grape juice when there is elevated fibrinogen levels.

Product availability: Healthprin (aspirin), green tea, ginkgo biloba, vitamin E, Mega EPA, folic acid, vitamin C, vitamin B6 and Herbal Cardiovascular Formula can be ordered by phoning 1-800-544-4440. Call for a list of offshore pharmacies if you are interested in obtaining the drug Bezafibrate.

Fibromyalgia

Fibromyalgia represents one of the most frequent musculoskeletal problems. This condition, associated with widespread pain, is characterized by a number of specific tender points, as well as such symptoms as tiredness, limb stiffness, depression and a lack of refreshing sleep. Patients suffering from fibromyalgia also can demonstrate temporo-mandibular disorders or muscular-fascial pain.

Sleep disturbances are more common in fibromyalgia patients. One study found that 55 percent of fibromyalgia patients suffered from sleep disturbances, and that these sleep disturbances were not caused by pain. Alleviating insomnia with anti-depressant medication, melatonin and/or prescription sleep-inducing drugs could alleviate pain.

Anti-depressant drugs have been used with varying degrees of success in treating fibromyalgia. One European study showed that the combination of monoamine oxidase (MAO)-inhibiting drugs, along with 5-hydroxytryptophan, significantly improved fibromyalgia syndrome, whereas other anti-depressant treatments yielded poorer benefits. The doctors who conducted this study stated that a natural analgesic effect occurred when serotonin levels and norepinephrine receptors were enhanced in the brain. The monoamine oxidase-inhibiting drugs did produce some side effects.

European doctors combine 5-hydroxytryptophan with a decarboxylase inhibitor in order to make it available to produce serotonin in the brain. It is difficult for Americans to get 5-hydroxytryptophan with a pharmaceutical decarboxylase inhibitor. The vitamin B6 Americans use also inhibits the ability of 5-hydroxytryptophan to enhance brain levels of serotonin.

A therapy for Americans to consider would be 3,000 mg a day of the amino acid l-tryptophan, which does not require a decarboxylase inhibitor to elevate serotonin in the brain. Since the FDA banned the sale of tryptophan in 1989, the drug Prozac may be an effective substitute. Some doctors suggest the use of Prozac specifically as a fibromyalgia therapy. Such nutrients as phenylalanine or tyrosine in doses of 1,500 mg a day could boost norepinephrine levels. Refer to the Phenylalanine And Tyrosine Precautions, in this book, before using this amino acid supplement.

The European anti-depressant drug S-adenosylmethionine (SAMe) has been shown in several published studies to be specifically effective as a therapy to reduce the chronic pain and depression associated with fibromyalgia. The suggested dose is 400 mg to 800 mg twice a day.

Epidemiological studies have shown that the tendency toward depression in patients with fibromyalgia may be a manifestation of a familial depressive spectrum disorder (alcoholism and/or depression in the family members), not simply a "reactive" depression secondary to pain and other symptoms.

Substantial overlap between chemical sensitivity, fibromyalgia and chronic fatigue syndrome exists. The latter two conditions often involve chemical sensitivity and may even be the same disorder. Those agents associated with symptoms and suspected of causing onset of chemical sensitivity with chronic illness include gasoline, kerosene, natural gas, pesticides (especially chlordane and chlorpyrifos), solvents, new carpet and other renovation materials, adhesives/glues, fiberglass, carbonless copy paper, fabric softener, formaldehyde and glutaraldehyde, carpet shampoos and other cleaning agents, isocyanates, combustion products (poorly vented gas heaters, overheated batteries, etc.), and medications (dinitrochlorobenzene for warts, intranasally packed neosynephrine, prolonged antibiotics and general anesthesia with petrochemicals, for example).

Multiple mechanisms of chemical injury that magnify response to exposures in chemically sensitive patients can include neurogenic inflammation, kindling and time-dependent neurologic sensitization and auto-immune activation.

A study of thyroid function showed that 63 percent of a group of fibromyalgia patients suffered from some degree of hypothyroidism. This percentage is much higher than for the general population. Fibromyalgia patients were shown either to suffer from a thyroid hormone deficiency or from cellular resistance to thyroid hormone. Refer to the Thyroid Deficiency protocol for suggestions that could correct a thyroid hormone defect as a possible underlying cause of fibromyalgia.

A study to ascertain the long-term natural history of fibromyalgia syndrome was conducted on a group of patients seen in an academic rheumatology referral practice. These patients were originally surveyed soon after onset of symptoms, and were again interviewed 10 years later. Of the original 39 patients, there were four deaths, and of the remaining 35 patients, 29 (83 percent) were re-interviewed. Mean age at the followup interview was 55 years, and mean duration of symptoms was 15.8 years.

All patients had persistence of the same fibromyalgia symptoms, although almost half (48 percent) had not seen a doctor for them in the last year. Moderate to severe pain or stiffness was reported in 55 percent of patients; moderate to a great deal of sleep difficulty was noted in 48 percent; and moderate to extreme fatigue was noted in 59 percent. These symptoms showed little change from earlier surveys. In 79 percent of the patients, medications still were being taken to control symptoms. Despite continuing symptoms, 66 percent of patients reported that symptoms were a little or a lot better than when first diagnosed. Fifty-five percent of patients said they felt well or very well in terms of symptoms, and only 7 percent felt they were doing poorly.

With the exception of sleep trouble, which was persistent, baseline survey symptoms correlated poorly with symptoms at the 10-year followup. The conclusion was that fibromyalgia symptoms last, on average, at least 15 years after illness onset. However, most patients experience some improvement in symptoms after fibromyalgia onset.

Refer also to the Depression, Chronic Fatigue Syndrome and Insomnia protocols.

Product availability: S-adenosylmethionine (SAMe), phenylalanine and tyrosine supplements are available by calling 1-800-544-4440.

Flu-Influenza Virus

Flu viruses temporarily disable most Americans every year, and at least 60,000 elderly Americans can die in a year when there is a flu epidemic. If you have the flu, there are alternative therapies that can shorten the duration of your illness and, if you are elderly, possibly save your life.

Ribavirin is a broad-spectrum, anti-viral drug that is especially effective against influenza-like viruses. Ribavirin is approved in almost every country in the world. When you first develop the symptoms of the flu, take 200 mg of ribavirin every three to four hours. In many cases, this can prevent the full development of the flu because of ribavirin's ability to interfere with influenza virus replication.

There also are herbal extracts that have anti-viral effects. When flu symptoms occur, it is suggested that you take echinacea liquid herbal extract at a dose of six full droppers in a small amount of water, followed by two full droppers every two waking hours until the 2-ounce bottle is empty. You also may want to consider taking 300 mg of astragalus extract, as well as four capsules a day of Sports Ginseng, a standardized extract containing both Korean and Siberian ginseng.

A new extract from the elderberry called Sambucol has been shown to keep the influenza virus from entering the cells. Sambucol should be taken in doses of one tablespoon four times a day.

DHEA is an adrenal hormone that has shown anti-viral and immune-boosting benefits. When flu symptoms occur, 100 mg of DHEA should be taken three times a day until flu symptoms subside. Refer to DHEA-Pregnenolone Precautions before taking DHEA. Melatonin has immune-enhancing benefits and possible anti-viral effects, and helps you get the sleep you need to fight the flu virus. Melatonin should be taken in doses of 10 mg before going to sleep for the duration of the flu attack.

Influenza and other infectious diseases tend to be more severe in older patients. Despite immunization, elderly people often lack the immune capacity to generate an antibody response to prevent infection from the influenza virus. As many as 69,000 Americans have died from influenza in a bad epidemic year. Biostim is a French drug that has been shown to prevent infectious diseases in the elderly. Biostim is used in Europe to boost immune function and treat certain infectious diseases.

An examination of the published literature reveals that, if Biostim were available in the United States, thousands of American lives could be saved every year. These studies also indicate that Biostim would dramatically reduce the need for antibiotic therapy, thereby saving untold millions of dollars in prescription drug costs.

A double-blind trial was conducted to evaluate the capacity of Biostim to diminish the frequency of infectious episodes in chronic bronchitis. The study duration was nine months. Of the 73 subjects selected, 38 received Biostim and 35 a placebo. By the ninth month, the duration in days of infectious episodes was 60 percent lower in the Biostim group, compared with the placebo group. The use of antibiotic therapy was reduced by 81 percent in the Biostim group, compared with the placebo group. Pre-winter administration of Biostim to subjects significantly diminished the frequency of infectious episodes, and thus the consumption of antibiotics.

In another study, 314 elderly subjects admitted to hospitals were given either Biostim or a placebo. The subjects were regularly examined every three months for one year. The incidence of acute infectious episodes was evaluated in both groups. The number of subjects with infection in the group receiving the Biostim were significantly lower than in the placebo group, compared with. In the group receiving the Biostim, the number of infectious episodes was reduced throughout the 12 months of the trial. Finally, there was a significant decrease in the duration of antibiotic therapy. Biostim was well-tolerated. This study showed that Biostim is effective in protecting elderly, and therefore fragile, subjects against respiratory infections.

An evaluation of the safety of Biostim given with an antibiotic to treat acute infections was performed in three double-blind, placebo-controlled studies on fragile institutionalized or hospitalized patients. Two of the studies showed that, in acute respiratory infections, Biostim is well-tolerated and resulted in a more rapid improvement. The third study showed that Biostim produced a more rapid improvement in the most severely ill patients. It was concluded that Biostim can be initiated safely during acute episodes occurring in subjects with recurrent respiratory infections, and that it results in a faster improvement of clinical symptoms.

High potency vitamin formulas such as Life Extension Mix and other nutrients cited in the Immune Enhancement protocol should be considered. Also refer to the Common Cold protocol for additional suggestions.

Product availability: Ribavirin can be obtained in Mexico, or you can call 1-800-747-0149 for a list of offshore suppliers who will mail it to you. If you already have the flu, it will take too long to obtain ribavirin by mail to be of any help; echinacea liquid herbal extract, elderberry (Sambucol) astragalus extract, Sports Ginseng, DHEA, melatonin and Life Extension Mix can be ordered for overnight delivery by phoning 1-800-544-4440. For Biostim, ask for a list of offshore suppliers who will mail-order these products to Americans for personal use.

Gingivitis

Gingivitis is characterized by inflammation, swelling, irritation and redness of the gums. If left untreated, it will result in tooth loss. Gingivitis is the most common cause of tooth loss. Modern dentistry has succeeded in preventing most problems associated with chronic gingivitis by encouraging daily flossing, regular brushing and professional teeth-cleaning every three to six months.

However, gingivitis can be an underlying symptom of diabetes, leukemia or a vitamin deficiency. While proper dental hygiene is still required for optimal oral health, vitamin supplements, coenzyme Q10 and green tea can alleviate the symptoms of gingivitis.

The standard dose of Life Extension Mix (three tablets, three times a day) can improve the health of your gums. Life Extension Mix provides more than 2,500 mg of vitamin C. Also, coenzyme Q10 in oil-filled capsules should be taken in 100- to 200-mg daily doses. Green tea beverages provide direct bacteria-killing, plaque-inhibiting effects for the gums. Standardized green tea capsules providing 200 mg a day of polyphenols can be used to help deliver gingiva-protecting nutrients.

For people suffering from chronic gingivitis, the regular use of Life Extension Mouthwash provides every nutrient shown to be of benefit topically for the health of your gums. One study showed that zinc and folic acid can inhibit gingivitis, and Life Extension Mouthwash contains the identical amount of zinc and folic acid used in this study. Life Extension Mouthwash also contains a chlorophyll extract, sanguinaria extract, vitamin E, aloe vera and caprylic acid. All contribute to the health and healing of the gums via different mechanisms.

Product availability: Life Extension Mouthwash, coenzyme Q10, Life Extension Mix and green tea capsules can be ordered by calling 1-800-544-4440.

Glaucoma

Glaucoma is a condition in which the pressure within the eye becomes elevated. If not brought under control, glaucoma will cause visual defects leading to blindness. Glaucoma is caused by blockage of the normal flow of fluid between the cornea and lens of the eye. Conventional ophthalmologists will prescribe eye drops that usually are highly effective in controlling intraocular pressure.

If conventional anti-glaucoma eye drops are not successful, or if you wish to attempt to address the underlying cause of glaucoma, it is suggested that you try the herbal extract forskolin at a dose of 10 to 60 mg a day. Forskolin lowers intraocular pressure by enhancing the energy cycles that are necessary to move fluid into and out of the eye. Check your blood pressure to make sure that forskolin is not causing low blood pressure.

CAUTION: If you have prostate cancer, do not use forskolin.

Hydergine also improves energy factors via the same mechanism as forskolin. A dose of 5 to 20 mg a day of Hydergine could be effective in lowering intraocular pressure. It is mandatory that you have regular intraocular pressure tests administered by an ophthalmologist if you are trying to use forskolin or Hydergine as a treatment for glaucoma.

Product availability: You can order forskolin by calling 1-800-544-4440. Call for a list of off-shore suppliers who sell high-potency Hydergine tablets by mail order for personal use, or ask your physician to prescribe Hydergine for you.

Hair Loss

Refer to the protocol on Balding.

Hearing Loss

Aging produces a consistent reduction in the ability to hear sounds. Deafness is a common ailment associated with normal aging. The drug Hydergine may help restore hearing in some cases of deafness. While the FDA has approved doses of only 3 mg a day of Hydergine, doses of 12 to 20 mg a day may be required to help restore hearing.

The best form of Hydergine to take is enterically coated liquid capsules made by Sandoz. These are expensive because they come only in 1 mg strength. Many people choose to obtain low-cost 5 mg Hydergine from overseas pharmacies.

Ginkgo biloba has helped some people with the hearing disorder tinnitus. Ginkgo provides a wide range of health benefits, including improving neurological function. People with hearing loss should consider taking 120 mg a day of ginkgo extract.

Product availability: Hydergine is a prescription drug in the United States. For a list of suppliers that sell low-cost, high-potency Hydergine from offshore pharmacies, phone 1-800-544-4440. You also can order pharmaceutical ginkgo biloba extract at that number.

Hemochromatosis

A genetic defect can predispose some people to build-up toxic levels of iron in their bodies. Conventional medicine's solution to this problem is to have these people donate blood regularly to purge their bodies of excess blood. (An interesting anti-aging and immune-boosting therapy involves the administration of one's own youthful blood during a state of disease or severe aging. If affordable, the Life Extension Foundation recommends that hemochromatosis patients have their blood frozen for future use.)

Iron is a catalyst for many enzymatic reactions as well as for massive free radical damage to cells. The chronic high iron levels from which hemochromatosis patients suffer predisposes them to a host of free-radical-generated diseases, including cancer and heart disease. It is crucial to inhibit these free radicals by consuming large amounts of antioxidants on a regular basis.

One problem that hemochromatosis patients must face is that the potent antioxidant vitamin C, when taken in the presence of iron-containing foods, can dramatically increase the absorption of iron from the digestive tract into the bloodstream. Therefore, hemochromatosis patients should take one 500-mg *buffered* vitamin C capsule three times a day between meals. Published findings demonstrate that in iron-overloaded plasma, vitamin C acts as a potent antioxidant against lipid peroxidation. Some doctors, on the other hand, suggest that hemochromatosis patients should avoid vitamin C altogether.

Hemochromatosis patients are at severe risk for developing liver damage. It has been suggested that lipid peroxidation plays an important role in hepatic damage caused by chronic iron overload. Vitamin E is an important lipid-soluble antioxidant that has been shown to be decreased in patients with hereditary hemochromatosis and in experimental iron overload. Iron loading has been shown to significantly decrease hepatic and plasma vitamin E, which can be overcome by Vitamin E supplementation. Free radical index markers increase three- to fivefold in the iron-loaded livers, but supplementation with Vitamin E has been shown to reduce these levels of free radical activity by at least 50 percent.

There is growing evidence that normal or only mildly increased amounts of iron in the liver can be damaging, particularly when it is combined with such other hepatotoxic factors as alcohol, certain drugs or chronic viral hepatitis. Iron enhances the pathogenicity of microorganisms, adversely affects the function of macrophages and lymphocytes, and enhances fibrogenic pathways, all of which may increase liver injury. Iron also may be a co-carcinogen or promoter of hepatocellular carcinoma.

It should be noted that copper overload induces similar free radical-induced damage as does iron overload. Iron-overload disease causes severe depletion of liver glutathione. Glutathione is an important antioxidant, and its depletion in iron overload causes additional free radical damage.

Hemochromatosis patients should take, with meals, a total of 800 IU of vitamin E, 400 micrograms of selenium, the complete vitamin B-complex including at least 800 micrograms of folic acid, 60 mg of zinc, 100 mg of grape seed-skin extract, 120 mg of ginkgo extract, 800 to 1,000 mg of garlic, 1,200 mg of N-acetylcysteine, 500 mg of alpha-lipoic acid, 300 IU of gamma tocopherol, and 3 mg of melatonin. Melatonin should be taken at bedtime only. The other nutrients should be taken in two or three divided doses.

A potent iron-chelating agent is green tea extract. Green tea is a potent antioxidant and helps to remove excess iron from the liver. Hemochromatosis patients should take four to 10 green tea extract capsules that provide at least 200 mg of active polyphenols per capsule. Hemochromatosis patients also may consider intravenous chelation therapy administered by a knowledgeable physician.

The prescription drug deferoxamine has been shown to reverse both the biochemical indicators and the clinical manifestations of iron overload over a two-year time period.

Nutritionist Carmen Fusco has successfully helped patients with the most severe form of hemochromatosis. Her regimen includes tea with every meal for the tannins that bind iron, and providing extra calcium because calcium competes with iron and prevents some of its absorption.

If a glass of wine is desired once the liver improves, red wine with the tannins and chromium found in the grape skins is preferrable to white wine.

Product availability: vitamin C, vitamin E, selenium, folic acid, zinc, grape seed-skin extract, N-acetylcysteine, garlic, ginkgo biloba, alpha-lipoic acid, B-complex, green tea, gamma tocopherol and melatonin can be ordered by calling 1-800-544-4440. Call for a list of physicians in your area who are knowledgeable in the administration of chelation therapy.

Hepatitis B

Hepatitis B is a viral disease characterized by inflammatory necrosis of the liver. It is most often spread by contact with contaminated blood via the sharing of unsterilized needles or sexual contact.

The symptoms of hepatitis include anorexia, malaise, flu-like conditions, nausea, vomiting, fever, hives, joint pain, dark urine and a distaste for tobacco. Jaundice often appears if the disease is well advanced. Liver-function blood testing and a specific test can determine if hepatitis B is active and causing liver damage.

The blood tests that monitor viral hepatitis liver damage include AST (SGOT), ALT (SGPT), alkaline phosphatase, and GGTP. The hepatitis B antibody test, together with the hepatitis surface antigen (HBsAg) test, can provide a definitive diagnosis. The presence of HBsAg refers to the viral surface coat.

Treatment by an infectious-disease specialist is essential. One-third of all people infected by this virus can expect total remission after two to four months of treatment with alpha interferon. Of the remaining two-thirds, 10 to 15 percent will become lifelong carriers of the disease. It is this group that is at greatest risk of hepatocellular carcinoma. Cirrhosis also is a great risk, and many of these patients will find themselves future candidates for liver transplants.

Hepatitis viruses have been shown to induce liver inflammation, cirrhosis and primary liver cancer via free radical attacks on liver cells. Antioxidant supplements, in addition to anti-viral therapies, are used to protect against the lethal consequences of hepatitis B and C.

In areas of China with high rates of hepatitis B and primary liver cancer, epidemiological surveys demonstrated that high levels of dietary selenium reduce liver-cancer incidence and hepatitis B infection. Animals studies showed that selenium supplementation reduced hepatitis B infection by 77.2 percent and pre-cancerous liver lesions by 75.8 percent. In a four-year trial on 130,471 Chinese, those who were given a selenium-spiked table salt showed a 35.1-percent reduction in primary liver cancer, compared with the group given salt without selenium.

A clinical study of 226 hepatitis B-positive people showed that a 200-microgram tablet a day of selenium reduced primary liver cancer incidences down to zero. Upon cessation of selenium supplementation, primary liver cancer incidences began to rise, indicating that viral hepatitis patients should take selenium on a continuous basis.

In Europe, isoprinosine, a powerful immune-stimulating drug that is unapproved in the U.S., has been found to be effective in treating hepatitis B. Also in Europe, the herb silybum marianum (milk thistle) has been given German Commission E status as a supportive agent in the treatment of inflammatory liver diseases (hepatitis and cirrhosis). In Japan, glycyrrhiza glabra (licorice root) has found widespread use in the treatment of hepatitis B. This herb has the ability to decrease serum liver enzymes, aspartate aminotransferase (AST) and alanine aminotransferase (ALT).

The Life Extension Foundation's protocol for hepatitis B includes:

1. The standard dose of alpha interferon (3 million IU injected subcutaneously, three times a week) for four months, prescribed by your infectious-disease physician. (Interferon is an FDA-approved therapy to treat hepatitis B. It works only in one-third of patients.) The drug ribavirin in the dose of 1,000 mg a day may be tried in conjunction with interferon therapy, even though most studies show ribavirin being effective against hepatitis C.

2. Isoprinosine at a dose of 2,000 to 3,000 mg per day, for two months on and two months off (continue for two rounds).

3. Milk thistle extract, 150 mg three times per day; licorice root extract, 500 mg three times a day; selenium, 800 micrograms a day; green tea extract, 1,200 mg of polyphenols in three divided doses to reduce serum iron levels that may facilitate liver injury.

4. The standard doses of Life Extension Mix and Life Extension Herbal Mix to further reduce free radical damage, along with 2,000 mg per day of garlic and 5,000 to 20,000 mg of vitamin C. Please note that some hepatitis patients cannot tolerate beta-carotene. If liver enzyme levels increase in response to Life Extension Mix, discontinue it and take most of the nutrients separately, avoiding vitamin A, beta-carotene and niacin. Beta-carotene has potent immune-boosting properties that can be beneficial for hepatitis B patients, but it may not be tolerated by some people.

5. High doses of green tea, garlic, and chelation therapy to reduce serum and liver iron levels to a minimum. Iron promotes hepatitis virus-induced liver injury and precludes successful treatment with interferon. Verify that liver iron levels have been reduced before starting interferon therapy.

Please refer to the Hepatitis C protocol for additional suggestions. A strong immune system can keep the hepatitis virus in long-term remission. For additional suggestions, refer to the Immune Enhancement protocol.

Product availability: Milk thistle extract, green tea extract, Life Extension Mix, Life Extension Herbal Mix, Kyolic garlic, vitamin C, licorice, selenium, glutathione, etc. can be ordered by phoning 1-800-544-4440. Call for a list of offshore companies that sell isoprinosine or ribavirin to Americans by mail for personal use. Interferon is a drug that should be prescribed by a knowledgeable physician.

Hepatitis C

Infection with the hepatitis C virus occurs from blood transfusions, needle sharing, working in a medical environment and sexual contact. Often, the infected individual does not know how he or she acquired this potentially lethal virus that has a high affinity for liver cells.

Hepatitis C used to be called non-A/non-B hepatitis and was not considered a significant health risk. There is now more research being conducted on hepatitis C than on any other cause of liver disease. New data indicate that those infected with the hepatitis C virus are likely to develop hepatocellular carcinoma, a primary cancer of the liver with a very low cure rate. If the hepatitis C victim does not develop liver cancer, there still is a great risk that the patient will develop cirrhosis of the liver, which may require a transplant. There also are other non-liver diseases associated with hepatitis C viral infection.

The hepatitis C virus does most of its damage by latching onto molecules of iron, and then delivering massive free-radical damage to liver cells. These free radicals can mutate DNA to cause hepatocellular carcinoma, and can kill large numbers of liver cells. Liver dysfunction causes havoc throughout the body. Successful eradication of the hepatitis C virus from the body requires that iron levels in the liver and blood be at very low levels, and thus it can be said that high stores of iron in the liver preclude successful therapy against the hepatitis C virus.

The blood test that can identify the hepatitis C virus and measure overall viral load is the polymerase chain reaction test (PCR). Standard tests to measure hepatitis C activity include the liver function tests SGOT, SGPT, GGTP and alkaline phosphatase. Hepatitis C antibody tests can accurately diagnose hepatitis C infection, but are not always precise in evaluating the success of treatments.

Hepatitis viruses have been shown to induce liver inflammation, cirrhosis and primary liver cancer via free-radical attacks on liver cells. Antioxidant supplements, in addition to anti-viral therapies, are used by scientists to protect against the lethal consequences of both hepatitis B and C.

In areas of China with high rates of hepatitis B and primary liver cancer, epidemiological surveys demonstrated that high levels of dietary selenium reduce liver-cancer incidence and hepatitis B infection. Animal studies showed that selenium supplementation reduced hepatitis B infection by 77.2 percent and precancerous liver lesions by 75.8 percent. In a four-year trial on 130,471 Chinese, those who were given a selenium-spiked table salt showed a 35.1-percent reduction in primary liver cancer, compared with the group given salt without selenium added.

A clinical study of 226 hepatitis B-positive people showed that one 200-microgram tablet a day of selenium reduced primary liver-cancer incidences down to zero. Upon cessation of selenium supplementation, primary liver-cancer incidences began to rise, indicating that viral hepatitis patients should take selenium on a continuous basis. selenium also appears to be effective in suppressing the hepatitis C virus.

In patients with hepatitis C, particularly those who are HIV-positive, a systemic depletion of glutathione is present, especially in the liver. This depletion may be a factor underlying the resistance to interferon therapy. This finding represents a biological basis for N-acetylcysteine (NAC) and glutathione supplements as adjuvant (assisting) therapies.

The FDA-approved therapy to treat hepatitis is a six-month regimen of alpha interferon. While hepatitis C patients see only a 20-percent response to interferon monotherapy, when the anti-viral drug ribavirin is combined with interferon the response rate improves by two- to threefold.

The most recent published study showed that, in hepatitis C patients who initially failed interferon therapy, the addition of ribavirin to a new round of interferon therapy produced a tenfold increase in the number of patients showing eradication of detectable hepatitis C virus.

The Life Extension Foundation's protocol for hepatitis C includes:

1. The standard dose of alpha interferon (3 million IU injected subcutaneously three times a week for six months) prescribed by an infectious-disease physician. Interferon is the FDA-approved therapy for treatment of hepatitis C. However, it works only in a minority of patients when used without ribavirin.

2. 1,000 to 1,200 mg a day of ribavirin (taken in three doses) for six months. Ribavirin is an unapproved drug that increases the effectiveness of interferon therapy by up to tenfold.

3. The standard doses of Life Extension Mix and Life Extension Herbal Mix. Please note that some hepatitis C patients encounter liver enzyme elevations in response to the moderate doses of vitamin A, niacin and beta-carotene in Life Extension Mix. If your liver-enzyme levels elevate after starting Life Extension Mix, discontinue it and take separately the other nutrients contained in Life Extension Mix. Beta-carotene possesses unique immune-enhancing benefits that could help suppress the hepatitis C virus.

4. High doses of green tea and garlic, as well as chelation therapy, to reduce serum and liver iron levels to a minimum. Iron promotes hepatitis virus-induced liver injury and precludes successful treatment with interferon. Verify that liver iron levels have been reduced before starting interferon therapy.

5. Liver-protecting nutrients and immune-boosting therapies such as milk thistle extract, 150 mg three times a day; 500 mg of licorice extract, three times a day; 2,000 mg a day of garlic; 800 micrograms a day of selenium; 1,200 mg a day of N-acetylcysteine; 500 mg a day of glutathione; and vitamin C ranging from 5,000 to 20,000 mg a day.

For hepatitis C patients who fail the above regimen, the intake of 30 grams a day of whey protein concentrate could boost liver glutathione levels to help protect liver cells against hepatitis C-induced free radical liver damage.

Also, a strong immune system can keep the hepatitis virus in long-term remission. For additional suggestions, refer to the Immune Enhancement protocols.

Product availability: Green tea, licorice, silymarin, garlic, vitamin C, selenium, Life Extension Mix and Life Extension Herbal Mix, etc., can be ordered by phoning 1-800-544-4440. Call for a list of offshore mail order companies that supply medications such as ribavirin to Americans for personal use.

HIV Infection (AIDS) (Opportunistic Infections)

Free radicals have been linked to much of the immune-system destruction caused by the human immunodeficiency virus (HIV). Recent studies show that HIV depletes cellular glutathione levels and is associated with free-radical injury to critical immune-system components. Scientific evidence shows that antioxidants can protect immune function, and that certain nutrients may prevent or slow the progression of HIV infection.

A major controversy has developed in the scientific community as to whether HIV is the only agent responsible for the decline in immune function clinically defined as acquired immunodeficiency syndrome (AIDS). In 1985, the Life Extension Foundation first proposed that the decline in immune function in HIV-positive individuals might be prevented or slowed by taking high-potency nutrient supplements. Since 1985, several hundred medical papers have provided evidence that the basic mechanisms involved in HIV-related immune system destruction are associated with deficiencies in vitamins, minerals and amino acids. Another conclusion that emerges from the scientific literature is that some people with healthy immune systems who test positive for HIV may never develop immune suppression or AIDS. They remain perfectly healthy in spite of having antibodies to the human immunodeficiency virus.

Antibody production occurs when the immune system is exposed to a foreign body, such as a virus. Having HIV antibodies shows you have been infected by HIV, but it does not necessarily mean that you will develop AIDS. What this tells us is that most people should be on a nutrient-supplement program, not only to protect against AIDS but also to protect against cancer, the common cold, influenza, auto-immune diseases, hepatitis B and C, and other diseases.

The Foundation's HIV treatment protocol is comprised of the following three elements:

1. Nutritional immune support
2. Hormonal immune-system support
3. European immune-boosting therapies

A critical part of this protocol is monthly blood monitoring to assess the effectiveness of whatever HIV-treatment choice(s) you make. Since many FDA-approved anti-viral drugs are toxic, regular blood tests can warn you against life-threatening organ damage by indicating toxicity before symptoms appear.

Among the nutrients that HIV patients should consider taking is the amino acid N-acetyl-cysteine (NAC). Much of the immunologic decline caused by HIV involves depletion of cellular glutathione levels, resulting in massive free-radical damage to immune-system cells throughout the body. An effective way of boosting cellular glutathione levels is to take N-acetylcysteine.

The suggested dose of NAC for those who are HIV-positive is 600 mg three times a day. Two to 3 grams of vitamin C should be taken with each 600-mg dose of NAC. For AIDS patients with severe liver impairment, NAC could become toxic if ingested over an extended period of time. We suggest that this small sub-group switch to 500 mg a day of pure glutathione instead of NAC.

Another glutathione precursor is the trace mineral selenium, which also counteracts potentially damaging free radicals and may inhibit chemicals that HIV requires for reproduction. The minimum dose of selenium is 300 micrograms daily, but HIV patients should consider taking 600 to 1,000 micrograms daily. There are many inexpensive selenium supplements on the market, but none are better than Super Selenium Complex, which includes three forms of elemental selenium to provide different health benefits to the body.

A nutrient that often is overlooked by those who are HIV-positive is the amino acid arginine, which enhances immune function via several different mechanisms, including stimulation of growth-hormone secretion. Arginine has been shown to be an effective way of preventing AIDS-related wasting syndrome. The suggested dose for HIV patients is 6 to 15 grams of arginine a day on an empty stomach, preferably at bedtime.

Arginine is available as a powder, but the most convenient way of taking it is as arginine caplets. Each caplet contains 1,200 mg of arginine, which enables a person to consume high doses of the amino acid without having to swallow a large number of capsules.

Another amino acid often overlooked by HIV-positive individuals is L-carnitine, which has been shown to boost immune function via several different mechanisms, to protect the heart against AZT-induced toxicity, and to enhance essential fatty acid and glucose uptake. High doses of L-carnitine have enhanced immunologic and metabolic functions in HIV patients who were deficient in L-carnitine. The suggested dose of L-carnitine for HIV patients is 2,400 mg a day in two divided doses on an empty stomach.

A popular supplement used by HIV-positive patients is coenzyme Q10. Studies indicate that coenzyme Q10 boosts immune function. In a pilot study in AIDS patients, coenzyme Q10 provided significant benefits. Coenzyme Q10 has been shown to be deficient in HIV-infected people. It is suggested that HIV patients take at least 200 mg a day of coenzyme Q10.

Studies indicate that AIDS patients suffer from severe malabsorption of vitamin B12 and have a severe vitamin-B12 deficiency. AIDS-related dementia has been reversed by the administration of vitamin B12. Some forms of AIDS dementia could be caused by a simple vitamin-B12 deficiency. Vitamin B12 is not absorbed well when taken orally. We suggest that those who are HIV-positive take vitamin-B12 tablets that dissolve under the tongue. Three 500-microgram sublingual vitamin-B12 tablets a day are suggested. If a blood test reveals a continuing vitamin-B12 deficiency, weekly vitamin-B12 injections should be considered.

In a study in the January-April 1995 issue of the *Yale Journal of Biology and Medicine*, AIDS patients were given 100,000 IU a day of beta-carotene. After four weeks of beta-carotene treatment, total lymphocyte counts rose by 66 percent and T-helper cells rose slightly. Six weeks after beta-carotene treatment, the immune-cell measurements returned to pretreatment levels.

While this study demonstrated no toxicity associated with high-dose beta-carotene supplementation, the Life Extension Foundation recommends against high-dose beta-carotene in AIDS patients who also have hepatitis. For some people with hepatitis, long-term use of beta-carotene could cause liver-enzyme elevation, indicating potential liver damage. Many people infected with HIV also have been infected with hepatitis B or C. HIV/AIDS patients who do not have hepatitis or other liver damage should consider taking 25,000 to 100,000 IU a day of beta-carotene. Healthy people seeking to boost overall immune function should consider 25,000 IU a day of beta-carotene, along with other complementary antioxidants.

It is known that murine (mouse) AIDS is functionally similar to human AIDS. A study was conducted to assess the effect of vitamin-E supplementation on the decrease of cellular immune functions following the development of murine AIDS. Vitamin-E supplementation suppressed the enlargement of spleen and the increased number of splenocytes following retrovirus infection. The decrease of natural killer cell (NK) activity shown in mice infected with the murine AIDS retrovirus also was partly improved by high vitamin-E diet.

Proliferation of splenic T-lymphocytes was significantly restored by a higher vitamin-E diet, compared with the control group. Further, vitamin-E supplementation increased production of gamma interferon (IFN-gamma) and suppressed production of tumor necrosis factor-alpha (TNF-alpha) from splenocytes. In addition, the high vitamin-E diet decreased the increased ratio of CD4 and CD8 single positive T-cells following the development of murine AIDS, which was almost equal to the levels of the uninfected control and high vitamin-E groups.

These results suggest that vitamin E supplementation normalizes the decrease of immune functions following the development of AIDS in mice.

Antioxidant defense status was investigated in HIV-infected patients by measuring serum selenium, glutathione peroxidase activity and glutathione concentrations, along with the assessment of the clinical stage and surrogate markers of HIV disease. The results showed that stages I to III of HIV disease are characterized by significant impairments of antioxidative defenses provided by selenium, glutathione peroxidase and glutathione.

In AIDS patients, chronic inflammation and elevated levels of cytokines seem to be associated with reduced levels of glutathione. Glutathione has been proposed as an inhibitor of HIV-1 replication. A study on mouse HIV-1 provided evidence that glutathione and N-acetylcysteine (NAC), but not L-cysteine, could inhibit the reverse transcriptase replication process of HIV-1. Glutathione depletion also has been shown to play a direct role in the obliteration of CD4 helper cells that cause immune dysfunction.

A survey was conducted on the use of nutrient supplements in 64 HIV-1 seropositive men and women, and on 33 seronegative controls participating in a study of heterosexual HIV-1 transmission. HIV-infected patients had lower mean blood concentrations of magnesium, total carotenes, total choline and glutathione, and higher concentrations of niacin, than did the controls. Further, 59 percent of HIV-positive patients had low concentrations of magnesium, compared with 9 percent of controls. Participants who took vitamin supplements had fewer low concentrations of antioxidants. The low magnesium concentrations were thought to be particularly relevant to HIV-related symptoms of fatigue, lethargy and impaired mental activity.

Serum selenium levels were determined cross-sectionally in 57 HIV-infected patients. The results showed a progressive reduction of serum selenium in HIV infection that was associated with the loss of CD4 helper cells, and with increased levels of markers of disease progression and inflammatory response.

Lymphocyte cell death (apoptosis) in HIV-infected individuals may play a role in T-cell depletion, and therefore favor progression to AIDS. In this study, the effects of short-term (five-day) intravenous treatment with L-carnitine on apoptosis of CD4 and CD8 cells from 10 AIDS patients was studied. L-carnitine administration has been shown to induce a strong reduction in the percentage of both CD4 and CD8 cells undergoing apoptosis. These results suggest that L-carnitine could prevent the death of CD4 and CD8 cells in AIDS patients.

Vitamin C (ascorbic acid) is required for normal host defense and functions. An analysis of vitamin-C uptake and its effects on virus production and cellular proliferation was performed. Exposure to high concentrations of vitamin C preferentially decreased the proliferation and survival of the HIV-infected cells, and caused decreased viral production. This study showed that high concentrations of vitamin C were preferentially toxic to HIV-infected host defense cell lines in vitro.

When plasma levels were measured for all antioxidant-micronutrients in subjects with HIV infection and in controls, it was observed that the HIV-infected subjects showed a significant depletion of all the carotenoids (lutein, lycopene, alpha-carotene, etc.) and vitamin C.

Another test studied the tendency in HIV patients to experience apoptosis (cell death) in immune cells. The presence of N-acetylcysteine (NAC), acetyl-L-carnitine or nicotinamide was able to prevent apoptosis in most cases. The scientists concluded that NAC, acetyl-L-carnitine and nicotinamide could be used, in addition to antiviral drugs, in treating HIV infection.

There are many other nutrients that appear to benefit those infected with HIV. Life Extension

Mix contains potent doses of 56 different disease-preventing nutrients that can be taken in a convenient, economical form. HIV-infected people should take three tablets of Life Extension Mix three times a day.

The immune-enhancing properties of certain herbal extracts are gaining considerable attention in the scientific literature. Herbal extracts are expensive because large quantities of bulk herbs have to be used to produce a relatively small amount of pharmaceutical herbal extract. In order to make the daily intake of disease-fighting herbs affordable, a powdered Life Extension Herbal Mix was designed incorporating 27 different herbs into one drink mix. The suggested daily dose is one to two tablespoons taken first thing in the morning. Some of the herbal extracts contained in Life Extension Herbal Mix may produce anti-viral activity in addition to immune-boosting properties.

Hormones synchronize immune function. An immune system that is not precisely synchronized will not function optimally. The Foundation's HIV Infection protocol works best in HIV-positive individuals with T-helper cells counts of 500 and above. HIV causes immune system destruction and desynchronization. Hormone-replacement therapies can protect and restore immune functions.

Researchers now believe that the AIDS virus replicates at a furious pace from the time of infection, creating as many as 2 billion new viruses a day. The reason there appears to be such a long incubation period between the time of infection and the development of AIDS symptoms is because the immune system is creating new anti-viral cells as quickly as the AIDS virus replicates. At some point, however, the AIDS virus overwhelms the ability of the immune system to produce anti-viral cells and the patient succumbs to immune suppression, eventual immune system destruction and, finally, death.

However, the knowledge that the immune system responds aggressively to fight the AIDS virus means that therapies that enhance the immune system could be effective AIDS therapies.

Preliminary evidence suggests that HIV infection can be slowed by the nightly intake of melatonin. Melatonin enhances the production of T-helper cells, the very cells lost to HIV infection. Melatonin also enhances the production of other immune system components known to be affected by HIV infection, including natural killer cells (NK), interleukin-2, -4, and -10, gamma interferon, eosinophils and red blood cells. In addition to enhancing the production of cells being killed by the AIDS virus, melatonin also may prevent HIV cellular destruction via its action as an antioxidant.

The latest evidence suggests that melatonin is even more effective than nutrient antioxidants in suppressing immune cell-killing free radicals generated by HIV. One study, conducted by Dr. Russel Reiter of the University of Texas, in Austin, indicated that melatonin may have a direct effect on HIV replication. For HIV to replicate, it needs a substance called nuclear factor kappa-B (NKF). Since the amount of NKF is reduced by 23 percent at night, Dr. Reiter sought to determine whether melatonin is responsible for the nightly decline in NKF. When he injected rats with melatonin during the day, he observed a 43-percent reduction of NKF binding activity. This finding suggests that melatonin may interfere with the division of HIV viruses by cutting off their supply of NKF.

Dr. George Maestroni, a pioneer in melatonin immunotherapy, conducted a pilot AIDS study in Italy whereby 11 HIV-infected people were given 20 mg of melatonin every night. After a month of treatment, the patients had a 35-percent increase in T-helper cells, a 57-percent increase in natural killer cells, and a 76-percent increase in lymphocyte production.

In spite of these remarkable findings, this line of research has not been pursued because melatonin is not a patentable drug that can generate billions of dollars of profits for the pharmaceutical giants.

However, melatonin appears to benefit AIDS patients in many other ways, including providing protection against AZT toxicity and the wasting syndrome. We suggest that HIV patients obtain the book *Melatonin*, by Dr. Russel Reiter and Jo Robinson. This book contains newly discovered findings about AIDS and melatonin.

The suggested dose of melatonin for HIV patients ranges from 3 to 30 mg nightly.

Studies have shown that HIV infection progresses only when serum levels of the hormone DHEA begin to decline. The speculation from these studies is that maintaining healthy blood levels of DHEA might prevent HIV infection from progressing to full-blown AIDS. DHEA now is used widely by HIV patients. Its beneficial action may not be due to any direct anti-viral effect, but rather to DHEA's ability to protect immune functions against a wide array of insults.

The Life Extension Foundation recommends that all HIV-infected patients and most people over 40 have their DHEA blood levels tested, and then take DHEA supplements to restore their serum DHEA levels to that of a healthy 21-year-old. An appropriate dosage for men is 25 mg, three times a day. For those with liver disease, DHEA capsules should be opened and held under the tongue for 10 to 20 minutes and then swallowed.

DHEA possibly can contribute to liver damage in people with hepatitis or cirrhosis. Before starting DHEA replacement therapy, refer to the DHEA-Pregnenolone Precautions in this book.

For those who can afford it, growth hormone therapy could be very beneficial for HIV-infected and AIDS patients. Growth hormone boosts immune function, is a protease inhibitor, and promotes anabolic cell renewal and muscle building.

T-cells are produced and mature in response to hormones secreted by the thymus gland. However, aging causes shrinkage of the thymus gland, and the resulting reduction in the production of thymic hormones is a major cause of the progressive age-related decline in immune function. HIV infection adversely affects hormone secretion from the thymus gland.

As noted in an earlier protocol, but which bears repeating in this context, Thymic Protein A has been shown in laboratory and animal experiments to cause the T-4 lymphocyte to mature, thereby initiating a specific cell-mediated immune response. This specific protein has been shown to be a stimulant in animal models for the production of interleukin-2. Interleukin-2 production by T-4 cells is the benchmark measurement for T-cell maturity and initiation of immune response.

The following is worth repeating verbatim:

A trial with 22 cats infected with feline immunodeficiency virus (FIV) concluded that Thymic Protein A enhances immune response to infectious agents measured serologically, diminishes disease symptoms, lengthens survival and increases lymphocyte values.

A daily dose of 4 micrograms of Thymic Protein A may make a major difference in longevity by strengthening the immune system through its T-cell "programming" role. The more T-cells that are functioning properly, the more immune response may be mounted against metastasized cancer cells.

It is well-known among oncologists that chemotherapy and radiation often will induce a serious drop in white blood count to dangerous levels, which may require an end to the therapy. Initial reports from those undergoing chemotherapy indicate that Thymic Protein A has maintained their total white blood count at acceptable levels during the therapy. Healthy people can take one packet of Thymic Protein A every day or every other day. Those whose treatment is dependent on a strong immune system may need three packets a day for several months.

Another product, Thymex, provides extracts of fresh, healthy tissue from the thymus and other glands that produce the disease-fighting cells of our immune system.

The primary ingredient in Thymex is immunologic tissue from the thymus gland. Also included in Thymex is tissue from the lymph nodes and spleen that produces the white blood cells that engage in life-or-death combat with invading organisms in our bloodstream under the "instruction" of the thymus gland.

Thymex is a synergistic formula that contains herbal activators and a full complement of natural homeopathic nutrients, in addition to fresh, healthy thymus, lymph and spleen tissues. Thymex is a professional formula normally dispensed through doctors' offices. Thymex has been extensively used to amplify the immune-potentiating effect of DHEA-replacement therapy. According to a physician most familiar with DHEA, thymus extract is required to obtain the immune system-boosting benefit of DHEA.

Another therapy to boost thymus-gland activity is isoprinosine. Isoprinosine is approved by almost every regulatory agency in the world except the Food and Drug Administration. In 1990, *The New England Journal Of Medicine* published findings that isoprinosine slows the progression of HIV infection. This report is one of hundreds of studies showing that isoprinosine boosts immune function in cancer patients, HIV patients and healthy people.

In 1985, the Life Extension Foundation recommended that HIV-infected people take isoprinosine to slow the decline in immune function that leads to full blown AIDS. Isoprinosine and other immune-boosting drugs work best when taken on an alternative-dosing schedule, two months on and two months off.

A French drug, Biostim, was studied with regard to its effect of modulating varying immune responses. In response to staph infection, Biostim therapy significantly increased the critical phagocytosis component of immune attack. Biostim also modulated synthesis of human polymorphonuclear granulocytes.

The immunological effects in aged humans was studied to see what specific immune components were affected by the oral administration of Biostim. The results showed significant restoration of cellular immunity, an increased percentage of CD3+, CD2+, CD4+ and HNKI+ immune cells, and increased phagocytic activity.

Preincubation of immune cells with Biostim resulted in augmentation of natural microbicidal activity. Non-specific activation of host defences may have a significant impact on the outcome of infections in the immunocompromized patient. Biostim was shown to be effective in increasing resistance to experimental infections in animals. Biostim also was shown to have anti-Candida effects.

Alveolar macrophages are issued from circulating monocytes and stand at the cross-road immune defenses of the lung. The effectiveness of Biostim in respiratory infections is due to its action on deep lung cells, and in particular alveolar macrophages. This compound has been shown to recruit cells (which is a sign of macrophage activation) to increase enzymatic activities, phagocytosis and to promote interleukine 1 secretion. These activities have been demonstrated in in-vitro studies as well as in animal and human studies.

Biostim is an immunomodulator of organic origin acting on cells of the immune system (B cells, T cells, phagocytic cells) and on mediators (IL1-CSF). Its mode of action has been explored by means of experimental Infections. The types of defense involved differ according to whether the experimental infection is caused by an extracellular or intracellular micro-organism. Candida albicans and Saccharomyces cerevisiae were used to produce fungal infections, while bacterial infections were obtained with Staph, E. coli, Strep. pneumoniae and other organisms. The influenza virus was used to produce a viral infection. In these experimental models, Biostim increased the survival time of the infected animals and reduced bacterial, fungal and viral proliferation. These effects were observed even in immunocompromised mice. These in-vitro and in-vivo studies have demonstrated that Biostim is effective whatever the type of body defense involved.

Here is an immune-boosting program for HIV patients to consider:

❖ **Isoprinosine Therapy** — 2,000 to 3,000 mg daily for two months. Repeat every other two months.

   After completing isoprinosine therapy, we suggest a two-month regimen of:

❖ **Thymus Therapy** — four Thymex capsules a day for two months, or one to three paks a day of Thymic Protein A. Thymus therapy should be taken when isoprinosine is not used.

Repeat isoprinosine and thymus therapies every other two months. Some doctors believe that Thymic Protein A should be taken every single day.

❖ **Biostim Therapy** — Three-month dosing schedule as follows: two tablets daily for eight days, then stop for three weeks; one tablet daily for eight days, then stop for three weeks; one tablet daily for eight days, then stop for nine months.

Proper levels of thyroid hormones are crucial for optimal immune function. Blood tests do not always accurately detect a thyroid-hormone deficiency. One method of determining if you are thyroid-deficient is to take your body temperature about 30 minutes before lunch. If your temperature is consistently below normal, you may want to take a thyroid hormone supplement. The TSH (thyroid stimulating hormone) test is extremely sensitive to both hypo- and hyperthyroid conditions, often showing subclinical disorders.

Popular prescription thyroid replacement drugs are Synthroid (synthetic thyroid hormone), Armour, Forest Pharmaceuticals (natural thyroid hormone) and Cytomel (T3 thyroid fraction). You must be careful not to overdose on thyroid hormone, so the advice of a knowledgeable physician is important when considering thyroid-hormone supplementation or replacement.

HIV infection causes excessive cortisol production from the adrenal glands that can decimate immune function. Therefore, it is crucial to suppress excessive cortisol production. There are 17 European studies showing that HIV causes some of its destruction of the immune system by stimulating excessive cortisol production. DHEA and melatonin may suppress cortisol levels.

Two tablets of the European procaine drug KH3, taken twice a day on an empty stomach, is suggested as the best way of suppressing elevated cortisol levels in cancer and AIDS patients. One or two tablets of KH3 can be taken first thing in the morning on an empty stomach, with the same dose taken an hour before dinner. It is difficult to test cortisol levels in the blood because adrenal surges of cortisol can occur erratically throughout the day. That's one reason why this important cause of immune-system destruction has largely been ignored by American doctors. However, a resting morning level of cortisol, taken before 9 a.m., may be quite significant in determining overall cortisol status in the body.

The FDA has approved four cytotoxic anti-viral drugs to slow the progression of HIV infection. These drugs are AZT, ddI, ddC and 3TC. There are additional cytotoxic anti-viral drugs that soon will be approved. There is enthusiasm in some parts of the AIDS community that various combinations of these anti-viral drugs could enable those with HIV infection and clinically diagnosed AIDS to maintain long-term remissions.

The published research shows that the proper combination of these anti-viral drugs and a protease inhibitor works far better than AZT alone. A combination of AZT and 3TC, along with one of the new, relatively non-toxic protease inhibitors, may be the ideal combination to try first in AIDS patients.

In several studies published in 1994, AZT was compared to a placebo with no difference in overall survival rates. In some cases, AZT caused an *increase* in mortality. Recognizing that AZT monotherapy is clearly not the solution to AIDS, some of the AIDS support groups are suggesting that aggressive combinations of almost every anti-viral drug available be tried in AIDS patients. These combination therapies can, in the short-term, produce a significant reduction in the PCR (viral load testing) and even an increase in CD4 (T-helper cells). Regular blood tests would be needed to monitor the toxicity of these anti-viral drugs to determine when to switch from one toxic combination to another.

Our concern is, if combination anti-viral therapy produces irreversible damage to the immune system, there could very well be no increase in survival, even though the therapy might kill a large number of HIV viruses and infected immune cells. It is interesting to note that, in two studies documenting the benefits of combination anti-viral drug and protease-inhibitor therapy, those who had never taken an anti-viral drug had higher survival rates than those who had previously taken AZT. One reason for the better effect on these "anti-viral virgins" was that not as much drug resistance to anti-viral drugs had developed in them. The use of AZT results in the development of drug-resistant strains of HIV within one to two years.

Another reason the "anti-viral virgins" did better is that their immune systems may not have been previously damaged by toxic drugs such as AZT and ddl. Since HIV is a slow-progressing disease, and since blood tests enable you to monitor the benefits of the Foundation's protocol, HIV patients may consider following a non-toxic protocol first before resorting to combination anti-viral drug and protease-inhibitor therapy. Other scientists believe that the toxic drug combination should be used as soon as HIV infection is diagnosed in order to try to eradicate the HIV from the body before too many viruses are produced.

Product availability: N-acetylcysteine, arginine, coenzyme Q10, Life Extension Mix, Life Extension Herbal Mix, melatonin, selenium, carnitine, vitamin B12, beta-carotene, DHEA, Thymic Protein A and Thymex are available by calling 1-800-544-4440. For access to drugs like isoprinosine and Biostim, ask for a list of offshore suppliers who will mail-order these products to Americans for personal use. Growth-hormone therapy is available from a few doctors in the U.S. and abroad. Call for a list of doctors who offer this therapy.

Hypertension
(High Blood Pressure)

There are many nutrients that may reduce or eliminate the need for anti-hypertensive medications. However, nutrients do not work immediately to lower blood pressure the way drugs do, so it is important to carry through nutritional blood pressure-lowering therapy over a period of four to 12 weeks. Also, physician cooperation is crucial if you are to reduce your intake of blood pressure-lowering drugs safely, and regular blood pressure monitoring is mandatory in order to determine if the nutritional regimen you are following is controlling your blood pressure.

The two nutrients best documented to control hypertension are garlic and coenzyme Q10. The amount of standardized garlic extract needed to lower blood pressure is 1,500 to 6,000 mg a day. The amount of coenzyme Q10 needed to lower blood pressure is 200 to 300 mg a day.

The coenzyme Q10 should be taken in a liquid oil capsule for optimal assimilation. After following this garlic/coenzyme Q10 regimen for four weeks, consult your physician about reducing the dosage of your anti-hypertensive medication. The objective is to be able to slowly reduce your intake of drugs as the natural anti-hypertensive effective of garlic/coenzyme Q10 begins to take effect. It is crucial to monitor your blood pressure closely, since the garlic/coenzyme Q10 combination does not work for everyone.

Some people have high blood pressure because they are deficient in certain minerals that keep blood pressure in balance. Anyone with elevated blood pressure should be taking 500 to 1,500 mg of elemental magnesium a day. About 80 percent of Americans are magnesium-deficient, and low levels of magnesium are associated with hypertension and arterial disease. Even if magnesium fails to lower your blood pressure, it can reduce the risk of complications, such as stroke.

Among the most popular types of anti-hypertensive drugs are calcium channel blockers. These drugs are sold under such trade names as Norvasc and Procardia. However, magnesium is nature's calcium-channel blocker. It inhibits excessive calcium infiltration into cells. Magnesium also is safe to take, with the only adverse side effect being diarrhea when too much is taken.

A potassium deficiency can cause high blood pressure in some people, so those with high blood pressure should consider taking 500 mg of potassium. Unlike magnesium, which is very safe, too much potassium can be lethal. A blood test can reveal if you need less or more potassium.

Supplemental calcium may help some women lower their high blood pressure.

High doses of fish oil concentrates have lowered blood pressure in some people. It requires eight to 10 capsules of Mega EPA capsules of fish oil to duplicate those studies. There are cardiovascular and other health benefits associated with taking fish oil, so if your gastrointestinal tract can tolerate such a high daily dose of fish oils, then you may lower your blood pressure and gain other benefits.

Some other blood pressure-lowering nutrients include vitamin C in doses of 3,000 to 10,000 mg, and the amino acid arginine in doses of 5,000 mg one to three times a day. Arginine can work synergistically with such ACE-inhibiting anti-hypertensive drugs as Vasotec, Capoten and Zestril (see more on ACE inhibitors later in this protocol). This is important for those with chronic hypertension who fail to respond to conventional or alternative therapies. Since the Life Extension Foundation's original recommendations about using arginine to treat hypertension were made in 1991, numerous new studies have been published indicating that arginine may be even more effective as an anti-hypertensive agent than was previously reported.

> **Warning**: If you'd like to see if any of the nutritional anti-hypertensive agents can help you reduce the dosage or replace your anti-hypertensive drugs, extreme caution is mandatory and physician cooperation is essential. You should reduce the dosage of your anti-hypertensive drug very slowly while increasing your intake of the nutrient supplement(s). Monitor your blood pressure on a daily basis. *If you do not exercise caution, an acute hypertensive event could occur, resulting in a stroke.*
>
> Our general precaution is, if you're going to attempt to use any of the nutrients the Foundation recommends to replace anti-hypertensive drugs, you must do so with the cooperation of your physician. You cannot assume that any nutrients will be able to replace a drug that already is effectively controlling your blood pressure. Daily blood-pressure monitoring is mandatory to ensure that the nutrient regimen you are following is really keeping your blood pressure under control.

If nutrients fail to keep your blood pressure under control, our favorite class of anti-hypertensive drugs are the ACE inhibitors. ACE stands for angiotensin-converting enzyme, which causes hypertension by constricting the arterial system. By blocking the angiotensin-converting enzyme, which is what ACE inhibitors do, the arterial system can be returned to a more youthful state of elasticity. Popular ACE-inhibiting drugs that have relatively few side effects are Capoten and Zestril.

One of the newest anti-hypertensive drugs is called Hyzaar. Ask your doctor about Hyzaar if you are not satisfied with the anti-hypertensive drugs you currently are using. Those with hypertension often have artery disease. See the Atherosclerosis protocol for additional suggestions.

Product availability: CoQ10, Mega EPA, garlic, vitamin C, Life Extension Mix, garlic, potassium, calcium, magnesium and arginine are available by calling 1-800-544-4440. Prescription drugs cited should be prescribed by a doctor who treats hypertension.

Hypoglycemia

Low blood sugar caused by excessive release of insulin from the pancreas can cause fatigue, weakness, loss of consciousness and even death. In hypoglycemia attacks, there is too much insulin and not enough blood sugar. Insulin can be partially neutralized by taking the amino acid cysteine along with vitamin B1 and vitamin C.

Hypoglycemics should start out with once-a-day doses of 500 mg of cysteine along with 250 mg of vitamin B1 and 1,500 mg of vitamin C. The second week, this dose should be administered twice a day, and by the third week it should be taken three times a day. The objective is to prevent hypoglycemic attacks by neutralizing excess insulin. Every hypoglycemic is slightly different, so the dosage ranges will vary from person to person.

Another possible cause of low blood sugar is the inability to release glycogen (stored sugar in the liver), secondary to vitamin B6 and chromium deficiency. Some hypoglycemics are helped by the daily administration of 100 to 250 mg of the vitamin B6 metabolite pyridoxal 5-phosphate and 200 micrograms of chromium.

Hypoglycemia may damage brain cells. When hippocampal brain-cell cultures are deprived of glucose, a massive release of lactate dehydrogenase (LDH) occurs, which is an indicator of neuronal death. The addition of pyridoxal 5-phosphate has been shown to inhibit the LDH release. When pyridoxal 5-phosphate is given before glucose deprivation, a more potent inhibitory effect on LDH release has been observed. Scientists have suggested that pyridoxal 5-phosphate protects neurons from glucose deprivation-induced damage. These scientists recommend that this pyridoxal 5-phosphate be used prophylactically to protect against brain-cell death induced by metabolic disorders such as hypoglycemia.

Product availability: The amino acid cysteine, vitamin B1, vitamin B6, pyridoxal 5-phosphate, vitamin C caps and chromium picolinate are available by calling 1-800-544-4440.

Immune Enhancement

The Life Extension Foundation's Immune Enhancement protocol is designed to enhance immune function in people who are aging, are receiving cancer chemotherapy, or who have chronic viral or bacterial infections.

The foundations for nutritional immunology emerged in the early 1800s with the finding that severe malnutrition would lead to thymic atrophy, and for most of that century, all evidence for a relationship between malnutrition and the immune system was based on anatomical findings. With the discovery of vitamins, it became evident that single essential nutrients each played an important role in maintaining immune function.

During the 1920s and 1930s, vitamin A became known as the "anti-infective" vitamin, and the first attempts were made to use vitamin A therapeutically during infectious illnesses. The first systematic studies of immuno-nutritional interrelationships in laboratory animals were initiated in 1947 by Abraham E. Axelrod and his students. Human studies followed soon thereafter, and by the late 1970s the field of nutritional immunology was well-established.

Studies published in the 1980s and 1990s clearly show specific immune-enhancing effects with the proper use of nutritional supplements, proteins, hormones and certain drugs.

Free radicals have been linked to immune-system damage caused by normal aging. A strong immune system is critical to the prevention of infection by viruses, fungi and bacteria. Cancer cells are thought to form regularly, and a vigilant immune response is required to kill or inactivate these transformed cells before they become malignant tumors. Members of the Life Extension Foundation have long been encouraged to follow a daily antioxidant regimen that protects against immune-suppressing free radicals.

The incidence of cancer and new infectious diseases has been increasing every year in the U.S. Many dangerous bacteria have become resistant to antibiotics that once kept them in check, and these bacteria are now a threat to our lives. However, scientific evidence shows that antioxidants can protect and enhance immune function.

The cornerstone of any program to boost immune function involves making sure that you are consuming every nutrient that has a role in maintaining a healthy immune system. The most convenient way of obtaining most of the nutrients needed for healthy immune function is to take three tablets, three times a day of the 56-ingredient Life Extension Mix. In addition, one capsule a day of Life Extension Booster provides added amounts of nutrients that protect immune system cells against damaging free radicals.

Just one of the 56 ingredients found in Life Extension Mix has shown a powerful effect in boosting natural killer (NK) cell activity in elderly men. In a placebo-controlled, double-blind study, the effects of 10 to 12 years of beta-carotene supplementation on NK cell activity was evaluated. No significant difference was seen in NK cell activity in the middle-aged group. Those elderly men, however, who were supplemented with beta-carotene had significantly greater NK cell activity than another group of elderly men receiving placebo. These results showed that long-term beta-carotene supplementation enhances NK cell activity in elderly men, which may be beneficial for immune viral and tumoral surveillance.

Immune dysfunctions and susceptibility to infections have been observed in zinc-deficient human subjects. A study investigated production of cytokines and characterized the T-cell subpopulations in three groups of mildly zinc-deficient subjects. These included head and neck cancer patients, healthy volunteers who were found to have a dietary deficiency of zinc, and healthy volunteers in whom a zinc deficiency was induced by dietary means.

This study showed that the zinc status affected cytokines levels. The production of interleukin-2 and gamma interferon were decreased even when the deficiency of zinc was mild. Natural killer cell activity also was decreased in zinc-deficient subjects. T-cell formation was decreased in mildly zinc-deficient subjects. This study shows the role that zinc plays in promoting specific immune responses.

The best-publicized study of the use of Vitamin E to boost immune function appeared in

The Journal of the American Medical Association, 1997, 277/17 (1380-1386). This double-blind, placebo-controlled study looked at healthy humans at least 65 years of age. Supplementation with Vitamin E for four months improved certain clinically relevant indexes of cell-mediated immunity. These results clearly showed that a level of Vitamin E greater than that currently recommended by the FDA enhanced certain clinically relevant in-vivo indexes of T-cell-mediated immune function in healthy elderly persons.

A powdered Life Extension Herbal Mix incorporates 27 different herbs into one daily drink. Many of these herbs have shown immune enhancing effects. The suggested daily dose is one tablespoon taken first thing in the morning.

Two of the herbal extracts contained in Life Extension Herbal Mix are echinacea and ginseng. In a controlled study, echinacea and ginseng were evaluated for their capacity to stimulate cellular immune function in normal individuals, as well as in patients with either chronic fatigue syndrome or acquired immunodeficiency syndrome (AIDS). Both echinacea and ginseng significantly enhanced NK function of all groups. Similarly, the addition of either herb increased other measurements of immune competence. This study showed that extracts of echinacea and ginseng enhance cellular immune function in normal individuals, as well as in patients with depressed cellular immunity.

Another herb extract found in Life Extension Herbal Mix is grape seed-skin extract. This extract contains a mixture of bioflavonoids called proanthocyanidins that exhibit significant antioxidative activity. The effects of the proanthocyanidins found in grape seed-skin extract on immune dysfunction were studied in mice. The proanthocyanidin enhanced in-vitro inter-leukin-2 production and natural killer cell cytotoxicity.

Other nutrients that have shown a positive effect on immune function include L-carnitine in doses of 1,800 to 2,400 mg a day, and coenzyme Q10 in doses of 100 mg to 300 mg a day.

Aging, cancer chemotherapy and infectious agents cause immune system destruction and desynchronization. The most effective hormone therapy to protect and improve immune function is melatonin, which enhances the production of T-helper cells, which are necessary to identify cancer cells, viruses, fungi and bacteria.

Melatonin enhances the production of other immune components, including natural killer cells, interleukin-2, interleukin-4, interleukin-10, gamma interferon and eosinophils. The latest evidence suggests that melatonin is even more effective than nutrient antioxidants in suppressing immune cell-killing free radicals.

Further, studies have documented that DHEA (dehydroepiandrosterone) has a beneficial role in maintaining healthy immune function. DHEA has been shown to protect mice from a variety of lethal infections. This includes, but is not limited to, infection from viruses, bacteria and the parasite Cryptosporidium parvum.

The Life Extension Foundation recommends that most people over 40 have their blood levels of DHEA tested, and then take supplemental DHEA accordingly to restore their serum DHEA levels to that of a healthy 21-year-old. This usually can be accomplished by taking 25 mg of DHEA three times a day for men, and 15 mg three times a day for women.

In addition, a product called Thymic Protein A has been shown in laboratory and animal experiments to cause the T-4 lymphocyte to mature, thereby initiating a specific cell-mediated immune response. Thymic Protein A has been shown to be a stimulant in animal models for the production of interleukin-2. Interleukin-2 production by T-4 cells is the benchmark measurement for T-cell maturity and initiation of immune response. A daily dose of 4 micrograms of this material may make a major difference in longevity by strengthening the immune system through its T-cell "programming" role. The more T-cells that are properly functioning, the more immune response may be mounted against metastasized cancer cells.

It is well-known among oncologists that chemotherapy and radiation often will induce a serious drop in white blood count to dangerous levels, which may require that the therapy be stopped. However, initial reports from those undergoing chemotherapy indicate that Thymic Protein A has maintained their total white blood count at acceptable levels during the therapy.

Healthy people can take one packet of Thymic Protein A every day or every other day. Those with disease whose treatment is dependent on a strong immune system may need three packets a day for several months.

A less-expensive thymic enhancing product is Thymex. Thymex provides extracts of fresh, healthy tissue from the thymus and other glands that produce the disease-fighting cells of our immune system.

The primary ingredient in Thymex is immunologic tissue from the thymus gland. Also included in Thymex is tissue from the lymph nodes and spleen that produce the white blood cells that engage in life-or-death combat with invading organisms in our bloodstream under the "instruction" of the thymus gland.

Thymex is a synergistic formula that contains herbal activators and a full complement of natural homeopathic nutrients, in addition to fresh, healthy thymus, lymph and spleen tissues. Thymex is a professional formula normally dispensed through doctors' offices. Thymex has been extensively used to amplify the immune-potentiating effect of DHEA-replacement therapy. According to a physician most familiar with DHEA, thymus extract is required to obtain the immune system-boosting benefit of DHEA.

T-cells mature in response to hormones secreted by the thymus gland. Aging causes a shrinkage of the thymus, and the resulting reduction in the production of thymic hormones is a major cause of the progressive decline in immune function that occurs with aging. By taking two to four capsules a day of Thymex, you can replace some of the thymic hormones lost to aging.

Aging, cancer and AIDS often generate sub-optimal levels of thyroid hormone production. Proper levels of thyroid hormones are crucial for optimal immune function. Blood tests do not always detect a thyroid hormone deficiency. However, a TSH (thyroid stimulating hormone) test is recommended. If your temperature 30 minutes before eating is consistently below normal, you may want to start taking a thyroid hormone supplement, as directed by your physician. Popular prescription thyroid replacement drugs are Synthroid (synthetic thyroid hormone, T4) and Cytomel (T3 thyroid hormone). You must be careful not to overdose on thyroid hormones, so the advice of a knowledgeable physician is important when considering thyroid hormone therapy.

Soy protein extract can boost thyroid output and eliminate the need for thyroid hormone replacement.

Aging, cancer and AIDS can stimulate excessive cortisol production from the adrenal glands, which decimates immune function. Thus, it is crucial to inhibit excessive cortisol production. As has been noted in the HIV Infection (AIDS) protocol, there are 17 European studies showing that HIV causes the destruction of the immune system by stimulating excessive cortisol production.

DHEA and melatonin may suppress cortisol levels. High doses of the European procaine drug KH3, taken at least twice a day, are suggested as the best way of suppressing elevated cortisol levels in cancer, AIDS and stressed-out patients. One to two tablets of KH3 can be taken first thing in the morning on an empty stomach, with the same dose taken again one hour before dinner on an empty stomach. It is difficult to test cortisol levels in the blood because adrenal surges of cortisol can occur erratically throughout the day. That's one reason why this important cause of immune-system destruction has been largely ignored by American doctors.

Influenza and other infectious diseases tend to be more severe in older patients. Despite immunization, elderly people often lack the immune capacity to generate an antibody response to prevent infection from the influenza virus. As many as 69,000 Americans have died from influenza in a bad epidemic year. Biostim is a French drug that has been shown to prevent infectious diseases in the elderly. Biostim is used in Europe to boost immune function and treat certain infectious diseases.

An examination of the published literature reveals that, if Biostim were available in the United States, thousands of American lives could be saved every year. These studies also indicate that Biostim would dramatically reduce the need for antibiotic therapy, thereby saving untold millions of dollars in prescription drug costs.

A double-blind trial was conducted to evaluate the capacity of Biostim to diminish the frequency of infectious episodes in chronic bronchitis. The study duration was nine months. Of the 73 subjects selected, 38 received Biostim and 35 a placebo. By the ninth month, the duration in days of infectious episodes was 60 percent lower in the Biostim group, compared with the placebo group. The use of antibiotic therapy was reduced by 81 percent in the Biostim group, compared with the placebo group. Pre-winter administration of Biostim to subjects significantly diminished the frequency of infectious episodes, and thus the consumption of antibiotics.

In another study, 314 elderly subjects admitted to hospitals were given either Biostim or a placebo. The subjects were regularly examined every three months for one year. The incidence of acute infectious episodes was evaluated in both groups. The number of subjects with infection in the group receiving the Biostim were significantly lower than in the placebo group, compared with. In the group receiving the Biostim, the number of infectious episodes was reduced throughout the 12 months of the trial. Finally, there was a significant decrease in the duration of antibiotic therapy. Biostim was well-tolerated. This study showed that Biostim is effective in protecting elderly, and therefore fragile, subjects against respiratory infections.

An evaluation of the safety of Biostim given with an antibiotic to treat acute infections was performed in three double-blind, placebo-controlled studies on fragile institutionalized or hospitalized patients. Two of the studies showed that, in acute respiratory infections, Biostim is well-tolerated and resulted in a more rapid improvement. The third study showed that Biostim produced a more rapid improvement in the most severely ill patients. It was concluded that Biostim can be initiated safely during acute episodes occurring in subjects with recurrent respiratory infections, and that it results in a faster improvement of clinical symptoms.

Here is an immune-boosting regimen for immune-compromised patients:

- ❖ **Thymic Protein A**: One to two 4-microgram packets under the tongue every day.
- ❖ **Biostim therapy**: Three-month dosing schedule as follows: 2 tablets daily for eight days, then stop for three weeks; one tablet daily for eight days, then stop for three weeks; one tablet daily for eight days, then stop for nine months. Repeat Biostim therapy once a year.

Whey protein concentrate dramatically raises glutathione levels. Glutathione protects immune cells and detoxifies harmful compounds in the body. Glutathione is intimately tied to immunity. Reduced glutathione levels have been associated with AIDS and other viral diseases, and raising glutathione levels appears to be one way of modulating immunity.

In a study, glutathione in animals was raised to higher-than-normal levels by whey protein better than other proteins, including soy. A study involving HIV-positive men fed whey protein concentrate found dramatic increases in glutathione levels, with most men reaching their ideal body weight. Whey protein improves immune function and fights infections. Immune response also was dramatically enhanced in animals fed whey protein concentrate when exposed to such immune challenges as salmonella, streptococcus pneumonia and cancer-causing chemicals. Again, this effect on immunity was not seen with other proteins.

Studies have examined the impact of whey protein concentrate on preventing or treating cancer. When different groups of rats were given a powerful carcinogen, those fed whey protein concentrate showed fewer tumors and a reduced pooled area of tumors (tumor mass index). The researchers found that whey protein offered "considerable protection to the host" over that of other protein. It should be noted that not all whey protein concentrates are created equal. Processing whey protein to remove the lactose and fats without losing its biological activity takes special care by the manufacturer. The protein must be processed under low temperature and low acid conditions so as not to "denature" the protein. Maintaining the natural state of the protein is essential to its biological activity.

Immune-suppressed patients should consider taking 30 grams a day of specially designed whey protein concentrate.

Product availability: Life Extension Mix, whey protein concentrate, Life Extension Booster, Thymex, Thymic Protein A, coenzyme Q10, carnitine, melatonin, Soy Power and DHEA are available by phoning 1-800-544-4440. Ask for a listing of offshore companies that sell Biostim and KH3.

Insomnia

Insomnia can be caused by a wide variety of factors, but for people over age 35 or 40, the most common cause of insomnia is deficiency of the hormone melatonin. Melatonin is the hormone released by the pineal gland that induces drowsiness, and enables the body to enter the deep-sleep patterns characteristic of youth.

After darkness, young pineal glands secrete melatonin slowly for about five hours to enable the body to enter the various stages of deep sleep, so people can feel revitalized and rejuvenated the next morning. Further, melatonin supplementation has been shown in many scientific studies to be the safest and most effective sleep-enhancing therapy in the world. While most people find that taking one 3-mg capsule of melatonin before bedtime helps to solve their sleep problems, some people still wake up too frequently during the night or too early in the morning, even after taking melatonin.

In order to duplicate the mechanisms by which the young pineal gland induces youthful sleep patterns, a formula called Natural Sleep has been developed. This formula contains two different melatonin delivery systems that work together to generate the same kind of secretion of melatonin that occurs naturally in young people.

Here is how Natural Sleep works: First, the Natural Sleep capsule bursts open in the stomach within five minutes after swallowing to provide immediate-release melatonin. That induces the drowsiness needed to get to sleep. Then, Natural Sleep gradually introduces tiny beadlets of sustained-release melatonin into your digestive tract, to enable you to stay asleep and avoid the nocturnal tossing and turning characteristic of age-related sleep disturbances.

Only pharmaceutical-grade melatonin is used in Natural Sleep. This is the identical form of melatonin used in the published studies documenting melatonin's insomnia-relieving properties.

Each capsule of Natural Sleep contains 2.5 mg of immediate-release melatonin plus 2.5 mg of sustained-release melatonin, for an average daily dose of 5 mg of melatonin. This is the average dose most people find effective to enable them to enjoy a complete night's rest every night.

Natural Sleep also contains vitamin B12 because of studies showing that it can normalize circadian rhythms, thereby enabling people to enter sleep without stress or tension. Also, chromium picolinate and chromium polynicotinate are included in the new formula to help lower blood sugar levels that can inhibit the ability to fall asleep. Niacinamide ascorbate, magnesium, calcium and inositol are included as well in Natural Sleep to help induce a state of relaxation.

Some people use the herb valerian to fall asleep. Valerian produces a drug-like hypnotic effect within the central nervous system similar to benzodiazepine drugs such as Valium and Halcion. Since valerian-containing products often are promoted as natural herbal remedies, the public mistakenly believes it is safe to take on a regular basis. Studies indicate, however, that there is a significant toxicity risk when taking valerian over an extended period of time. Since a tolerance effect occurs with valerian due to its Valium-like properties, people often need to take greater and greater amounts of it as time goes by in order to continue to obtain the desired hypnotic (sleep-inducing) effect. Further, the chronic use of valerian could result in permanent liver damage along with potential central nervous system impairment.

The Life Extension Foundation has thoroughly investigated the use of herbal insomnia remedies such as valerian, hops and passion flower, and found that they have an unacceptable risk of toxicity with long-term use.

Natural Sleep does not contain any potentially toxic herbal extracts. Insomnia often is a lifelong affliction, requiring the continuous need for nightly self-medication. The ingredients in Natural Sleep have been thoroughly investigated for long-term safety, and can be taken for an indefinite period of time without any risk of toxicity or tolerance.

Depression often is an underlying cause of insomnia. For alternate suggestions to FDA-approved antidepressant drugs, refer to the Depression protocol in this book.

Product availability: To order Natural Sleep or other melatonin products, call 1-800-544-4440.

Jet Lag

Jet lag is caused by disruption of the body's circadian rhythm cycle because of a rapid move to a new time zone. The body's circadian rhythm is controlled by the release of the pineal hormone melatonin, which has been shown to alleviate jet lag in several studies by synchronizing biological rhythms. One study showed that melatonin was a well-tolerated remedy for jet lag on long-haul flights.

Another study looked at the effects of melatonin during the rapid deployment of Army aviation personnel across time zones. The soldiers suffered the combined insult to their systems of going on missions beginning immediately upon arrival, which resulted in desynchronization of physiological and cognitive performance rhythms. The benefits of melatonin (10 mg) in maintaining stable sleep/wake cycles of Army air crews was tested during a training mission involving rapid deployment to the Middle East and night operations. Cognitive performance was tested before and after travel. Activity rhythms were recorded continuously for 13 days. Melatonin treatment advanced both bed times and rise times, and maintained sleep durations between seven and eight hours. Placebo treatment mostly was associated with longer advances in rise times than bed times, resulting in shorter sleep durations (five to seven hours).

Upon awakening, the melatonin group exhibited significantly fewer errors (mean 7.5) than the placebo group (mean 14.5) in a dual task-vigilance test. This study demonstrated the value of melatonin for the prevention not only of sleep disruptions but also of cognitive degradation, even in uncontrolled sleeping environments characteristic of military deployments.

The best way of using melatonin to alleviate jet lag is to take one 3-mg capsule of melatonin the night before you leave, and another 3 mg capsule on the first night you go to sleep in your new destination. The melatonin will adjust your circadian rhythm to the new time zone, and you should wake up feeling as if you were home. If you are able to sleep on the plane, taking melatonin at that time could enable you to arrive at your new destination fully refreshed.

Product availability: Pharmaceutical-grade melatonin supplements in a wide range of potencies are available by calling 1-800-544-4440.

Kidney Disease

The kidney has a pivotal role in maintaining taurine balance throughout the body. Taurine has been shown to concentrate in a unique pattern along the specialized cells of the kidneys (nephrons) and to protect against experimentally induced lipid peroxidation of the renal tubular and glomerular cells.

The beneficial effects of taurine on kidney function may be due to its antioxidant actions. Researchers have suggested that clinical trials be done to determine the usefulness of taurine as an adjunct (assisting) therapy in the treatment of progressive glomerular disease and diabetic nephropathy. Suggested supplementation with taurine is 1,000 mg, two to three times a day.

High levels of homocysteine can be especially damaging to the kidney. Homocysteine can be lowered by taking 800 micrograms of folic acid, 300 micrograms of vitamin B12, and 500 mg of TMG (trimethylglycine, also known as betaine) twice a day. At least 150 mg of vitamin B6 also should be taken throughout the day for optimal homocysteine reduction. Kidney dialysis patients often require higher levels of such homocysteine-lowering nutrients as folic acid and vitamin B12.

Free-radical damage has been implicated as a major cause of renal failure. Vitamin E has been shown to restore urinary filtration and flow to rats with severe kidney disease by suppressing free radicals that cause tubulointerstitial injury. The suggested dose is 800 to 1,200

IU a day of Vitamin E succinate.

For kidney stones, take about 2,000 mg a day of magnesium to inhibit calcium oxalate formation. Kidney stone patients should always have a blood test to measure serum calcium and parathyroid hormone to make sure they are not suffering from hyperparathyroidism.

Refer to the Acetaminophen (Tylenol) Poisoning protocol to learn about a common cause of kidney disease.

Refer to the Diabetes protocols if you are diabetic.

Product availability: Taurine, Vitamin E succinate and magnesium are available by phoning 1-800-544-4440.

Learning Disorders

Refer to Age-Associated Mental Impairment (Brain Aging) or Attention Deficit Disorder (ADD) protocols.

Leukemia-Lymphoma (and Hodgkin's Disease)

Cancers of the blood-forming organs and lymph tissues respond better to conventional chemotherapy than most forms of cancer. The rate of cure of Hodgkin's lymphoma using chemotherapy has been reported to be between 70 and 80 percent. It should be noted that there are many forms of leukemia and lymphoma, so each treatment regimen has to be based on the specific type of disease that has been diagnosed.

Alternative cancer therapies should be used with caution when treating leukemia or lymphoma because many alternative therapies boost immune cell function, which could speed the proliferation of leukemia and lymphoma cancer cells. Nevertheless, there are specific alternative therapies that may be effective in treating certain forms of leukemia and lymphoma.

A vitamin-A analog drug called Vesanoid has been approved for promyelocytic leukemia. This drug inhibits leukemia cell division and helps cells to mature into normal cells. We recommend that leukemia and lymphoma patients ask their oncologists to consider prescribing Vesanoid, even though it has been approved for only one form of leukemia.

If your doctor will not prescribe Vesanoid because the FDA has not approved it for your type of cancer, we suggest that you use 100,000 to 300,000 IU a day of water-soluble vitamin A liquid. Monthly blood tests are needed to guard against the possibility of vitamin A liver toxicity.

Important: Refer to the Symptoms of Vitamin A Toxicity, in Appendix A.

Vitamin D3 and its analogs can induce certain leukemia and lymphoma cells to differentiate into normal cells. The Life Extension Foundation suggests that leukemia/lymphoma patients take 4,000 to 6,000 IU of vitamin D3 a day on an empty stomach. Vitamin D3 may enhance the anti-proliferative effects of vitamin A and vitamin A analog drugs. Data show vitamin D3 derivatives inhibit myeloma cell growth in comparison with conventional drugs used to treat multiple myeloma.

Vitamin D3 derivatives 1) induce arrested growth of human myeloma cells; 2) induce apoptosis (programmed cell death) in synergy with the conventional drugs and immune cytokines; 3) downregulate the expression receptor on malignant plasma cells; and 4) inhibit the deleterious side effects of conventional drugs that can up-regulate cancer cell gene expression.

This strongly suggests that specific vitamin D3 analogs could be of value in the treatment of multiple myeloma, especially in association with the conventional drug dexamethasone. Even though vitamin A drugs can induce complete remissions in patients with acute promyelocytic leukemia, the duration of response is short, and further therapy with this agent is less effective, suggesting the development of drug resistance. Researchers are overcoming this drug resistance problem by using retinoic acid in combination with other agents that can induce differentiation, such as vitamin D3 or its analogs. Monthly blood tests to monitor serum calcium and liver and kidney function should be done to protect against vitamin D3 toxicity. The recommended doses of vitamin D3 are high, and physician monitoring is suggested.

All-trans-retinoic acid is an effective vitamin analog drug that has been shown to reduce mortality and significantly prolong the disease-free survival in acute promyelocytic leukemia. It also appears to be effective against other leukemias. When combined with alpha interferon, all-trans-retinoic acid appears to be effective in patients with chronic myeloid leukemia. A side effect of this therapy is the induction of thrombosis (blood clotting inside blood vessels). Thrombosis could be inhibited by low molecular weight heparin or possibly by the nutrients listed in the Thrombosis Prevention Protocol.

Chronic lymphocytic leukemia (CLL) patients have not responded well to vitamin A and vitamin D3 analog drug therapies. CLL patients should still consider supplementation with vitamin A and vitamin D3 because of the documented benefits these nutrients have against a wide range of cancer cells.

Curcumin, widely used as a spice and coloring agent in food, possesses potent antioxidant, anti-inflammatory and anti-tumor promoting activities. Curcumin has been found to induce apoptotic cell death in promyelocytic leukemia. The antioxidants N-acetylcysteine (NAC), L-ascorbic acid, alpha-tocopherol, catalase and superoxide dismutase all may effectively prevent curcumin-induced apoptosis. Therefore, if a leukemia patient is going to take the recommended 2,000 mg of curcumin a day with a heavy meal, he or she should avoid antioxidant supplements.

Soy genistein, vitamins A and D3, and conventional therapies do not appear to interfere with curcumin-induced apoptosis.

Do not take curcumin if you have biliary tract obstruction.

Soy extracts with a high concentration of genistein inhibit leukemia/lymphoma cell proliferation by interfering with protein tyrosine kinase, the enzyme that cancer cells need for replication. Genistein is a specific inhibitor of protein tyrosine kinase. The growth inhibition associated with genistein strongly supports the use of genistein for bone marrow purging in many forms of leukemia.

Do not take soy extract when undergoing radiation therapy because the genistein in soy can interfere with the ability of the radiation to kill cancer cells.

The Life Extension Foundation has preliminary evidence about the types of cancer that soy extract may be effective against, and the types of cancer which it may be less effective against.

Genistein has produced significant cell growth inhibition in many types of cancer. A study was conducted to examine the effects of genistein on cancer cell growth factors such as protein kinase C. Genistein suppresses protein kinase C activity and the subsequent growth stimulating incorporation of thymidine into cancer cells.

An investigation into the effects of soy genistein on the growth and differentiation of human melanoma cells showed that genistein significantly inhibited cell growth. Some studies suggest that genistein may enhance the efficacy of certain chemotherapy regimens.

Cancer patients whose tumor cells have a mutant p53 oncogene are far more likely to benefit from soy extract supplementation. Only a pathology examination of the actual cancer cells can determine p53 status. An immuno-histochemistry test can help to determine the p53 status of tumor cells. The following laboratory can perform this new test:

IMPATH Laboratories
1010 Third Avenue, Suite 203
New York, N.Y. 10021
Phone: 1-800-447-5816

IMPATH Laboratories measures mutant p53. If the test is positive, you have mutant p53 and are *more* likely to benefit from soy extracts. If the test is negative, this indicates that you have functional p53 and are *less* likely to benefit from soy extracts. The Foundation realizes that many cancer patients seeking to use soy supplements may find it difficult to have an immuno-histochemistry test performed to ascertain p53 status.

The most concentrated soy extract product available is called Mega Soy Extract. The suggested dose for cancer patients is five 700-mg capsules of Mega Soy Extract four times a day. This provides the optimal daily dose of approximately 2,800 mg of standardized genistein. Genistein is rapidly metabolized within the body, which makes it necessary for cancer patients to take Mega Soy Extract in four divided doses spaced evenly throughout the day.

Soy genistein may inhibit an enzyme that normally recycles cyclooxygenases in the colon. This may lead to excess levels of Cox-2 (cyclooxygenase 2) in the colon. Cox-2 causes excess production of prostaglandin E2, which in turn can promote cancer growth, stimulate angiogenesis and induce immunosuppression. Colon cancer patients taking soy supplements should consider taking an aspirin with their heavy meal every day to inhibit Cox-2. Other Cox-2 inhibitors include a daily dose of fish oil concentrate containing 2,400 mg of EPA and 1,800 mg of DHA, 2,000 mg of ginger extract and 6,000 mg a day of garlic. For some cancers, inhibition of Cox-2 can be an effective adjuvant therapy in and of itself.

In a study on chronic myelogenous leukemia (CML) , the continuous exposure to genistein induced a statistically significant and dose-dependent suppression of CML colony formation. Genistein caused a 50 percent inhibition of CML and normal progenitors. Analysis of nuclear DNA fragmentation showed that preincubation of CML with genistein induced significant evidence of apoptosis. These observations show that genistein is capable of exerting a strong antiproliferative effect on this type of leukemia, probably through an apoptotic (programmed cell death) mechanism.

Cancer patients undergoing radiation therapy should not take soy supplements one week before, during, and one week after being treated. Soy inhibits protein kinase C activity in cancer cells. Since cancer cells use protein kinase C for energy production, inhibiting this enzyme is usually desirable. Radiation therapy, on the other hand, depends on protein kinase C to help generate free radicals that kill cancer cells. It's possible, therefore, that large amounts of genistein in cancer cells could protect them against radiation-induced free radical-mediated destruction.

Since all cancer therapies produce individual responses, the Foundation recommends that all cancer patients have monthly blood tumor marker tests to determine if the therapies they are using are working or not. If, for instance, tumor markers were to continue to elevate 30 to 60 days after initiating soy extract supplementation, discontinue its use and seek another therapy immediately.

We cannot overemphasize the importance of monthly blood testing for all cancer patients. Every patient responds differently to both conventional and alternative cancer therapies. The results of blood tests provide critically important data to evaluate the effectiveness of these therapies. Some of the blood tests commonly used in defining progression or regression of leukemia include CBC with differential, immune cell differentiation, and the leukemia profile.

CAUTION: Some doctors are under the impression that leukemia, Hodgkin's disease, and lymphoma patients should avoid melatonin until more is known about its effects on these forms of cancer. If melatonin is tried in these types of cancer, tumor blood markers should be watched closely for any sign that melatonin is promoting tumor growth.

The Life Extension Foundation recommends that leukemia/lymphoma patients use these alternative therapies in addition to conventional therapy.

Product availability: Water-soluble vitamin A liquid, vitamin D3 caps and Mega Soy Extract are available by phoning 1-800-544-4440. Vesanoid is a prescription drug that should be prescribed by your oncologist or hematologist.

Liver (Cirrhosis)

Liver degeneration can be caused by chronic alcohol (ethanol) intake, viral disease, FDA-approved drugs, malnutrition, congestive heart failure and various hepatic toxins. Cirrhosis of the liver occurs when too many liver cells break down and become infiltrated with non-functioning fat cells.

It is possible to regenerate a degenerated liver if extraordinary therapies are followed and the underlying cause of the cirrhosis is eliminated.

Free radicals directly cause liver injury and fibrosis. Vitamin E and related compounds appear to be the most reasonable antioxidants to protect against oxidative damage to the liver. Specific therapies to help protect against free radicals and regenerate the liver include a daily regimen of 500 mg of vitamin B1, 75 mg of vitamin B2, 1,500 mg of vitamin B5, 200 mg of vitamin B6, 1,500 mg of choline, 1,600 micrograms of folic acid, 500 mg of vitamin C, 800 IU of vitamin E, 300 micrograms of selenium and 100 mg of coenzyme Q10.

CAUTION: Avoid niacin, vitamin A and beta-carotene as these nutrients can be harmful to a severely damaged liver.

Also, acetyl-L-carnitine should be taken in two daily doses of 1,000 mg each, along with two daily doses of 600 mg each of N-acetylcysteine. Green tea in a dose of four to 10 standardized 100-mg capsules a day can be used to lower toxic levels of iron that may be generating dangerous free radicals in the liver. Five to 10 grams of arginine and 2,000 mg a day of glutamine may help to lower toxic ammonia levels in the blood caused by a defective liver, if there is at least a 20-percent reserve capacity remaining. Arginine also can help facilitate liver regeneration.

An important therapy to help restore liver function and prevent chronic encephalopathy involves the branched-chain amino acids. This includes twice-daily administration of 1,200 mg of leucine, 600 mg of isoleucine, and 600 mg of valine.

Silymarin has been proven to protect the liver via several identified mechanisms. Long term treatment is able to reduce mortality even in patients with established alcoholic liver cirrhosis. According to the published data available today, silymarin treatment, at a dose of about 300 mg a day, should be applied to all patients suffering from alcoholic liver disease.

Type II diabetes patients with liver cirrhosis often suffer severe diabetic complications. Treatment with silymarin has been shown to reduce the lipoperoxidation of cell membranes and insulin resistance, thus significantly decreasing the need for exogenous insulin administration.

In addition, the European antidepressant drug S-adenosylmethionine (SAMe) has potent liver regeneration properties. Suggested dose is four to eight 200-mg tablets of SAMe throughout the day until normal liver function is restored. Regular blood tests for liver function are required to assess the effectiveness of whatever therapy is being used.

Ethanol damages the liver by the generation of free radicals and by depressing an enzyme required to convert methionine into SAMe. An alcohol-induced depletion of SAMe can be bypassed by SAMe supplementation, which restores hepatic SAMe levels and significantly attenuates ethanol-induced liver injury. Supplementation with 400 to 800 mg twice a day of SAMe may be able to reverse alcoholic cirrhosis. For those alcoholics who cannot afford the high price of SAMe, supplementation twice a day with 500 mg of trimethylglycine (TMG, also known as betaine), 800 micrograms of folic acid and 500 micrograms of vitamin B12 could facilitate natural liver synthesis of SAMe. Phosphatidylcholine supplementation at 2,000 mg a day may protect against alcohol-induced septal fibrosis, cirrhosis and lipid peroxidation.

Anemia is a frequent complication in patients with cirrhosis, and folate deficiency is significantly more common in alcoholic patients. Iron deficiency should be ruled out if anemia is present, but supplementation with excess iron must be done with caution as excess iron can cause severe iron damage. There is growing evidence that normal or only mildly increased amounts of iron in the liver can be damaging, particularly when they are combined with such other hepatotoxic factors as alcohol, porphyrogenic drugs, or chronic viral hepatitis. Iron enhances the disease-producing abilities of viruses, adversely affects immune function and enhances fibrogenic pathways, all of which may increase liver injury due to iron. Iron also may be a co-carcinogen or promoter of hepatocellular carcinoma, even in patients without hepatitis C or cirrhosis.

A deficiency of vitamin B1 may directly cause alcoholic cirrhosis. One study attributed vitamin B1 (thiamine) deficiency as a greater risk factor for liver cell death than heavy alcohol consumption.

For specific anti-viral therapies to help eradicate hepatitis B or hepatitis C, refer to our Hepatitis B and Hepatitis C protocols.

Product availability: SAMe, vitamin B1, vitamin B2, vitamin B5, vitamin B6, folic acid, choline, vitamin C, vitamin E, coenzyme Q10, acetyl-L-carnitine, N-acetylcysteine, green tea, arginine, curcumin, silymarin and the branched-chain amino acid complex can be ordered by phoning 1-800-544-4440.

Lupus

Lupus is thought to be caused by autoimmune reactions. Refer to the Life Extension Foundation's Autoimmune Disease protocol. Lupus patients should exercise extreme caution when attempting any new medical therapy as there is a chance the condition could be made worse.

Macular Degeneration (Dry)

Dry macular degeneration is characterized by a deficiency of blood flow to some parts of the eye, causing atrophy and a slow loss of vision.

Nutrients that may improve micro capillary circulation in the eye include ginkgo biloba at 120 mg a day, grape seed-skin extract at 150 mg a day, and bilberry extract at 150 mg a day.

A double-blind case-controlled study showed that those with macular degeneration had decreased intake of vitamin E, magnesium, zinc, vitamin B6 and folic acid. This study identified 14 specific antioxidant components that could stabilize, but not improve, dry macular degeneration when consumed for a period of 1.5 years. Supplementation with the Life Extension Mix and Life Extension Booster formulas provide these specific antioxidant components. Also, Life Extension Mix and Booster contain other nutrients, such as lutein, which have been shown to prevent wet macular degeneration.

Hydergine in doses of 4 to 5 mg a day and higher has shown benefit in treating dry macular degeneration. The following antioxidant nutrients also should be considered: alpha-lipoic acid, 500 mg a day; and glutathione, 500 mg a day.

The daily application of the vitamin A-based Viva Drops can provide antioxidant protection to the lens of the eye. Also, wrap-around UV-blocking sunglasses provide significant protection against UV sun rays. Exposure to sunlight without wearing UV blocking sunglasses is a risk factor in developing macular degeneration.

Cigarette smoking among women has been shown to increase the risk of macular degeneration by 2.4-fold, compared with women who never smoked. Those who quit smoking still had a twofold increased risk relative to those who had never smoked. Even among those who had quit smoking for 15 or more years, little reduction in risk was shown, compared with current smokers. Cigarette smoking has been determined to be an independent and avoidable risk factor for age-related macular degeneration among women.

The standard daily dose of Life Extension Mix — three tablets, three times a day — provides adequate levels of vitamin B-complex, zinc and other nutrients that are crucial for ocular function.

Anyone with dry macular degeneration also should refer to the Wet Macular Degeneration protocol, since those with dry macular degeneration are at a high risk of developing the more-debilitating wet macular degeneration.

Product availability: Ginkgo biloba extract, proanthocyanidins (grape seed-skin extract), bilberry extract, selenium, alpha-lipoic acid, glutathione, zinc, Life Extension Mix, Viva Drops and wrap-around sunglasses can be obtained by calling 1-800-544-4440.

Macular Degeneration (Wet)

Wet macular degeneration is characterized by an overgrowth of leaky blood vessels into the retina of the eye. When these blood vessels rupture, they cause severe visual loss, usually leading to blindness. However, those who eat a large amount of spinach and collard greens have very low rates of wet macular degeneration.

The phytochemicals that protect against wet macular degeneration are lutein and zeaxanthin. Life Extension Mix and Chloroplex both contain lutein. Those with early-stage wet macular degeneration also should use a product called Lutein Plus, which provides potent concentrations of both zeaxanthin and lutein. One tablespoon a day of Lutein Plus vegetable powder is suggested to prevent or slow the progress of wet macular degeneration.

The overgrowth of new blood vessels in the eye is called angiogenesis. Soy contains the phytochemical genistein, which has anti-angiogenesis properties. Those with wet macular degeneration may want to take two 700-mg capsules, two times a day, of Mega Soy Extract in order to obtain enough genistein to possibly inhibit blood-vessel growth in the eye.

Also, there are several new anti-angiogenesis drugs being developed, primarily to treat cancer. An FDA advisory panel has approved thalidomide to treat leprosy. Thalidomide is an extremely potent anti-angiogenesis drug that could slow or possibly stop the progression of wet macular degeneration. It would be legal for doctors to prescribe thalidomide to treat wet macular degeneration, even though it only will be officially approved to treat leprosy.

CAUTION: Thalidomide causes severe birth defects and must not be used by pregnant women or women who may become pregnant.

Free radical damage has been implicated in the development of wet macular degeneration. Zinc, vitamin C and Vitamin E deficiencies have been found in many people who develop wet macular degeneration. It should be noted that these vitamins have not yet been shown to slow the progression of the disease once it has been clinically manifested. The daily dose of Life Extension Mix — three tablets, three times a day — will provide broad-spectrum antioxidant protection against free radical damage to the eye. An additional 30 mg of zinc also should be considered.

Product availability: Lutein powder, Mega Soy Extract, Life Extension Mix, zinc, Lutein Plus and wrap-around UV blocking sunglasses are available by phoning 1-800-544-4440.

Medical Testing Protocols

The Life Extension Foundation has advocated regular medical testing since 1983 for the purpose of optimizing your personal life extension program. Regular blood testing enables you to detect:

1. Abnormalities that may predispose you to diseases that are treatable if caught at an early stage, such as cancer, diabetes and cardiovascular disease.

2. Toxicities that could be counteracted to prevent organ damage—for example, liver damage caused by hepatotoxic drugs, vitamin A, iron overload, etc.—by adjusting your nutrient-drug intake.

3. Hormone imbalances—e.g., DHEA deficiency or cortisol overload—that can accelerate your rate of aging if not corrected.

4. Other imbalances that could be adjusted to enable you to become healthier, more energetic, sexier and stronger.

Here are some of the important tests that can be used to assess your health and longevity, and the results you should strive to attain:

❖ **Glucose: Optimal level should be under 100.**

A consistent effect of calorie restriction is a reduction in serum glucose levels to within a normal range. Calorie restriction is the only documented method of extending maximum life span. Calorie-restricted people often have serum glucose levels between 70 and 80. When glucose levels are greater than 100, accelerated aging can occur via several mechanisms.

Glucose-lowering nutrients include 200 micrograms of chromium picolinate with every meal, and/or 7.5 mg of vanadyl sulfate three times a day, and/or four decaffeinated green tea capsules with every meal, and/or fiber supplements. If your glucose level is too high, you should have your thyroid hormone level checked. If it is too low, you should consider low-dose thyroid hormone under a doctor's supervision. Another method of improving thyroid function is to take 6 to 30 grams of a highly concentrated soy extract, which can help to normalize your thyroid hormone levels.

❖ **Iron: Optimal level should be under 100.**

Iron is a catalyst for free radical activity that increases the risk of heart disease, Alzheimer's disease, cancer and a host of degenerative diseases. Low iron levels have been shown to protect against cancer and heart disease in large human populations.

Iron-lowering nutrients include four decaffeinated green tea capsules and/or four garlic/EDTA capsules with every meal, and/or the undergoing of a series of intravenous chelation (metal-removing) treatments under the care of a physician, and/or the donating of a pint of blood to yourself for future use.

❖ **Cholesterol: Optimal LDL cholesterol level below 120. Optimal HDL cholesterol level above 50.**

Oxidized LDL cholesterol adheres to the inner linings of arteries, a condition which contributes to atherosclerosis. It also promotes abnormal arterial clotting. HDL cholesterol removes excess fat and other types of cholesterol from the arterial system.

Nutrients that favorably alter cholesterol levels—i.e., lower dangerous LDL cholesterol and elevate HDL cholesterol—include 200 micrograms of chromium picolinate twice a day, 30 grams a day of soluble fiber, 1,000 to 3,000 mg a day of niacin with meals, and 2,000 mg a day and higher of vitamin C. Herbal extracts such as curcumin and gugulipid have dose-related cholesterol-lowering effects.

❖ **Triglycerides: Optimal triglyceride level is below 100.**

Triglycerides combine a fatty acid and glycerol. Elevated triglyceride levels predispose a person to atherosclerosis and abnormal platelet aggregation. Nutrients that may lower elevated triglyceride levels include high doses of fish oil, garlic and niacin.

Why Blood Tests Are Not Used Regularly

The high cost and inconvenience of regular blood testing prevents many people from being tested as often as they should be. Another problem with blood testing is that different labs often produce varying readings from the same blood specimen, making the results of regular testing difficult to interpret.

The Life Extension Foundation receives blood-test results for evaluation from members who sometimes use different laboratories every time they are tested. In many cases, the member is not even aware that different laboratories had been used in testing.

Another problem is that commercial testing laboratories seldom perform the unique tests that Foundation members request, which means, for example, that a lab technician may be doing his first-ever DHEA serum test on your blood.

In order to standardize the methods used for all blood tests, the Life Extension Foundation has made an arrangement with a nationwide testing laboratory to perform all basic blood testing. For specialized tests to measure DHEA, growth hormone and cortisol , the Foundation has contracted with a reputable specialty laboratory which has been performing these unique tests for 15 years.

Here are descriptions and discount prices for the most popular blood tests:

Blood Chemistry/Complete Blood Count

This testing panel includes LDL, HDL, total cholesterol, triglycerides, iron, glucose, liver and kidney function, and many more important tests.

These tests detect blood changes that may predispose you to a wide range of degenerative diseases. They also provide information to assess whether or not the drugs and nutrients you may be taking are causing liver, kidney or heart damage.

We suggest that this battery of tests be performed annually. If a serious abnormality is detected, such as elevated glucose, cholesterol or iron, testing should be repeated more often to determine the benefits of whatever therapy you are using to correct the potentially life-shortening abnormality.

Member price $37.00, non member price $55.00.

Fibrinogen

Elevated levels of fibrinogen predispose you to arterial clotting that can cause a heart attack or a stroke. Elevated fibrinogen may be at least as great a risk factor for coronary artery disease as elevated LDL cholesterol. Optimal fibrinogen levels should be under 300.

Fibrinogen-lowering nutrients include bromelain in doses of 250 to 1,000 mg twice a day, and/or eight fish oil capsules a day, and/or beta-carotene in doses of 25,000 IU to 100,000 IU a day, and/or vitamin C in doses exceeding 2,000 mg a day, and/or taking a European drug called Bezafibrate.

Member price $37.00, non member price $55.00.

Prostate Specific Antigen (PSA)

The PSA test is more than 80-percent accurate in detecting prostate cancer and measuring the effectiveness of prostate cancer therapies.

The Life Extension Foundation believes that men over 40 should have a PSA test annually. And men over 60 should have this test every six months. Individuals with prostate cancer should have a PSA test every 30 days in order to measure the efficacy of the prostate cancer therapy they are using.

Member price $40.00, non member price $60.00.

Immune Cell Subset Tests

For people with cancer, HIV infection, chronic herpes outbreaks, hepatitis, autoimmune disorders and other diseases that suppress immune function, or who have declining immune function due to normal aging, the immune cell subset test shows your T-helper to T-suppressor cell ratio, your total T-helper cell count, and natural killer cells. This information can be used to help develop an immune system-boosting program that could put these diseases into long-term remission.

The immune cell subset test should be repeated several months after the initiation of such immune-boosting therapies as isoprinosine, melatonin, gamma linolenic acid (GLA) and DHEA, with the objective of restoring your immune system to normal, healthy function.

Member price $210.00, non member price $315.00.

Hormone and Cancer Profiles

If you are considering hormone-replacement therapy, we suggest that you take one or more of the tests below. Low DHEA levels can be raised to youthful levels by taking DHEA. We suggest, after you take your initial DHEA sulfate test to determine the dosage you need, further DHEA testing be done three weeks and six months after commencing DHEA-replacement therapy and every six months thereafter.

Men who take DHEA or pregnenolone should have a PSA test done because DHEA may elevate testosterone levels, which can cause existing prostate cancer cells to hyperproliferate. DHEA and pregnenolone usually are contraindicated in men with prostate cancer. However, some scientists favor its limited use in prostate cancer patients.

Men (and women, to a lesser extent) should consider testing to determine if DHEA is elevating their testosterone levels, which in turn could produce an anti-aging effect. Women (and men to a lesser extent) should consider testing for total estradiol to see if DHEA is elevating their estrogen levels, which might reduce or eliminate their need for estrogen replacement therapy, and which may become undesirably elevated in men.

Ovarian and breast cancer patients should consider that DHEA supplementation may increase estrogen levels in some individuals, and that estrogen may be a contributing factor to these disorders. In this respect, the estrogen receptor-blocking properties of melatonin may prevent estrogen from causing such a problem.

New findings indicate that growth hormone plays an important role in maintaining many functions of youth, including the formation of new bone matrix and the maintenance of normal protein synthesis in brain cells. Hence, there is the test for IGF-1 (somatomedin-C).

Aging is associated with the excess secretion of cortisol from the adrenal glands. Cortisol is a glucocorticoid hormone that suppresses immune function, inhibits healthy brain-cell metabolism, promotes atherosclerosis, and accelerates aging. The drawback of cortisol testing is that it needs to be done twice in the same day, around 9 a.m. and 4 p.m., to obtain reliable results.

Cortisol reducing therapies include:

1. vitamin C (at least 4 grams a day)
2. Aspirin

3. DHEA- or pregnenolone-replacement therapy

4. Double doses of the procaine formulas KH3 or GH3

If you have elevated cortisol , we suggest trying several of the therapies above and then repeating the cortisol test monthly until you find the right combination of therapies to reduce your cortisol levels adequately.

	Member Price	Non-Member Price
DHEA Sulfate	$ 51.00	$ 77.00
Free Testosterone (men and women)	$ 78.00	$112.00
Estradiol	$ 68.00	$102.00
Total Progesterone	$ 68.00	$102.00
Ovarian Cancer Marker (CA 125)	$ 77.00	$115.00
Breast Cancer Marker (CA 27.29)	$ 77.00	$115.00
Gastric Pancreatic Marker (CA 19.9)	$ 77.00	$115.00
Somatomedin-C (IGF-1) (growth hormone marker)	$159.00	$238.00
Cortisol (x1)	$ 40.00	$ 60.00

Cancer Profile

Emil Schandl, Ph.D., a clinical biochemist and oncobiologist with the Center for Metabolic Disorders and American Metabolic Testing Laboratories, has developed a battery of blood tests designed to predict your risk of developing cancer (CA) long before symptoms occur. This CA Profile includes the HCG and HCG b hormones, PHI (phosphohexose isomerase) and GGTP (g-glutamyl transpeptidase) enzymes, CEA (carcinoembrionic antigen), TSH (thyroid stimulating hormone), and DHEA-S (dehydroepiandrosterone, the "anti-stress, immunity, and longevity hormone"). Dr. Schandl also suggests a PTH (parathyroid hormone) test to evaluate calcium status in the bones.

The CA Profile yields 90 positives out of 100 pathologically established malignancies. Because of its capacity to foretell the development of cancer years before a tumor is apparent, a positive finding is a serious warning sign of a developing cancer. The CA Profile test also can be used to monitor the response of cancer patients to various therapies . . . an increasing or decreasing value of a tumor marker may indicate the futility or benefits of a therapy.

Also, the CA Profile can be combined with specific cancer tests, such as the PSA, CA 27.29 (to detect breast cancer), CA 125 (to detect ovarian cancer), and CA 19.9 (for pancreatic or gastric cancer) to provide the most complete picture of your risk and/or the status of almost every cancer.

	Member Price	Non-Member Price
Cancer Profile	$233.00	$331.00
PTH (parathyroid hormone)	$ 84.00	$126.00

Cancer may actually be the number-one killer of humans on the North American continent. Whereas there is no certain cure for cancer, it may be preventable. Fortunately, in most cases, treatments and therapies can successfully extend life for many years. It is essential for cancer patients and their physicians to know how a person is responding to therapy. Biochemical tests are the quickest and most sensitive heralds in this respect.

Persons who appear to be healthy may be harboring growing, developing cancer cells without any physical signs or symptoms. In other words, no diagnosis can be made by X-rays or other established methods. The importance of early diagnosis, made possible by biochemical tests, cannot be over-emphasized.

The CA Profile, together with a chemistry profile (SMAC or similar), CBC with differential and platelet count, PTH for the evaluation of calcium metabolism, PSA for men over 40, or CA 125 and CA 27.29 for women, and CA 19.9 for both genders, is the most comprehensive evaluation available for prevention, early detection and therapeutic monitoring of metabolic disorders.

Dr. Schandl has tested thousands of patients. The results of these tests not only indicate whether or not cancer is present, but also measure the fluctuating conditions of the patient. Obviously this capacity is essential for assessing the effectiveness of the therapy instituted. This possible early diagnosis may add years of precious human life via prompt attention to the developing problem.

Even though our scientists consider the CA Profile to be the most comprehensive of its kind, a negative score does not entirely rule out the presence of cancer. It does, however, provide a reasonable degree of confidence.

The blood usually carries messages of ill health before such a condition could be detected by any other method. However, it should be mentioned that the final, definitive diagnosis for cancer is tissue/cell examination by a pathologist. The CA Profile is a very powerful tool as a part of a diagnostic work-up. A positive value may suggest, sometimes strongly, the presence or the process of developing a cancer. The tests, in general, are not organ-specific.

The CA Profile tests are the following:

HCG	May be elevated in cancer, stress related to cancer, a developing cancer, or pregnancy. Normal: less than one mlU/mL; gray up to 3.0.
PHI	May be elevated above 42 in cancer, developing cancer, active AIDS, other viral

disease, or acute heart, liver or muscle disease. Normal: less than 42 U/L.

GGTP
May be elevated above 41 U/L in females and 53 U/L in males in diseases of the liver, pancreas and the biliary system.

TSH
Thyroid stimulating hormone, for thyroid and oxygen metabolism. Normals: 0.3-5.0 mcIU/mL.

DHEA-S
Adrenal anti-stress, immunity, and longevity hormone; low or zero in most cancer patients. Normal: F 35-430 micro-grams/dL, M 80-560 micrograms/dL. Results must be interpreted in reference to a person's age.

CEA
Carcinoembrionic antigen is elevated in just about all malignancies. Normals: less than 2.5 ng/mL.

Tests Also Recommended:

PSA
For men over the age of 40 to detect prostate cancer. Normals: less than 4.0 ng/mL. However, PSA values between 3.0 and 4.0 ng/mL or above should be verified by a free PSA test.

PTH
Parathyroid hormone, for the detection of calcium depletion from the bones, e.g., osteoporosis. Normals: 12-72 pg/mL.

CA 125
A sensitive marker for residual epithelial carcinomas of the ovary. Normals are less than 35 U/mL.

CA 27.29
A sensitive breast cancer marker. Normals: less than 32 U/mL.

CA 19.9
A sensitive test for gastric/pancreatic can-cer. Normals are less than 37 U/mL.

Somatomedin C (IGF 1)
Human youth/longevity/growth hormone.

A Letter From Dr. Schandl

"I designed the CA Profile while in the nuclear medicine department of a large hospital. My work was to inject people with radioactive substances for the performance of various scans: brain, bone, liver, kidney, heart, lung, etc. I felt very uncomfortable making people radioactive for the tests, touching the radioactive materials, and having to be near the radiated, injected people.

"The doses used were well within acceptable limits by all regulatory agencies. However, I have always maintained there is no such thing as safe radiation. So, having an excellent background in clinical chemistry, radiation biology, biochemistry, biology, genetics and enzymology, I composed the CA Profile. It is made up of various tests. It is not invasive or radioactive. It requires no radioactive substances nor any X-rays, CAT scan radiation or even nuclear magnetic imaging (MRI). MRI involves speedy resonance of hydrogen atom protons due to an induced electromagnetic field, which is 3,000 to 25,000 times that of our Earth's own field.

"No surgical manipulations are used. Most commonly used diagnostic modalities can potentially cause cancer themselves. A recent issue concerning mammograms is an example. There also is considerable information on the carcinogenic effects of high-energy, high-frequency magnetic (or any) radiation.

"The CA Profile is simply composed of blood tests. The only invasiveness is the prick of a needle. To assure specimen stability, samples must be handled strictly as instructed. Tests are performed weekly and results reported on Mondays. Early detection and monitoring of cancers is thus reliably achieved. The CA Profile is being used by many doctors in the U.S., as well as in Europe, Canada, South America, the Philippines and the Atlantic island communities.

"Many years of experience show the accuracy value can be as high as 92 percent. This means if there are 100 established cases with active cancer, 92 will yield positive results. Do not forget, however, the absolute final diagnosis is a biopsied specimen; that is, a tissue pathology. A positive test result may warrant a complete change of lifestyle through metabolic therapy. An M.D., D.O., chiropractor, podiatrist, dentist or acupuncture physician can order the tests."

Sincerely yours in health,

Dr. Emil K. Schandl

How To Order Blood Tests

You can order blood tests by mail by calling 1-800-208-3444. All tests must be pre-paid unless the tests are covered by Medicare or other insurance, and you have submitted the Advanced Beneficiary Notice. As soon as you place your order, you will be sent a package with information regarding the location of the nearest blood-drawing stations, a Request for Phlebotomy form, a bullet tube (if required), and a postage-paid return envelope or overnight UPS label with envelope if you are ordering specialized tests.

You should take the Request for Phlebotomy form to any of the blood drawing stations in your area (you are not limited to these facilities). There is a drawing fee, usually $5 to $10. A phlebotomist will draw the appropriate specimens of your blood; then you ship your specimen(s) to the Foundation. We will send the specimen to the designated laboratory for testing. You (or your physician) will then be mailed your test results. These results will show if you have any abnormalities. If the results show abnormalities, you should make sure you show these results to your personal physician, who can determine if you have any serious problems and what you can do about them.

If longevity risk factors, such as glucose, iron, cholesterol, fibrinogen, or other tests such as the CA Profile are abnormal—slightly elevated or below normal, for example—you can take nutritional steps to reverse the trend. You can repeat the test in 45 to 60 days, and then chart your progress in improving your health and your chances of living longer in good health.

For a professional test interpretation and a personal biochemical/nutritional program by Dr. Schandl, please call 1-800-208-3444.

Important notes:

1. Remember, if you intend to bill your tests to an insurance company or to Medicare, you need to submit a completely filled out insurance claim form and Advanced Beneficiary Notice form, your M.D. or D.O.'s UPIN number, the diagnostic code for each test ordered, your name, address and phone number, and the prescription for the tests. Other licensed practitioners of the healing arts who can order blood tests are chiropractors, podiatrists, dentists and acupuncture physicians. The Foundation cannot do mail-order blood testing paid by Medicare or other types of insurance without a health-care practitioner first ordering the test and the Advanced Beneficiary Notice filled out.

2. Blood testing is an important and exacting science. Interpretations depend on the knowledge and expertise of trained clinical scientists. Therefore, it is recommended that you work closely with your physician or other qualified health professional for a satisfactory outcome.

Product availability: To order mail-order blood tests, phone 1-800-208-3444.

Meningitis

Meningitis is an acute, life-threatening inflammatory condition caused by a pathogen that requires immediate conventional medical care.

Refer to the Bacterial Infections protocol. Also, see the Immune Enhancement protocol and the HIV Infection protocol.

Menopause

Menopause, which involves the natural cessation of menstruation, is an event stemming from the lack of ovarian function and the subsequent curtailment of ovarian hormone secretion. During menopause, menstrual patterns change dramatically, estrogen levels fall and FSH (follicle-stimulating hormone) and LH (luteinizing hormone) levels increase. During this time, 65 percent of the requests for treatment are due to night sweats, and 45 percent are due to psychological syndromes.

The primary symptoms of menopause are:

- ❖ Vasomotor: Hot flashes, palpitations, spontaneous sweating, panic attacks and the inability to sleep.

- ❖ Psychological: Anxiety, mood swings, depression, poor memory and lack of concentration.

- ❖ Urogenital: Sexual organ atrophy, dyspareunia (pain during sex), trigonitis and frequent and urgent urination.

- ❖ Skeletal: Osteoporosis, vertebral crush fractures and femoral neck fractures. Symptoms usually begin well into menopause.

- ❖ Cardiovascular: Ischemic heart disease and/or cerebrovascular disease. Symptoms usually begin well into menopause.

The average age for those seeking treatment for menopause is 44. Currently, the most prescribed hormone replacement therapy is Premarin, a form of estrogen that alleviates some of the symptoms of menopause . . . and increases, at the same time, the risk of hormone-dependent cancers.

Here is the Foundation's protocol for the treatment of menopause and post-menopause symptoms:

1. Safe estrogen and progesterone replacement therapy using soy extracts, pregnenolone and/or DHEA. Pregnenolone is converted into both estrogen and progesterone in the body. DHEA also can convert to estrogen.

2. For some women, supplementation with estriol or TriEst (which contains 80 percent estriol, the safe form of estrogen) is needed.

3. High potency vitamin and mineral supplementation.

For further information on female hormone replacement therapy, refer to the Estrogen Replacement Therapy protocol.

Product availability: Pregnenolone, soy extracts and progesterone cream are available by calling 1-800-544-4440. When calling the Foundation, ask for a listing of offshore companies that sell estriol and TriEst.

Menstrual Disorders (Premenstrual Syndrome)

Premenstrual syndrome refers to a combination of symptoms that occur two to 14 days before the onset of menstruation, and which may be caused by nutritional and/or hormonal factors. There are many symptoms that vary from person to person, and they may increase in severity with age because of declining progesterone levels.

Many factors contribute to the severity of PMS other than age, including heredity, diet, progesterone deficiency, stress, and very frequently the ingestion, intentional or otherwise, of synthetic hormones. Some women apply ¼ to ½ teaspoon of natural progesterone cream topically to their skin 14 days before their periods to reduce PMS discomfort.

The symptoms of PMS can be alleviated by avoiding synthetic hormones, either in the form of birth control pills or the even more dangerous hormones found in dairy and meat. For example, cows bred for milk production are given large amounts of hormones and antibiotics to increase their production, and animals bred for their meat are injected with massive doses of hormones to increase their weight for sale, and are fed diets with pesticide-laced grains.

Exercise has shown benefits in lessenging PMS symptoms. Exercise enables bones to retain their youthful density by creating the bone-forming cells known as osteoblasts. (Progesterone also is involved in the formation of bone-forming osteoblasts.) Exercise releases tension, and increases endorphin levels which lessen pain and increases one's sense of well-being. It also maximizes metabolism, and increases energy and the ability to deal with stress.

Diet is a major player in reducing the symptoms of PMS. A low-fat, high complex-carbohydrate, high soy-protein diet has been shown to enhance general health, ward off diseases and significantly reduce the symptoms of PMS. Soy is the best source of protein, especially for women, because it provides natural estrogens that are converted in our bodies into other hormones as needed. One tablespoon a day of a high-genistein soy powder is suggested for help in alleviating PMS and to prevent breast cancer.

We know that too much fat is dangerous, but the essential fatty acids (EFA) are, yes, essential in the natural production of hormones. EFAs help us maintain healthy weight and improve cardiovascular health, skin, hair and nail appearance. It also helps improve the elasticity and texture of the skin, and thus improves self-image. A poor or declining appearance can lead to depression, stress, anxiety and a decline in health.

Nutritional supplements are very important. Some women report that 200 to 300 mg of vitamin B6, starting two weeks before their periods, can alleviate some PMS symptoms. There are high-potency multi-vitamin supplements recommended by gynecologists for the specific purpose of alleviating PMS. Life Extension Mix is comparable to these doctor-recommended formulas. The suggested dose is three tablets three times a day of Life Extension Mix.

Extra calcium and magnesium also can alleviate PMS symptoms. The Mineral Formula For Women (four to six capsules a day) provides an excellent source of the calcium and magnesium women need to ward off the symptoms of PMS. And Udo's Choice Flax Oil provides the best combination of omega-3 and omega-6 essential fatty acids. One to two tablespoons a day is suggested.

Product availability: Mineral Formula For Women, Life Extension Mix and Udo's Choice Flax Oil can be obtained by phoning 1-800-544-4440.

Migraine

Migraine headaches can be relieved in some people by taking 10 to 40 mg of the beta-blocking drug propranolol. However, those with very low blood pressure, congestive heart failure and asthma should *avoid* this class of drugs.

An herbal extract called feverfew has been used successfully in Europe to prevent migraine headaches. The recommended dose is one capsule daily, with each capsule containing a minimum of 600 micrograms of the active ingredient parthenolide.

Another European anti-migraine therapy is hyperforat, an extract from the herb St. John's wort. The suggested dose of St. John's wort is one 300-mg tablet (standardized to contain 0.3 mg of hypericin) twice a day.

Also, the regular use of the hormone melatonin has been reported to reduce the incidence of migraine attacks and cluster headaches. The suggested dose is 3 to 10 mg a night for people over 40. Younger people may need only 500 micrograms to 1 mg of melatonin every night.

Newly approved conventional drugs now are providing more migraine suffers with relief. The most effective of these drugs is Imitrex, which can knock out an impending migraine headache before it can get going. Imitrex is an expensive prescription drug available in oral and injectable forms.

Warning: Imitrex may have dangerous side effects in the middle aged and the elderly.

Product availability: Propranolol and Imitrex are drugs that need to be prescribed by your doctor. Mygracare (feverfew), St. John's wort and melatonin can be ordered by phoning 1-800-544-4440.

Multiple Sclerosis (MS)

Multiple sclerosis is a debilitating disease caused by the loss of the protective, insulating myelin sheath covering the nerve fibers in the brain, spinal cord and peripheral nervous system. Muscle weakness, numbness, visual disturbances and multiple disabilities characterize this disease.

There are several theories to explain what causes the destruction of the myelin sheath in MS patients. Some doctors believe it is an autoimmune attack. Others believe a virus may be involved in myelin sheath destruction. Dr. Emil Schandl published a paper in the *American Journal of Clinical Nutrition* that presented a strong correlation between MS and exposure to carbon monoxide from automobile exhaust, fossil fuel-utilizing heating devices and cigarette smoking, as well as vitamin-B6 deficiency. A smoker has little hope of recovering from MS because of the constant high level of carbon monoxide that cigarette smoking produces. This also means that MS patients should avoid second-hand cigarette smoke and carbon monoxide exposure whenever possible.

The Life Extension Foundation's protocol for MS is based partially on the work of Dr. Hans Neiper of Germany, who has used for many years high-potency nutrient supplements to treat multiple sclerosis. The FDA has banned the importation of Dr. Neiper's MS nutrient formulas, but the Foundation has attempted to follow his recommendations.

To help correct autoimmune disorders and protect against free radical injury to the myelin sheath, the 56-ingredient Life Extension Mix should be taken in doses of four tablets three times a day. In addition, one capsule of Life Extension Booster should be taken daily; men also should take six capsules of Mineral Formula For Men, and women should take six capsules of Mineral Formula For Women. These formulas contain important minerals that have helped both men and women MS patients.

To protect the myelin sheath against a deficiency of essential fatty acids, eight capsules a day of Mega EPA fish oil and five capsules a day of Mega GLA borage oil should be taken. These oils help to suppress autoimmune reactions and provide the building blocks to help rebuild the myelin sheath.

Hydergine (5 to 20 mg a day), and/or acetyl-L-carnitine (1,000 mg twice a day), and/or alpha-lipoic acid (500 mg twice a day) should be taken to provide myelin sheath protection and energy enhancement to the nerve fibers. Also, coenzyme Q10 in doses of 100 mg three times a day can be especially important for MS patients. Coenzyme Q10 should be taken in oil-filled capsules for maximum assimilation. The addition of 100 to 250 mg of vitamin B6 in the form of pyridoxal phosphate, and 1,000 micrograms of sublingual (taken under the tongue) vitamin B12 could be beneficial.

Product availability: Life Extension Mix, Life Extension Booster, Mineral Formula For Men, Mineral Formula For Women, Mega EPA, Mega GLA, acetyl-L-carnitine, alpha-lipoic acid, coenzyme Q10, pyridoxal 5-phosphate and vitamin B12 are available by phoning 1-800-544-

4440. Call for a list of overseas pharmacies that sell high-potency Hydergine to Americans for personal use.

Muscle Building

Aging causes a progressive catabolic (breaking-down) effect on muscle tissue that results in muscle atrophy and a general weakening of the entire body. The underlying causes of muscle wasting are well-documented in the scientific literature. One cause of muscle atrophy is the age-associated breakdown of carbohydrate metabolism that precludes the efficient use of insulin and glucose to rebuild muscle mass.

Therapies that can restore youthful carbohydrate metabolism include 200 micrograms of chromium picolinate with every meal, 5 to 15 grams of the amino acid arginine on an empty stomach, and thyroid-replacement hormone when indicated. DHEA and growth hormone can restore aged muscles to a youthful anabolic state. Men normally take 50 to 75 mg of DHEA a day. Women usually need only 25 to 50 mg of DHEA a day. The dose of growth-hormone replacement is based on serum levels of somatomedin C, a growth-hormone metabolite. The normal dose to restore growth hormone to youthful levels is 2 to 4 IU, injected subcutaneously three times a week. Growth hormone should be used only under physician supervision.

For those who can afford human growth-hormone therapy, it can result in a marked anabolic effect on muscle mass in older people. For a referral to a physician with expertise in administering growth hormone replacement therapy, call the Life Extension Foundation at 1-800-544-4440. Refer to the DHEA-Pregnenolone Precautions for complete information about DHEA.

Estrogen is an important anabolic hormone in women. Some women find that DHEA provides benefits similar to estrogen, since DHEA favorably cascades down into estrogen in most women. Woman who are interested in estrogen therapy should refer to the Life Extension Foundation's Estrogen Replacement Therapy protocol in this book.

The age-associated decline in cellular energy production is another cause of muscle atrophy. A cell-energy enhancing program would include the daily intake of 1,000 to 2,000 mg of acetyl-L-carnitine, 100 to 300 mg of coenzyme Q10, one tablespoon of Udo's Choice flax oil, and the standard dose of the 56-ingredient multi-nutrient Life Extension Mix. Also, the amino acid glutamine is used by many body builders in the dose of 2,000 mg a day. Glutamine is especially important for aging humans in order to maintain muscle mass.

Many body builders take a large number of supplements to generate an anabolic effect, so as to build muscle mass. The most efficient way of taking most of the nutrients used by body builders is to take three heaping scoops of Optifuel powder by Twinlab. Optifuel provides the full range of amino acids and other anabolic nutrients. It must be used in conjunction with an exercise program for maximum results.

A popular product used by body builders is creatine. In a survey conducted by the magazine *Muscle Media 2000* (September 1996), 83 percent of respondents said they used creatine. Creatine has quickly become the favorite among athletes. It's one of the few supplements for athletes that has legitimate research studies backing its benefits.

Creatine is naturally produced within our bodies, and therefore it is not a foreign compound. Creatine is a natural by-product of liver, kidney and pancreas metabolism.

While arginine and glycine are precursors to creatine, they require many enzymatic steps in order for these amino acids to significantly elevate creatine levels in the body. In addition, it is difficult to get an appropriate amount of creatine from food. For example, to get 6 grams of creatine, you would have to consume approximately 3 pounds of fresh, uncooked steak (*Clin Sci*, 1992 Sept., 83:3, 367-74).

Consumers can choose from various forms of creatine, including creatine phosphate, creatine monohydrate, creatine citrate and now the creatine-based mixtures. The most stable and cost-effective form is creatine monohydrate. Don't use creatine phosphate because it is de-phosphorylated by enzymes as soon as it enters the gut. A Canadian company is marketing creatine citrate, which is a citrate salt form of creatine. There's no scientific information on creatine citrate at this time, but some clinical trials are being conducted.

Researchers note that insulin may open the gates for creatine entry into the muscles. This explains why many trainers recommend consuming creatine with sugar water or grape juice, which unlike fructose offers high glycemic-index carbohydrates. This is analogous to a fuel-injection effect for creatine.

Aging is characterized by a decline in protein synthesis that results in progressive weakening throughout the body as more cells fail to divide into fresh new cells. Creatine monohydrate supplementation is a cost-effective method of protecting and enhancing protein synthesis throughout the body.

Product availability: Chromium picolinate, Life Extension Mix, Optifuel, acetyl-L-carnitine, coenzyme Q10, DHEA, arginine, creatine monohydrate and Udo's Choice Oil Blend can be ordered by phoning 1-800-544-4440. Thyroid hormone and growth-hormone replacement therapy should be prescribed by your doctor.

Muscular Dystrophy

Muscular dystrophy is a group of diseases characterized by weakness and wasting of skeletal muscle tissue, without the breakdown (primarily demyelination) of nerve tissue. Each type of muscular dystrophy is different with regard to the group of muscles affected and the rate of progression of the disease.

A recent study showed significant benefits when muscular dystrophy patients were given high doses of coenzyme Q10. The recommended dose of coenzyme Q10 is one 100-mg oil-filled capsule three times a day.

Vitamin E and selenium deficiencies have been shown to be a direct cause of muscular dystrophies in animal studies. Muscular dystrophy patients should consider taking 400 IU of Vitamin E three times daily, and 200 micrograms of selenium two to three times a day.

Subacute degeneration of the spinal cord can be caused by a vitamin-B12 deficiency. Studies suggest that demyelination of the posterior part of the spinal cord and peripheral axonal degeneration might be related to vitamin-B12 deficiency. Muscular dystrophy patients should consider taking 2,000 micrograms of vitamin B12 in sublingual tablet form. There are many ancillary health benefits to vitamin-B12 supplementation.

The results of a controlled human study showed a significant increase of free radicals, nitric oxide, arginine, tryptophan, noradrenaline and homocysteine in multiple sclerosis patients. This same study showed low levels of aspartate, glutamate, dopamine and vitamin B12.

Based on this study, muscular dystrophy patients should *avoid* arginine (which promotes nitric oxide formation) along with phenylalanine, tyrosine and caffeine (which promotes noradrenalin). Muscular dystrophy patients should supplement with 2,000 mg a day of l-glutamine, 250 mg a day of aspartic acid, along with the homocysteine-lowering nutrients folic acid, 800 micrograms a day; vitamin B6, 100 mg a day; vitamin B12, 2,000 micrograms a day; and trimethylglycine (TMG), 500 mg day. Boosting dopamine levels could be accomplished with low doses of deprenyl (one 5-mg tablet twice a week), or high doses KH3 (two to three tablets a day).

An interesting study showed that gamma interferon could stimulate a calcium influx intracellular process that triggered muscular dystrophy activity. This study adds credence to the role played by autoimmunity in muscular dystrophy. Since melatonin may boost gamma-interferon production, those with muscular dystrophy may want to avoid melatonin. Muscular dystrophy patients may want to consider the calcium-channel blocking drug Nimotop (nimodipine). This FDA-approved prescription drug is specific to the central nervous system and significantly inhibits calcium infiltration into brain cells. The dose would be 30 mg three times a day.

S-adenosylmethionine (SAMe) is involved in numerous methylation reactions involving remyelination of nerves and neurotransmitter metabolism. For enhancing methylation, muscular dystrophy patients who can afford SAMe may consider taking 800 mg a day. The methylation-enhancing nutrients folic acid, vitamin B12 and TMG may work as well as SAMe and cost a lot less.

Experimental autoimmune encephalomyelitis (EAE) in mice is an autoimmune disease believed to be a model for human muscular dystrophy. In one study, EAE was completely prevented by the administration of vitamin D3. The researchers showed that vitamin D3 also could prevent the progression of EAE when administered at the first appearance of the disability symptoms. Further, withdrawal of vitamin D3 resulted in a resumption of the progression of EAE, and a deficiency of vitamin D resulted in an increased susceptibility to EAE. The scientists concluded that vitamin D3 or its analogs are potentially important for treatment of muscular dystrophy. Muscular dystrophy patients may consider taking around 1,000 IU of vitamin D3 once a day.

Muscular dystrophy patients also should refer to the Life Extension Foundation's Muscle Building and Catabolic Wasting protocols for additional suggestions.

Product availability: Coenzyme Q10, vitamin D3, vitamin E, SAMe, TMG and selenium are available by calling 1-800-544-4440.

Myasthenia Gravis

Myasthenia gravis is a disease characterized by periodic muscle weakness, primarily involving muscles that are connected directly to the cranial nerves. The disease is caused by an autoimmune attack on the acetylcholine receptor, resulting in a defect in the transmission of nerve signals from nerve fibers to muscles. Anything that interferes with the interaction between acetylcholine and its receptors will block neuro-muscular transmission.

In myasthenia gravis, the interaction between acetylcholine and its receptor is prevented by antibodies in the serum. These auto antibodies bind to the acetylcholine receptors and cause destruction at the tips of the folds of the muscle where the receptors are concentrated. Correcting this hyper-autoimmunity antibody production is a crucial step in gaining control over the disease.

Conventional medicine treats myasthenia gravis by suppressing the immune system with toxic corticosteroid drugs, and in extreme cases by surgically removing the entire thymus gland. However, the thymus gland is the master gland of immunity, and removing this gland severely weakens the body's ability to fight infections and cancer. Also, a primary conventional treatment for myasthenia gravis involves the use of drugs that boost acetylcholine levels by inhibiting an enzyme called cholinesterase. Cholinesterase degrades acetylcholine into choline and acetate, thus reducing the amount of acetylcholine available to interact with muscle receptors. Anti-cholinesterase drugs inhibit the degradation of acetylcholine, and are thus an important conventional treatment.

Mainstream scientists have not yet conducted studies to explore the relationship between nutrition, nutritional therapies and myasthenia gravis. However, there are nutritional therapies that appear to play an important role in the functioning and maintenance of muscle tissue.

To boost the levels of the neurotransmitter acetylcholine using dietary supplements, five capsules a day of Cognitex (which includes choline and synergistic co-factors) is suggested.

Essential fatty acids have been shown to be effective in suppressing many autoimmune diseases. Since myasthenia gravis is caused by an autoimmune attack on the acetylcholine receptor affecting normal neuromuscular transmission, myasthenia gravis patients should consider taking six to eight capsules a day of Mega EPA, a fish oil concentrate that provides a potent dose of the omega-3 fatty acids, and five capsules a day of Mega GLA to provide the critical omega-6 fatty acid gamma linolenic acid (GLA). Fish oil also may directly facilitate nerve conductivity. The lipotropic agent inositol is required to utilize the fatty acids; 1,000 to 2,000 mg a day could be helpful. Free radical damage should be reduced by taking three tablets, three times a day, of Life Extension Mix.

To improve the transmission of nerve signals, 400 mg of alpha-lipoic acid should be taken twice a day. Vitamin D3 at a dose of 1,000 IU a day could help with calcium ion exchange, which is needed for nerve conduction. Also, Hydergine can be prescribed by your physician in the range of 5 to 20 mg a day, and deprenyl at a dose of 5 mg twice a week.

High-dose intravenous immune globulin (IVIg) has emerged as a conventional therapy for various neurologic diseases. Although expensive, IVIg has become a first-line or adjunctive therapy in the treatment of diverse autoimmune diseases, including myasthenia gravis. IVIg therapy has received Food and Drug Administration approval for use as a maintenance treatment of patients with primary humoral (blood-based) immunodeficiencies, and as therapy for acute or chronic autoimmune thrombocytopenic purpura.

In controlled clinical trials, IVIg has been effective in treating chronic inflammatory demyelinating polyneuropathy. IVIg also has produced improvement in several patients with myasthenia gravis, but had a variable or unsubstantiated benefit in some patients.

Therapeutic plasma exchange has been advocated in several neurologic disorders, but clinical trials assessing the efficacy of plasma exchange have come to controversial conclusions. A conference on the subject concluded that plasma exchange is a promising new mode of treatment of several neurologic diseases, including myasthenia gravis.

Nerve-conduction failure can be caused by demyelinated nerve fibers. The role of demyelination of nerve fibers has not been fully established in myasthenia gravis, but some studies point to demyelinating diseases that have similarities to myasthenia gravis. Preliminary data shows that drugs that prolong the action potentials of demyelinated and unmyelinated fibers can facilitate nerve conduction.

One such drug is called 4 aminopyridine, a potassium-channel blocking agent. 4 aminopyridine has been used in Britain with beneficial effects in the treatment of myasthenia gravis. The essential fatty acids (Mega EPA and Mega GLA) that have been shown to suppress autoimmune attacks also help to protect the myelin sheath, and therefore could provide additional benefit in the treatment of myasthenia gravis.

Myasthenia gravis can be a difficult problem to manage, so those with moderate to severe disease do best if treated by an experienced specialist. Life-threatening respiratory-muscle involvement occurs in about 10 percent of cases.

Product availability: The essential fatty acids Mega EPA and Mega GLA, along with alpha-lipoic acid, vitamin D3, vitamin E, choline, inositol, Cognitex, vitamin D3 and Life Extension Mix can be ordered by calling 1-800-544-4440. Your doctor can prescribe Hydergine and deprenyl. If you want to order these products by mail from low-cost offshore pharmacies, call 1-800-544-4440 to ask for a list of companies that ship medicines to Americans for personal use only. The conventional drugs used to treat myasthenia gravis are potentially toxic, and must be monitored by an experienced physician.

Nails

Nails are composed of a protein called keratin, woven together by the sulfur-containing the amino acid cysteine.

When nails don't grow properly or have other abnormalities, it often is caused by a nutritional deficiency.

Here are the known nutritional factors affecting the nails:

1. A lack of vitamin A and calcium causes dryness and brittleness.
2. A vitamin-B deficiency causes fragility with horizontal and vertical ridges.
3. A vitamin-B12 deficiency leads to rounded and curved nails.
4. A lack of protein, folic acid and vitamin C causes hangnails.
5. A lack of "friendly bacteria" (lactobacillus) leads to fungus under and around the nails.
6. A deficiency in hydrochloric acid contributes to splitting nails.
7. Low iron can cause "spoon" nails and/or vertical ridges.

In a placebo-controlled, double-blind clinical study, 60 patients with reduced nail quality without biotin deficiency were treated over a period of six months with a daily dose of 2,500 micrograms of oral biotin. The changes in nail quality were documented technically by measuring the swelling behavior of nail keratin after incubation with NaOH, the trans-onychial water loss, as well as by clinical judgment of the investigator and the patients themselves. All evaluation parameters showed improvement of nail quality.

We suggest the following:

- ❖ Life Extension Mix — Three tablets, three times a day, with food.
- ❖ Biosil — six drops orally per day (provides silica, a building block of nails).
- ❖ Designer Protein — two servings per day.
- ❖ L-cysteine — 1,500 mg per day.
- ❖ Biotin — 2,500 micrograms a day.

Product availability: Life Extension Mix, Biosil, Designer Protein, L-cysteine and biotin can be ordered by calling 1-800-544-4440.

Neuropathy

Neuropathies involve inflammation and wasting of the nerves, often manifested in severe chronic pain and weakness. Neuropathies can be caused by diabetes, fatty acid imbalance, blood-supply disruption to the nerves, poisoning, side effects from FDA-approved drugs, free radicals, viruses, bacteria and other factors.

Diabetes mellitus is associated with defective essential fatty acid desaturation. In experimental models, essential fatty-acid desaturation contributes to reductions in peripheral nerve-conduction velocity and blood flow. This fatty-acid imbalance may be corrected by dietary supplementation with supplements that contain gamma-linolenic acid (GLA), such as borage oil. In animal studies, significant improvements in blood flow and nerve-conduction velocity were observed in response to omega-6 oil supplementation.

Oxidative stress is present in the diabetic state. Antioxidant enzymes are reduced in peripheral nerves and are further reduced in diabetic nerves. The mechanism of oxidative stress appears primarily to be due to the processes of nerve ischemia (reduced blood flow) and hyperglycemia -induced oxidation. Alpha-lipoic acid is a potent antioxidant that prevents lipid peroxidation in vitro and in vivo. Alpha-lipoic acid has been shown to prevent the deficits in nerve conduction and nerve blood flow. Also, alpha-lipoic acid restores reduced glutathione levels in nerves and reduces lipid peroxidation.

Scientists believe that alpha-lipoic acid is potentially beneficial for human diabetic sensory neuropathy. In Germany, alpha-lipoic acid is sold as a prescription drug for the treatment of various neuropathies. The benefits and safety of alpha-lipoic acid were studied in a three-week double-blind placebo-controlled trial in 328 Type II diabetic patients with peripheral neuropathy. Patients were randomly assigned to treatment with intravenous infusion of alpha-lipoic acid, using three doses of either 100 mg, 600 mg or 1,200 mg, or placebo.

The response rates after 19 days on alpha-lipoic acid were 70.8 percent at 1,200 mg of alpha-lipoic acid, 82.5 percent at 600 mg, and 65.2 percent at 100 mg. The response rate for the placebo group was 57.6 percent. These findings substantiate the benefits of intravenous treatment with alpha-lipoic acid using a dose of 600 mg a day over three weeks, benefits that are superior to placebo in reducing symptoms of diabetic peripheral neuropathy without causing significant adverse reactions.

In another study, 28 out of 33 patients (84.8 percent) who previously were treated with alpha-lipoic acid for peripheral polyneuropathy showed further improvement after combination with both alpha-lipoic acid and vitamin B5 (pantothenic acid). The theoretical basis for this improvement is that both substances intervene at different sites and thus are more effective than each substance alone. In an overview, scientists pointed out that glutathione, the most important thiol antioxidant, cannot be directly administered, whereas alpha-lipoic acid can. In vitro, animal and preliminary human studies indicate that alpha-lipoic acid may be effective in numerous neurodegenerative disorders, including neuropathies.

Nerve conduction and perfusion deficits in diabetic rats have been corrected by antioxidants and gamma linolenic acid (GLA) supplements. A deficit in sciatic nutritive endoneurial blood flow was corrected by 34.8 percent with GLA therapy, and by 24.8 percent with free radical scavenger therapy. When both treatments were combined, a flow improvement of 72.5 percent was observed. This study showed a synergistic effect of antioxidant and omega-6 essential fatty acid (GLA) combination treatment against diabetic neuropathy.

Fish oil concentrate (EPA) was shown to improve the clinical symptoms (coldness, numbness) as well as the vibration perception-threshold sense of the lower extremities. A significant decrease of serum triglycerides also was noted by EPA administration. The results of this study suggest that EPA has significant beneficial effects on diabetic neuropathy and serum lipids, as well as on other diabetic complications such as nephropathy and macroangiopathy.

Rats treated daily with acetyl-L-carnitine for 16 weeks showed an improvement in nerve conduction velocity. Treatment of hyperglycemic rats with acetyl-L-carnitine was associated with increased nerve conduction velocity, myelin width, and large myelinated fibers. In a prevention study with acetyl-L-carnitine, the nerve conduction defect was 73 percent prevented and structural abnormalities attenuated. Intervention with acetyl-L-carnitine resulted in a 76-percent recovery of the conduction defect, and corrected neuropathologic changes. Acetyl-L-carnitine treatment promoted nerve-fiber regeneration, which was increased twofold compared with nontreated diabetic rats.

A comparison was made of the benefits of a novel essential fatty acid derivative, ascorbyl gamma linolenic acid, with that of gamma-linolenic acid in correcting diabetic neurovascular deficits. Conduction velocity was corrected by 39.8 percent with gamma-linolenic acid, 87.4 percent with ascorbyl gamma-linolenic acid, and 66.8 percent with a combintation of gamma-linolenic acid plus ascorbate. Corresponding ameliorations of the nutritive blood flow deficit were 44 percent with gamma linolenic acid, 87.4 percent with ascorbyl gamma-linolenic acid, and 65.7 percent with gamma linoleic acid plus ascorbate.

Since ascorbyl gamma linoleic acid is not commercially available, those with neuropathy should take 1,500 mg a day of GLA, along with 500 mg a day of ascorbyl palmitate and an additional 3,000 mg a day of ascorbates (vitamin C).

The effects of treatment with the glutathione precursor N-acetylcysteine on nerve conduction, blood flow, maturation and regeneration was studied in diabetic mature rats. The deficits in sciatic motor conduction velocity and endoneurial blood flow were largely corrected by N-acetylcysteine treatment during the second month.

Nutrients used to treat neuropathies are alpha-lipoic acid at a dose of 500 mg twice a day, acetyl-L-carnitine at a dose of 1,000 mg twice a day, and N-acetylcysteine at a dose of 600 mg twice a day. Essential fatty acids are recommended at a dose of five capsules a day of

Mega GLA borage oil (300 mg GLA per capsule) and five capsules a day of Mega EPA (400 mg EPA per capsule) fish oil concentrate.

To suppress free radical injury to nerve fibers, take the 56-ingredient Life Extension Mix at a dose of three tablets three times a day. Life Extension Mix contains a relatively high level of pantothenic acid.

DHEA may be of help in some cases of neuropathy. Refer to the DHEA-Pregnenolone Precautions and dosage suggestions before using DHEA.

Product availability: Acetyl-L-carnitine, alpha-lipoic acid, Mega EPA, Mega GLA, DHEA and Life Extension Mix can be ordered by calling 1-800-544-4440.

Obesity

The Life Extension Foundation does not have a permanent cure for obesity, but we offer several innovative therapies that can make the success of various drugs, psychiatric care, and other obesity therapies more effective. Refer to the Foundation's Weight Loss protocols to find therapies that enhance the benefits of an anti-obesity program.

Organic Brain Syndrome

Refer to the Life Extension Foundation's protocols for Alzheimer's disease.

Osteoporosis

Osteoporosis is characterized by the loss of bone density to the point that small holes appear in the bones. It can cause pain (especially in the lower back), fractured bones, loss of body height and bone deformity.

Osteoporosis occurs because of hormonal imbalances that interfere with bone-forming cells, called osteoblasts, which pull calcium, magnesium and phosphorous from the blood in order to build bone mass. Osteoblasts require the hormone progesterone. The other hormones that promote bone-forming osteoblasts are DHEA, melatonin, growth hormone and vitamin D3.

To maintain youthful bone-forming capability during and after menopause, women should be on progesterone-replacement therapy. The most effective progesterone therapy may be a topical natural progesterone cream. Pre-menopausal women should use ¼ to ½ teaspoon daily, starting on the 15th day of their menstrual cycle and continuing until the end of the menstrual cycle. Post-menopausal women should use ¼ to ½ teaspoon of topical progesterone cream once daily. Those with severe osteoporosis should use ½ teaspoon morning and night for the first jar of natural progesterone cream, then ¼ teaspoon morning and night for the second jar.

Natural progesterone cream should be applied to different areas of the skin with each application to prevent saturation of the fat cells in any one area of the body. It should be rubbed on the wrists, the face, the breasts, the underarms and thighs.

Pregnenolone is a hormone that breaks down into DHEA, progesterone, estrogen and testosterone. Women may be able to get some or all of the combined benefits of topically applied progesterone cream and estrogen/DHEA/testosterone replacement by taking 50 to 200 mg a day of pregnenolone.

DHEA can stimulate osteoblast activity and boost estrogen levels to help prevent bone loss. Most women use 15 mg of DHEA three times a day. Refer to the DHEA-Pregnenolone Precautions before using DHEA or pregnenolone.

Estrogen is beneficial for bones because it promotes the action of osteoclasts, which remove dead portions of demineralized bone. DHEA and/or soy extracts may provide enough estrogen to maintain youthful osteoclast activity.

Based upon records of dietary soy consumption in Japan, where breast cancer rates are very low, the typical daily phytoestrogen intake from soy has been estimated at 50 mg per person. By contrast, the typical Western diet has been estimated to provide only two to three mg a day of the phytoestrogen genistein. Not only are certain cancer levels lower in those who consume soy, but menopausal symptoms and the incidence of osteoporosis are reduced. One study shows that soy isoflavones promote an anabolic effect on bone density in post-menopausal women by binding to an estrogen receptor in bone.

A new soy supplement called Mega Soy Extract provides 110 mg of soy phytoestrogens in just two capsules. This is more than twice the amount in the typical Japanese diet. Since the phytoestrogen genistein is water-soluble, it is suggested that one capsule of Mega Soy Extract be taken in the morning and one in the evening. Some women seeking to use Mega Soy Extract as an estrogen-replacement therapy may take two to three capsules twice a day.

Women over the age of 35 or 40 should consider taking melatonin, in the range of 500 micrograms to 6 mg every night, to help prevent osteoporosis and reduce the carcinogenic risks associated with estrogen-replacement therapy. Refer to the protocol on Estrogen Replacement Therapy for more information.

Blood tests can help to determine optimal individual dosing of these hormone-replacement therapies.

Calcium supplementation is one part of an osteoporosis prevention and treatment program. The Life Extension Foundation recommends that women take between 1,000 and 2,000 mg of elemental calcium along with 600 to 1,000 mg of elemental magnesium every day, plus about 1,000 IU of vitamin D3 to ensure optimal calcium absorption.

The inability to absorb calcium is a major reason that calcium therapy fails to prevent or slow the progression of osteoporosis. Vitamin D3 taken with calcium will normally promote absorption and assimilation of calcium into the bone matrix. Vitamin D3 also has been shown to promote the production of IGF-I and other growth factors in osteoporotic patients, which improves osteoblast (bone-building) function.

Calcitriol and calcitonin are FDA-approved drugs that can facilitate calcium absorption if vitamin D3 is not effective. One study showed that the addition of calcitonin (administered intramuscularly) to calcium supplementation not only inhibited bone loss but significantly increased bone mass in fractured forearm bones. Another study showed that the drug calcitriol corrects the malabsorption of calcium.

Higher amounts of vitamin D3 also have been shown to normalize calcium malabsorption that occurs as result of aging. Patients taking calcitriol should be monitored for serum and urine calcium response to the drug. As is common with most FDA-approved drugs, dangerous side effects are a significant risk. Prescription of calcitriol for the treatment of osteoporosis should be reserved for physicians and their patients with a special interest in the treatment of metabolic bone disease. The taking of high doses of vitamin D3 also should be under physician supervision.

A woman can obtain potent doses of elemental bone-building minerals calcium and magnesium, as well as vitamin D3, by taking six to ten capsules of the Mineral Formula For Women, along with the standard dose of Life Extension Mix every day. Life Extension Mix provides other vitamins and minerals required to maintain youthful bone density.

A number of women take calcium tablets, but calcium is a strong binding agent that often is difficult to break down in the digestive tract. Calcium capsules, on the other hand, burst open in the stomach within five minutes for quick absorption into the bloodstream.

For those with severe osteoporosis, higher amounts of calcium and vitamin D3 may be required, along with a six-month regimen of growth hormone-replacement therapy. A parathyroid hormone (PTH) test must be performed to see if calcium is leaving the bones—that is, if the process of bone demineralization is occurring. An elevated parathyroid hormone level indicates the possibility of osteoporosis, secondary to calcium deficiency. You can order blood tests by mail by calling 1-800-544-4440.

Effective alternatives to estrogen drugs are natural estrogens derived from plants. Refer to the Estrogen Replacement Therapy protocols for more information.

Exercise may be an effective therapy for osteoporosis. A study was performed to evaluate the effectiveness of the exercises for the treatment of postmenopausal osteoporosis. Both back extension and posture exercises lasting for one hour were undertaken twice a week, as well as fast walking exercises for one hour three times a week. At the end of the study, women who added exercise to their medical therapy increased spinal bone density by 4.4 percent, while women receiving only bone-restoring medicines showed an increase in spinal bone density of just 1.6 percent.

Recent investigations and clinical studies suggest that essential fatty acids and antioxidant nutrients influence bone formation. In animals, bone modeling appears to be optimal when omega-3 and omega-6 fatty acids are supplied in the diet. These studies support the role that dietary fatty acids and antioxidants play in reducing the severity of diseases involving bone-density loss. Vitamin E was reported to increase bone formation rate and to restore collagen synthesis.

Bone-density loss occurs in response to a wide range of conditions, including major surgery, glucocorticoid drugs, liver cirrhosis, Crohn's disease, cystic fibrosis, hormone deficiencies and normal aging. Numerous studies show that supplementation with high doses of calcium and vitamin D is an effective method for the prevention and treatment of osteoporosis that is induced by these bone-stripping conditions. Low doses of calcium generally are not shown to be effective. While osteoporosis and vitamin-D deficiency are common in patients with a wide range of degenerative diseases, therapies to prevent bone loss and treat established osteoporosis often are not utilized by conventional medicine.

Product availability: Progesterone cream, DHEA, pregnenolone, Natural Estrogen, Mineral Formula For Women, vitamin D3, Life Extension Mix and melatonin can be obtained by calling 1-800-544-4440. If you need growth hormone-replacement therapy, ask for doctors who have expertise in this area. Call the Life Extension Foundation at 1-800-544-4440 for information on blood testing.

Pain

The Life Extension Foundation's fundamental protocol for pain management is to eradicate the underlying cause of chronic pain. You should, therefore, first consider the specific condition causing your pain (such as arthritis, for example) and refer to the protocol for this condition.

For general pain relief, some people find that boosting brain levels of the endorphins can provide natural pain suppression. This approach isn't an effective way of dealing with acute (short-term, severe) pain, but is the safest method of alleviating chronic (long-lasting) pain. By taking 500 mg of the nutrient amino acids dl-phenylalanine or tyrosine two to three times a day, you can raise your brain endorphin levels to reduce, and perhaps eliminate, chronic pain of almost any type.

Melatonin is a potential therapy for the treatment of diseases with pain and abnormal immune responses. The effects and mechanisms of melatonin on inflammation and immunoregulation have been studied systematically. Melatonin showed significant analgesic effects in animal studies. Melatonin also was shown to enhance the pain-suppressing effects of analgesics. Further studies showed that melatonin could enhance the functions of T and B lymphocytes and macrophages in vitro and in adjuvant (assisting) arthritis treatment. In animal studies, melatonin was shown to inhibit the swelling of the hindpaw.

These factors suggest that melatonin possesses marked anti-inflammatory, immunoregulatory, and analgesic effects that may be related to the system of opiate modulation. Use melatonin cautiously when treating autoimmune disease such as rheumatoid arthritis. Some scientists have speculated that melatonin could worsen the severity of an autoimmune disease.

For nighttime pain relief, 3 to 10 mg of melatonin should be taken before bedtime. Melatonin should be used only at night before bedtime, not during the day.

CAUTION: Before starting on such a pain-management program, refer to our Phenylalanine And Tyrosine Precautions.

Refer to the Migraine protocol for more information on melatonin's pain-relieving properties. Also refer to the Arthritis or Fibromyalgia protocols if these diseases are an underlying cause of your particular pain.

Product availability: Dl-phenylalanine, melatonin and tyrosine are available by calling 1-800-544-4440.

Parathyroid (Hyperparathyroidism)

Too much parathyroid hormone is clinically defined as hyperparathyroidism. The excess parathyroid hormone pulls calcium from the bones, which overloads the blood system with excessive amounts of calcium. Many long-term degenerative diseases have been linked to this type of calcium imbalance.

A standard blood-chemistry test can reveal elevated calcium levels caused by hyperparathyroid disease. Only a PTH (parathyroid hormone) blood test can effectively diagnose hyperparathyroidism. If your blood test is high in calcium and parathyroid hormone, it may be an indication of hyperparathyroidism. People who do not have regular blood tests usually find out they have hyperparathyroidism when a bone suddenly breaks, a kidney stone develops, or when their kidneys fail altogether.

Surgery is necessary when there is a parathyroid tumor that causes the overproduction of parathyroid hormone. There are diagnostic procedures (MRI, CT scan, sonography) to determine if the excess parathyroid hormone is caused by a tumor or by a vitamin D3/calcium deficiency.

The first step in countering parathyroidism is to take 1,000 IU of vitamin D3 every day, along with 2,000 mg of elemental calcium. This much calcium and vitamin D3 will act as a signal to your parathyroid glands to stop producing so much parathyroid hormone. When your bloodstream is loaded with calcium, your parathyroid glands will no longer have to pull it from your bones to guarantee proper calcium metabolism. Many people undergo surgery to remove one or more parathyroid glands when, in fact, all they need to do is take calcium and vitamin D3.

Studies show that glucocorticoid-induced osteoporosis is associated with the development of secondary hyperparathyroidism. Alternate-day therapy with corticosteroid drugs can't prevent bone loss. Supplementation of calcium and vitamin D has been shown to be an effective method for prevention and treatment.

Primary hyperparathyroidism is the most prevalent cause of hypercalcemia (high calcium in the blood). The advent of blood screening has resulted in earlier detection that has changed the clinical presentation of primary hyperparathyroidism. As many as 80 percent of patients do not have any sign or symptom, such as kidney stones, that can be attributed solely to the disease. Improvement in blood assays for parathyroid hormone has allowed for accurate biochemical diagnosis in more than 90 percent of cases. Neck exploration is the conventional treatment of choice for those with signs, symptoms or complications associated with primary hyperparathyroidism. Medical therapy is indicated in patients who either cannot undergo surgery because of medical contraindication, have unresectable parathyroid carcinoma, or who simply refuse surgery.

Estrogen-replacement therapy potentially may be an alternative form of therapy to surgery in elderly women with primary hyperparathyroidism. In one study, estrogen-replacement therapy appeared as effective as parathyroidectomy (combined with either calcitriol or calcium supplements) for the treatment of osteoporosis in elderly postmenopausal women showing primary hyperparathyroidism symptoms.

In treating hemodialysis patients suffering from uremic hyperparathyroidism, the addition of the drug calcitonin to vitamin D3 therapy may inhibit bone resorption and increase bone mineral density. Dialysis patients often suffer from uncontrolled serum phosphate levels that preclude successful treatment with vitamin D3. Blood levels of phosphate should be carefully monitored in dialysis patients.

Calcium-alpha-ketoglutarate is known as a highly effective phosphate binder in hemodialysis patients. Also, alpha-ketoglutarate has been shown to improve metabolic alterations. A study investigated the effect of long-term phosphate-binding therapy with calcium-alpha-ketoglutarate to determine whether phosphate accumulation is the main reason of secondary hyperparathyroidism in kidney dialysis patients. Calcium ketoglutarate was prescribed to 14 patients in a mean dosage of 4.5 grams a day (which provided 975 mg of elemental calcium) for a period of 36 months. Serum phosphate levels continuously dropped whereas serum calcium levels increased to normal levels. Intact parathyroid hormone continuously normalized in all patients. The present data show that long-term treatment with calcium-alpha-ketoglutarate normalizes secondary hyperparathyroidism by simultaneously binding phosphate and correcting the calcium/phosphate ratio in serum without vitamin-D treatment.

Product availability: Vitamin D3 and an encapsulated calcium-mineral formula called Mineral Formula For Women can be ordered by phoning 1-800-544-4440.

Parkinson's Disease

For every decade we live past age 40, we lose an average of about 10 percent of our dopamine-producing brain cells. Once 80 percent of these brain cells have died, Parkinson's disease often is diagnosed. Parkinson's disease is characterized by uncontrolled muscle tremors, rigidity, depression, weakness and an unsteady gait.

Studies have shown that if healthy people take antioxidants throughout most of their lives, their risk of acquiring Parkinson's disease is reduced considerably. However, when Parkinson's patients are given Vitamin E by itself there is no slowdown in disease progression. Since Parkinson's patients already have sustained massive damage to crucial brain cells, aggressive multiple therapies are required to have a chance of significantly slowing the natural progression of the disease.

The Life Extension Foundation's protocol for Parkinson's disease is based on studies showing that low doses of several drugs work better than high doses of a single drug. The Foundation receives updates from its members about the benefits or lack of benefits of the therapies it recommends. We would appreciate hearing from Parkinson's patients, their families or doctors about the effects of our Parkinson's disease protocol.

The 14 components that comprise this protocol are suggested because of evidence of their safety and benefits in treating the multiple underlying neurological disorders linked to the disease.

1. Bromocriptine — Take the lowest effective dose to begin with, usually 1.25 mg a day. May be withheld until later in the disease phase.

2. Sinemet CR (controlled release) and/or Sinemet (L-dopa plus a dopa decarboxylase inhibitor) — Take lowest effective dose to begin with. Some doctors withhold Sinemet until later in the progression of the disease in order to give the Parkinson's patient more time to benefit from Sinemet before its effects wear off.

3. Amantadine — Take lowest effective dose to begin with, usually 300 mg a day.

4. Deprenyl — Take lowest effective dose to begin with, between 1.25 and 5 mg a day. Deprenyl dosing has been significantly reduced based on studies showing that high doses of deprenyl may be detrimental to Parkinson's patients.

5. Hydergine — 10 to 20 mg every day.

6. Acetyl-L-carnitine — 1,000 mg twice a day.

7. Phosphatidylserine — 200 mg twice a day.

8. NADH — 5 to 10 mg twice a day.

9. DHEA — 100 mg three times a day, and/or pregnenolone at 50 mg three times a day. Pregnenolone is a DHEA precursor. Refer to the DHEA-Pregnenolone Precautions before taking DHEA or pregnenolone.

10. Coenzyme Q10 — 100 mg three times a day.

11. Life Extension Mix — three tablets, three times a day. Avoid if taking Sinemet because the vitamin B6 in Life Extension Mix may prevent L-dopa from reaching the brain. Take other antioxidants in place of Life Extension Mix that do not contain vitamin B6.

12. Melatonin — 3 to 10 mg every night at bedtime.

13. Life Extension Booster — one capsule twice a day.

14. Human growth hormone — 2 IU daily, by injection.

This protocol attempts to cover the many neurological problems, neurochemical imbalances and hormonal deficiencies associated with Parkinson's disease. While the drug therapies and some of the hormone therapies in this protocol have to be carefully monitored, the nutrient therapies can be used safely on a regular basis to help protect and improve overall neurological functions.

Product availability: DHEA, melatonin, pregnenolone, acetyl-L-carnitine, Life Extension Mix, Life Extension Booster, NADH, Cognitex, phosphatidylserine and coenzyme Q10 can be ordered by phoning 1-800-544-4440. A neurologist should carefully prescribe the other medications. Call 1-800-544-4440 if you need a referral to a physician knowledgeable in the use of growth-hormone therapy.

Phenylalanine and Tyrosine Precautions

There are some people who cannot use the amino acid phenylalanine. This includes those born with a genetic deficiency that prevents them from metabolizing phenylalanine (Phenylketonuria, or PKU), those with high blood pressure, and people with cancer. Phenylalanine and tyrosine can promote cancer cell division, especially malignant melanoma.

Phobias

Phobias are common. Surveys have shown that more than half of those surveyed admit to having one or more phobias. People become phobic when the adrenal glands release large amounts of adrenaline and the brain releases its own form of adrenaline called norepinephrine, an excitatory neurotransmitter that stimulates cells in the brain and other parts of the body. Epinephrine initiates its effects by binding to beta-adrenergic sites on the cell membrane.

By taking a beta-blocking drug before a phobia-inducing event (such as public speaking, flying in an airplane, meeting new people, etc.), the excess adrenaline and norepinephrine will not create the anxiety, shaking, heart palpitations, sweating and queasy stomach that characterize a phobia. The first beta-blocking drug was propranolol, and it has more than 30 years of clinical use to document its safety.

Propranolol is available in low-cost generic form. The suggested dose is 10 to 40 mg of propranolol before a phobia-inducing event. People with very low blood pressure, certain forms of congestive heart failure, and asthma should not take propranolol or other beta-blocking drugs. Nutritionally, vitamin B3 (niacin) and calcium may be beneficial.

Conventional doctors often prescribe selective serotonin reuptake inhibitor (SSRI) drugs such as Prozac, Zoloft or Paxil in the treatment of anxiety, phobias, and obsessive-compulsive symptoms. It is argued that a serotonergic dysfunction may underlie such non-psychotic disorders as anxiety, and affective and compulsive-obsessive disorders. While the SSRIs are safer than such tranquilizers as Xanax and Valium, there are concerns in the life extension community about long-term side effects, such as serotonin overload.

Product availability: Propranolol is a prescription drug. For a listing of knowledgeable physicians in your area who will prescribe propranolol to treat phobia, call 1-800-544-4440. Vitamin B3 (niacin) is available by calling 1-800-544-4440.

Pregnenolone Precautions

Since pregnenolone is converted into DHEA within the body, some of our precautions for DHEA may apply to pregnenolone. For some people, pregnenolone may raise DHEA serum levels to reduce the need for DHEA supplementation.

Women may experience an increase in progesterone after taking pregnenolone, which may eliminate the need for natural progesterone cream and progestin drugs. Proper blood testings of various hormones will reveal the likely metabolic pathway in each individual. Refer to DHEA-Pregnenolone Precautions for more information.

Premenstrual Syndrome

Refer to the Menstrual Disorders-Premenstrual Syndrome (PMS) protocol.

Prevention Protocols

If you are healthy now, and want to stay that way, The Life Extension Foundation has designed protocols that incorporate the best documented disease-preventing nutrients and hormones.

The Foundation's Prevention Protocols consist of the top ten most important supplements for the average person to take every day to reduce the risk of contracting the degenerative diseases of aging. Remember, Prevention Protocols are for healthy people. Those seeking to treat an existing disease should refer to the other protocols in this book.

The following Prevention Protocols are listed in order of importance:

Recommendation Number 1: Life Extension Mix
(Multi Vitamin-Mineral-Herbal-Amino Acid Formula)

Dosage: Breakfast—three tablets; lunch—three tablets; dinner—three tablets

Life Extension Mix is a super-potent formula containing 56 different vegetable extracts, vitamins, minerals, amino acids, herbal extracts and other unique antioxidants that cannot be found in any other multi-nutrient product.

Life Extension Mix saves people time and money by combining the most popular nutrient supplements into one product, thus enabling most people to eliminate the need to take many separate bottles of B-complex, vitamins C and E, mineral supplements, etc.

The Life Extension Foundation mandates that the ingredients in Life Extension Mix come only from pharmaceutical-grade suppliers such as Roche and Nutrition 21. These premium companies charge more for their vitamin C, selenium, etc., but the pharmaceutical purity of these nutrients greatly exceeds the lower-cost generic versions that are so prevalent in the vitamin industry.

Life Extension Mix is the cornerstone of a comprehensive supplement program because it provides so many different disease-preventing nutrients. If you are on a budget, Life Extension Mix will provide you with more disease-preventing nutrients per dollar spent than any other product on earth.

Recommendation Number 2: Life Extension Booster

Dosage: One capsule daily with a meal

Some nutrients are so well-documented to prevent disease, that many people want to take even higher amounts than are contained in Life Extension Mix. The Life Extension Booster contains many important nutrients that cannot fit into the tightly packed Life Extension Mix formula.

Life Extension Booster is designed to be a convenient, low-cost method of obtaining the most important disease-preventing nutrients in just one capsule.

While a member pays an average of $9.76 a month for the Life Extension Booster, the cost of taking these pharmaceutical-grade ingredients separately would be much higher.

Recommendation Number 3: Coenzyme Q10

Dosage: 30 to 100 mg daily with meals

One of the most researched disease-preventing nutrients is coenzyme Q10 (CoQ10).

The Life Extension Foundation was the first organization to introduce CoQ10 to the American public, and since then, hundreds of new studies on CoQ10 have appeared in the scientific literature documenting the multiple life-extension benefits of this versatile nutrient.

CoQ10 absorbs into the bloodstream much better when it is in an oil-base. For this reason, we suggest that CoQ10 be taken as a separate oil-based supplement.

Most dry powder CoQ10 supplements absorb only into the bloodstream at about half the rate of oil-based CoQ10. Since CoQ10 is a relatively expensive product, it makes sense to take it in an oil base. CoQ10 is available in 30-mg and 100-mg softgel capsules in which the CoQ10 is dissolved in tocotrienol-rich rice bran oil.

Recommendation Number 4: Melatonin

Dosage: 500 mcg to 6 mg at bedtime

For people over age 40, melatonin may be the most effective overall disease-preventing agent available, yet it is very inexpensive.

Melatonin has been shown in hundreds of published studies to reduce the risk of numerous degenerative diseases, boost immune function, inhibit cancer cell proliferation and slow aging.

Many people take an average of 3 mg per night of melatonin to sleep better. If you are over 40 and sleep fine, we suggest taking only a 500-microgram capsule of melatonin at bedtime. People over age 50 may consider higher doses of melatonin for disease prevention.

Recommendation Number 5: Trimethylglycine (TMG)

Dosage: One tablet daily with meals

Trimethylglycine (TMG) provides a unique biological effect that makes it a critical component of a disease-prevention program. TMG facilitates youthful methylation metabolism. Published research shows three specific benefits of enhancing methylation:

1. Methylation lowers dangerous homocysteine levels, thus lowering the risk of heart disease and stroke.

2. Methylation produces SAMe, which may have potent anti-aging effects, and has been shown to alleviate depression, remylenate nerve cells, improve Alzheimer's and Parkinson's disease patients, and protect against alcohol-induced liver injury.

3. Methylation protects DNA. Protecting DNA may slow cellular aging.

Enhancing methylation improves health and slows premature and, perhaps, normal aging.

Published research shows that methylation is related to a variety of disease states, including cardiovascular disease, cancer, liver disease and neurological disorders.

TMG should be taken with co-factors vitamin B12 and folic acid. If you take Life Extension Mix and Life Extension Booster, you will get these co-factors.

Trimethylglycine (TMG) is the most effective methylation enhancing agent known.

Recommendation Number 6: Cognitex, Ginkgo and other Neurological-Enhancing Nutrients

Dosage: Five Cognitex capsules early in the day. One 120 mg ginkgo cap early in the day.

Brain aging is a leading cause of disease, disability and death in the elderly. Healthy people seeking to slow down brain aging often notice cognitive enhancing effects in response to Cognitex and ginkgo.

The quest to slow brain aging is the reason most people contact the Life Extension Foundation. While the antioxidants found in Life Extension Mix and Life Extension Booster protect against free radical damage to brain cells, there are other mechanisms of brain cell aging that may be prevented by nutrients such as phosphatidylserine, choline, pregnenolone and other components of the Cognitex formula.

Life Extension Herbal Mix (Recommendation Number 9), contains ginkgo extract, so if you take Life Extension Herbal Mix, it is not necessary to take additional ginkgo.

Recommendation Number 7:
For Men—Saw Palmetto Extract

Dosage: One capsule in the morning and one capsule in afternoon with meals

Prostate enlargement is an inevitable consequence of aging for most men. An extract from the saw palmetto berry may prevent benign prostatic hypertrophy and possibly reduce the risk of prostate cancer in males.

For Women—Mineral Formula for Women

Dosage: Five to nine capsules, preferably before bedtime

Osteoporosis is a common consequence of aging for women. In order to prevent bone loss, calcium supplements are often used. The problem is that osteoporosis is caused by a wide range of nutrient deficiencies, including magnesium, vitamin D3, and the hormones DHEA and progesterone.

For calcium to prevent bone loss, adequate amounts of vitamin D3 and progesterone have to be available so that calcium, magnesium and phosphorous will be incorporated into the bone matrix.

Calcium tablets often fail to break down in the digestive tract, which is why the Mineral Formula for Women is in capsule form. Mineral Formula for Women capsules burst open within five minutes of swallowing, making the minerals and vitamin D3 immediately available for absorption into the bloodstream for incorporation into the bone.

Mineral Formula for Women contains forms of calcium that have been shown to help prevent bone loss.

Recommendation Number 8: Garlic

Dosage: Two capsules a day with heaviest meal

Garlic is one of the better-documented disease-preventing nutrients. Published studies have shown that garlic prevents cancer, boosts immune function, and protects against many forms of cardiovascular disease.

Garlic is not contained in the Life Extension Herbal Mix because it would adversely effect the taste of the product. The garlic supplement we recommend most is a high-allicin, odor-suppressed garlic extract made by PureGar. Garlic can help neutralize dietary carcinogens, which is why we recommend it be taken with the heaviest meal of the day.

Recommendation Number 9: Life Extension Herbal Mix

Dosage: One tablespoon early in the day, with or without food

Numerous published studies show that specific herbal extracts can prevent a wide range of degenerative diseases and boost cognitive function.

Life Extension Herbal Mix contains some of the best-documented herbals, including green tea extract, gingko extract, grape-seed extract, bilberry extract, licorice extract and ginseng extract, along with 21 other disease-fighting phytochemicals such as chlorella and soy.

The cost of taking these herbal extracts in capsule form is around $100 a month, but Foundation members can save 60 percent by taking all of these herbals together in one good-tasting herbal drink mix.

Herbal extracts are expensive because a large quantity of organic plant has to be used to produce a minute quantity of the pharmaceutical extract.

Some members take only Life Extension Herbal Mix several times a week in order to reduce the monthly cost.

Recommendation Number 10: Mega Soy Extract

Dosage: Two capsules a day. For women taking Mega Soy Extract as an estrogen-replacement therapy, take two to three capsules a day.

Based upon records of dietary soy consumption in Japan, where breast cancer rates are very low, the typical daily phytoestrogen intake from soy has been estimated at 50 mg per person. By contrast, the typical Western diet has been estimated to provide only two to three mg a day of the phytoestrogen genistein. Not only are certain cancer levels lower in those who consume soy, but menopausal symptoms and the incidence of osteoporosis are reduced. One study shows that soy isoflavones promote an anabolic effect on bone density in post-menopausal women by binding to an estrogen receptor in bone.

A new soy supplement called Mega Soy Extract provides 110 mg of soy phytoestrogens in just two capsules—more than twice the amount in the typical Japanese diet. Since the phytoestrogen genistein is water-soluble, it is suggested that one capsule of Mega Soy Extract be taken in the morning and one in the evening.

Recommendation Number 11: Aspirin

Dosage: One heart-shaped tablet (¼ aspirin) a day with a heavy meal

The greatest cause of death and disability is an abnormal clot that develops inside an artery to cause a heart attack or a thrombotic stroke.

While many of the nutrients included in the Prevention Protocols will reduce the risk of an abnormal blood clot forming inside a blood vessel, it is still beneficial for most people to take just 81 mg of aspirin with the heaviest meal of the day.

Low-dose aspirin prevents blood clots from forming inside of arteries by a unique mechanism that is well-documented in the scientific literature.

Product availability: Life Extension Mix, Life Extension Booster, coenzyme Q10, melatonin, TMG, Cognitex, ginkgo, saw palmetto extract, Mineral Formula for Women, garlic, Life Extension Herbal Mix, Mega Soy Extract, aspirin (Healthprin) can be ordered by phoning 1-800-544-4440.

Prostate Cancer (Early Stage)

Unlike most forms of cancer, early stage prostate cancer is almost completely controllable with total hormone-blocking therapy. The drugs used to contain early stage prostate cancer are FDA-approved, yet a recent survey showed that only a small percentage of urologists are using hormone-blocking therapy properly in treating early stage prostate cancer patients. The published scientific literature has confirmed the failure of radical prostatectomy (surgical removal of the prostate) and external beam radiation therapy to produce an acceptable percentage of long-term, disease-free survival. The severe long-term side effects of these two extensively used conventional therapies are well-documented.

In lieu of radical surgery or external beam radiation, prostate cancer patients may want to consider the Life Extension Foundation's early stage protocols that incorporate combined testosterone and prolactin blockade for temporary control of most prostate cancers. Innovative natural therapies are implemented immediately upon the initiation of hormone-blocking drug therapies.

The goal is to give these natural therapies an opportunity to keep the PSA (prostate specific antigen) measurement at a non-detectable level after the discontinuation of three to nine months of combined testosterone and prolactin blockade. Intermittent hormone-blockade drug therapy is advised for almost all prostate cancer patients, since this greatly enhances the time before prostate cancer cells become androgen-independent.

If your PSA level is less than 11, the odds are that the cancer is confined to the prostate sack. Even if your PSA is greater than 11, there still is a good chance that the combination of FDA-approved hormone-blocking therapy, along with our innovative cancer-treatment protocols, can result in long-term remission. You should institute a three- to nine-month course of complete hormone blockade by using the FDA-approved drug Casodex, and then receive a pellet implant of FDA-approved Lupron a week later. This combination therapy should reduce your PSA level to less than 1 after only a few months. Casodex is taken every day and the Lupron pellets should be re-administered every three months.

When taking Casodex, it should first be taken orally for one week prior to the an injection of Lupron. Many urologists do not know that Lupron causes a temporary prostate cancer cell flare-up if Casodex (or flutamide) is not first given one week prior to Lupron's administration.

For many years, the Foundation has advocated that prostate cancer patients first try three to nine months of complete hormone blockade before considering any permanent therapies. The rationale is to shrink the prostate-cancer volume by inhibiting testosterone production and blocking testosterone receptor sites on prostate cells. Testosterone is responsible for most prostate cancer-cell proliferation. Blocking testosterone will cause an elevated PSA blood reading to drop to virtually zero within two months. The reduced PSA is indicative of a significant drop in prostate cancer cell activity. The prostate specific antigen test is an extremely accurate measure of prostate cancer cell activity. Peer-reviewed studies show that hormone-blocking therapy instituted before aggressive therapy significantly increases your chances of a cure.

Studies have shown that prolactin also may be involved in prostate growth. A rising serum level of prolactin indicates progression in patients with advanced prostate cancer.

The presence of prolactin receptors in prostate cancer cells may facilitate the entry of testosterone into prostate cells. Since testosterone-blocking therapies do not completely eliminate testosterone from the blood, it is conceivable that prolactin could carry a small amount of residual testosterone into the prostate cells and cause cancer growth. Thus, suppressing prolactin secretion with relatively safe prescription drugs appears to be another method of slowing the progression of prostate cancer.

In a study in the *European Journal of Cancer* (Vol 31A, No. 6, 1995), the use of a prolactin-suppressing drug (bromocriptine) with flutamide and orchiectomy (surgical removal of the testes) resulted in a 61-percent suppression of primary prostate growth, compared with only a 48-percent reduction with orchiectomy and flutamide alone. After 36 months, 40 percent of the group receiving bromocriptine and orchiectomy/flutamide experienced disease progression, compared with 60 percent in the orchiectomy/flutamide-only group. Most prostate cancer patients, understandably, prefer taking the drug Lupron instead of undergoing testicle removal, and in fact, Lupron may be more effective than orchiectomy.

Prostate cancer patients should have their prolactin levels checked via a blood test. If your prolactin levels are elevated, you should consider one of the following prescription-drug regimens prescribed by a physician:

- ✔ Bromocriptine, 5 mg one to two times a day; or
- ✔ Pergolide, 0.25 mg to 0.5 mg twice a day; or
- ✔ Dostinex, 0.5 mg twice a week.

Check your prolactin levels again in 30 days to make sure the drug you choose is, in fact, suppressing prolactin release into your blood from the pituitary gland.

Dostinex is the newest and cleanest drug to use. Dostinex has fewer side effects than the older drugs, is more effective in suppressing prolactin, and requires dosing only twice a week.

The Foundation has been recommending only a three- to nine-month course of Casodex (or flutamide) and Lupron therapy. Prolactin suppression therapy may be continued longer. During this period, it is suggested that innovative natural cancer-control therapies be incorporated to see if long-term remission can be achieved.

In many cases, the PSA stays low after hormone-blocking therapy has been discontinued. If the PSA level does increase again to between 6 and 20, the prostate-cancer patient is encouraged either to go on another three- to nine-month hormone-blocking regimen and alter his natural cancer control regimen, or seek out a permanent solution such as enhanced radioactive seed implantation or cryoablation therapy.

When a permanent remission is sought, it is critical that the prostate-cancer patient have undetectable levels of PSA by previously being on the three- to nine-month hormone blocking therapy regimen. An opposite view comes from doctors who perform enhanced radioactive seed implantation, who have said they do not want too much prostate-cancer shrinkage to occur in response to hormone-blocking therapy because they find they cannot find any tumor tissue to implant the seeds into.

If a person continuously stays on hormone-blocking therapy, after two to four years the prostate cancer cells will mutate to a new form of cancer cell that will not need testosterone to proliferate. Thus, once the cancer cells become "androgen-independent," the prostate cancer is usually out of control and will freely metastasize throughout the body.

In a study published in the *Journal of Steroid Biochemistry and Molecular Biology* (May 1996), prostate cancer in mice was treated with either continuous hormone-blocking therapy or the intermittent hormone-blocking regimen recommended by the Life Extension Foundation. The results showed that five to six cycles of intermittent hormone blockade were possible before the prostate-cancer cells mutated to a form that did not need testosterone to proliferate. There was an initial 66-percent greater time period of prostate cancer cell control in the intermittent group compared, with the group receiving continuous hormone blockade. In the late term of the study, the mice on intermittent hormone-blocking therapy had an astounding 3.78-fold reduction in their PSA levels, compared with the mice receiving continuous hormone-blocking therapy.

This study showed that continuous hormone-blocking therapy accelerates the rate at which prostate-cancer cells become resistant to testosterone blocking therapy, and that intermittent hormone blockade significantly increases the length of effectiveness of hormone-blocking therapy in the long-term treatment of prostate cancer.

What follows is a brief description of the Foundation's alternative protocols for treating early stage prostate cancer that should be implemented before, during and after combined hormone-blockade therapy:

Prostate cancer patients usually take five 700-mg capsules of Mega Soy Extract three to four times a day. Mega Soy Extract provides pharmaceutical doses of soy isoflavones such as genistein.

Cancer cells use the enzyme protein kinase as a growth factor. Soy genistein is a potent inhibitor of protein kinase activity. The effects of protein kinase inhibitors on human prostate cell growth have been extensively investigated.

Incidences of prostate cancer are high in the Western world, compared with countries in Asia where soy is consumed as part of the normal diet. Soy phytochemicals such as genistein are abundant in the plasma of people living in areas with low cancer incidence.

These phytochemicals protect against cancer via several different mechanisms, including interacting with intracellular enzymes, regulating protein synthesis, controlling growth-factor action, inhibiting malignant-cell proliferation, inducing differentiation, deterring cancer cell adhesion and inhibiting angiogenesis. Animal experiments provide evidence suggesting that both lignans and isoflavonoids in soy may prevent the development of cancer.

Genistein may prevent the expression of metastasic capacity in hormone-dependent cancers. Studies have shown that genistein inhibits proliferation and expression of the invasive capacity of prostatic cancer cells with different invasive potentials. In a cell-culture system, genistein appears to be cytotoxic and inhibitory of prostate cancer cell proliferation.

Genistein's protein-tyrosine kinase inhibiting effects have been identified as a cancer-prevention mechanism. The consumption of soy is associated with a low incidence of clinical metastatic prostate cancer, even in the face of a sustained high incidence of organ-confined prostate cancer. A study examined genistein's effect upon cell adhesion as one possible mechanism by which it could be acting as an anti-metastatic agent. A morphogenic analysis revealed that genistein caused cell flattening in a way that prevented metastatic adhesion of prostate cancer cell lines.

CAUTION: Do not take any soy genistein product 10 days prior, during, or three weeks after any form of radiation therapy. Genistein may protect cancer cells against radiation-induced death.

Additional natural therapies include 4,000 IU of vitamin D3, four saw palmetto/pygeum extract capsules, and as much of the Foundation's Cancer Treatment protocol, in this book, as possible. The Foundation especially recommends that prostate-cancer patients take four to 10 decaffeinated green tea extract capsules each day.

Epidemiological data suggest that vitamin D3, obtained from dietary sources and sunlight exposure, protects against mortality from prostate cancer. The most active vitamin D metabolite, vitamin D3 inhibits the growth and differentiation of several human prostate cancer cell lines.

Permixon (saw palmetto extract) is a drug used in the treatment of benign prostatic hyperplasia. A study of permixon's androgenic and anti-androgenic effects in the prostatic cell lines showed that it has a clear anti-androgenic action. Pygeum extract also has been shown to specifically inhibit prostate-cell proliferation by inhibiting protein kinase C enzyme activity.

Prostate cancer patients should take a PSA test every 30 days, before and after hormone-blocking therapy is discontinued, to see if the innovative cancer therapies are keeping the prostate cancer under control. Serum calcium blood tests also are suggested to make sure that the relatively high daily doses of vitamin D3 are not causing toxicity.

There are many prostate cancer patients following the Foundation's protocols with success. Individuals have personal decisions to make, based on a wide range of factors, regarding how they are going to deal with their prostate cancer in the long run. Every prostate cancer patient should consider three to nine months of complete hormone blockade before attempting any form of permanent therapy, such as surgery, radiation, cryoablation, radioactive seeds, etc. For some prostate-cancer patients, complete hormone-blocking therapy results in a long-term remission without the need of incorporating any additional therapies.

For those seeking a permanent remission, there is a therapy that combines enhanced ultrasound guided radioactive seed implantation and conformal external beam radiation aimed only at the implanted seeds in the prostate and seminal vesicle tissue. The seeds provide a greater amount of cancer cell-killing radiation directly to prostate-cancer cells, while serving as an easy target for conformal external beam radiation therapy. Since the external radiation beam hits only the areas that have been "seeded," the long-term complication of rectal and bladder radiation damage is largely avoided, and the areas identified as having cancer cells are intensely irradiated.

As noted, during radiation therapy it is crucial that all soy supplements be discontinued since soy produces a specific mechanism that can protect cancer cells from radiation-induced death. Discontinue soy at least 10 days before radiation, during radiation, and for at least three weeks afterward.

During radiation therapy, the use of high doses of antioxidants will protect healthy cells from free radical-induced radiation damage.

The combination of enhanced ultrasound radioactive seeding with precision external beam therapy is available at the clinic of Dr. Frank A. Critz in Decatur, Ga. Dr. Critz's phone number is 404-320-1550. This therapy also has been instituted at the University of Miami (Fla.) Medical School, and may be available in other hospitals.

The following represents the latest findings about conventional diagnosis and treatment of prostate cancer:

1. Tests to measure PSA density and percent of free PSA were performed on men with total PSA levels ranging from 4.1 to 10. In those with benign prostate disease, the median PSA density was 0.14, compared with 0.19 in prostate cancer patients. The median percent of free PSA was 18.9 in benign cases, compared with 10.1 in prostate cancer cases. This study showed that the use of PSA fractionated testing could detect at least 95 percent of prostate cancers and reduce the need for biopsies by 26.9 percent in men who did not have prostate cancer. These PSA fractioned tests are expected to become more widely available in the near future.

2. A significant false-negative rate for initial transrectal ultrasound guided prostate was shown in a study of 130 men. Needle biopsies of the prostate gland missed 23.8 percent of cancer cells detected by a second needle biopsy. The doctors who conducted the study suggested that repeat biopsies be done for patients in whom the initial biopsy is negative. The Life Extension Foundation interprets this study to validate greater use of the PSA fractionated tests showing free PSA and PSA density, in order to rule out men who do not need a biopsy at all.

3. Prostate tumors that recur locally after radical prostatectomy (surgical removal of the prostate) appear to have a higher proliferative rate, compared with the tumors removed during the radical surgery. Tumor proliferative rates were measured in 26 patients. Before radical prostatectomy, the mean pro-

liferation labeling index was 2.96. After surgical removal of the prostate gland, the mean labeling index increased to 6.47—a 64-percent increase in cancer-cell proliferation. Anyone contemplating prostate cancer therapy should obtain the latest information about the Life Extension Foundation's Prostate Cancer protocol on our web site: **http://www.lef.org**.

4. A randomized trial of 415 patients with locally advanced prostate cancer showed an 85-percent disease-free survival after five years in patients receiving Zoladex and external beam radiation therapy, compared with only a 48-percent disease free survival rate in patients receiving external beam radiation therapy alone. Zoladex is an FDA-approved drug that functions in a similar way as Lupron to suppress testosterone secretion. This study adds to the growing number of studies showing hormone blockade as an effective prostate cancer therapy, either by itself or in assisting other therapies. The Life Extension Foundation's protocol suggests additional hormone-blocking therapies be used along with Zoladex or Lupron.

5. A total of 200 cases were analyzed to determine accuracy of staging (determining the distinct phases) of prostate cancer. The addition of magnetic resonance imaging (MRI) was shown to enhance tumor-staging accuracy.

6. 3-D conformal radiotherapy was shown to cause few serious long-term side effects, compared with those expected from external beam radiation therapy. When 3-D conformal radiotherapy was used as a primary therapy, patients with a PSA greater than 10 at diagnosis had a significantly shorter period of disease-free survival, compared with patients whose PSA was less than 10. Patients with Gleason scores of 7 and above also had a significantly lower disease-free survival period.

7. Vitamin D3 was shown to induce prostate cancer cell apoptosis (programmed cell death) via several mechanisms. One newly identified action of vitamin D3 on prostate cancer cells was the translocation of the androgen receptor, thus making these cells less susceptible to proliferation stimulation by testosterone.

8. Hormone-blockade therapy was shown to reduce prostate volume by about 30 percent. Prostate cancer cells responded much more favorably to hormone-blocking therapy than non-cancerous prostate cells. The results suggest that hormone blockade downsizes, and in some cases down stages, prostate cancer cells. Down staging of prostate cancer cells could result in a significant long-term remission.

9. Statistically significant rises in PSA levels were observed in men who had undergone cardiac surgery. The doctors speculated this was caused by a lack of blood flow to the prostate gland during surgery, resulting in ischemic

damage to prostate cells that caused them to secrete PSA.

10. A study looked at patients with a mean age of 63 and a mean PSA of 8.6. Forty-six percent were found to have organ-confined prostate cancer, 25 percent had infiltration of cancer cells into the fatty sack containing the prostate gland, and 7 percent had seminal vesicle involvement. At surgery, 46 percent had positive margins, indicating that the cancer had spread beyond the prostate gland. When these patients were sub-grouped, those with a PSA under 10 were much more likely to have organ-confined disease.

11. There was a 27-percent failure rate at five years in men whose PSA was between 8 and 15, and with Gleason scores between 2 and 7 who were treated with external beam radiation alone. The doctors concluded that hormone-blocking therapy may have prevented this high failure rate in these men who had a relatively early stage of prostate cancer.

12. When CT evaluation of prostate tumor volume is performed, an enhancement of visualization occurred in 15 of 16 patients when intravesical contrast was used. Without the use of intravesical contrast, significant underestimating of the tumor volume occurred, which could lead to treatment failure.

13. The free radical-generating fatty acid called arachidonic acid was shown to stimulate prostate cancer cell growth. The molecular pathway of arachidonic stimulation involved the inflammatory enzyme 5-lipooxygenase. Lipooxygenase also is involved in the formation of abnormal blood clots (thrombosis). Nutrients that specifically inhibit 5-lipooxygenase include garlic. Drugs that are beneficial include ibuprofen and aspirin. Fish oil supplements in high doses have been shown to suppress arachidonic acid formation.

14. Prostaglandins are synthesized from arachidonic acid by the enzyme cyclooxygenase. A particularly dangerous prostaglandin is PGE2, which is involved in many chronic inflammatory diseases. The administration of PGE2 to prostate, breast and colon-cancer cells resulted in increased cellular proliferation. An ibuprofen derivative called flurbiprofen inhibited PGE2-induced prostate cancer cell growth. Aspirin, ibuprofen and fish oil are several available agents that inhibit PGE2 synthesis.

15. In advanced, hormone-refractory (not readily yielding to treatment) prostate cancer, the chemotherapy drug mitoxantrone, in combination with a prednisone or hydrocortisone, showed clinical benefits in 35 to 40 percent of patients. Quality of life improvements where noted with less toxicity encountered, compared with traditional chemotherapy drugs. The administration of mitoxantrone, however, did not result in increased survival compared to corticosteroid drugs being used alone.

16. As many as 80 percent of 80-year-old men were shown to have prostate cancer cells present at autopsy, but only 10 percent of them will ever be diagnosed with it, and only 3 percent will ever die from it.

17. Pygeum africanum extract, sold under the trade name Tadenan as a drug in Europe, is used to treat the urinary symptoms of BPH. In a study conducted in rats, pygeum extract was specifically shown to inhibit the benign proliferation of prostate cells. One mechanism of suppression of prostate cell growth was the inhibition of protein kinase C, an enzyme involved in both benign and malignant cell over-proliferation. Soy genistein also is a potent inhibitor of protein kinase C.

18. Doctors report on a patient whose prostate cancer had become hormone-refractory. Flutamide withdrawal, along with the addition of hydrocortisone, has resulted in a 46-month period of total remission. There is currently no evidence of prostate cancer in this patient. Repeat biopsies that had previously showed positive are now negative. The doctors believe that this one case, and the results of previous published studies, indicate that flutamide withdrawal and hydrocortisone therapy is an option for the hormone-refractory disease in the advanced-state prostate cancer patient.

19. A total of 274 men completed questionnaires about their quality of life after radical prostatectomy and external beam radiation. The conclusions from the questionnaires showed that men who had undergone these radical conventional therapies experienced difficulty long after treatment. In this study, the prostatectomy group fared worse as far as sexual and urinary functions, whereas the radiation therapy group experienced more bowel dysfunction.

20. Prostate cancer was detected in 22 percent of men 50 years or older whose PSA reading was between 2.6 and 4. All cancers detected were clinically localized. This study indicates that PSA readings greater than 2.6 may represent a 22-percent risk of prostate cancer. The use of a free PSA test would help determine which of these men whose PSA readings were greater than 2.6 had prostate cancer; such a test could thus reduce the number of unnecessary biopsies.

21. In men with PSA levels greater than 10, and/or Gleason scores equal to or greater than 7, only 60 to 84 percent were free of PSA-measured disease progression three years after conventional therapy. This study indicated the need for adjuvant (assisting) therapies such as hormone blockade.

22. Over a five-year period, prostate cancer patients whose family members also had the disease had a relapse-free survival rate of only 29 percent, compared with relapse-free survival rate of 59 percent in similarly staged prostate cancer patients whose family members did not have prostate cancer. These

findings show that familial prostate cancer may be more aggressive than non-familial forms, and that standard clinical and pathological measurements may not adequately predict this course.

23. In men with advanced metastasized prostate cancer (stage D1 and D2) who were previously untreated, combination therapy utilizing Lupron, flutamide, and pharmaceutically administered suramin produced an overall positive response rate of 67 percent. There were three complete responses in this trial of 48 patients. There were 18 deaths reported in this group.

24. A new term, "anti-androgen withdraw syndrome," has been coined to deal with prostate cancer patients who become refractory (resistant) to hormone-blockade treatment. It appears that upon withdrawal of flutamide, Casodex, and other similar drugs, the PSA level goes sharply down. The doctors advocate a trial of anti-androgen withdrawal therapy prior to the initiation of toxic therapies.

25. If combined hormone therapy begins to fail—that is, if the PSA level starts to elevate or symptoms of disease progression occur—substituting Casodex for flutamide, or visa versa, may buy additional time before hormone-blockade therapy is no longer effective.

26. It may be possible to reduce the dosage of flutamide and still receive the same benefits while minimizing potential side effects. Those who have been on flutamide one to two years may consider reducing the dose to one 125-mg tablet every eight hours, or eliminating it altogether.

27. Dihydrotestosterone may be five times more potent in promoting prostate cancer cell growth than testosterone. Some doctors are using low-dose Proscar drug therapy in varying combinations with other hormone-blocking therapies. Proscar may be a more specific inhibitor of dihydrotestosterone than saw palmetto extract. While saw palmetto has been shown to work equally as well or better than Proscar in treating BPH, saw palmetto may interfere with benign prostate cell growth by mechanisms other than direct dihydrotestosterone suppression. More studies are needed to validate the benefits of Proscar in treating prostate cancer.

Product availability: Mega Soy extract, Soy Power, green tea extract, vitamin D3 capsules, PC Spes and saw palmetto/pygeum extract can be ordered by phoning 1-800-544-4440.

Prostate Cancer
(Metastasized/Late Stage)

Refer to the Life Extension Foundation's basic Cancer Treatment protocol and the Prostate Cancer (Early Stage) protocol for treatment suggestions. Initiate prolactin-suppression drug therapy if prolactin levels in the blood are even slightly elevated. After prostate cancer cells have become androgen-independent, the withdrawal from flutamide or Casodex can result in a temporary but significant reduction in PSA tumor markers and clinical symptoms of the disease.

The survival rate of stage D3 prostate cancer patients is poor. Reports have suggested the existence of humoral (in the blood) and cell-mediated immunity against prostate cancer tumor-associated antigens. These observations prompted a group of doctors to treat stage D3 prostate cancer patients with an in vitro-produced transfer factor able to transfer protection against bladder and prostate cancer infiltration. Fifty patients entered this study and received one intramuscular injection of two to five units monthly of specific transfer factor. The followup, ranging from one to nine years, showed that complete remission was achieved in two patients, partial remission in six, and no progression of metastatic disease in 14. The median survival was 126 weeks, higher than the survival rates reported in the literature for patients of the same stage. The Life Extension Foundation is investigating several different transfer factors.

Management of prostate cancer that has spread outside of the prostate capsule is a difficult problem. Innovative, non-toxic approaches to the disease are required. New, relatively non-toxic vitamin-D3 analogs have recently been synthesized. Published studies report that vitamin D3 and vitamin-Λ compounds have marked anti-proliferative effects on prostate cells.

Genistein has been proposed as an effective agent to prevent the expression of metastasic capacity in hormone-dependent cancers. A study assessed the benefits of genistein in inhibiting the proliferation and expression of the in vitro invasive capacity of prostatic cells with different invasive potential. In a cell-culture system, genistein appeared to be cytotoxic and inhibitory of prostate cancer cell proliferation.

Hypocalcemia is a common but frequently unrecognized complication of prostatic cancer. In patients with prostatic carcinoma, calcium levels are an indicator of early changes in calcium homeostasis (natural stability). Some advanced prostate-cancer patients show extensive bony metastases and osteomalacia. Improvement in a patient's symptoms and normalization of serum calcium and phosphorus have occurred after treatment with vitamin D3 drugs.

PC Spes is a new herbal therapy for treating prostate cancer at various stages. PC Spes consists of a combination of eight herbal extracts, and has been in development for 10 years. There are 400 people taking the product, and the manufacturer reports that 75 percent of prostate cancer patients show improvements in their condition and reduction in PSA. The less severe the case, the better the results. Minimum dose is one 320-mg capsule three times a day. Most prostate cancer patients take about nine capsules a day for two or three months, and then reduce the dose to three to six capsules a day. Up to 12 capsules a day for one to two months have been used by advanced prostate cancer patients.

A few non-statistically significant cases of thrombosis have been reported in users of PC Spes. Some literature has reported that PC Spes works by enhancing immune function and boosting estrogen levels. However, a review of the molecular mechanisms of action of PC Spes on prostate cancer cells indicates that it functions as a specific suppressor of prostate cancer cell growth by modulating cell regulatory protein molecules, and that it may induce cancer-cell apoptosis (programmed cancer cell death). Anyone taking PC Spes should carefully follow the Foundation's Thrombosis Prevention protocol.

For referrals to doctors experienced in using combined hormone blockade, cryo-ablation therapy, seed implantation, etc., call The Educational Center for Prostate Patients at 516-997-1777 or PAACT at 616-453-1477.

Prostate Enlargement (Benign Prostatic Hypertrophy)

The benign enlargement of the prostate gland affects most men over the age of 60. The enlarged prostate blocks the flow of urine from the bladder, which can produce mild to severe urinary obstruction. The inability to completely evacuate the bladder is especially troublesome at night. Men with prostate enlargement often complain about having to get up multiple times throughout the night to urinate. Benign prostate disease can mean a higher risk of prostate cancer in the future. Thus, the Life Extension Foundation's protocol to shrink enlarged benign prostate glands also is designed to reduce the risk of prostate cancer.

One cause of prostate enlargement is overproduction of a hormone metabolite called dihydrotestosterone (DHT), which is considered a prime culprit in the development of benign prostate enlargement and, possibly, prostate cancer. The stimulating nature of dihydrotestosterone in the development of prostate disease is well-documented, since castration before age 40 prevents prostate enlargement and prostate cancer. Additionally, castration is a proven therapy to reverse both benign and malignant prostate disease. These findings strongly suggest that strategies to reduce DHT levels would prevent many forms of prostate disease.

The evidence that DHT is a cause of prostate disease comes from observations in 1974 that men with low blood levels of DHT maintain normal muscle mass, libido and a small prostate, compared with men with average DHT levels who suffer from enlarged prostates, frontal hair recession, diffuse beard growth and acne. It appears that DHT is responsible for many of life's undesirable ills affecting males. Testosterone is converted into DHT by the enzyme 5-alpha reductase, which increases as men grow older, causing elevated DHT production, decreased serum testosterone, and enlargement of the prostate gland. When the action of 5-alpha reductase is blocked, dramatic reductions in DHT levels occur.

The reduction in DHT production via inhibition of 5-alpha reductase produces normalization of prostate volume and improvements in urinary and sexual function in men suffering from benign prostatic hypertrophy. Additionally, a decline in DHT could impact favorably on hairline recession, acne and excess facial hair. In females, testosterone is produced in the adrenal glands, and blocking dihydrotestosterone could be especially effective in ridding the patient of unwanted facial hair. By reducing serum DHT levels and displacing DHT and testosterone from prostate cells, the proliferation of prostate cells is inhibited, resulting in a reduction in prostate volume and, in most cases, relief from the symptoms of prostate enlargement.

For many years, the Foundation has recommended the European drug Permixon as an effective therapy for benign prostatic hypertrophy. Permixon is a standardized extract from the saw palmetto berry. Permixon was used in Europe to treat benign prostate enlargement almost 20 years before the FDA approved an equally expensive drug called Proscar.

In lieu of the Permixon drug, Americans are able to purchase high-quality saw palmetto extracts as low-cost dietary supplements. These saw palmetto extracts are identical to Permixon. Saw palmetto has been shown to significantly reduce total prostate weight and volume, even in the presence of hormones that promote prostate growth.

Studies have shown that saw palmetto produces significant improvement in those with prostate enlargement, resulting in the following clinical benefits:

- ❖ Reduction of nocturnal urinary urgency
- ❖ Increased urinary flow rate
- ❖ Reduced residual volume in the bladder
- ❖ Reduction in uncomfortable urination symptoms

A paper in *Current Therapies, Research, Clinical Experience* reports on a Belgian study involving 505 men with benign prostate disease. The results showed that saw palmetto improved urinary flow, reduced residual urinary volume and prostate size, and improved quality of life after only 45 days of treatment. After 90 days, 88 percent of the patients and treating physicians considered the treatment effective. In addition, the study showed for the first time that saw palmetto does not mask the PSA (prostate specific antigens) score as Proscar has been shown to do. The researchers concluded by stating, "The extract of saw palmetto appears to be an effective and well-tolerated pharmacologic agent in treating urinary problems accompanying benign prostatic hypertrophy."

For most men, two saw palmetto extract capsules a day will shrink an enlarged prostate gland to provide relief from benign prostate disease. If this is not successful, a combination of saw palmetto extract and another European prostate medication, pygeum, will provide relief in most cases. Pygeum inhibits prostate-cell proliferation and produces an anti-edema effect that can shrink enlarged prostate glands significantly.

Although more than 80 percent of men report improvement after using saw palmetto and/or pygeum extracts, some prostate enlargement often remains that continues to interfere with urinary flow and bladder evacuation.

An herbal extract called urtica dioica has been shown to reduce the symptoms of benign prostatic hypertrophy by 86 percent after three months of use. The urtica dioica extract is approved by the German government in combination with saw palmetto extract to treat the symptoms of benign prostate disease. In January 1998, the Life Extension Foundation introduced Americans to the identical urtica dioica extract used in Germany to treat benign prostate enlargement. The urtica extract comes in an herbal formula that also contains pharmaceutical extracts of saw palmetto and pygeum.

What follows is a review of how saw palmetto, pygeum and urtica extracts treat benign prostatic hypertrophy:

- ❖ Enlargement of the prostate gland, which occurs in most men with advancing age, is accompanied by reduced urinary flow and increased residual urine volume. Hormonal imbalances are known to be a major cause of age-related prostate disorders, but other factors have been identified as culprits that create urinary impairment.

- ❖ Phytosterol extracts from saw palmetto interfere with conversion of testosterone to dihydrotestosterone. New studies are showing that saw palmetto reduces smooth-muscle contraction, thereby relaxing the bladder and sphincter muscles that cause urinary urgency.

- ❖ Pygeum originally was shown to reduce prostate swelling (edema) and block dihydrotestosterone binding to prostate cells. New studies show that pygeum also interferes with protein kinase C activity to inhibit the proliferation of prostate cells. Rapidly growing benign and malignant cells both require the protein kinase C enzyme. Soy genistein is one of the most potent inhibitors of protein kinase C, a primary mechanism by which soy helps to prevent cancer and slows the growth of some existing cancers.

- ❖ Added to this herbal arsenal against enlarged prostate is the urtica dioica extract. One study showed that, after eight weeks of treatment with four capsules of urtica extract, there was an 82-percent improvement or total elimination of disorders associated with prostate enlargement. Another study showed that patients suffering from prostate enlargement with stage one to three hyperplasia (which can lead to prostate cancer) improved 86 percent after three months treatment with standardized urtica extract.

- ❖ After learning the results of these studies, researchers at St. Luke's/Roosevelt Hospital in New York conducted a study to discover the mechanism by which standardized urtica extract relieves the symptoms of benign prostate hyperplasia (excess cell proliferation). In their study, published in 1995, these scientists showed that urtica extract inhibits the binding of a testosterone-related protein to its receptor site on prostate cell membranes.

❖ Prostate cells grow out of control when the hormone metabolite dihydrotestosterone binds to prostate cell membranes, a process that induces the prostate cells to start dividing. If cell membrane receptors are blocked, the dihydrotestosterone cannot latch onto the cell. Urtica extract appears to work by preventing the binding of testosterone metabolites to membrane receptor sites on prostate cells.

While saw palmetto and urtica dioica are approved drugs in Germany for the treatment of benign prostate enlargement, pygeum and saw palmetto are approved throughout Europe. Urtica may be new to Americans, but it has been safely and successfully used in Germany for more than a decade.

Be careful from whom you buy your prostate-shrinking herbal extracts. Some companies sell saw palmetto "berry" capsules at very low prices. Saw palmetto berries do not provide the standardized fatty acid sterols needed for therapeutic benefits. What's surprising is that there are major name-brand supplement companies that sell both standardized saw palmetto extract and saw palmetto berry capsules. These commercial companies know there are no prostate benefits from taking saw palmetto berry capsules, but they sell them anyway just to offer a lower-priced product.

The Foundation believes it is immoral to sell a supplement whose name ("saw palmetto") implies therapeutic benefits, but which doesn't actually deliver such benefits.

The first standardized herbal formula sold in America that contains saw palmetto, pygeum and urtica extracts is called Natural Prostate Formula. The extracts in this exclusive formula are the exact same pharmaceutical-grade, standardized extracts used in these studies.

For the 10 to 20 percent of men who do not obtain sufficient benefit from the saw palmetto, pygeum and urtica extracts, the addition of the prescription drug Hytrin has proven beneficial.

For those for whom all nutrient and drug therapies fail, testosterone blockade for three months of prostate cell receptor sites with the drug Casodex may provide significant prostate-gland shrinkage. Casodex is not approved by the FDA to treat benign prostatic hypertrophy, but your doctor can legally prescribe it.

The FDA-approved drug Lupron dramatically suppresses testosterone production. Lupron is used to treat prostate cancer, but has been shown to be beneficial in shrinking enlarged prostate glands when all other non-surgical therapies have failed. Lupron is injected at a doctor's office and will last for three months. Make sure your doctor prescribes the standard dose of Casodex or flutamide one week prior to receiving the Lupron injection in order to protect against the temporary testosterone surge that can occur immediately after Lupron is administered.

Avoid the surgical procedure known as transurethral resection. It involves the insertion of a device into the urethra, and the grinding away of part of the prostate gland. Many painful side effects can occur as a result of this procedure, and it also appears to increase the risk of having a heart attack later in life. A study was conducted on 811 men who, between 1983 and 1992, underwent transurethral resection of the prostate. Fifty-two patients developed a first-time heart attack after the procedure. A pre-operative low blood hemoglobin concentration in the range of 100 to 129 g/l was associated with double the risk of a first-time heart attack. The acute heart attack risk was even greater in men who had already suffered one heart attack. The normal range for serum hemoglobin is 130 to 165 g/l. If your hemoglobin is below this, you may face a doubled risk of developing an acute heart attack in later life if you undergo the transurethral resection. Other studies confirm this.

There is an alternative procedure that appears to benefit those with severe benign prostatic hypertrophy, and which should be available soon in most cities. A study was done to investigate the long-term outcome of patients treated with lower energy transurethral microwave thermotherapy. After three years of followup, the previous application of lower energy transurethral microwave thermotherapy showed significant improvements in 52 percent of the patients with severe benign prostate enlargement. This therapy was used by alternative doctors for years, and is now being used by some conventional urologists.

Based upon records of dietary soy consumption in Japan, where prostate cancer rates are very low, the typical daily isoflavone intake has been estimated at 50 mg per person. By contrast, the typical Western diet has been estimated to provide only two to three mg a day of genistein. Soy phytoestrogens such as genistein may counteract some of the effects of dihydrotestosterone, and therefore may be helpful in treating benign prostate enlargement.

A soy supplement called Mega Soy Extract provides 110 mg of soy phytoestrogens in just two capsules, more than twice the amount in the typical Japanese diet. Since the phytoestrogen genistein is water-soluble, it is suggested that one capsule of Mega Soy Extract be taken in the morning and one in the evening. Some men with severe prostate enlargement may double this dose if lower doses do not provide benefits within 60 days.

Scientists have published papers indicating that the consumption of soy phytoestrogens may significantly reduce prostate cancer risk. Since men with benign prostate disease are at a greater risk for eventually developing prostate cancer, the use of high-potency soy supplements is highly recommended.

Since men with benign prostate growth are at an increased risk of developing prostate cancer, the PSA and free-PSA blood tests should be considered every six months. The free-PSA test helps to determine if a moderately elevated PSA (with levels of 4 to 10) is indicative of early stage prostate cancer.

Product availability: Saw palmetto extract, Mega Soy Extract, Natural Prostate Formula and saw-palmetto/pygeum extract are available by calling 1-800-544-4440. Hytrin, Lupron and Casodex are drugs that can be prescribed by your doctor.

Pulmonary Insufficiencies

Refer to the Emphysema And Chronic Obstructive Pulmonary Disease protocol.

Retinopathy

Diseases of the eye, diagnosed as retinopathies, often are caused by nutrient deficiencies. Diabetic retinopathy, for example, has been shown to be caused by a deficiency of vitamin B6. In order to rule out a nutritional deficiency as a cause of retinopathy, it is suggested that three tablets, three times a day, of Life Extension Mix be taken for 10 weeks. Life Extension Mix contains 56 high-potency nutrients, including the complete B-complex vitamins that are often deficient in patients with retinopathy.

A newborn rat model of retinopathy was used to test the hypothesis that a lack of the antioxidant superoxide dismutase (SOD) contributes to the retinal damage. Delivery of SOD to the retina via long-circulating liposomes proved beneficial, suggesting that restoration and/or supplementation of antioxidants in retinal tissue is a potentially valuable therapeutic strategy.

In another study, the antioxidant activity was investigated in the lens and vitreous of diabetic and nondiabetic subjects. Glutathione peroxidase activity and ascorbic acid levels, known to exert important antioxidant functions in the eye compartment, were found to be significantly decreased in the lens of diabetic patients, especially in the presence of retinal damage. This study indicated that oxidative damage is involved in the onset of diabetic eye complications, in which the decrease in free radical scavengers was shown to be associated with the oxidation of vitreous and lens proteins.

Activities of enzymes that protect the retina from reactive oxygen species were investigated in diabetic rats known to develop retinopathy. Diabetes significantly decreased the activities of glutathione reductase and glutathione peroxidase in the retina. Activities of two other important antioxidant defense enzymes—superoxide dismutase (SOD) and catalase—also were decreased (by more than 25 percent) in retinas of diabetic rats.

Administration of supplemental vitamins C and E for two months prevented the diabetes-induced impairment of the antioxidant defense system in the retina. This study showed that diabetes causes significant impairment of this defense system, and antioxidant supplementation can help alleviate the subnormal activities of antioxidant defense enzymes.

A study was carried out on 60 oxygen-treated premature infants and their mothers to assess retinopathy. The results showed the signs of an acute oxidative stress in all 60 oxygen-treated infants. The concentrations of methionine-cysteine in the plasma, as well as blood selenium levels, were significantly lower in the prematures suffering from moderate retinopathy than in the other oxygen-treated prematures without retinopathy. The same tendency was seen in the mothers. Vitamin E treatment of retinopathy infants seemed to have a positive effect against the development of retinopathy of prematurity. The close correlation found between the antioxidant capacity of the mothers and babies suggests that the supplementation of feeding with sulfur-containing amino acids (methionine, cysteine) and folic acid during pregnancy would improve the antioxidant capacity of premature infants. An antioxidant cocktail of selenium plus vitamin E, given to high-risk mothers (high risk factors including advanced age, smoking, and pregnancy-induced hypertension) before delivery might be useful in the prevention of retinopathy in premature infants.

The effect of propionyl-L-carnitine, an analogue of L-carnitine, was examined in rats with laboratory-induced diabetes. These findings showed a potential therapeutic value of propionyl-L-carnitine for diabetic retinopathy. Until propionyl-L-carnitine becomes available, taking 2,000 mg a day of acetyl-L-carnitine should be considered by those with retinopathy.

Glycation (glycosylation) of proteins has been shown to play a prominent role in the development of many diseases related to diabetes, including atherosclerosis, cataract formation and retinopathy. This process also occurs as a result of general aging. Investigations have been conducted to explore the possibility of preventing glycation by use of pyruvate and alpha-keto glutarate. The results demonstrate that both these compounds are effective in preventing the initial glycation reaction, as well as the formation of eye disease.

Both pyruvate and alpha-keto glutarate also inhibit the generation of high molecular weight aggregates associated with cataract formation. The preventive effects appear to be due to competitive inhibition of glycation by the keto acids and the antioxidant properties of these compounds. These agents might be useful in preventing glycation-related protein changes and consequent tissue pathological manifestations associated with cataract, diabetes and normal aging.

Diabetics should consider taking 650 mg of ornithine alpha-ketoglutarate three times a day. The best form of pyruvate is calcium pyruvate. A 500-mg capsule of calcium pyruvate provides 405 mg of elemental pyruvic acid. One to three capsules a day of calcium pyruvate is suggested. The formation of advanced glycation products and free radicals has been implicated in the development of diabetic complications. Strategies for the prevention of diabetic complications, therefore, should aim to prevent both the effects of glycation and oxidative stress.

A lack of vitamin B12 may damage the optic nerve. Studies have suggested that marginal vitamin deficiency plays an indirect but important role in the development of diabetic complications. The use of 1,000 to 3,000 mg a day of niacin might decrease lipoprotein(a), which could help prevent diabetic retinopathy.

The drug aminoguanidine in the dose of 300 mg a day can specifically inhibit glycosylation, as can the nutrients keto-glutarate and pyruvate. The most effective antioxidant protection can be obtained by taking three tablets, three times a day, of the Life Extension Mix antioxidant formula, along with one capsule a day of the Life Extension Booster formula.

Product availability: Life Extension Mix, Life Extension Booster, and acetyl-L-carnitine can be ordered by calling 1-800-544-4440. Aminoguanidine is available from European suppliers.

Seasonal Affective Disorder (SAD)

Research is being conducted to understand a depressive state that occurs when the days get shorter. The early loss of sunlight in the winter appears to induce chemical changes in the brain that bring on depression.

In some people, melatonin makes the symptoms of seasonal affective disorder (SAD) worse. These people should stop melatonin or reduce its dosage during the times of the year when darkness appears early in the day.

Some people take prescription antidepressants such as Prozac only during the time of the year they are affected by seasonal affective disorder. Prozac's mechanism of action is to selectively inhibit serotonin reuptake. There is evidence that serotonergic dysregulation is involved in SAD.

A safer way of boosting serotonin levels is to ingest 2,000 to 3,000 mg of the amino acid tryptophan each night. The clinical use of l-tryptophan has been specifically shown to benefit SAD patients and to improve their response to light therapy.

Bright light therapy is an effective treatment for seasonal affective disorder. Bright lights have been used as adjuncts (assisting therapies) in the pharmacological treatment of other types of depressive illness. Standard morning light therapy regimen often consists of exposure of 10,000-lux cool-white fluorescent light for 30 minutes. About 66 percent of SAD patients respond to light therapy. Light therapy also appears to be an effective treatment for pediatric SAD. Some research indicates that the serotonin system might be involved in the mechanism of action of light therapy. In patients who do not respond to light therapy, the addition of tryptophan has resulted in significant reduction of mean depression scores of SAD.

Refer to the Foundation's protocol for Depression. People who are afflicted with SAD should consider the Foundation's natural protocols before resorting to conventional antidepressant drugs.

Skin Aging

The most important thing to do to prevent skin aging is to protect your skin from exposure to ultraviolet (UV) light. That means wearing a sunscreen every time you go outdoors. If you look at the skin in areas of your body not exposed to the sun, you'll see that it is far more youthful than your face and hands, which are chronically bombarded with UV light.

The oral intake of antioxidants, especially the proanthocyanidin flavonoid found in grape seed-skin extract, can boost the production of collagen and elastin. Grape seed-skin extract also provides broad-spectrum protection against damaging free radicals that cause proteins in the skin to crosslink and form wrinkles.

Vitamin C taken orally and applied topically enhances collagen production and protects against free radicals. The average dose of grape seed-skin extract to protect against skin aging is 200 mg a day, along with several thousand milligrams of vitamin C. The grape seed-skin extract we recommend contains 50 mg of pharmaceutical-grade extract, along with 250 mg of vitamin C from buffered calcium ascorbate.

Skin plays an important role in immunity. Boosting the health of the skin increases the natural rate of cell renewal and repair. Epidermal growth factors encourage young cells to replace old cells in the upper layers of the skin. The stimulation of epidermal growth factors is one of the mechanisms responsible for the anti-aging effects of the prescription drug Retin-A.

Aging causes the skin to lose such moisturizing components as NaPCA, lactic acid and hyaluronic acid, required for skin cells to retain moisture. Replacing these natural moisturizing factors topically can produce a youthful, moistening effect in dry, aged skin. Skin damaging free radicals can be suppressed by the topical application of such antioxidants as vitamin E, vitamin C and EDTA.

A well-documented mechanism of skin aging is the accumulation of dead cells at the surface of the skin. Young skin rapidly produces fresh skin cells that move to the surface to replace old, damaged cells, but aged skin forms a natural glue that binds to dead skin cells and prevents them from sloughing off.

The topical application of alpha-hydroxy fruit acids can gently remove dead cells at the surface of aged skin and more quickly expose the young cells underneath. The effects of the daily application of alpha-hydroxy fruit acids are to reduce the appearance of fine lines and enlarged pores, and expose more youthful appearing skin cells. The topical application of RNA and yeast cell wall extracts can stimulate greater production of youthful skin cells, thus increasing the appearance-enhancing effect of the alpha-hydroxy acids.

You can purchase many different commercial products at very high prices that can provide, individually, these well-documented anti-aging factors, or you can obtain all of them in a product called Rejuvenex, which includes alpha-hydroxy fruit acids, the complete moisturizing complex, cell-renewing nutrients such as retinyl palmitate, RNA, a special yeast cell wall extract, topical antioxidant vitamins, epidermal growth factors, and a light sunscreen to protect against daily indoor and outdoor ultraviolet light exposure.

For those seeking a highly potent alpha-hydroxy skin product, a formula designed by Durk Pearson and Sandy Shaw called Look & Feel provides high concentrations of all the alpha-hydroxy fruit acids that have shown an anti-wrinkling effect.

In a double-blind randomized study, the topical application of melatonin suppressed UV-induced erythema, a marker of skin aging damage. A distinct dose-response relationship was observed between the topical dose of melatonin and the degree of UV-induced erythema. The scientists suggested that the topical application of melatonin might open a new approach in the prevention and control of free radical-influenced skin diseases.

Product availability: Rejuvenex, proanthocyanidins (grape seed-skin extract), vitamin C and Look & Feel can be ordered by phoning 1-800-544-4440.

Stress

Refer to the Life Extension Foundation's Anxiety protocol.

Stroke (Hemorrhagic)

Twenty percent of strokes are caused by a rupture in an artery of the brain. Blood flow is disrupted to the area of the brain normally served by the ruptured artery, which usually results in paralysis or death. Hemorrhagic stroke can be caused by high blood pressure, an aneurysm in a brain artery, or an overdose of blood-thinning medication.

The acute treatment for hemorrhagic stroke is different from the treatment for stroke caused by a blood clot. That is why a CAT scan has to be done in a hospital setting to determine whether an apparent stroke has been caused by a ruptured artery or by an arterial blood clot.

When a hemorrhagic stroke occurs, blood-thinning agents like aspirin and ginkgo biloba have to be avoided. A hemorrhagic stroke not only deprives a portion of the brain of blood, but also causes massive free radical injury from the iron-rich blood that saturates brain cells.

The emergency room doctor should immediately administer 10 mg of Hydergine sublingually and 10 mg of Hydergine orally. Liquid Hydergine should be avoided in treating hemorrhagic stroke because of its high alcohol content. Hydergine is a powerful antioxidant that helps to protect brain cells from free radical injury and death. More importantly, Hydergine protects brain cells from oxygen deprivation and improves their ability to utilize oxygen, something that is critical when there is a disruption of blood supply to an area of the brain.

In Europe, Hydergine is administered on an acute-care basis to prevent permanent brain damage due to stroke. Since the FDA has not approved Hydergine for acute stroke, most emergency room doctors are reluctant to prescribe it. You (or your medical surrogate) should insist on Hydergine being administered when symptoms of an acute stroke are present. Hydergine should be readily available from the hospital pharmacy.

What will not be available from the hospital pharmacy are such European medications as piracetam, which can protect brain cells against injury and death after interruption of blood flow. The administration of 4,800 mg of piracetam orally may provide considerable protection against permanent neurologic injury.

Hemorrhagic stroke is very common in the Chinese population. A study of Chinese patients with hemorrhagic stroke showed that 50 percent of the patients had previously diagnosed hypertension, but only 20 percent of these patients regularly took their antihypertensive medication. This study concluded that better management of hypertension would help reduce the incidence of hemorrhagic stroke.

To learn about therapies that may strengthen the arteries in the brain to prevent hemorrhagic stroke, refer to the Life Extension Foundation's protocol on treating Cerebral Vascular

Disease.

To learn about therapies that might help to restore neurological function lost to a hemorrhagic stroke, refer to the Life Extension Foundation's protocol for Age-Associated Mental Impairment (Brain Aging).

Product availability: You can order high-potency Hydergine tablets and piracetam from offshore suppliers who ship to Americans for personal use. Some people keep Hydergine in their medicine cabinet for emergency administration in case of a heart attack, stroke or accident. Many people take Hydergine and piracetam every day to help prevent neurological aging. For a list of offshore sources for these drugs, phone 1-800-544-4440.

Stroke (Thrombotic)
(also Transient Ischemic Attack)

Eighty percent of strokes are caused by a blood clot that forms in an artery in the brain. The blood clot blocks the flow of blood to a portion of the brain, resulting in paralysis or death. A stroke caused by a blood clot is called a thrombotic stroke, as opposed to stroke caused by a breakage in a cerebral artery, which is called a hemorrhagic stroke.

Underlying risk factors for thrombotic stroke are cerebral atherosclerosis, hypertension, excessive blood-clotting factors such as homocysteine, fibrinogen and LDL cholesterol, heart valve defects, diabetes and aging. More than 400,000 Americans suffer thrombotic strokes yearly. When a thrombotic stroke occurs, it is crucial to dissolve the blood clot that is blocking the artery in the brain.

The FDA has approved a clot-busting drug called t-PA. You should insist that the emergency room doctor administer the drug t-PA (sold under the brand name Activase) immediately in order to dissolve the clot that is preventing blood from reaching a portion of your brain. T-PA stands for tissue plasminogen activator. It is a natural clot-dissolving substance produced by the body.

T-PA has saved the lives of hundreds of thousands of heart attack victims. In the latest study, 30 percent more stroke victims were able to regain full use of their faculties after receiving T-PA. However, the FDA took eight years to approve t-PA as a treatment for thrombotic stroke, even as t-PA was being used in progressive emergency rooms in the U.S. as an unapproved drug to treat thrombotic stroke. Even today, patients may encounter severe resistance from emergency room doctors who are reluctant to administer it, even if a patient's life is at stake.

While t-PA can dissolve the blood clot that causes blood-vessel blockage, there are other complications that occur during a thrombotic stroke that have to be addressed if permanent brain damage is to be prevented. Any interruption in blood flow causes an oxygen imbalance that results in massive free radical damage. It is critically important to have antioxidants in your bloodstream when t-PA is administered to reduce the free radical damage that will occur when blood flow is restored.

The most potent antioxidant that hospital pharmacies normally stock is Hydergine. You should insist that the emergency room doctor administer 10 mg of Hydergine sublingually, and another 10 mg of Hydergine orally in liquid form. Hydergine is a powerful antioxidant that reduces free radical damage. Hydergine will increase the amount of oxygen delivered to the brain, enhance the energy metabolism of brain cells, and protect brain cells against both the low and high oxygen environments that thrombotic stroke victims often encounter.

Hydergine is used routinely in Europe as a treatment for stroke, but, as noted, most emergency room doctors in the U.S. are reluctant to prescribe it because the FDA does not recognize its value in preventing brain-cell death. Paralyzed stroke victims consume billions of health-care dollars every year, and the reason most thrombotic stroke victims are permanently paralyzed is that the FDA has stopped patients from being treated with medications to prevent brain-cell death.

If you have access to the European drug piracetam when stroke symptoms occur, brain-cell damage can be prevented, or at least mitigated. The recommended dose is 4,800 mg of piracetam administered immediately. If you know a thrombotic stroke is occurring, large quantities of antioxidant vitamins and herbs such as ginkgo biloba would be of benefit.

The problem is, if it's a brain hemorrhage (hemorrhagic stroke) instead of a blood clot (thrombotic stroke), these nutrients could cause additional cerebral bleeding. Magnesium in an oral dose of 1,500 mg is a safe nutrient to relieve arterial spasm, a common problem in thrombotic stroke. If you take high-potency antioxidant nutrients at least three times a day, your chances of fully recovering from a thrombotic stroke would be vastly improved.

Preventing new blood clots in cerebral vessels is critical in preventing another thrombotic stroke. The choice of anti-thrombotic agents depends on the specific type of stroke—thrombosis, embolism or hemorrhage. Anti-platelet agents are considered most beneficial in thrombotic stroke, and anti-coagulants are most effective in cardioembolic stroke; antithrombotic agents are generally contraindicated in hemorrhagic stroke.

An analysis of 18 trials documented a 23-percent reduction in stroke risk with anti-platelet agents. Low-dose aspirin is the conventional anti-platelet agent of choice for stroke prevention, although nutrients such as fish oil and garlic may produce similar and more broad-spectrum anti-thrombotic benefits. The drug ticlopidine is the most effective anti-platelet agent, but its adverse-effect profile restricts its use. Here again, nutrients such as gingko and green tea extracts may be as effective, and are free of side effects.

Anti-coagulants are highly effective for preventing cardioembolic stroke, but their effectiveness in non-cardioembolic stroke is uncertain. If the complete thrombosis prevention protocol is followed, the need for anti-coagulant drugs like Coumadin and heparin may be reduced. The use of thrombotic risk factor blood testing can help your physician reduce or eliminate your dose of anti-coagulant medications.

WARNING: Never change your anti-coagulation medication without physician approval.

Sudden death could occur if the thrombosis prevention protocol is used without physician guidance.

Mild hyperhomocysteinemia, due to genetic or environmental factors, is now recognized as a risk factor for premature arterial disease, including thrombotic stroke. The nutrients contained in the Atherosclerosis protocol can dramatically lower homocysteine levels.

Remember, stroke is an emergency. Thrombotic stroke is similar to heart attack caused by coronary artery occlusion. The mechanism of damage is loss of blood supply to the tissue, which can result in irreversible brain-cell damage if blood flow is not restored quickly. Public education is needed to emphasize the warning signs of stroke.

A patient should seek medical help immediately, using an ambulance or other emergency transport system. Therapy geared toward minimizing the damage from an acute stroke should be started without delay in the emergency room. This includes measures to protect brain tissue, support perfusion pressure, and minimize cerebral edema. Strategies for improving recovery also should begin immediately. Basic research has opened the door to new therapies aimed at re-establishing blood flow and limiting tissue damage. Trials in progress are testing the usefulness of neuroprotective agents used in Europe, antioxidant agents, anti-inflammatory agents, low molecular-weight heparin, thrombolytic drugs (like t-PA), and angioplasty.

If you already suffer from brain-cell damage caused by a previous thrombotic stroke, please refer to the Life Extension Foundation's protocol on treating Age-Associated Mental Impairment. These therapies can help restore circulation and energy levels of cells effected by a stroke or transient ischemic attack.

To learn how to prevent a stroke or transient ischemia attacks, refer to the Atherosclerosis, Hypertension and Thrombosis Prevention protocols.

Product availability: If you want to keep Hydergine and piracetam in your medicine cabinet for emergency use during a heart attack, stroke or accident, phone 1-800-544-4440 for a list of offshore pharmacies that will ship these products by mail to Americans for personal use. Many people take Hydergine and piracetam every day to prevent brain-cell injury due to normal aging.

Surgical Precautions

Refer to the Life Extension Foundation's Anesthesia And Surgery Precautions protocol.

Thrombosis Prevention
(Preventing Blood Clots in Blood Vessels)

One of the leading causes of death in the Western world is the formation of an abnormal blood clot (thrombus) in a blood vessel.

If a clot occurs in a coronary artery, a person can have a heart attack. If the clot occurs in an artery in the brain, a person can have a stroke. Clots that form anywhere inside the vascular system can travel elsewhere in the body, causing lethal damage in the lungs (pulmonary embolism), kidneys, and other parts of the body. Cancer patients are especially vulnerable to disability and death from abnormal clot formation inside the blood vessels.

Conventional medicine prescribes drugs like Coumadin and heparin to reduce the risk of abnormal blood clotting (thrombosis), but these drugs block only about 33 percent of the coagulation cascade. As a result, people who are taking prescription anti-coagulant drugs often die from a heart attack or stroke caused directly by the formation of a blood vessel clot, even though they properly took their medicine. Prescription anti-coagulation drugs do not effectively deal with the many factors that have been identified as directly causing blood clots to form inside of blood vessels.

Some common thrombotic risk factors are:

- ❖ Atrial fibrillation
- ❖ Heart valve replacement
- ❖ Cigarette smoking
- ❖ Atherosclerosis
- ❖ Some forms of cancer
- ❖ Heart attack, thrombotic stroke, carotid stenosis
- ❖ Diabetes
- ❖ Cold weather
- ❖ Aging

The mechanisms that cause abnormal clots to form inside blood vessels have been extensively studied and documented, yet conventional medicine fails to recognize and recommend supplements that could prevent many people from dying of heart attacks, strokes and other diseases caused by abnormal blood clotting inside blood vessels.

In order for the reader to understand how many different thrombotic mechanisms exist, here is a partial list of contributing factors of blood clotting inside a vessel. Any one of the following could cause a life-threatening blood clot:

- ✔ Elevated homocysteine
- ✔ Oxidized LDL cholesterol
- ✔ Platelet activating factor (PAF)
- ✔ Elevated fibrinogen

✔ Excess platelet free-radical activity
✔ Elevated thromboxane A2, prostaglandin E2, lipooxygenase, and/or cyclooxygenase
✔ Thrombin activating factor
✔ Deficiency of tissue plasminogen activator (tPA)
✔ Hyper-aggregation of red blood cells and loss of red blood cell fluidity
✔ Increased blood viscosity (blood becomes too thick)
✔ Increased total platelet (thrombocyte) count
✔ Increased red blood cell protein kinase activity (PKC)
✔ Inflammation of arterial wall
✔ Atherosclerotic plaque
✔ Elevated triglycerides
✔ Increased platelet adhesion
✔ Collagen-induced platelet aggregation
✔ Arachidonic acid-induced platelet aggregation
✔ Adenosine diphosphate (ADP) induced platelet aggregation
✔ Epinephrine-induced platelet aggregation
✔ Serotonin-induced platelet aggregation

When you see how many different factors are involved in the clotting process, you may understand why conventional anti-coagulation drugs can only provide partial protection against the lethal effects of thrombosis.

People who take vitamin supplements are getting some protection against thrombosis. Published studies show that people taking vitamin supplements have reduced incidences of heart attack, stroke and a host of other diseases related to thrombosis.

For those with significant thrombotic risk factors, the Life Extension Foundation has designed a comprehensive anti-thrombotic supplement protocol. What is not known is how these nutrients interact with prescription anti-coagulant drugs like heparin and Coumadin (warfarin). For example, there are no published studies where these nutrients have been combined with anti-coagulant drugs to see whether the blood becomes too thin. For those who want to take some or all of the Foundation's Anti-Thrombotic Protocols, weekly prothrombin (PT) blood tests are recommended. The four monthly or semi-monthly combination of blood tests to help precisely measure thrombotic risk are:

1. Partial thromboplastin time (PTT)
2. Fibrinogen
3. D-Dimer of fibrin
4. Prothrombin

There are specific nutrients that have been identified that may lower the risk of thrombosis. These nutrients provide many other health benefits, and many people already take these supplements to maintain overall good health.

WARNING: Never change your anticoagulation medication without physician approval. Sudden death could occur if the Thrombosis Prevention Protocol is used without physician guidance.

What follows is a protocol that provides optimal protection against the many factors that have been identified in published studies to cause thrombosis:

- ❖ **Life Extension Booster (take one capsule, three times a day)**

    This multi-nutrient supplement provides potent doses of homocysteine-lowering folic acid and vitamin B12; vitamin E to protect against free radical induced platelet aggregation and LDL cholesterol oxidation; grape skin extract containing some of the components of red wine that have been shown to protect against thrombosis via well-defined mechanisms; and ginkgo to inhibit platelet activating factor (PAF), thrombin activating factor, platelet adhesion, and excess blood viscosity.

- ❖ **Garlic with EDTA (take four capsules a day with a heavy meal)**

    One of the best-documented blood thinning nutrients is garlic. It specifically protects against collagen induced-, arachidonic acid induced-, ADP-induced-, and epinephrine-induced platelet aggregation. Garlic inhibits cyclooxygenase and lipooxygenase-induced thromboxane A2 synthesis. EDTA is so effective in inhibiting blood clotting that it is used in laboratories to keep blood samples from clotting in test tubes.

- ❖ **Fish oil (take two capsules, three times a day with meals)**

    The fatty acids EPA and DHA extracted from fish oil protect against inflammatory platelet aggregation (prostaglandin E2), lower triglyceride levels by 35 percent, may lower fibrinogen levels, and provide many of the other anti-clotting properties of garlic.

- ❖ **Aspirin (take ¼ aspirin tablet a day with a heavy meal)**

    The specific benefit of aspirin is inhibition of cyclooxygenase-2 and thromboxane A2, two primary culprits in the formation of an abnormal blood clot. There are other anti-clotting effects attributed to aspirin. **Doctors tell Coumadin patients to avoid aspirin.**

- ❖ **Vitamin C (take two 1,000-mg capsules three times a day with meals)**

    Vitamin C lowers fibrinogen levels. If fibrinogen levels are below 300, less vitamin C can be taken.

- ❖ **PABA (take one 500-mg capsule, three times a day)**

    This nutrient is especially recommended for cancer patients seeking to reduce their risk of thrombosis.

❖ **Life Extension Mix (take three tablets three times a day)**

> This multi-nutrient formula provides vitamin B6 to suppress homocysteine via a different pathway than folate/vitamin B12. Contains many nutrients that have been shown to protect against thrombosis.

AVOID: Drugs that may increase blood serotonin levels, such as 5-hydroxytryptophan (5-HTP) and dexfenfluramine.

CONSIDER: One glass of red wine a day. Red wine boosts serum levels of tissue plasminogen activator (tPA), a potent clot-busting natural substance. Also consider drinking green tea or taking one green tea extract capsule a day that provide at least 200 mg of polyphenols per capsule.

CAUTION: As noted, it is not known how the nutrients in the Foundation's Anti-Thrombotic Protocol interact with anti-coagulation prescription drugs such as Coumadin and heparin. It is suggested that patients on physician prescribed anti-coagulation drugs slowly introduce the nutrients included in the Anti-Thrombotic Protocol. Weekly blood tests are suggested to make sure the blood is not becoming too thin.

The use of low-molecular weight heparin has proved superior to regular heparin and Coumadin in certain medical conditions. This is an extremely expensive drug, but ask your doctor to consider prescribing low molecular weight heparin if you can afford it, or if you can convince your insurance company to pay for it.

Cancer Patients

In patients affected with different tumors, disorders concerning blood clotting are frequently observed. The biological processes leading to coagulation are probably involved in the mechanisms of metastasis. About 50 percent of all cancer patients, and up to 95 percent of those with metastatic disease, show some abnormalities—a prethrombotic state—in the coagulation-fibrinolytic system. Thromboembolic complications are seen in up to 11 percent of cancer patients, and hemorrhage occurs in about 10 percent. Thromboembolism and hemorrhage, as a whole, are the second most common cause of death after infection.

In a recently published study, subclinical changes in the coagulation-fibrinolytic system were frequently detected in lung cancer patients. Five conventional and one new test of blood coagulation—that is, platelet count (P), prothrombin time (PT), partial thromboplastin time (PTT), fibrinogen (F) and D-Dimer of fibrin (DD)—were prospectively recorded in a series of 286 patients with new primary lung cancer. A pre-thrombotic state (depicted by a prolongation of PT, PTT and increase of D-Dimer of fibrin) was significantly associated with an adverse outcome.

Anticoagulant treatment of cancer patients, particularly those with lung cancer, has been reported to improve survival. These interesting, although preliminary, results of controlled trials lent some support to the argument that activation of blood coagulation plays a role in the natural history of tumor growth. Recently, two studies compared the effectiveness of standard heparin with low molecular weight heparin (LMWH) in the treatment of deep vein thrombosis (DVT). In both studies, mortality rates were lower in the patients randomized to LMWH. The analysis of these deaths reveals a striking difference in cancer-related mortality.

Cancer-related mortality with standard heparin was 31 percent versus 11 percent with low molecular weight heparin. This difference cannot solely be attributed to thrombotic or bleeding events. Since large numbers of cancer patients were included in the studies, it seems unlikely that ones with more advanced tumors were present in the standard heparin group. While it also is possible that standard heparin increases cancer mortality, such an adverse effect has not been previously reported. These considerations suggest that low molecular weight heparin might exert an inhibitory effect on tumor growth. If your oncologist will not test for thrombotic risk factors, contact the Life Extension Foundation at 1-800-544-4440.

WARNING: Never change your anticoagulation medication without physician approval. Sudden death could occur if the Thrombosis Prevention Protocol is used without physician guidance.

Product availability: Low-dose aspirin, Life Extension Booster and Mix, garlic with EDTA, and highly concentrated fish oil capsules are available by calling 1-800-544-4440.

Thyroid Deficiency

Many people over age 40 are thyroid-deficient, but blood tests fail to detect this subtle hormonal deficiency that can be a cause of weight gain, fatigue, immune impairment, adult-onset diabetes and premature aging.

One way of detecting thyroid deficiency is to take your temperature about 30 minutes before lunch for seven days. If your temperature is consistently below 98.6 degrees F, you may be thyroid-deficient. Drugs that can be prescribed to treat severe thyroid deficiency include Cytomel, Synthroid and Armour.

Natural therapies that may correct thyroid deficiency include 1 mg a day of iodine, 500 to 1,000 mg of the amino acid tyrosine, 3 mg of melatonin at bedtime, one capsule two timtes a day of Mega Soy Extract, and DHEA-replacement therapy. An appropriate dose for men is 25 mg of DHEA three times a day; an appropriate dose for women is 15 mg of DHEA three times a day. Refer to DHEA-Pregnenolone Precautions before beginning DHEA therapy.

Correcting a thyroid deficiency can slow down some of the degenerative diseases associated with normal aging and help you lose weight. Natural therapies boost youthful levels of thyroxine, which is safer than replacing it with drugs such as Synthroid.

Product availability: Melatonin, tyrosine, Mega Soy Extract powder or tablets, and DHEA are available by calling 1-800-544-4440. Thyroid medication should be prescribed by a knowledgeable physician.

Tinnitus

Chronic ringing in the ears, a frequent complaint of the elderly, is clinically diagnosed as tinnitus. Published studies have shown that 120 to 240 mg a day of pharmaceutical-grade ginkgo extract can alleviate tinnitus, though some earlier studies failed to show benefits.

A controlled study showed that ginkgo extract caused a statistically significant decrease in behavioral manifestation in the animal model of tinnitus. The most recent human study showed that, in patients suffering from cerebrovascular insufficiency (a common problem associated with normal aging), ginkgo extract produced a significant improvement in the symptoms of vertigo, tinnitis, headache and forgetfulness.

If ginkgo does not work, try 10 to 15 mg a day of Hydergine, or 20 to 40 mg a day of vinpocetin, as there is evidence that these neurologic-enhancing therapies can alleviate tinnitus in some people.

Carmen Fusco notes she has had excellent results with niacin/niacinamide in relatively high doses, along with 25 mg of zinc gluconate twice a day. If the tinnitus is a recent duration, complete improvement is possible. If of long duration, the ringing of the ears can be diminished with these nutrients in most people.

Product availability: To order pharmaceutical ginkgo biloba extract, phone 1-800-544-4440. Ask for a list of offshore suppliers who will ship high-potency Hydergine and vinpocetin to Americans for personal use.

Trauma

Permanent injury or death due to trauma is often caused by free radicals generated when the tissues of the body are physically disrupted. This is well-documented in spinal cord injury cases where the free radical damage that occurs immediately after the injury is what causes permanent paralysis.

Antioxidants should be immediately administered to most victims of trauma to protect against free radical injury. Trauma involving massive bleeding may preclude the use of antioxidants such as ginkgo that could accelerate hemorrhaging.

To protect brain cells against oxygen deprivation or permanent damage from direct trauma to the head, 10 mg of sublingual Hydergine should be immediately administered along with 10 mg of Hydergine LC capsules. If piracetam is available, 4,800 mg of piracetam should be administered to further protect against brain damage.

In laboratory studies where two groups of animals were exposed to the same traumatic force, animals given high doses of vitamin C died less frequently than animals not given vitamin C. Antioxidants appear to protect against many forms of permanent damage inflicted by trauma.

The hormone pregnenolone has been shown to protect against paralysis from spinal cord injury in laboratory animals. The immediate administration of 400 mg of pregnenolone, along with 800 IU of vitamin E, to a spinal injury patient might be advisable. Vitamin E could speed the bleeding process, so do not use Vitamin E if excessive bleeding is occurring.

Vitamin E administration has been shown to reverse free radical damage induced by trauma and to reverse the effects of lipid peroxidation after trauma. The administration of Vitamin E has been shown to therapeutically protect against reduced T-cell membrane fluidity and suppressed T-cell functions. A vitamin E-enriched diet has been shown to protect the brains of mice against brain-circulatory injury. Also, diabetic rats experience a delay in corneal healing when deficient in vitamin E. Trauma patients should consider supplementing with 800 IU a day of vitamin E.

Product availability: vitamin C, vitamin E and pregnenolone can be ordered by calling 1-800-544-4440. Call for a list of offshore companies that sell high-dose Hydergine and piracetam to Americans for personal use.

Urinary Tract Infections

Chronic urinary tract infections cause discomfort to many people, especially women. The over-prescribing of antibiotics to treat recurring urinary tract infections often results in chronic yeast infections. The urinary tract is vulnerable to chronic bacterial infection because of the ability of bacteria to bind to the wall of the bladder and urethra.

Studies document that drinking eight glasses of cranberry juice twice a day can eradicate most urinary tract infections. As long as the cranberry juice is continued, the infections are not likely to return. One way that cranberry juice works is to prevent bacteria from adhering to the linings of the urinary tract.

Cranberry juice has developed into a simple, non-drug means to reduce or treat urinary tract infections. Studies suggests that bacterial infections (bacteriuria) and the associated influx of white blood cells into the urine (pyuria) can be reduced by nearly 50 percent in elderly women who drink 300 mL of cranberry juice cocktail each day.

Laboratory studies have attempted to account for the effectiveness of cranberry juice. Microscopic studies have focused on urine acidification and bacteriostasis. One study showed that the common Escherichia coli bacteria's adherence was inhibited by 75 percent or more in more than 60 percent of the clinical isolates.

When cranberry cocktail was given to mice in the place of their normal water supply for a period of 14 days, the adherence of E. coli bacteria to urinary wall cells was reduced by approximately 80 percent. Anti-adherence activity also could be detected in human urine. Fifteen of 22 subjects showed significant anti-adherence activity in the urine one to three hours after drinking 15 ounces of cranberry cocktail.

In urostomy patients, urinary wall skin problems are common and may stem from alkaline urine. Cranberry juice appears to acidify urine and has bacteriostatic properties, and is widely recommended for the reduction of urinary tract infections. A recent study showed that drinking cranberry juice could help to prevent and/or improve skin complications for urostomy patients. It also showed that cranberry juice resulted in improvements of skin conditions and a reduction in skin complications in patients with severe urinary wall disease.

Most people would find it difficult to drink 16 8-ounce glasses of cranberry juice a day, but there is a dietary supplement called Cranex Cranberry Juice Concentrate that provides the equivalent of eight 8-ounce glasses of cranberry juice in just one capsule. That means that people predisposed to urinary tract infections need to take only two capsules to consume the active ingredients in 16 glasses of cranberry juice.

Product availability: You can order Cranex Cranberry Juice Concentrate by calling 1-800-544-4440.

Valvular Insufficiency/Heart Valve Defects

There are many causes of heart valve defects and degeneration, including congenital defects, bacterial infections, drug toxicities and age-associated aortic valve stenosis (narrowing). Since heart-valve diseases are anatomical in nature, it is difficult to address an existing valve defect from a nutritional or drug standpoint.

The most common serious heart-valve defect is called aortic stenosis. Aortic stenosis is usually an age-related disease that consists of the aortic valve progressively narrowing and restricting the amount of blood that is able to be pumped by the ventricle. The result is ventricular enlargement, as the heart muscle has to pump harder to force blood through the narrowing aortic valve.

Valvular heart disease is most easily diagnosed by Doppler echocardiography. This noninvasive diagnostic technique makes it possible to measure blood flow and to evaluate the extent of valve defects. The color Doppler echocardiography gives the physician a better survey of the severity of valve disease, and the spectral Doppler provides an exact analysis and quantification of the valve defect and the degree of stenosis.

Cardiac disability and death from congestive heart failure will result if the aortic valve cannot be re-opened or replaced. Valve-replacement surgical procedures currently are the only effective long-term therapy. Regrettably, this surgical procedure also has numerous potential long-term side effects, especially in elderly people who so often need an aortic-valve replacement. The potential development of non-surgical therapies to correct aortic-valve stenosis offers some hope of an alternative to valve-replacement surgery.

Apolipoproteins are protein variations of the LDL cholesterol molecule. There is evidence that the deposition of apolipoprotein A, B and E on the aortic valve creates a binding site for calcium. Aortic valve stenosis is often described as a calcification process. Fibrinogen may also deposit on aortic valves to bind calcium. Studies also implicate a chronic inflammatory process that promotes calcium infiltration into the aortic valve.

Preventing or slowing the progression of aortic-valve disease may involve lowering of homocysteine, fibrinogen, and apolipoproteins A, B and E in the blood. Regular blood tests to guard against hypercalcemia (too much calcium in the blood), and supplementation with magnesium to possibly inhibit excess calcification of the aortic valve should be considered. Long-term anti-inflammatory therapy with non-steroidal anti-inflammatory drugs (aspirin, ibuprofen or prescription drugs) may be considered under physician supervision. Nutrients that safely suppress many chronic inflammatory reactions include fish oil, borage oil, curcumin and ginger. Refer to the Fibrinogen and Atherosclerosis protocols for suggestions on lowering homocysteine, fibrinogen and apolipoprotein levels.

Since narrowed and/or leaky heart valves keep blood from being efficiently pumped, and thus place a strain on the heart muscle, we suggest you follow the Congestive Heart Failure And Cardiomyopathy protocol. The nutrients in this protocol will help strengthen the contractile strength of the heart muscle, but will do nothing to alleviate or correct the underlying anatomical valvular defect.

Vertigo

Vertigo involves feelings of dizziness, faintness and the inability to maintain normal balance in a sitting or standing position. There are many causes of vertigo, including ear infection, ear surgery or accidental injury to the ear.

If conventional medicine is unable to diagnose and treat vertigo, you may want to consider taking medications that can correct a neurological deficit that may be causing your vertigo. Some people have found that 5 to 10 mg a day of Hydergine can be an effective therapy for vertigo. Other people have successfully used 2,400 to 4,800 mg of piracetam a day for this condition. A third option is to take 20 to 40 mg of vinpocetin a day.

In the most recent human study, ginkgo extract was shown to improve the symptoms of vertigo, tinnitis, headache and forgetfulness in people suffering from a cerebral circulatory deficit. The reduction of blood circulation to the brain is a common problem in aging humans, and this circulatory deficit can cause many of the neurological disease states, including vertigo.

Piracetam has been shown in several published studies to alleviate vertigo through diverse effects in the brain. In a recent multi-center, double-blind, placebo-controlled study, piracetam was administered in a dose of 800 mg, three times daily, for eight weeks. The study group consisted of 143 middle-aged and elderly outpatients who had suffered from vertigo for at least three months, had experienced at least three episodes per month, and experienced vertigo severe enough to disrupt daily life. Tolerance to piracetam was good, with few drug-related adverse events occurring. The findings showed that piracetam alleviated vertigo by reducing the frequency of episodes, the severity of malaise, imbalance between episodes, and the duration of vertigo-induced incapacity.

Product availability: To obtain high-potency Hydergine, piracetam or vinpocetin, phone 1-800-544-4440 for a list of offshore suppliers who ship these products to Americans for personal use.

Weight Loss

Weight gain associated with aging is one of the most significant health problems in the Western world. And weight loss is one of its biggest challenges.

Obesity is an underlying risk factor for hypertension, adult-onset diabetes, heart disease, cancer and stroke, and is a major cause of the overall loss of energy experienced by so many people.

More Americans are overweight now than ever before. In the 1980s, Americans gained an average of 8 pounds each, yet consumption of diet drinks and low-fat foods was much higher than in the previous decade.

Recently, "lite" versions of almost every processed food on the market have been consumed by Americans obsessed with losing weight. Yet, despite diet manipulation, vigorous exercise and the use of diet drugs, the fat epidemic continues unabated. The media blame high fat consumption for America's overweight problem, but the facts are that previous generations often consumed higher percentages of dietary fat than many overweight people today. Could a widespread deficiency of a specific nutrient be a major factor in causing the excess body fat in many people? Let's take a look at one hypothesis.

Conjugated linoleic acid (CLA) is a component of beef and milk that has been shown to reduce body fat in both animals and humans. CLA is essential for the transport of dietary fat into cells where it is used to build muscle and produce energy. Fat that is not used for anabolic energy production is converted into new stored fat cells. There are published research findings about how dietary CLA reduces body fat, but first let's take a look at why many Americans are now deficient in CLA compared with their parents.

The primary dietary sources of CLA are beef and milk, and Americans are eating less beef and drinking less whole milk in order to reduce their dietary intake of saturated fat. People often drink non-fat milk, but it's the *fat content of the milk* that contains CLA. Since skim milk contains virtually no CLA, those seeking to lose weight who use skim milk are depriving themselves of a potential source of this fat-reducing nutrient.

Now, here's where the real problem occurs. In 1963, the CLA percentage in milk was as high as 2.81 percent. By 1992, the percentage of CLA in dairy products seldom exceeded one percent. The reason for the sharp reduction in milk CLA was because of changing feeding patterns. Cows that eat natural grass produce lots of CLA. Today's "efficient" feeding methods rely far less on natural grass. For example, grass-fed Australian cows have three to four times as much CLA in their meat as do American cows.

So, health-conscious Americans are avoiding beef and whole milk because these foods are high in fat, and when people *do* consume beef or milk, they are consuming very little CLA because of CLA-deficiency in today's cows. Thus, most Americans have inadequate amounts of CLA in their diet, and this CLA deficit may be at least partially responsible for the epidemic of overweight people of all ages that now exists.

Encouraging Results with CLA

How significant is CLA in preventing excess accumulation of body fat? The results to date are preliminary, but extremely encouraging.

Athletes are taking CLA to push glucose into their muscle cells and connective tissues instead of letting it turn into fat. CLA has been shown to reduce protein degradation in both humans and animals.

CLA is required to maintain optimal function of the phospholipid membranes of cells. Healthy cell membranes will allow fat, protein and carbohydrates to flow into active cells such as muscle, connective tissue and organ cells, instead of being stored passively in fat cells. A deficiency of CLA can inhibit fat from entering muscle cells, which can result in excessive accumulation of body fat.

CLA has been studied in different species of animals, and the results consistently show that CLA reduces the percentage of body fat. An abstract from the 1996 Environmental Biology Conference showed that rats, after 28 days of being supplemented with CLA, showed a 58-percent reduction in body fat, compared with the control animals which did not receive CLA. In addition, the percentage of muscle was greater in the CLA group; CLA did not induce weight loss, since muscle weighs more than fat.

In July 1997, the results of the first human study on CLA were released by the Medstat Research Ltd. group of Lillesterom, Norway. This three-month preliminary study involved 20 healthy volunteers. Half the group was given six 500-mg CLA capsules a day, and the other half received identical-looking placebo capsules. The subjects were asked not to alter their diet or lifestyle; 18 of the 20 subjects completed the study protocol. The results showed that the people in the CLA group experienced a 15 to 20 percent reduction of average body fat, compared with the placebo group. In the CLA group, the initial body fat percentage was 21.3 percent at the beginning of the study, and only 17 percent body fat after three months on CLA capsules. In contrast, the placebo group started with an average of 22 percent body fat, and three months later recorded an average of 22.4 percent body fat.

CLA received widespread media attention in the early 1990s when it was identified as a component of red meat that helps prevent cancer. Further research showed that CLA is a potent anti-cancer agent, an anti-catabolic agent and, through a unique mechanism, a fat metabolizing agent. CLA is one of the substances the FDA is investigating for disease prevention. New studies are appearing about the ability of CLA to prevent cancer, and possibly function as an adjuvant (assisting) cancer therapy. CLA appears to be especially effective in preventing breast cancer.

Using CLA to reduce body fat may reduce your risk of getting cancer. Compare this to FDA-approved diet drugs that were removed from the market after being linked to heart-valve degeneration.

A deficiency of CLA in our diet may be a major factor in causing Americans to gain so many fat pounds. CLA is a potent antioxidant, but appears to prevent cancer via other mechanisms of action.

A dose of six 500-mg capsules of 70-percent CLA, taken in the morning on an empty stomach, may be an effective part of an overall weight-loss program. The studies indicate that it usually takes about three weeks before body-fat loss occurs in response to CLA supplementation.

CLA inhibits fat storage by enhancing the ability of cell membranes (other than fat cells) to open up and allow the absorption of fats and other nutrients. CLA promotes the growth of muscles by letting nutrients into active muscle cells. That's why CLA has become such a popular supplement among body builders. The fat-reducing mechanism of CLA involves the rejuvenation of cell membranes in the muscles and connective tissues to allow fats to enter freely in order to generate energy and growth. This anabolic effect could provide anti-aging benefits in the elderly, but there have been no studies to date to investigate this.

Chitosan: The Fat-Magnet

Let's turn our attention to another therapy that can induce, independent of CLA, weight loss—chitosan.

Chitosan is a fiber that binds to fat molecules in the gut to prevent dietary fat from being absorbed into the bloodstream. Fat in the blood readily converts into body fat. The best way of using chitosan is to take between 1,500 and 3,000 mg of chitosan immediately before a meal that contains fat. Drink at least 8 ounces of water with the chitosan. The chitosan capsules will burst open in your stomach within five minutes and be available to absorb dietary fat in your stomach and intestine before the fat can be absorbed into your bloodstream. The fat bound to the chitosan is then carried out of your body in the feces. Studies show that chitosan absorbs 44 percent more dietary fat on average than any other fiber tested.

Chitosan is now available in 500-mg capsules, thus making it much easier to consume the optimal amount of chitosan needed to bind to the dietary fat contained in a typical high-fat meal. Those seeking to lose weight should take three to six 500-mg chitosan capsules before each fatty meal. This dose also should help to reduce LDL cholesterol by binding to bile acids secreted by the liver into the intestine, and preventing their reabsorption into the bloodstream.

In addition, studies show that ascorbic acid (vitamin C) helps dissolve the chitosan that is in the stomach and intestine into a fat-absorbing gel. When ascorbic acid was given with chitosan to rats, far more fat was trapped and excreted in the feces than when chitosan was given without ascorbic acid. It is important to take pure ascorbic acid to enhance the fat absorbing effects of chitosan. Buffered ascorbate will not work.

The most significant human study using chitosan was published in the August-October 1994 issue of the journal *ARM Medicina-Helsinki*. In this study, 30 moderately obese patients were given chitosan, while members of a control group on the identical diet received a placebo. Within four weeks, the chitosan group lost an average of 15 pounds, while members of the control group lost only 5.5 pounds. This study confirmed the findings of a previous uncontrolled human study conducted in Norway.

Take three to six 500-mg chitosan capsules and one 1,000 mg ascorbic acid capsule right before a high-fat meal.

CAUTION: Do not take chitosan and CLA together. The chitosan will absorb the CLA and prevent it from getting into the bloodstream. Do not take coenzyme Q10 rice bran oil capsules, Mega EPA, Mega GLA or flax oil with chitosan, since these important oils also will become trapped in the chitosan and be unavailable for absorption. It is best to take your essential fatty acid oil supplements all together first thing in the morning if you are going to use chitosan throughout the day to absorb dietary fat.

The Role of Thyroid Deficiency

We tend to put on weight as we grow older in part because aging impairs our ability to metabolize carbohydrates. Since most food is eventually broken down into glucose (blood sugar), the age-related decline in our ability to metabolize glucose is a significant cause of degenerative disease and excessive weight gain associated with aging.

One cause of impaired carbohydrate metabolism is sub-clinical thyroid deficiency. Blood tests are not always reliable in diagnosing this condition. A study found that 18 percent of elderly people who were initially diagnosed as having normal thyroid levels were later found to have significant thyroid deficiency after undergoing extensive testing. Many physicians believe that most people over 40 suffer from a sub-clinical thyroid deficiency that contributes to their weight gain.

The thyroid gland secretes hormones involved in cellular energy expenditure. When you go on a diet, there is a decrease in thyroid-hormone secretion that causes your body's metabolic rate to slow down. This decrease occurs because your thyroid gland thinks you are starving and tries to conserve energy until you find more food to eat.

Everyone who has ever dieted knows about the rebound effect . . . how your body resists losing weight while you "starve yourself," but then puts the weight back on with devastating quickness after you eat a little more. This is why dieting is such a miserable way to try to lose weight. Now you know why—it's because your thyroid gland fights you all the way by reducing your energy efficiency in order to keep you from losing weight.

This biological mechanism involving the thyroid gland, which evolved over hundreds of thousands of years to counter the very real risk of starvation, is what sabotages you in today's world of plenty when you deliberately eat less in an attempt to lose weight.

To give you an idea how your thyroid gland dictates how much you weigh, consider the fact that, when the thyroid produces too much thyroid hormone, the most common clinical symptom is the significant loss of weight. The name for the disease caused by an overactive thyroid gland is hyperthyroidism, and in 76 to 83 percent of cases, the patient's first complaint to their doctor is about how much weight they've been losing!

On the other hand, clinical studies have consistently shown that dieting produces a *decline* in thyroid output, resulting in a severe reduction in resting energy expenditure. This reduced metabolic rate prevents cells from burning calories to produce energy. If the cells do not take up glucose to produce energy, the sugar is stored as fat within the body. The only way dieting can produce significant long-term weight loss is for the cells to take up glucose for conversion into energy rather than into body fat.

One way of boosting thyroid function in order to lose weight and fight fatigue is to take supplemental thyroid hormone. People who have serious thyroid hormone deficiency should take it under the care of a doctor, but for most people the adverse side effects of supplementation with thyroid hormone outweigh the benefits.

While there are studies showing that thyroid-supplementation promotes weight loss in some people, it also can kill you. Excessive thyroid hormone can cause rapid heart rate and atrial fibrillation—the abnormal, chaotic quivering of a heart chamber—that could lead to a heart attack or stroke. The problem is not thyroid deficiency per se, but that people become thyroid-deficient in response to dieting. In short, thyroid-hormones drugs don't always work and can be dangerous.

Later in this protocol, we're going to reveal a safe and effective, natural way of boosting your thyroid function without having to take thyroid hormone.

There are several reasons why thyroid hormone supplementation hasn't consistently produced weight loss in clinical studies:

1. Commercially available thyroid supplements may not provide all the thyroid hormones needed to restore optimal carbohydrate metabolism. When safe doses of thyroid supplements are given to dieters, their resting energy expenditure still does not approach their pre-diet level, even though measurable serum levels of thyroid hormone are up to 130-percent higher than pre-diet levels.

2. The thyroid supplements currently on the market have been tested only by themselves in clinical studies. When only one therapy is tested at a time without producing dramatic results, the therapy is considered useless. But thyroid deficiency is only one factor that works against successful weight loss in response to dieting.

3. Normal diets do not provide optimal levels of minerals; dieting can cause severe deficiencies of chromium and magnesium, for example. These deficiencies cause insulin-resistance, which is a major factor in carbohydrate metabolic disorders. Chromium and magnesium must be present if thyroid hormone is to work synergistically with insulin, in order to drive glucose into the cells for energy production.

4. There are other hormones, such as DHEA and pregnenolone, that boost the effect of thyroid hormone on carbohydrate metabolism.

The scientific evidence shows that dieting induces a thyroid-deficient state that slows the body's metabolic rate. If body weight is to be controlled by diet, something must be done to safely boost thyroid hormone to near pre-diet levels.

Research Abounds on Soy Protein

There are more than 80 years of scientific research to document the ability of soy protein to lower blood fat levels. A study in the August 3, 1995, issue of *The New England Journal of Medicine* showed that soy protein lowered LDL cholesterol by 12.9 percent and triglycerides by 10.5 percent. *One mechanism by which soy reduces blood fats is by boosting thyroid hormone levels.* An added benefit: studies show that thyroid hormone burns up harmful LDL cholesterol globules in the blood.

Because of the many documented health benefits from soy intake, the Life Extension Foundation suggests that anyone seeking to lose weight safely through dieting should take 6 to 30 grams a day of soy protein concentrate. Soy protein not only boosts thyroid hormone levels to burn sugar calories, it also contains an amino acid complex that helps spare the body's protein stores, which are often broken down in response to dieting. The phyto-estrogens and essential fatty acids in soy further help to promote weight loss.

The Life Extension Foundation has recommended soy protein concentrates to cancer patients for many years. Soy protein extracts contain eight to 10 times more of the active ingredients of soy than conventional soy extracts. Some of these ingredients are cancer-preventing phytoestrogens, such as genistein.

Soy protein powder has a light, pleasant-tasting nutty flavor. If you consume 6 to 30 grams of Soy Power in water, you may be able to skip a meal because the soy protein, which contains essential fatty acids, and the soy fiber have a satiating effect.

The isoflavones (especially genistein) contained in soy protein extracts have potent cancer prevention effects, especially against breast and prostate cancer. Cancer patients often take high doses of soy protein extract as an adjuvant (assisting) therapy because of studies showing that the genistein inhibits cancer cell proliferation via several well-established mechanisms. And, as noted, soy protein also has been shown to lower cholesterol, possibly via its thyroid hormone stimulating effect.

Soy intake is associated with significant reductions in the risk of many forms of cancer and in blood fat levels. Many Foundation members already are taking supplemental soy to reduce their risk of cancer, especially breast and prostate cancer.

The optimal method of taking soy protein extract is to take one to two heaping tablespoons (20 to 40 grams) of the powder each day. Soy extract capsules are available, but may not provide the full spectrum of soy constituents needed to boost tyroid hormone output.

Magnesium and Chromium

While thyroid hormone plays a definite role in weight management, the scientific literature makes it clear that both magnesium and chromium also are required to break down the cellular insulin resistance that causes higher-than-normal blood sugar levels.

Overweight people usually suffer from insulin impairment that prevents the proper cell uptake of carbohydrates (sugars). Excessive serum glucose is converted into body fat unless this insulin resistance is broken down and the cells are able to regain youthful carbohydrate metabolism. Chromium has received widespread publicity for its ability to lower serum glucose levels by potentiating insulin sensitivity. Studies have shown that chromium supplementation results in a slight reduction in body fat and an increase in lean body mass. Niacin improves the metabolic-enhancing effect of chromium picolinate.

To improve the fat-reducing effects of dieting, the Foundation now suggests that one capsule of this new chromium picolinate be taken with every meal to facilitate youthful carbohydrate metabolism. The importance of taking a chromium capsule with each meal is illustrated in animal studies in which chromium was given throughout the day in order to lower serum glucose levels. When you consume food, your serum glucose levels rise significantly unless your cells are sensitized to insulin. Chromium will help sensitize your cells to insulin by helping to lower your blood sugar levels.

You should not take more than three 200-mg chromium capsules a day. Always take antioxidant supplements like Vitamin E when you take chromium, to protect against free radical activity. At least 30 mg of niacin should be contained in each 200-microgram chromium picolinate capsule.

While chromium has received the most media attention, the scientific literature shows that magnesium plays an even more important role in regulating carbohydrate metabolism. Magnesium is involved in a number of enzymatic reactions required for cells to uptake and metabolize glucose. Magnesium deficiency causes insulin resistance and elevated blood sugar levels.

About 80 percent of Americans are magnesium-deficient. When they go on a diet, they become severely deficient in magnesium, which causes the insulin resistance that contributes to the failure of the diet. Life Extension Mix contains high amounts of magnesium. For those going on a calorie-restricted diet, it is suggested that at least one 500-mg magnesium capsule a day be taken in addition to the full dose Life Extension Mix.

The Anabolic Hormone DHEA

Hormone deficiencies are a cause of age-associated weight gain. DHEA has kept old animals remarkably thin, but has not worked this well in humans. Nevertheless, many older people taking DHEA report anabolic muscle gain and fat loss. DHEA has been shown to boost insulin growth factor (IGF-1) in humans, and the increase in this youth factor may be responsible for the fat reduction and anabolic effects seen in some elderly people. The main benefits to people over 40 in restoring DHEA levels to a youthful state includes immune enhancement, protection against neurological disease and memory loss, reductions in risks of certain cancers, alleviation of depression, and protection against osteoporosis.

For people over 35 years of age, DHEA-replacement therapy is suggested as part of an overall weight management program. The average dose of DHEA for men should be 25 mg of DHEA, three times a day. Women need only 15 mg of DHEA, three times a day.

CAUTION: Refer to the DHEA-Pregnenolone Precautions protocol before taking DHEA.

Most dieters need help in taking off pounds. They need dietary aids to jump-start the weight-loss process to give them the encouragement they need to stay on the program long enough to succeed. That's why we recommend nutrients that fight diseases while taking off pounds. Nutrients make you look and feel better while you're losing weight, and it's easy to continue to take them year-after-year to stay healthy and fit.

Here is a re-capitulation of the disease-fighting nutrients we recommend for weight loss:

❖ Chitosan

Chitosan is a fiber that binds to fat molecules in the gut to inhibit dietary fat from being absorbed into the bloodstream. Fat in the blood readily converts into body fat. The best way of using chitosan is to take between 1,500 and 3,000 mg of chitosan immediately before a meal that contains fat. Drink at least 8 ounces of water with the chitosan. The chitosan capsules will burst open in your stomach within five minutes and be available to absorb dietary fat in your stomach and intestine before the fat can be absorbed into your bloodstream. The fat bound to the chitosan is then carried out of your body in the feces. Studies show that chitosan absorbs 44 percent more dietary fat on average than any other fiber tested.

The recommended dosage also should help to reduce harmful LDL cholesterol by binding to bile acids secreted by the liver into the intestine and preventing their reabsorption into the bloodstream.

CAUTION: Do not take chitosan and CLA together. The chitosan will absorb the CLA and prevent it from getting into the bloodstream. Do not take CoQ10 Rice Bran Oil capsules, Mega EPA, Mega GLA, or flax oil with chitosan; they also will become trapped in the chitosan and be unavailable for absorption. Take your essential fatty acid oil supplements all together first thing in the morning if you are going to use chitosan throughout the day to absorb dietary fat.

❖ Conjugated Linoleic Acid

CLA inhibits fat storage by enhancing the ability of cell membranes (other than fat cells) to open up and allow the absorption of fats and other nutrients. CLA promotes the growth of muscles by letting nutrients into active muscle cells. The fat-reducing mechanism of CLA involves the rejuvenation of cell membranes in the muscles and connective tissues to allow fats to enter freely in order to generate energy and growth. This anabolic effect could provide anti-aging benefits in the elderly. Remember, do not take with chitosan, as the chitosan will absorb the CLA before it can get into your bloodstream. Take six 500-mg capsules of CLA every day to duplicate successful fat-loss clinical studies.

❖ Chromium and Magnesium

Insulin resistance prevents serum glucose from entering cells. If glucose cannot get into the cells to produce energy, it will be stored in the body as fat. chromium picolinate and magnesium have been shown to help break down cellular insulin resistance. For chromium to be effective in the body, it needs to have niacin present. Many health-conscious people receive supplemental niacin with their B-complex formula, but Prolongevity's chromium supplement contains 30 mg of niacin in addition to 200 micrograms of chromium picolinate in each capsule. This small amount of niacin does not usually produce a niacin "flush," but does ensure that niacin will be available to work with chromium to reduce serum glucose levels by breaking down insulin resistance. The published studies actually show that magnesium is more effective than chromium in breaking down insulin resistance.

Magnesium deficiency is another cause of excess weight gain in Americans. chromium can lower cholesterol levels as well as serum glucose levels. Magnesium can protect against heart attacks and stroke. Taking these supplements to help lose weight may provide significant life extension benefits in addition to weight loss. Take at least 500 mg of elemental magnesium every day. One 200-microgram capsule of chrominum picolinate should be taken with each meal.

❖ **Soy Protein**

A deficiency of thyroid hormone can slow down metabolic actions in the body and cause weight gain. Consumption of soy protein can boost the body's natural secretion of thyroid hormone, thereby increasing the body's metabolic rate. Thyroid hormone also is necessary to drive glucose into the cells. The isoflavones (especially genistein) contained in soy protein extracts have potent cancer-prevention effects, especially against breast and prostate cancer. Cancer patients often take high doses of soy protein extract as an adjuvant (assisting) therapy because of studies showing that the genistein inhibits cancer cell proliferation via several well-established mechanisms. Soy protein also has been shown to lower cholesterol, possibly via its thyroid hormone stimulating effect. Take 20 to 40 grams of soy protein extract powder once a day.

❖ **DHEA**

Almost everyone gains weight as they grow older. One cause of age-related weight gain is the progressive decline in the body's levels of the hormone DHEA. Many older people who take DHEA report muscle gain and fat loss. Other benefits to people over 40 in restoring DHEA to youthful levels include improved immune function, protection against memory loss, relief of depressive symptoms, protection against osteoporosis, and reduction in the risk of certain cancers. Refer to the DHEA-Pregnenolone Precautions protocol before taking DHEA

The Weight-Loss Regimen

Those seeking significant fat-loss effects should commit to a two to three month program that would involve the following schedule:

First thing in the morning:

- ✔ Six CLA capsules (some people need only four CLA capsules)
- ✔ One DHEA capsule (take with an antioxidant like Life Extension Mix)
- ✔ One chromium picolinate-niacin capsule
- ✔ One heaping tablespoon of soy protein powder (soy can be taken at another time of the day if desired)

Five minutes before lunch:

- ✔ Six 500-mg chitosan capsules with an eight ounce glass of water (some people need only three chitosan capsules)
- ✔ One 1,000-mg ascorbic acid capsule
- ✔ One chromium picolinate-niacin capsule
- ✔ One DHEA capsule

Five minutes before dinner:

- ✔ Six 500-mg chitosan capsules with an eight ounce glass of water (some people need only three chitosan capsules)
- ✔ One 1,000-mg ascorbic acid capsule
- ✔ One chromium picolinate-niacin capsule
- ✔ One 500-mg magnesium capsule

Product availability: chromium picolinate with niacin, soy protein extracts, magnesium, chitosan and DHEA can be ordered by phoning 1-800-544-4440.

Wound-Healing
(Surgical Wounds, Trauma, Burns)

There is strong evidence that at least two nutrients and one juice — the amino acid arginine, the trace metal zinc, and the juice from the aloe vera plant — can enhance wound-healing significantly. The typical western diet contains about 5 grams a day of arginine, mainly from meat, fish, poultry and dairy products. Under normal conditions, 5 grams a day of arginine is barely enough to maintain tissue viability.

It is well-documented that, following traumatic injury, there is a significantly increased need for arginine for a variety of metabolic functions. Animal studies have demonstrated that, following surgical trauma, dietary supplementation with arginine results in an increase in nitrogen retention and increased body weight, both of which are essential for successful recovery from traumatic injury.

Arginine is a substrate for protein synthesis, creatine synthesis and polyamine synthesis, involved in the control of cell division. Arginine also is involved in a metabolic pathway in which it is converted into nitric oxide.

Studies in patients undergoing gall bladder surgery have shown that taking 15 grams per day of arginine for three days significantly reduces nitrogen excretion, compared with patients receiving conventional nutritional support. In patients with gastrointestinal malignancies undergoing surgery, 25 grams a day of arginine (for seven days) improved their nitrogen balance five to seven days after surgery.

In a study published in the journal *Surgery*, 85 patients with gastrointestinal malignancies receiving dietary supplementation with arginine, omega-3 fatty acids and RNA showed major improvement in nitrogen balance, compared with patients receiving a standard nutritional regimen. Patients in the arginine group recovered more rapidly and were discharged sooner from the hospital.

Studies have shown that arginine speeds wound healing via several different mechanisms.

In a clinical study in the August 1990 issue of *Surgery*, scientists recruited 36 healthy volunteers from medical and non-medical hospital personnel. None of the subjects suffered from diabetes, smoked, or took drugs known to impair wound healing. The 36 subjects were randomly placed into three groups of equal size. Group one received 100 mL/day of an aromatic syrup as a placebo. Group two received 30 grams of arginine aspartate in 100 mL of aromatic syrup (the equivalent of 17 grams/day of free arginine). Group three received 30 grams of arginine hydrochloride in 100 mL of aromatic syrup (the equivalent of 24.8 grams/day of free arginine). All supplements were taken throughout the day for two weeks. Immediately prior to the study, and on days seven and 14, peripheral blood was drawn for analysis after an overnight fast.

On the first day of the study, and after receiving a local anesthetic, all the subjects underwent the creation of a "standard wound" (5 centimeter long, one millimeter in diameter). A catheter was inserted into the wound with one end sutured and left protruding from the skin. The wound then was covered with an occlusive, transparent dressing which was changed during the study as needed.

The primary finding of the study was that in both arginine groups, there was a significant increase in the amount of reparative collagen synthesized at the site of the wound. The scientists concluded, "To our knowledge, this is the first instance in which collagen synthesis has been shown to be enhanced to 'supranormal' levels." In the same study, there also was marked enhancement in the activity and effectiveness of peripheral T-lymphocytes in the bloodstream.

Other studies in animals have shown that dietary supplementation with arginine increases the weight of the thymus, which is the master gland of immunity, and reduces shrinkage of the thymus after trauma and in normally aging animals. The benefits of arginine for thymic function also have been demonstrated by its ability to restore thymic endocrine function by increasing blood levels of thymulin, one of the hormones secreted by the thymus gland.

Growth hormone plays a critical role in modulating the action of the immune system, and is essential for muscle growth and development. One of the primary reasons that the functioning of the immune system and muscular strength decline dramatically as we grow older is the progressive decline in growth hormone secretion with advancing age. There is evidence that arginine's ability to improve both wound healing and immune-system function are related to its ability to stimulate the release of growth hormone.

The role of copper in healing was first observed by a German physician, Dr. Rademacher, who noted that broken bones seemed to heal faster when patients were given a copper salt during convalescence. Since then, the need for copper in the biosynthesis of bone and connective tissues has been established. The Life Extension Foundation does not recommend copper as a dietary supplement because of the preponderance of evidence that long-term excessive copper intake generates too much free radical activity throughout the body. The evidence makes it clear that, while copper is important for health and wound healing, it is potentially harmful if its intake is excessive. On the other hand, the therapeutic, short-term use of copper to enhance wound healing in localized injury sites is both reasonable and appropriate.

To accelerate wound healing, the Foundation recommends 10 to 22 grams of supplemental arginine a day, along with 90 mg of zinc and 8 mg of copper. Extra amounts of vitamin C also are very important for proper functioning of enzyme protocollagen hydroxylase, which is essential for wound healing. Glutamine in the dose of 2,000 mg a day appears promising. Supplemental nutrients obtained by taking three tablets of Life Extension Mix three times a day can aid in wound-healing.

Refer to the Catabolic Wasting and Muscle Building protocols for additional suggestions on accelerating wound healing.

Product availability: You can obtain premium-grade arginine powders, tablets and capsules, zinc, aloe vera, copper, vitamin C and Life Extension Mix by phoning 1-800-544-4440.

Yeast Infections

For suggestions on treating chronic yeast infections, refer to the Life Extension Foundation's protocol on Candida (Fungal, Yeast) Infections.

Avoiding Vitamin A Toxicity

Based upon hundreds of published studies, the Life Extension Foundation has recommended vitamin A analog drugs to cancer patients. For the many cancer patients who cannot gain access to vitamin A analogs because the FDA classifies them as "unapproved new drugs," the Foundation has recommended the use of water-soluble vitamin A liquid drops.

The dosage range of vitamin A liquid drops that cancer patients have been using is 100,000 to 200,000 IU a day. The Foundation has cautioned that these high doses could produce toxicity if taken over extended periods of time, yet cancer patients often are forced to risk some degree of toxicity to obtain an effective dose of vitamin A.

Anyone taking very high doses of vitamin A for cancer or any other reason should do so under the care of a physician, and should be on the lookout for symptoms of vitamin A toxicity. The following are common symptoms of vitamin A overdose that should be watched for in cancer patients taking high doses of any vitamin A product:

✔ Headache
✔ Dizziness
✔ Blurred vision
✔ Joint pain
✔ Dry lips
✔ Scaly, dry skin
✔ Excessive hair loss

Blood tests showing elevated liver enzymes may be a sign of a vitamin A overdose. If any of these symptoms appear, discontinue using vitamin A until the symptoms disappear, and then resume vitamin A therapy at a much lower dosage. The cancer patient faces a dilemma in attempting to use the maximum dose of vitamin A to fight his or her cancer, while trying to avoid vitamin A toxicity.

Those with thyroid cancer should avoid vitamin A.

Therapy Caveats

Remember, the information in this book is not intended to replace the attention or advice of a physician or other health care professional. Anyone who wishes to embark on any dietary, drug, exercise, or other lifestyle change intended to prevent or treat a specific disease or condition should consult with, and seek clearance and guidance from, a qualified health care professional. The book offers general suggestions based upon scientific evidence, not specific advice or recommendations. Patients need to be treated in an individual manner by their own personal physician, and the information in this book must not be considered a substitute for the individual attention of a personal physician.

There are a number of caveats individuals should be aware of when considering certain therapies, or when they are suffering from specific problems. They include, but are not limited to, the following:

Adrenal diseases. Some adrenal diseases such as Addison's disease involve under-production of cortisol. This is a potentially acute, life-threatening condition that requires expert physician intervention.

Arginine. For a minority of Type II diabetics, arginine can elevate blood sugar by neutralizing insulin. Therefore, any diabetic who is contemplating using arginine or Powermaker II (Sugar-Free) should check their blood sugar with a glucometer every time they take an arginine supplement during the first three weeks.

Also, some nutritionists are concerned about the use of high-doses of arginine in cancer patients. Arginine promotes cellular growth, and the concern is that this amino acid could cause cancer cells to grow faster. Scientific studies, however, show arginine provides beneficial effects to cancer patients. Only one study on breast cancer patients hinted at a risk for arginine supplementation.

Muscular dystrophy patients should avoid arginine, which promotes nitric oxide formation.

Bee products. Bee products should not be administered to children under the age of three.

Beta-carotene. When suffering from a damaged liver, avoid niacin, vitamin A and beta-carotene, since these nutrients can be harmful for this condition. Also, the Life Extension Foundation recommends against high doses of beta-carotene in AIDS patients who have hepatitis.

Caffeine. Those with cardiac arrhythmias should avoid caffeine, heavy alcohol intake and dietary saturated fats.

Also, muscular dystrophy patients should avoid caffeine, which promotes noradrenalin hyper secretion.

Coumadin. It is not known how nutrients recommended by the Foundation to avoid thrombosis interact with anti-coagulation prescription drugs such as Coumadin and heparin. It is suggested that patients on physician-prescribed anti-coagulation drugs introduce these nutrients very slowly. Weekly blood tests are suggested to make sure the blood is not becoming too thin.

Curcumin. Do not use curcumin if you have biliary tract obstruction, because curcumin could eliminate the flow of bile excretion through the bile duct. High doses of curcumin on an empty stomach can cause stomach ulceration.

Deprenyl. High doses of deprenyl may be detrimental to Parkinson's disease patients, especially when taking L-dopa.

Depression. Anyone suffering from clinical depression of any type should be under the care of a physician.

DHEA. Those with prostate cancer should avoid DHEA. Generally, it is a good idea to use any hormone with caution and under the direction of a competent physician.

Fish oil concentrates. Extreme caution should be exercised by those with leaky blood vessels when taking essential fatty acids in the form of fish oil concentrates, such as Mega-EPA, because they inhibit blood-clotting. There is a chance that a cerebral hemorrhage could occur because of the blood-thinning effects these nutrients can produce. Blood tests that measure clotting time can be used to make sure these nutrients are not reducing the clotting factors in your blood too much.

Forskolin. Do not use forskolin if you have prostate cancer or low blood pressure. If you are going to use forskolin or any other alternative therapy to replace drugs that strengthen heart muscle contraction, then extreme caution is mandatory and physician cooperation essential. Tests should be conducted to make sure forskolin and other nutrients are maintaining sufficient cardiac output.

If you'd like to see if forskolin can replace your anti-hypertensive drugs, extreme caution is mandatory and physician cooperation essential. You should reduce the dosage of your anti-hypertensive drug very slowly, while increasing your intake of forskolin and monitoring your blood pressure on a daily basis. If you do not exercise caution, an acute hypertensive event could occur, resulting in a stroke.

Garlic. Garlic taken in high doses—for example, 6,000 mg to 8,000 mg to lower cholesterol—can cause stomach irritation if taken on an empty stomach.

Genistein. Do not take soy extract when undergoing radiation therapy because the genistein in soy can interfere with the ability of radiation to kill cancer cells.

Glutamine. Some nutritionists are concerned about the use of high-doses of glutamine in cancer patients. Glutamine promotes cellular growth, and the concern is that this amino acid could cause cancer cells to grow faster. Scientific studies, however, show glutamine provides beneficial effects to cancer patients.

Gingko. Trauma involving massive bleeding may preclude the use of antioxidants such as ginkgo that could accelerate hemorrhaging.

Herparin. It is not known how nutrients recommended by the Foundation to avoid thrombosis interact with anti-coagulation prescription drugs such as Coumadin and heparin. It is suggested that patients who are on physician-prescribed anti-coagulation drugs introduce these nutrients very slowly. Weekly blood tests are suggested to make sure the blood is not becoming too thin.

Hodgkin's disease. See melatonin.

Hops. See valerian.

Hydergine. Liquid Hydergine should be avoided in treating hemorrhagic stroke because of its high alcohol content.

Hypertension. The Foundation's general precaution is, if you're going to attempt to use any of the nutrients the Foundation recommends to replace anti-hypertensive drugs, you *must* do so with the cooperation of your physician. You cannot assume that any nutrients will be able to replace a drug that is effectively controlling your blood pressure. Daily blood pressure monitoring is mandatory to ensure that the nutrient regimen you are following is keeping your blood pressure under control.

Imitrex. A drug used to block migraine headaches, Imitrex may have dangerous side effects in the middle aged and the elderly.

Interleukin-2. While melatonin is strongly recommended for breast cancer patients, interleukin-2, which often is combined with melatonin, should be avoided by breast cancer patients. Interleukin-2 may promote breast cancer cell division.

Leukemia. Alternative cancer therapies should be used with caution when treating leukemia or lymphoma because most alternative therapies boost immune-cell function, which could speed the proliferation of leukemia and lymphoma cancer cells. Also, see melatonin, below.

Lupus. Lupus patients should exercise extreme caution when attempting any new medical therapy, since there is a chance the condition could be made worse.

Lymphoma. Alternative cancer therapies should be used with caution when treating leukemia or lymphoma because most alternative therapies boost immune cell function, which could speed the proliferation of leukemia and lymphoma cancer cells. Also, see melatonin, below.

KH3. People allergic to procaine (the active ingredient in KH3) or who are on sulfa drugs should not take KH3.

Melatonin. Some doctors are under the impression that leukemia, Hodgkin's disease and lymphoma patients should avoid melatonin until more is known about its effects on these forms of cancer. If melatonin is tried in these types of cancer, tumor blood markers should be watched closely for any sign that melatonin is promoting tumor growth.

Since melatonin may boost gamma interferon production, those with multiple sclerosis may want to avoid melatonin.

Use melatonin cautiously when treating autoimmune diseases such as rheumatoid arthritis. Some scientists have speculated that melatonin could worsen the severity of an autoimmune disease.

Niacin. When suffering from a severely damaged liver, avoid niacin, vitamin A and beta-carotene, as these nutrients can be harmful for these conditions.

Pain. Before starting on a pain management program, please refer to the Phenylalanine Precautions in this book.

Passion flower. See valerian.

Phenylalanine or tyrosine. There are some people who are genetically sensitive to phenylalanine and cannot take it. Hypertensive people should use phenylalanine with caution because it can elevate blood pressure in people who already have high blood pressure. Cancer patients should avoid taking extra phenylalanine and tyrosine because these amino acids can contribute to cancer cell proliferation.

Muscular dystrophy patients should avoid phenylalanine and tyrosine.

Pregnenolone. See DHEA-Pregnenolone Precautions in this book.

Procaine. People allergic to procaine (the active ingredient in KH3) or who are on sulfa drugs should not take KH3.

Propranolol. People with very low blood pressure, or certain forms of congestive heart failure and asthma should not take propranolol or other beta-blocking drugs.

St. John's wort. When using St. John's wort, avoid prolonged sunlight exposure, since the active ingredient hypericin may make the skin more sensitive to UV light.

Shark liver oil. Do not take shark liver oil for more than 30 days because it may cause the overproduction of blood platelets.

Soy extract. Do not take soy extract when undergoing radiation therapy because the genistein in soy can interfere with the ability of the radiation to kill cancer cells.

Sulfa drugs. People allergic to procaine (the active ingredient in KH3) or who are on sulfa drugs should not take KH3.

Thalidomide. Users are cautioned that thalidomide — which may be useful in treating wet macular degeneration — causes severe birth defects and must never be used by pregnant women, or women who may become pregnant.

Thyroid hormone therapy. You must be careful not to overdose on thyroid hormones. The advice of a knowledgeable physician is important when considering thyroid hormone therapy.

Tyrosine. See Phenylalanine or tyrosine.

Valerian. Some people use the herb valerian to fall asleep. Valerian produces a drug-like hypnotic effect within the central nervous system similar to benzodiazepine drugs such as Valium and Halcion. Since valerian-containing products often are promoted as natural herbal remedies, the public mistakenly believes they are safe to take on a regular basis. Studies indicate, however, that there is a significant toxicity risk when taking valerian over an extended period of time. Since a tolerance effect occurs with valerian because of its Valium-like properties, people often need to take greater and greater amounts of it as time goes by in order to continue to obtain the desired hypnotic effect. The chronic use of valerian could result in permanent liver damage along with potential central nervous system impairment. The Life Extension Foundation has thoroughly investigated the use of herbal insomnia remedies such as valerian, hops and passion flower, and found that they have an unacceptable risk of toxicity with long-term use.

Vitamin A liquid drops. The dosage range of vitamin A liquid drops that cancer patients have been using is between 100,000 and 200,000 IU a day. The Foundation has cautioned that these high doses could produce toxicity if taken over extended periods of time. See Appendix A for details.

Vitamin B6. Since high doses of vitamin B6 taken chronically may cause peripheral nerve damage, high doses (500 mg a day and higher) should only be used when a blood test documents the failure of folic acid, vitamin B12 and TMG to lower homocysteine levels. Never take high doses of vitamin B6 without also taking the other B-complex vitamins.

Vitamin D3. Monthly blood tests to monitor serum calcium and parathyroid hormone levels should be done to protect against vitamin D3 toxicity.

In addition, underlying kidney disease precludes high-dose vitamin D3 supplementation.

Vitamin E. Vitamin E can speed the bleeding process, so do not use vitamin E if excessive bleeding is occurring.

References

The Life Extension Foundation's protocols are based on sound scientific research. Here are pertinent references from studies worldwide that support the protocols in this book. Those readers who are interested in particular protocols, and wish to know more about the underpinnings of the Foundation's protocol recommendations and the original science on which they are based, can use these references to find abstracts of the papers cited here online through a computer database such as MEDLINE, or the papers themselves at a medical library. Also, the abstracts for these references can be accessed at the Foundation's web site, **www.lef.org**.

Acetaminophen (Tylenol) Poisoning
Acute And Chronic

Pearls, pitfalls, and updates in toxicology. Emergency Medicine Clinics of North America (USA), 1997, 15/2 (427-450)

Refining the level for anticipated hepatotoxicity in acetaminophen poisoning. Journal of Emergency Medicine (USA), 1996, 14/6 (691-695)

Outpatient N-acetylcysteine treatment for acetaminophen poisoning: An ethical dilemma or a new financial mandate? Veterinary and Human Toxicology (USA), 1996, 38/3 (222-224)

Management of acetaminophen toxicity. American Family Physician (USA), 1996, 53/1 (185-190)

[Recommendations for treatment of paracetamol poisoning. Danish Medical Society, Study of the Liver]. Ugeskr Laeger (DENMARK) Nov 25 1996, 158 (48) p6892-5

Factors responsible for continuing morbidity after paracetamol poisoning in Chinese patients in Hong Kong. Singapore Med J (SINGAPORE) Jun 1996, 37 (3) p275-7

[Clinical-toxicological case (1). Dosage of N-acetylcysteine in acute paracetamol poisoning]. Schweiz Rundsch Med Prax (SWITZERLAND) Aug 2 1996, 85 (31-32) p935-8

Acute renal failure due to acetaminophen ingestion: a case report and review of the literature. J Am Soc Nephrol (UNITED STATES) Jul 1995

Acute hepatic and renal toxicity from low doses of acetaminophen in the absence of alcohol abuse or malnutrition: evidence for increased susceptibility to drug toxicity due to cardiopulmonary and renal insufficiency. Hepatology (UNITED STATES) May 1994

Protective effect of oral acetylcysteine against the hepatorenal toxicity of carbon tetrachloride potentiated by ethyl alcohol. Alcohol Clin Exp Res (UNIT-

References

ED STATES) Aug 1992

Cholestyramine as an antidote against paracetamol-induced hepato- and nephrotoxicity in the rat. Toxicol Lett (NETHERLANDS) May 1989

Relation of analgesic use to renal cancer: population-based findings. Natl Cancer Inst Monogr (UNITED STATES) Dec 1985

Acetaminophen-induced depletion of glutathione and cysteine in the aging mouse kidney. Biochem Pharmacol (ENGLAND) Jul 7 1992

Cysteine isopropylester protects against paracetamol-induced toxicity. Biochem Pharmacol (ENGLAND) Feb 4 1992

Fatal acetaminophen poisoning with evidence of subendocardial necrosis of the heart. J Forensic Sci (UNITED STATES) May 1991

Intrinsic susceptibility of the kidney to acetaminophen toxicity in middle-aged rats. Toxicol Lett (NETHERLANDS) Jun 1990

Glutathione enhancement in various mouse organs and protection by glutathione isopropyl ester against liver injury. Biochem Pharmacol (ENGLAND) Jun 15 1990

A comparison of the protective effects of N-acetyl-cysteine and S-carboxymethylcysteine against paracetamol (acetaminophen)-induced hepatotoxicity. Toxicology (NETHERLANDS) Nov 1983

Acetaminophen hepatotoxicity. An alternative mechanism. Biochem Pharmacol (ENGLAND) Jul 1 1983, 32 (13) p2053-9

Glutathione Metabolism and Its Role in Hepatotoxicity. Pharmacologic Therapy, 1991;52:287-305

Overdose of Extended-Release Acetaminophen. New England Journal of Medicine, July 20, 1995;196

Acute renal failure due to acetaminophen ingestion: a case report and review of the literature. J Am Soc Nephrol (UNITED STATES) Jul 1995

Acute hepatic and renal toxicity from low doses of acetaminophen in the absence of alcohol abuse or malnutrition: evidence for increased susceptibility to drug toxicity due to cardiopulmonary and renal insufficiency. Hepatology (UNITED STATES) May 1994

Protective effect of oral acetylcysteine against the hepatorenal toxicity of carbon tetrachloride potentiated by ethyl alcohol. Alcohol Clin Exp Res (UNITED STATES) Aug 1992

Cholestyramine as an antidote against paracetamol-induced hepato- and nephrotoxicity in the rat. Toxicol Lett (NETHERLANDS) May 1989

Relation of analgesic use to renal cancer: population-based findings. Natl Cancer Inst Monogr (UNITED STATES) Dec 1985

Acetaminophen-induced depletion of glutathione and cysteine in the aging mouse kidney. Biochem Pharmacol (ENGLAND) Jul 7 1992

Cysteine isopropylester protects against paracetamol-induced toxicity. Biochem Pharmacol (ENGLAND) Feb 4 1992

Fatal acetaminophen poisoning with evidence of subendocardial necrosis of the heart. J Forensic Sci (UNITED STATES) May 1991

Intrinsic susceptibility of the kidney to acetaminophen toxicity in middle-aged rats. Toxicol Lett (NETHERLANDS) Jun 1990

Glutathione enhancement in various mouse organs and protection by glutathione isopropyl ester against liver injury. Biochem Pharmacol (ENGLAND) Jun 15 1990

A comparison of the protective effects of N-acetyl-cysteine and S- carboxymethylcysteine against paracetamol (acetaminophen)-induced hepatotoxicity. Toxicology (NETHERLANDS) Nov 1983

Acetaminophen hepatotoxicity. An alternative mechanism. Biochem Pharmacol (ENGLAND) Jul 1 1983, 32 (13) p2053-9

Glutathione Metabolism and Its Role in Hepatotoxicity. Pharmacologic Therapy, 1991;52:287-305

Overdose of Extended-Release Acetaminophen. New England Journal of Medicine, July 20, 1995;196

Adrenal Disease

Adrenocortical insufficiency. Clinical Enocrinology Metab (ENGLAND) Nov 1995, 14 (4) p947-76

Changes in serum concentrations of conjugated and unconjugated steroids. J Clin Endocrinol Metab (UNITED STATES) Oct 1994, 79 (4) p1086-90

Ovarian suppression with triptorelin and adrenal stimulation with adrenocorticotropin in functional hyperadrogenism: role of adrenal and ovarian cytochrome P450c17 alpha. Fertil Steril (UNITED STATES) Sep 1994, 62 (3) p521-30

Pattern of plasma dehydroepiandrosterone sulfate levels in humans from birth to adulthood: evidence for testicular production. J Clin Endocrinol Metab (UNITED STATES) Sep 1978, 47 (3) p572-7

Adrenal function and ascorbic acid concentrations in elderly women. Gerontology (SWITZERLAND) 1978, 24 (6) p473-6

Age-Associated Mental Impairment (Brain Aging)

Cognition enhancers in age-related cognitive decline. Drugs Aging (NEW ZEALAND) Apr 1996, 8 (4) p245-74

Ginkgo biloba extract (EGb 761) independently improves changes in passive avoidance learning and brain membrane fluidity in the aging mouse. Pharmacopsychiatry (GERMANY) Jul 1996, 29 (4) p144-9

Neuronal actions of dehydroepiandrosterone. Possible roles in brain development, aging, memory, and affect. Ann N Y Acad Sci (UNITED STATES) Dec 29 1995, 774 p111-20

Effects of CDP-choline treatment on neurobehavioral deficits after TBI and on hippocampal and neo-cortical acetylcholine release. J Neurotrauma (UNITED STATES) Mar 1997, 14 (3) p161-9

Potentiation by DSP-4 of EEG slowing and memory impairment in basal forebrain-lesioned rats. Eur J Pharmacol (NETHERLANDS) Feb 26 1997, 321 (2) p149-55

Cholinergic neurotransmission and synaptic plasticity concerning memory processing. Neurochem

Res (UNITED STATES) Apr 1997, 22 (4) p507-15

Nutritional status and cognitive functioning in a normally aging sample: a 6-y reassessment. Am J Clin Nutr (UNITED STATES) Jan 1997, 65 (1) p20-9

The neurosteroid dehydroepiandrosterone sulfate (DHEAS) enhances hippocampal primed burst, but not long-term, potentiation. Neurosci Lett (IRELAND) Jan 5 1996, 202 (3) p204-8

The neuroprotective properties of the Ginkgo biloba leaf: a review of the possible relationship to platelet-activating factor (PAF). J Ethnopharmacol (IRELAND) Mar 1996, 50 (3) p131-9

Relations of vitamin B-12, vitamin B-6, folate, and homocysteine to cognitive performance in the Normative Aging Study. Am J Clin Nutr (UNITED STATES) Mar 1996, 63 (3) p306-14

Piracetam and fipexide prevent PTZ-kindling-provoked amnesia in rats. Eur Neuropsychopharmacol (NETHERLANDS) Nov 1996, 6 (4) p285-90

Nootropics: preclinical results in the light of clinical effects; comparison with tacrine. Crit Rev Neurobiol (UNITED STATES) 1996, 10 (3-4) p357-70

Piracetam and aniracetam antagonism of centrally active drug-induced antinociception. Pharmacol Biochem Behav (UNITED STATES) Apr 1996, 53 (4) p943-50

Effects of nicotinamide on central cholinergic transmission and on spatial learning in rats. Pharmacol Biochem Behav (UNITED STATES) Apr 1996, 53 (4) p783-90

Piracetam. An overview of its pharmacological properties and a review of its therapeutic use in senile cognitive disorders. Drugs Aging (NEW ZEALAND) Jan 1991, 1 (1) p17-35

Memory-enhancing effects in male mice of pregnenolone and steroids metabolically derived from it. Proc Natl Acad Sci U S A (UNITED STATES) Mar 1 1992, 89 (5) p1567-71

Piracetam elevates muscarinic cholinergic receptor density in the frontal cortex of aged but not of young mice. Psychopharmacology (Berl) (GERMANY, WEST) 1988, 94 (1) p74-8

Habituation of exploratory activity in mice: effects of combinations of piracetam and choline on memory processes. Pharmacol Biochem Behav (UNITED STATES) Aug 1984, 21 (2) p209-12

Profound effects of combining choline and piracetam on memory enhancement and cholinergic function in aged rats. Neurobiol Aging (UNITED STATES) Summer 1981, 2 (2) p105-11

Interaction between psychological and pharmacological treatment in cognitive impairment. Life Sci (ENGLAND) 1994, 55 (25-26) p2057-66

Impairment of learning and memory in shuttle box-trained rats neonatally injected with 6-hydroxy-dopamine. Effects of nootropic drugs. Acta Physiol Pharmacol Bulg (BULGARIA) 1993, 19 (3) p77-82

Latency of memory consolidation induced in mice by piracetam, a nootropic agent. Indian J Exp Biol (INDIA) Nov 1993, 31 (11) p898-901

Elevated corticosteroid levels block the memory-improving effects of nootropics and cholinomimetics. Psychopharmacology (Berl) (GERMANY) 1992, 108 (1-2) p11-5

A trial of piracetam in two subgroups of students with dyslexia enrolled in summer tutoring. J Learn Disabil (UNITED STATES) Nov 1991, 24 (9) p542-9

Aldosterone receptors are involved in the mediation of the memory-enhancing effects of piracetam.

References

Brain Res (NETHERLANDS) Aug 6 1990, 524 (2) p203-7

Pharmacological restoration of scopolamine-impaired memory. Acta Physiol Pharmacol Bulg (BUL-GARIA) 1985, 11 (3) p37-43

Gerontopsychological studies using NAI ('Nurnberger Alters-Inventar') on patients with organic psy-chosyndrome (DSM III, Category 1) treated with centrophenoxine in a double blind, comparative, ran-domized clinical trial. Arch Gerontol Geriatr (NETHERLANDS) Jul 1989, 9 (1) p17-30

[Characteristics of the action of psychostimulants on learning and memory in rats]. Biull Eksp Biol Med (USSR) Aug 1988, 106 (8) p161-3

Centrophenoxine: effects on aging mammalian brain. J Am Geriatr Soc (UNITED STATES) Feb 1978, 26 (2) p74-81

Centrophenoxine activates acetylcholinesterase activity in hippocampus of aged rats. Indian J Exp Biol (INDIA) May 1995, 33 (5) p365-8

On the role of intracellular physicochemistry in quantitative gene expression during aging and the effect of centrophenoxine. A review. Arch Gerontol Geriatr (NETHERLANDS) Nov-Dec 1989, 9 (3) p215-29

Neuronal lipopigment: a marker for cognitive impairment and long- term effects of psychotropic drugs [see comments]. Br J Psychiatry (ENGLAND) Jul 1989, 155 p1-11

Age-related change in the multiple unit activity of the rat brain parietal cortex and the effect of cen-trophenoxine. Exp Gerontol (ENGLAND) 1988, 23 (3) p161-74

[Effect of centrophenoxine, piracetam and aniracetam on the monoamine oxidase activity in different brain structures of rats]. Farmakol Toksikol (USSR) May-Jun 1988, 51 (3) p16-8

[Comparative neurophysiological study of the nootropic drugs piracetam and centrophenoxine]. Farmakol Toksikol (USSR) Nov-Dec 1987, 50 (6) p17-20

Fluidizing effects of centrophenoxine In vitro on brain and liver membranes from different age groups of mice. Life Sci (ENGLAND) Dec 1 1986, 39 (22) p2089-95

Studies on the effect of iron overload on rat cortex synaptosomal membranes. Biochim Biophys Acta (NETHERLANDS) Nov 7 1985, 820 (2) p216-22

Alterations of the intracellular water and ion concentrations in brain and liver cells during aging as revealed by energy dispersive X- ray microanalysis of bulk specimens. Scan Electron Microsc (UNITED STATES) 1985, (Pt 1) p323-37

Alterations in the molecular weight distribution of proteins in rat brain synaptosomes during aging and centrophenoxine treatment of old rats. Mech Ageing Dev (SWITZERLAND) Dec 1984, 28 (2-3) p171-6

Study on the anti-hypoxic effect of some drugs used in the pharmacotherapy of cerebrovascular dis-ease. Methods Find Exp Clin Pharmacol (SPAIN) Nov 1983, 5 (9) p607-12

Inability to deactivate the sympathetic nervous system in patients with brainstem infarction; correction of the disorder by centrophenoxine administration. Neurol Psychiatr (Bucur) (ROMANIA) Oct-Dec 1983, 21 (4) p425-39

Participation of adrenergic mechanisms in brain acetylcholine release produced by centrophenoxine. Acta Physiol Pharmacol Bulg (BULGARIA) 1979, 5 (4) p21-6

References

Acetyl-L-Carnitine: chronic treatment improves spatial acquisition in a new environment in aged rats. J Gerontol A Biol Sci Med Sci (UNITED STATES) Jul 1995, 50 (4) pB232-36

[Effects of L-acetylcarnitine on mental deterioration in the aged: initial results]. Clin Ter (ITALY) Mar 31 1990, 132 (6 Suppl) p479-510

Effect of acetyl-L-carnitine on conditioned reflex learning rate and retention in laboratory animals. Drugs Exp Clin Res (SWITZERLAND) 1986, 12 (11) p911-6

The effects of acetyl-l-carnitine on experimental models of learning and memory deficits in the old rat. Funct Neurol (ITALY) Oct-Dec 1989, 4 (4) p387-90

Alzheimer dementia and reduced nicotinamide adenine dinucleotide (NADH)-diaphorase activity in senile plaques and the basal forebrain. Neurosci Lett (NETHERLANDS) Jan 7 1985, 53 (1) p39-44

Effects of phosphatidylserine in Alzheimer's disease. Psychopharmacol Bull (UNITED STATES) 1992, 28 (1) p61-6

Nootropic drugs and brain cholinergic mechanisms. Prog Neuropsychopharmacol Biol Psychiatry (ENGLAND) 1989, 13 Suppl pS77-88

Effects of phosphatidylserine in age-associated memory impairment. Neurology (UNITED STATES) May 1991, 41 (5) p644-9

Memory effects of standardized extracts of Panax ginseng (G115), Ginkgo biloba (GK 501) and their combination Gincosan (PHL-00701). Planta Med (GERMANY) Apr 1993, 59 (2) p106-14

[Activity of Ginkgo biloba extract on short-term memory]. Presse Med (FRANCE) Sep 25 1986, 15 (31) p1592-4

Piracetam. An overview of its pharmacological properties and a review of its therapeutic use in senile cognitive disorders. Drugs Aging (NEW ZEALAND) Jan 1991, 1 (1) p17-35

Memory-enhancing effects in male mice of pregnenolone and steroids metabolically derived from it. Proc Natl Acad Sci U S A (UNITED STATES) Mar 1 1992, 89 (5) p1567-71

Piracetam elevates muscarinic cholinergic receptor density in the frontal cortex of aged but not of young mice. Psychopharmacology (Berl) (GERMANY, WEST) 1988, 94 (1) p74-8

Habituation of exploratory activity in mice: effects of combinations of piracetam and choline on memory processes. Pharmacol Biochem Behav (UNITED STATES) Aug 1984, 21 (2) p209-12

Profound effects of combining choline and piracetam on memory enhancement and cholinergic function in aged rats. Neurobiol Aging (UNITED STATES) Summer 1981, 2 (2) p105-11

Interaction between psychological and pharmacological treatment in cognitive impairment. Life Sci (ENGLAND) 1994, 55 (25-26) p2057-66

Impairment of learning and memory in shuttle box-trained rats neonatally injected with 6-hydroxy-dopamine. Effects of nootropic drugs. Acta Physiol Pharmacol Bulg (BULGARIA) 1993, 19 (3) p77-82

Latency of memory consolidation induced in mice by piracetam, a nootropic agent. Indian J Exp Biol (INDIA) Nov 1993, 31 (11) p898-901

Elevated corticosteroid levels block the memory-improving effects of nootropics and cholinomimetics. Psychopharmacology (Berl) (GERMANY) 1992, 108 (1-2) p11-5

A trial of piracetam in two subgroups of students with dyslexia enrolled in summer tutoring. J Learn Disabil (UNITED STATES) Nov 1991, 24 (9) p542-9

Aldosterone receptors are involved in the mediation of the memory-enhancing effects of piracetam. Brain Res (NETHERLANDS) Aug 6 1990, 524 (2) p203-7

Pharmacological restoration of scopolamine-impaired memory. Acta Physiol Pharmacol Bulg (BUL-GARIA) 1985, 11 (3) p37-43

Gerontopsychological studies using NAI ('Nurnberger Alters-Inventar') on patients with organic psychosyndrome (DSM III, Category 1) treated with centrophenoxine in a double blind, comparative, randomized clinical trial. Arch Gerontol Geriatr (NETHERLANDS) Jul 1989, 9 (1) p17-30

[Characteristics of the action of psychostimulants on learning and memory in rats] Biull Eksp Biol Med (USSR) Aug 1988, 106 (8) p161-3

Centrophenoxine: effects on aging mammalian brain. J Am Geriatr Soc (UNITED STATES) Feb 1978, 26 (2) p74-81

Centrophenoxine activates acetylcholinesterase activity in hippocampus of aged rats. Indian J Exp Biol (INDIA) May 1995, 33 (5) p365-8

On the role of intracellular physicochemistry in quantitative gene expression during aging and the effect of centrophenoxine. A review. Arch Gerontol Geriatr (NETHERLANDS) Nov-Dec 1989, 9 (3) p215-29

Neuronal lipopigment: a marker for cognitive impairment and long- term effects of psychotropic drugs [see comments] Br J Psychiatry (ENGLAND) Jul 1989, 155 p1-11

Age-related change in the multiple unit activity of the rat brain parietal cortex and the effect of centrophenoxine. Exp Gerontol (ENGLAND) 1988, 23 (3) p161-74

[Effect of centrophenoxine, piracetam and aniracetam on the monoamine oxidase activity in different brain structures of rats] Farmakol Toksikol (USSR) May-Jun 1988, 51 (3) p16-8

[Comparative neurophysiological study of the nootropic drugs piracetam and centrophenoxine] Farmakol Toksikol (USSR) Nov-Dec 1987, 50 (6) p17-20

Fluidizing effects of centrophenoxine in vitro on brain and liver membranes from different age groups of mice. Life Sci (ENGLAND) Dec 1 1986, 39 (22) p2089-95

Studies on the effect of iron overload on rat cortex synaptosomal membranes. Biochim Biophys Acta (NETHERLANDS) Nov 7 1985, 820 (2) p216-22

Alterations of the intracellular water and ion concentrations in brain and liver cells during aging as revealed by energy dispersive X- ray microanalysis of bulk specimens. Scan Electron Microsc (UNITED STATES) 1985, (Pt 1) p323-37

Alterations in the molecular weight distribution of proteins in rat brain synaptosomes during aging and centrophenoxine treatment of old rats. Mech Ageing Dev (SWITZERLAND) Dec 1984, 28 (2-3) p171-6

Study on the anti-hypoxic effect of some drugs used in the pharmacotherapy of cerebrovascular disease. Methods Find Exp Clin Pharmacol (SPAIN) Nov 1983, 5 (9) p607-12

Inability to deactivate the sympathetic nervous system in patients with brainstem infarction; correction of the disorder by centrophenoxine administration. Neurol Psychiatr (Bucur) (ROMANIA) Oct-Dec 1983,

21 (4) p425-39

Participation of adrenergic mechanisms in brain acetylcholine release produced by centrophenoxine. Acta Physiol Pharmacol Bulg (BULGARIA) 1979, 5 (4) p21-6

Acetyl-L-Carnitine: chronic treatment improves spatial acquisition in a new environment in aged rats. J Gerontol A Biol Sci Med Sci (UNITED STATES) Jul 1995, 50 (4) pB232-36

[Effects of L-acetylcarnitine on mental deterioration in the aged: initial results] Clin Ter (ITALY) Mar 31 1990, 132 (6 Suppl) p479-510

Effect of acetyl-L-carnitine on conditioned reflex learning rate and retention in laboratory animals. Drugs Exp Clin Res (SWITZERLAND) 1986, 12 (11) p911-6

The effects of acetyl-l-carnitine on experimental models of learning and memory deficits in the old rat. Funct Neurol (ITALY) Oct-Dec 1989, 4 (4) p387-90

Alzheimer dementia and reduced nicotinamide adenine dinucleotide (NADH)- diaphorase activity in senile plaques and the basal forebrain. Neurosci Lett (NETHERLANDS) Jan 7 1985, 53 (1) p39-44

Effects of phosphatidylserine in Alzheimer's disease. Psychopharmacol Bull (UNITED STATES) 1992, 28 (1) p61-6

Nootropic drugs and brain cholinergic mechanisms. Prog Neuropsychopharmacol Biol Psychiatry (ENGLAND) 1989, 13 Suppl pS77-88

Effects of phosphatidylserine in age-associated memory impairment. Neurology (UNITED STATES) May 1991, 41 (5) p644-9

Memory effects of standardized extracts of Panax ginseng (G115), Ginkgo biloba (GK 501) and their combination Gincosan (PHL-00701). Planta Med (GERMANY) Apr 1993, 59 (2) p106-14

[Activity of Ginkgo biloba extract on short-term memory] Presse Med (FRANCE) Sep 25 1986, 15 (31) p1592-4

Alcohol-Induced Hangover: Prevention

Reduction of lower motor neuron degeneration in wobbler mice by N-acetyl-L-cysteine. Journal of Neuroscience (USA), 1996, 16/23 (7574-7582)

Role of oxidative stress and antioxidant therapy in alcoholic and nonalcoholic liver diseases. Adv Pharmacol (UNITED STATES) 1997, 38 p601-28

Protective action of ascorbic acid and sulfur compounds against acetaldehyde toxicity: implications in alcoholism and smoking. Agents Actions (SWITZERLAND) May 1975, 5 (2) p164-73

Sulfur amino acid metabolism in hepatobiliary disorders. Scand J Gastroenterol (NORWAY) May 1992, 27 (5) p405-11

[Severe somatic complications of acute alcoholic intoxication]. Rev Prat (FRANCE) Oct 15 1993, 43 (16) p2047-51

[The therapeutic approach in optic neuropathy due to methyl alcohol]. Oftalmologia (ROMANIA) Jan-Mar 1991, 35 (1) p39-42

Alcohol and brain damage. Hum Toxicol (ENGLAND) Sep 1988, 7 (5) p455-63

Acute ethanol poisoning and the ethanol withdrawal syndrome. Med Toxicol Adverse Drug Exp (NEW ZEALAND) May-Jun 1988, 3 (3) p172-96

Clinical signs in the Wernicke-Korsakoff complex: a retrospective analysis of 131 cases diagnosed at necropsy. J Neurol Neurosurg Psychiatry (ENGLAND) Apr 1986, 49 (4) p341-5

Thiamine status of institutionalised and non-institutionalised aged. Int J Vitam Nutr Res (SWITZER-LAND) 1977, 47 (4) p325-35

[Vitamin B 1 deficiency in chronic alcoholics and its clinical correlation]. Schweiz Med Wochenschr (SWITZERLAND) Oct 23 1976, 106 (43) p1466-70

Effect of S-adenosyl-L-methionine administration on red blood cell cysteine and glutathione levels in alcoholic patients with and without liver disease. Alcohol Alcohol (ENGLAND) Sep 1994, 29 (5) p597-604

Glutathione prevents ethanol induced gastric mucosal damage and depletion of sulfhydryl compounds in humans. Gut (ENGLAND) Feb 1993, 34 (2) p161-5

Effects of amino acids on acute alcohol intoxication in mice--concentrations of ethanol, acetaldehyde, acetate and acetone in blood and tissues. Arukoru Kenkyuto Yakubutsu Ison (JAPAN) Oct 1990, 25 (5) p429-40

A possible protective role for sulphydryl compounds in acute alcoholic liver injury. Biochem Pharmacol (UNITED STATES) Aug 15 1977, 26 (16) p1529-31

Protection against toxic effects of formaldehyde in vitro, and of methanol or formaldehyde in vivo, by subsequent administration of SH reagents. Physiol Chem Phys (UNITED STATES) 1976, 8 (6) p543-50

"N-Acetylcysteine for Lung Cancer Prevention." Nico Chest May 1995;107(5):1437-1441.

"S-Adenosylmethionine and the Liver." The Liver: Biology and Pathobiology, 3rd Edition, 1994; 27:461-470

Protective action of ascorbic acid and sulfur compounds against acetaldehyde toxicity: implications in alcoholism and smoking. Agents Actions (SWITZERLAND) May 1975, 5 (2) p164-73

Sulfur amino acid metabolism in hepatobiliary disorders. Scand J Gastroenterol (NORWAY) May 1992, 27 (5) p405-11

[Severe somatic complications of acute alcoholic intoxication] Rev Prat (FRANCE) Oct 15 1993, 43 (16) p2047-51

[The therapeutic approach in optic neuropathy due to methyl alcohol] Oftalmologia (ROMANIA) Jan-Mar 1991, 35 (1) p39-42

Alcohol and brain damage. Hum Toxicol (ENGLAND) Sep 1988, 7 (5) p455-63

Acute ethanol poisoning and the ethanol withdrawal syndrome. Med Toxicol Adverse Drug Exp (NEW ZEALAND) May-Jun 1988, 3 (3) p172-96

Clinical signs in the Wernicke-Korsakoff complex: a retrospective analysis of 131 cases diagnosed at necropsy. J Neurol Neurosurg Psychiatry (ENGLAND) Apr 1986, 49 (4) p341-5

Thiamine status of institutionalised and non-institutionalised aged. Int J Vitam Nutr Res (SWITZER-

LAND) 1977, 47 (4) p325-35

[Vitamin B 1 deficiency in chronic alcoholics and its clinical correlation] Schweiz Med Wochenschr (SWITZERLAND) Oct 23 1976, 106 (43) p1466-70

Effect of S-adenosyl-L-methionine administration on red blood cell cysteine and glutathione levels in alcoholic patients with and without liver disease. Alcohol Alcohol (ENGLAND) Sep 1994, 29 (5) p597-604

Glutathione prevents ethanol induced gastric mucosal damage and depletion of sulfhydryl compounds in humans. Gut (ENGLAND) Feb 1993, 34 (2) p161-5

Effects of amino acids on acute alcohol intoxication in mice—concentrations of ethanol, acetaldehyde, acetate and acetone in blood and tissues. Arukoru Kenkyuto Yakubutsu Ison (JAPAN) Oct 1990, 25 (5) p429-40

A possible protective role for sulphydryl compounds in acute alcoholic liver injury. Biochem Pharmacol (UNITED STATES) Aug 15 1977, 26 (16) p1529-31

Protection against toxic effects of formaldehyde in vitro, and of methanol or formaldehyde in vivo, by subsequent administration of SH reagents. Physiol Chem Phys (UNITED STATES) 1976, 8 (6) p543-50

N-Acetylcysteine for Lung Cancer Prevention. Nico Chest May 1995;107(5):1437-1441.

S-Adenosylmethionine and the Liver. The Liver: Biology and Pathobiology, 3rd Edition, 1994; 27:461-470

Allergies

The effect of gamma-linolenic acid on clinical status, red cell fatty acid composition and membrane microviscosity in infants with atopic dermatitis. Drugs Exp Clin Res. 1994. 20(2). P 77-84

Fatty acid compositions of plasma lipids in atopic dermatitis/asthma patients. Arerugi. 1994 Jan. 43(1). P 37-43

Autoimmune disease and allergy are controlled by vitamin C treatment. IN VIVO (Greece), 1994, 8/2 (251-258)

Immune senescence and adrenal steroids: Immune dysregulation and the action of dehydroepiandrosterone (DHEA) in old animals. EUR. J. CLIN. PHARMACOL. (Germany), 1993, 45/SUPPL. 1 (S21-S23)

Omega-3 fatty acids in respiratory diseases: A review. J. AM. COLL. NUTR. (USA), 1995, 14/1 (18-23)

Vitamin C and the genesis of autoimmune disease and allergy (Review). In Vivo (Greece), 1995, 9/3 (231-238)

Is Linus Pauling, a vitamin C advocate, just making much ado about nothing? IN VIVO (Greece), 1994, 8/3 (391-400)

Asthma and vitamin C. ANN. ALLERGY (USA), 1994, 73/2 (89-99)

The effect of vitamin C infusion treatment on immune disorders: An invitation to a trial in AIDS patients (Review). INT. J. ONCOL. (Greece), 1994, 4/4 (831-838)

Chromium dermatitis and ascorbic acid. CONTACT DERMATITIS (DENMARK), 1984, 10/4 (252-253)

Colds and vitamin C. IRISH MED.J. (IRELAND), 1975, 68/20 (511-516)

Vitamin C metabolism and atopic allergy. CLIN.ALLERGY (ENGLAND), 1975, 5/3 (317-324)

Alzheimer's Disease

Brain aging and Alzheimer's disease, 'Wear and tear' versus 'Use it or lose it'. Swaab D.F., NEUROBIOL. AGING (USA), 1991, 12/4 (317-324), Netherlands Institute for Brain Research, Meibergdreef 33, 1105 AZ Amsterdam Netherlands

Immunohistochemical localization of advanced glycation end products, pentosidine, and carboxymethyllysine in lipofuscin pigments of Alzheimer's disease and aged neurons. Horie K.; Miyata T.; Yasuda T.; Takeda A.; Yasuda Y.; Maeda K.; Sobue G.; Kurokawa K., Biochemical and Biophysical Research Communications (USA), 1997, 236/2 (327-332), K. Kurokawa, Institute of Medical Sciences, Tokai University School of Medicine, Isehara, Kanagawa 259-11 Japan

Neuroanatomical aspects of neurotransmitters affected in Alzheimer's disease. Emson P.C.; Lindvall O., BR. MED. BULL. (ENGLAND), 1986, 42/1 (57-62), MRC Neurochemical Pharmacology Unit, Cambridge UNITED KINGDOM

Non-cholinergic neurotransmitter abnormalities in Alzheimer's disease. Rossor M.; Iversen L.L., BR. MED. BULL. (ENGLAND), 1986, 42/1 (70-74), Institute of Neurology, London UNITED KINGDOM

Changes in nerve cells of the nucleus basalis of Meynert in Alzheimer's disease and their relationship to ageing and to the accumulation of lipofuscin pigment. Mann D.M.A.; Yates P.O.; Marcyniuk B., MECH. AGEING DEV. (IRELAND), 1984, 25/1-2 (189-204), Department of Pathology, University of Manchester, Manchester M13 9PT UNITED KINGDOM

Physical basis of cognitive alterations in Alzheimer's disease: synapse loss is the major correlate of cognitive impairment. Terry RD; Masliah E; Salmon DP; Butters N; DeTeresa R; Hill R; Hansen LA; Katzman R, Ann Neurol (UNITED STATES) Oct 1991, 30 (4) p572-80, Department of Neurosciences, University of California-San Diego, La Jolla 92093-0624.

Synapse loss in frontal cortex biopsies in Alzheimer's disease: correlation with cognitive severity. DeKosky ST; Scheff SW, Ann Neurol (UNITED STATES) May 1990, 27 (5) p457-64, Department of Neurology, Lexington Veterans Administration, Medical Center, KY.

Neurofibrillary tangles but not senile plaques parallel duration and severity of Alzheimer's disease. Arriagada PV; Growdon JH; Hedley-Whyte ET; Hyman BT, Neurology (UNITED STATES) Mar 1992, 42 (3 Pt 1) p631-9, Department of Pathology, Massachusetts General Hospital, Harvard Medical School, Boston 02114.

Biochemical and anatomical redistribution of tau protein in Alzheimer's disease. Mukaetova-Ladinska EB; Harrington CR; Roth M; Wischik CM, Cambridge Brain Bank Laboratory, University of Cambridge Department of Psychiatry, England, Am J Pathol (UNITED STATES) Aug 1993, 143 (2) p565-78

Functional studies of Alzheimer's disease tau protein. Lu Q; Wood JG, Department of Anatomy and Cell Biology, Emory University School of Medicine, Atlanta, Georgia 30322, J Neurosci (UNITED STATES) Feb 1993, 13 (2) p508-15

References

Tau protein and the neurofibrillary pathology of Alzheimer's disease. Goedert M, Medical Research Council, Laboratory of Molecular Biology, Cambridge, UK, Trends Neurosci (ENGLAND) Nov 1993, 16 (11) p460-5

Dorothy Russell Memorial Lecture. The molecular pathology of Alzheimer's disease: are we any closer to understanding the neurodegenerative process? Smith C; Anderton BH, Department of Neuroscience, Institute of Psychiatry, London, UK, Neuropathol Appl Neurobiol (ENGLAND) Aug 1994, 20 (4) p322-38

Gene dose of apolipoprotein E type 4 allele and the risk of Alzheimer's disease in late onset families. Corder EH; Saunders AM; Strittmatter WJ; Schmechel DE; Gaskell PC; Small, GW; Roses AD; Haines JL; Pericak-Vance MA, Department of Medicine, Joseph and Kathleen Bryan Alzheimer's Disease Research Center, Duke University Medical Center, Durham, NC 27710, Science (UNITED STATES) Aug 13 1993, 261 (5123) p921-3

Immunodetection of the amyloid P component in Alzheimer's disease. Duong T.; Pommier E.C.; Scheibel A.B., Department of Anatomy and Cell Biology, UCLA Medical School, Los Angeles, CA 90024-1763 USA, ACTA NEUROPATHOL. (Germany, Federal Republic of), 1989, 78/4 (429-437)

Blood brain barrier dysfunction in acute lead encephalopathy: a reappraisal. Bouldin T.W.; Mushak P.; O'Tuama L.A.; Krigman M.R., Dept. Pathol., Univ. North Carolina Sch. Med., Chapel Hill, N.C. 27514 USA, ENVIRONM.HLTH PERSPECT. (USA), 1975, Vol.12 (81-88)

Can blood-brain barrier play a role in the development of cerebral amyloidosis and Alzheimer's disease pathology [editorial; comment]. Zlokovic B, Neurobiol Dis (UNITED STATES) 1997, 4 (1) p23-6

Development and in vitro characterization of a cationized monoclonal antibody against beta A4 protein: a potential probe for Alzheimer's disease. Bickel U; Lee VM; Trojanowski JQ; Pardridge WM, Department of Medicine, UCLA School of Medicine 90024, Bioconjug Chem (UNITED STATES) Mar-Apr 1994, 5 (2) p119-25

Beta-Amyloid precursor protein gene in squirrel monkeys with cerebral amyloid angiopathy. Levy E; Amorim A; Frangione B; Walker LC, Department of Pharmacology, New York University Medical Center, NY 10016, USA, Neurobiol Aging (UNITED STATES) Sep-Oct 1995, 16 (5) p805-8

Therapeutic approaches related to amyloid-beta peptide and Alzheimer's disease. Schenk DB; Rydel RE; May P; Little S; Panetta J; Lieberburg I; Sinha S, Athena Neurosciences, Inc., South San Francisco, California 94080, USA, J Med Chem (UNITED STATES) Oct 13 1995, 38 (21) p4141-54

Molecular mechanisms of Alzheimer's disease. Simons M., Monchgasse 9, D-69117 Heidelberg Germany, Fortschritte der Medizin (Germany), 1995, 113/31 (31-32)

Neuropathy in Waldenstrom's macroglobulinemia. Coimbra J.; Costa A.P.; Pita F.; Rosado P.; Bigotte De Almeida L., Servico de Neurologia, Hospital Garcia de Orta, Almada Portugal, Acta Medica Portuguesa (Portugal), 1995, 8/4 (253-257)

Advanced glycation endproducts in ageing and Alzheimer's disease. Munch G.; Thome J.; Foley P.; Schinzel R.; Riederer P., Germany, Brain Research Reviews (Netherlands), 1997, 23/1-2 (134-143)

Changes in biomechanical properties, composition of collagen and elastin, and advanced glycation endproducts of the rat aorta in relation to age. Bruel A.; Oxlund H., A. Bruel, Dept. of Connective Tissue Biology, Institute of Anatomy, University of Aarhus, DK-8000 Aarhus C Denmark, Atherosclerosis (Ireland), 1996, 127/2 (155-165)

Physiological production of the beta-amyloid protein and the mechanism of Alzheimer's disease. Selkoe D.J., Center for Neurological Diseases, Harvard Medical School, Brigham and Women's Hospital, Boston, MA 02115 USA, TRENDS NEUROSCI. (United Kingdom), 1993, 16/10 (403-409)

Aluminum, iron, and zinc ions promote aggregation of physiological concentrations of beta-amyloid peptide. Mantyh P.W.; Ghilardi J.R.; Rogers S.; DeMaster E.; Allen C.J.; Stimson E.R.; Maggio J.E., Molecular Neurobiology Laboratory, Veterans Administration Medical Ctr., Minneapolis, MN 55417 USA, J. NEUROCHEM. (USA), 1993, 61/3 (1171-1174)

Acetyl-L-carnitine: A drug able to slow the progress of Alzheimer's disease? Carta A.; Calvani M., Department of Neurological Research, Sigma-Tau, Pomezia, Rome 00040 Italy, ANN. NEW YORK ACAD. SCI. (USA), 1991, 640/- (228-232)

Clinical and neurochemical effects of acetyl-L-carnitine in Alzheimer's disease. Pettegrew J.W.; Klunk W.E.; Panchalingam K.; Kanfer J.N.; McClure R.J., University of Pittsburgh, Western Psychiatric Institute/Clinic, A710 Crabtree Hall/GSPH, 130 DeSoto Street, Pittsburgh, PA 15261 USA, NEUROBIOL. AGING (USA), 1995, 16/1 (1-4)

Vitamin E protects nerve cells from amyloid beta protein toxicity. Behl C; Davis J; Cole GM; Schubert D, Salk Institute for Biological Studies, San Diego, CA 92186-5800, Biochem Biophys Res Commun (UNITED STATES) Jul 31 1992, 186 (2) p944-50

The lipid peroxidation product, 4-hydroxy-2-trans-nonenal, alters the conformation of cortical synaptosomal membrane proteins. Subramaniam R; Roediger F; Jordan B; Mattson MP; Keller JN; Waeg G; Butterfield DA, Department of Chemistry, Center of Membrane Science, University of Kentucky, Lexington 40506, U.S.A., J Neurochem (UNITED STATES) Sep 1997, 69 (3) p1161-9

Deleterious network: a testable pathogenetic concept of Alzheimer's disease. Ying W

Department of Physiology, School of Medicine, University of New Mexico, Albuquerque, USA. Gerontology (SWITZERLAND) 1997, 43 (4) p242-53

Oxidative stress hypothesis in Alzheimer's disease. Markesbery WR, Sanders-Brown Center on Aging, Lexington, KY 40536-0230, USA, Free Radic Biol Med (UNITED STATES) 1997, 23 (1) p134-47

Amyloid precursor protein, copper and Alzheimer's disease. Multhaup G

ZMBH Center for Molecular Biology, University of Heidelberg, Germany, Biomed Pharmacother (FRANCE) 1997, 51 (3) p105-11

Oxidative-stress associated parameters (lactoferrin, superoxide dismutases) in serum of patients with Alzheimer's disease. Thome J; Gsell W; Rosler M; Kornhuber J; Frolich L; Hashimoto E; Zielke B ; Wiesbeck GA; Riederer P, Department of Psychiatry, University of Wurzburg, Germany, Life Sci (ENGLAND) 1997, 60 (1) p13-9

Methodologic aspects of a population pharmacodynamic model for cognitive effects in Alzheimer patients treated with tacrine. Holford NH; Peace KE, Department of Pharmacology and Clinical Pharmacology, University of Auckland, New Zealand, Proc Natl Acad Sci U S A (UNITED STATES) Dec 1 1992, 89 (23) p11466-70

Implications of the study population in the early evaluation of anticholinesterase inhibitors for Alzheimer's disease. Cutler NR; Sramek JJ; Murphy MF; Nash RJ, California Clinical Trials, Beverly Hills 90211, Ann Pharmacother (UNITED STATES) Sep 1992, 26 (9) p1118-22

References

A double-blind, placebo-controlled multicenter study of tacrine for Alzheimer's disease. The Tacrine Collaborative Study Group [see comments]. Davis KL; Thal LJ; Gamzu ER; Davis CS; Woolson RF; Gracon SI; Drachman DA ; Schneider LS; Whitehouse PJ; Hoover TM; et al, Mount Sinai Medical Center, New York, NY 10029-6574, N Engl J Med (UNITED STATES) Oct 29 1992, 327 (18) p1253-9

A controlled trial of tacrine in Alzheimer's disease. The Tacrine Study Group [see comments]. Farlow M; Gracon SI; Hershey LA; Lewis KW; Sadowsky CH; Dolan-Ureno J, Center for Alzheimer's Disease and Related Disorders, Indiana University Medical Center, Indianapolis, JAMA (UNITED STATES) Nov 11 1992, 268 (18) p2523-9

Effect of oestrogen during menopause on risk and age at onset of Alzheimer's disease [see comments]. Tang MX; Jacobs D; Stern Y; Marder K; Schofield P; Gurland B; Andrews H; Mayeux R, Gertrude H Serglevsky Center, Columbia University, New York, NY 10032, USA, Lancet (ENGLAND) Aug 17 1996, 348 (9025) p429-32

Use of phosphatidylserine in Alzheimer's disease. Amaducci L.; Crook T.H.; Lippi A.; Bracco L.; Baldereschi M.; Latorraca S.; Piersanti P.; Tesco G.; Sorbi S., Dept. of Neurologic/Psychiatric Sci., S.M.I.D. Center, University of Florence, 50123 Florence Italy, ANN. NEW YORK ACAD. SCI. (USA), 1991, 640/- (245-249)

Abnormalities of energy metabolism in Alzheimer's disease studied with PET. Heiss W.-D.; Szelies B.; Kessler J.; Herholz K., Max-Planck-Inst. Neurol. Forschung, Universitatsklinik fur Neurologie, Joseph-Stelzmann-Str. 9, D-5000 Koln 41 Germany, ANN. NEW YORK ACAD. SCI. (USA), 1991, 640/- (65-71)

Contrasting patterns of protein phosphorylation in human normal and Alzheimer brain: Focus on protein kinase C and protein F1/GAP-43. Florez J.C.; Nelson R.B.; Routtenberg A., Department of Neurobiology and Physiology, Northwestern University, Evanston, IL 60208 USA, EXP. NEUROL. (USA), 1991, 112/3 (264-272)

Drug treatment of Alzheimer's disease. Cooper J.K., University of California Davis Medical Center, 2221 Stockton Blvd, Sacramento, CA 95817 USA, ARCH. INTERN. MED. (USA), 1991, 151/2 (245-249)

Clinical trial of indomethacin in Alzheimer's disease. Rogers J.; Kirby L.C.; Hempelman S.R.; Berry D.L.; McGeer P.L.; Kaszniak A.W.; Zalinski J.; Cofield M.; Mansukhani L.; Willson P.; Kogan F., Sun Health Research Institute, P.O. Box 1278, Sun City, AZ 85372 USA, NEUROLOGY (USA), 1993, 43/8 (1609-1611)

Inflammatory mechanisms in Alzheimer's disease. Eikelenboom P.; Zhan S.-S.; Van Gool W.A.; Allsop D., Department of Psychiatry, PCA Valeriuskliniek, Valeriusplein 9, 1075 BG Amsterdam Netherlands, TRENDS PHARMACOL. SCI. (United Kingdom), 1994, 15/12 (447-450)

Inflammatory mechanisms in Alzheimer's disease: Implications for therapy. Aisen P.S.; Davis K.L., Department of Psychiatry, Mount Sinai School of Medicine, Box 1230, One Gustave L. Levy Place, New York, NY 10029 USA, AM. J. PSYCHIATRY (USA), 1994, 151/8 (1105-1113)

Brain interleukin-1beta in Alzheimer's disease and vascular dementia. Cacabelos R.; Alvarez X.A.; Fernandez-Novoa L.; Franco A.; Mangues R.; Pellicer A.; Nishimura T., Institute for CNS Disorders, P.O. Box 733, 15080 La Coruna Spain, METHODS FIND. EXP. CLIN. PHARMACOL. (Spain), 1994, 16/2 (141-151)

The role of estrogen in the treatment of Alzheimer's disease. Neurology (USA), 1997, 48/5 SUPPL. 7

(S36-S41)

Pharmacotherapy in Alzheimer's dementia: Treatment of cognitive symptoms Results of new studies. Fortschritte der Neurologie Psychiatrie (Germany), 1997, 65/3 (108-121)

Therapy of dementia - Neurologic and psychiatric aspects. Wiener Medizinische Wochenschrift (Austria), 1996, 146/21-22 (546-548)

The clinical potential of Deprenyl in neurologic and psychiatric disorders. (Austria), 1996, -/48 (85-93)

Modulation of gene expression rather than monoamine oxidase inhibition: (-)-Deprenyl-related compounds in controlling neurodegeneration. Neurology (USA), 1996, 47/6 SUPPL. 3 (S171-S183)

Neuroendocrine aspects of the menopause and hormone replacement therapy. Journal of Cardiovascular Pharmacology (USA), 1996, 28/SUPPL. 5

A 1-year multicenter placebo-controlled study of acetyl-L-carnitine in patients with Alzheimer's disease. Neurology (USA), 1996, 47/3 (705-711)

Monoamine oxidase B inhibitors. Current status and future potential. CNS Drugs (New Zealand), 1996, 6/3 (217-236)

Drug treatment of Alzheimer's disease. Effects on caregiver burden and patient quality of life. Drugs Aging (NEW ZEALAND) Jan 1996, 8 (1) p47-55

Orally active NGF synthesis stimulators: potential therapeutic agents in Alzheimer's disease. Behav Brain Res (NETHERLANDS) Feb 1997, 83 (1-2) p117-22

Calcium homeostasis and reactive oxygen species production in cells transformed by mitochondria from individuals with sporadic Alzheimer's disease. J Neurosci (UNITED STATES) Jun 15 1997, 17 (12) p4612-22

The search for disease-modifying treatment for Alzheimer's disease. Neurology (UNITED STATES) May 1997, 48 (5 Suppl 6) pS35-41

Molecular basis of Alzheimer's disease. Am J Health Syst Pharm (UNITED STATES) Jul 1 1996, 53 (13) p1545-57; quiz 1603-4

Functional studies of new drugs for the treatment of Alzheimer's disease. Acta Neurol Scand Suppl (DENMARK) 1996, 165 p137-44

Treatment of Alzheimer's disease: future directions. Acta Neurol Scand Suppl (DENMARK) 1996, 165 p128-36

Acetyl-L-carnitine restores choline acetyltransferase activity in the hippocampus of rats with partial unilateral fimbria-fornix transection. Int J Dev Neurosci (ENGLAND) Feb 1995, 13 (1) p13-9

Acetyl-L-carnitine arginyl amide (ST857) increases calcium channel density in rat pheochromocytoma (PC12) cells. J Neurosci Res (UNITED STATES) Feb 15 1995, 40 (3) p371-8

Neurite outgrowth in PC12 cells stimulated by acetyl-L-carnitine arginine amide.

Neurochem Res (UNITED STATES) Jan 1995, 20 (1) p1-9

Effects of acetyl-L-carnitine treatment and stress exposure on the nerve growth factor receptor (p75NGFR) mRNA level in the central nervous system of aged rats. Prog Neuropsychopharmacol Biol Psychiatry (ENGLAND) Jan 1995, 19 (1) p117-33

Acetyl-L-carnitine treatment increases nerve growth factor levels and choline acetyltransferase activity in the central nervous system of aged rats. Exp Gerontol (ENGLAND) Jan-Feb 1994, 29 (1) p55-66

Acetyl-L-carnitine affects aged brain receptorial system in rodents. Life Sci (ENGLAND) 1994, 54 (17) p1205-14

Stimulation of nerve growth factor receptors in PC12 by acetyl-L-carnitine. Biochem Pharmacol (ENGLAND) Aug 4 1992, 44 (3) p577-85

Culture of dorsal root ganglion neurons from aged rats: effects of acetyl-L-carnitine and NGF. Int J Dev Neurosci (ENGLAND) Aug 1992, 10 (4) p321-9

Acetyl-L-carnitine enhances the response of PC12 cells to nerve growth factor. Brain Res Dev Brain Res (NETHERLANDS) Apr 24 1991, 59 (2) p221-30

Effect of acetyl-L-carnitine on forebrain cholinergic neurons of developing rats. Int J Dev Neurosci (ENGLAND) 1991, 9 (1) p39-46

Nerve growth factor binding in aged rat central nervous system: effect of acetyl-L-carnitine. J Neurosci Res (UNITED STATES) Aug 1988, 20 (4) p491-6

Nootropics: preclinical results in the light of clinical effects; comparison with tacrine. Crit Rev Neurobiol (UNITED STATES) 1996, 10 (3-4) p357-70

[Neuroprotective therapy of Alzheimer's disease?]. Dtsch Med Wochenschr (GERMANY) Nov 29 1996, 121 (48) p1515

Prescribing practice with cognition enhancers in outpatient care: are there differences regarding type of dementia?--Results of a representative survey in lower Saxony, Germany. Pharmacopsychiatry (GERMANY) Jul 1996, 29 (4) p150-5

Coenzyme nicotinamide adenine dinucleotide: new therapeutic approach for improving dementia of the Alzheimer type. Ann Clin Lab Sci (UNITED STATES) Jan-Feb 1996, 26 (1) p1-9

Deprenyl reduces neuronal apoptosis and facilitates neuronal outgrowth by altering protein synthesis without inhibiting monoamine oxidase. J Neural Transm Suppl (AUSTRIA) 1996, 48 p45-59

Protection of the aged substantia nigra of the rat against oxidative damage by (-)-deprenyl. Br J Pharmacol (ENGLAND) Apr 1996, 117 (8) p1756-60

Different mechanisms regulate phosphatidylserine synthesis in rat cerebral cortex. Mol Cell Biochem (NETHERLANDS) Mar 1997, 168 (1-2) p41-9

Relationships between phosphatidylcholine, phosphatidylethanolamine, and sphingomyelin metabolism in cultured oligodendrocytes. J Neurochem (UNITED STATES) Mar 1997, 68 (3) p1252-60

Effect of phosphatidylserine on the binding properties of glutamate receptors in brain sections from adult and neonatal rats. Brain Res (NETHERLANDS) Nov 18 1996, 740 (1-2) p337-45

Pharmacological effects of phosphatidylserine enzymatically synthesized from soybean lecithin on brain functions in rodents. J Nutr Sci Vitaminol (Tokyo) (JAPAN) Feb 1996, 42 (1) p47-54

Aluminum facilitation of iron-mediated lipid peroxidation is dependent on substrate, pH and aluminum and iron concentrations. Arch Biochem Biophys (UNITED STATES) Mar 15 1996, 327 (2) p222-6

Influence of vitamin B12 on brain methionine adenosyltransferase activity in senile dementia of the Alzheimer's type. J Neural Transm Gen Sect (AUSTRIA) 1996, 103 (7) p861-72

Dementia and subnormal levels of vitamin B12: effects of replacement therapy on dementia. J Neurol (GERMANY) Jul 1996, 243 (7) p522-9

Is metabolic evidence for vitamin B-12 and folate deficiency more frequent in elderly patients with Alzheimer's disease? J Gerontol A Biol Sci Med Sci (UNITED STATES) Mar 1997, 52 (2) pM76-9

Effects of hormone replacement therapy on serum amyloid P component in postmenopausal women. Maturitas (IRELAND) Mar 1997, 26 (2) p113-9

Dehydroepiandrosterone and diseases of aging.

Drugs Aging (NEW ZEALAND) Oct 1996, 9 (4) p274-91

Dehydroepiandrosterone (DHEA) increases production and release of Alzheimer's amyloid precursor protein. Life Sci (ENGLAND) 1996, 59 (19) p1651-7

[Change of serum amyloid P component concentrations in women]. Nippon Sanka Fujinka Gakkai Zasshi (JAPAN) Jul 1996, 48 (7) p481-7

Serum dehydroepiandrosterone (DHEA) and DHEA-sulfate (DHEA-S) in Alzheimer's disease and in cerebrovascular dementia. Endocr J (JAPAN) Feb 1996, 43 (1) p119-23

Melatonin prevents death of neuroblastoma cells exposed to the Alzheimer amyloid peptide. J Neurosci (UNITED STATES) Mar 1 1997, 17 (5) p1683-90

[Melatonin. Hormone or wonder drug?]. Med Monatsschr Pharm (GERMANY) Mar 1996, 19 (3) p69-75

Daily rhythm of serum melatonin in patients with dementia of the degenerate type. Brain Res (NETHERLANDS) Apr 22 1996, 717 (1-2) p154-9

Alzheimer's disease: new horizons in diagnosis and treatment. Iowa Med (UNITED STATES) May-Jun 1997, 87 (5) p199-201

Cognitive enhancers in theory and practice: studies of the cholinergic hypothesis of cognitive deficits in Alzheimer's disease. Behav Brain Res (NETHERLANDS) Feb 1997, 83 (1-2) p15-23

The presence of leuko-araiosis in patients with Alzheimer's disease predicts poor tolerance to tacrine, but does not discriminate responders from non-responders. Age Ageing (ENGLAND) Jan 1997, 26 (1) p25-9

Characteristics of the binding of tacrine to acidic phospholipids. Biophys J (UNITED STATES) May 1996, 70 (5) p2185-2194

A risk-benefit assessment of tacrine in the treatment of Alzheimer's disease. Drug Saf (NEW ZEALAND) Jan 1997, 16 (1) p66-77

[A clinic for the study of dementia--110 consecutive patients]. Ugeskr Laeger (DENMARK) Feb 24 1997, 159 (9) p1246-51

Developing treatment guidelines for Alzheimer's disease and other dementias. J Clin Psychiatry (UNITED STATES) 1996, 57 Suppl 14 p37-8

New therapeutic approaches to Alzheimer's disease. J Clin Psychiatry (UNITED STATES) 1996, 57

Suppl 14 p30-6

Novel anticholinesterase and antiamnesic activities of dehydroevodiamine, a constituent of Evodia rutaecarpa. Planta Med (GERMANY) Oct 1996, 62 (5) p405-9

An enriched-population, double-blind, placebo-controlled, crossover study of tacrine and lecithin in Alzheimer's disease. The Tacrine 970-6 Study Group. Dementia (SWITZERLAND) Sep-Oct 1996, 7 (5) p260-6

Amnesia induced in mice by centrally administered beta-amyloid peptides involves cholinergic dysfunction. Brain Res (NETHERLANDS) Jan 15 1996, 706 (2) p181-93

Evaluation of tacrine hydrochloride (Cognex) in two parallel-group studies. Acta Neurol Scand Suppl (DENMARK) 1996, 165 p114-22

[Should Alzheimer disease be treated with tacrine? Review of the literature]. Tidsskr Nor Laegeforen (NORWAY) Sep 30 1996, 116 (23) p2791-4

Maximizing function in Alzheimer's disease: what role for tacrine? Am Fam Physician (UNITED STATES) Aug 1996, 54 (2) p645-52

Effects of estrogen replacement therapy on response to tacrine in patients with Alzheimer's disease. Neurology (UNITED STATES) Jun 1996, 46 (6) p1580-4

Determination of aluminium in samples from bone and liver of elderly Norwegians. J Trace Elem Med Biol (GERMANY) Apr 1996, 10 (1) p6-11

[Therapy approaches in cerebral cognitive deficits--neuropsychiatric aspects]. Wien Med Wochenschr (AUSTRIA) 1996, 146 (21-22) p546-8

[Effectiveness of brief infusions with Ginkgo biloba Special Extract EGb 761 in dementia of the vascular and Alzheimer type]. Z Gerontol Geriatr (GERMANY) Jul-Aug 1996, 29 (4) p302-9

Proof of efficacy of the ginkgo biloba special extract EGb 761 in outpatients suffering from mild to moderate primary degenerative dementia of the Alzheimer type or multi-infarct dementia. Pharmacopsychiatry (GERMANY) Mar 1996, 29 (2) p47-56

Isolated cerebral and cerebellar mitochondria produce free radicals when exposed to elevated CA2+ and Na+: implications for neurodegeneration. J Neurochem (UNITED STATES) Aug 1994, 63 (2)

Isoprenoids (coQ10) in aging and neurodegeneration. Neurochem Int (ENGLAND) Jul 1994, 25 (1) p35-8

Therapy for Alzheimer 's disease. Symptomatic or neuroprotective? Mol Neurobiol (UNITED STATES) Aug-Dec 1994, 9 (1-3)

The mystery of Alzheimer 's disease and its prevention by melatonin. Med Hypotheses (ENGLAND) Oct 1995, 45 (4) p339-40

Chrono-neuroendocrinological aspects of physiological aging and senile dementia. Chronobiologia (ITALY) Jan-Jun 1994, 21 (1-2) p121-6

Overview of clinical trials of hydergine in dementia. ARCH. NEUROL. (USA), 1994, 51/8 (787-798)

Combined cholinergic precursor treatment and dihydroergotoxine mesylate in Alzheimer 's disease. IRCS MED. SCI. (ENGLAND), 1983, 11/12 (1048-1049)

References

Hydergine treatment and brain functioning (CNV rebound) in Alzheimer 's patients: Preliminary findings. PSYCHOPHARMACOL. BULL. (USA), 1981, 17/3 (202-206)

Single-case study of clinical response to high-dose ergot alkaloid treatment for dementia. Preliminary report. GERONTOLOGY (SWITZERLAND), 1981, 27/1-2 (76-78)

Analyses of energy metabolism and mitochondrial genome in post-mortem brain from patients with Alzheimer 's disease. J. NEUROL. (Germany), 1993, 240/6 (377-380)

Muscle biopsy in Alzheimer's disease: Morphological and biochemical findings

CLIN. NEUROPATHOL. (Germany), 1991, 10/4 (171-176)

Growth hormone secretion in Alzheimer's disease: Studies with growth hormone-releasing hormone alone and combined with pyridostigmine or arginine. DEMENTIA (Switzerland), 1993, 4/6 (315-320)

Selegiline: A review of its clinical efficacy in Parkinson's disease and its clinical potential in Alzheimer's disease. CNS Drugs (New Zealand), 1995, 4/3 (230-246)

Age-related memory decline and longevity under treatment with selegiline. LIFE SCI. (USA), 1994, 55/25-26

Long-term effects of phosphatidylserine, pyritinol, and cognitive training in Alzheimer's disease. A neuropsychological, EEG, and PET investigation. DEMENTIA (Switzerland), 1994, 5/2 (88-98)

Abnormalities of energy metabolism in Alzheimer's disease studied with PET. ANN. NEW YORK ACAD. SCI. (USA), 1991, 640/- (65-71)

Effects of phosphatidylserine in Alzheimer's disease. USA PSYCHOPHARMACOL. BULL. (USA), 1992, 28/1 (61-66)

Effect of phosphatidylserine on cerebral glucose metabolism in Alzheimer's disease. DEMENTIA (Switzerland), 1990, (197-201)

Decreased methionine adenosyltransferase activity in erythrocytes of patients with dementia disorders. Sweden European Neuropsychopharmacology (Netherlands), 1995, 5/2 (107-114)

Folate, vitamin B12 and cognitive impairment in patients with Alzheimer's disease. ACTA PSYCHIATR. SCAND. (Denmark), 1992, 86/4 (301-305)

Alzheimer's Disease: A ?cobalaminergic? hypothesis. MED. HYPOTHESES (United Kingdom), 1992, 37/3 (161-165)

Vitamin B12 and folate concentrations in serum and cerebrospinal fluid of neurological patients with special reference to multiple sclerosis and dementia. J. NEUROL. NEUROSURG. PSYCHIATRY (United Kingdom), 1990, 53/11 (951-954)

Vitamin B12 levels in serum and cerebrospinal fluid of people with Alzheimer's disease. ACTA PSYCHIATR. SCAND. (Denmark), 1990, 82/4 (327-329)

Alzheimers disease/alcohol dementia: Association with zinc deficiency and cerebral vitamin B12 deficiency. J. ORTHOMOL. PSYCHIATRY (CANADA), 1984, 13/2 (97-104)

Carnitine and acetyl-L-carnitine content of human hippocampus and erythrocytes in Alzheimer's disease. Journal of Nutritional and Environmental Medicine (United Kingdom), 1995, 5/1 (35-39)

Advances in the pharmacotherapy of Alzheimer's disease. EUR. ARCH. PSYCHIATRY CLIN. NEU-

References

ROSCI. (Germany), 1994, 244/5 (261-271)

Clinical and neurochemical effects of acetyl-L-carnitine in Alzheimer's disease. NEUROBIOL. AGING (USA), 1995, 16/1 (1-4)

Neuroprotective activity of acetyl-L-carnitine: Studies in vitro. NEUROSCI. RES. (USA), 1994, 37/1 (92-96)

Acetyl-L-carnitine and Alzheimer's disease: Pharmacological beyond the cholinergic sphere. ANN. NEW YORK ACAD. SCI. (USA), 1993, 695/- (324-326)

Acetyl-L-carnitine: A drug able to slow the progress of Alzheimer's disease? ANN. NEW YORK ACAD. SCI. (USA), 1991, 640/- (228-232)

Pharmacokinetics of IV and oral acetyl-L-carnitine in a multiple dose regimen in patients with senile dementia of Alzheimer Type. EUR. J. CLIN. PHARMACOL. (Germany), 1992, 42/1 (89-93)

Double-blind, placebo-controlled study of acetyl-l-carnitine in patients with Alzheimer's disease. CURR. MED. RES. OPIN. (United Kingdom), 1989, 11/10 (638-647)

The pharmacotherapy of Alzheimer's disease based on the cholinergic hypothesis: An update. Neurodegeneration United Kingdom),1995, 4/4 (349-356)

Aniracetam: A new nootropic drug with excellent tolerance for mild to moderate cognitive impairment in elderly people. DRUGS TODAY (Spain), 1994, 30/1 (9-24)

Auditory and visual event-related potentials in patients suffering from Alzheimer's dementia and multiinfarct dementia, before and after treatment with piracetam. FUNCT. NEUROL. (Italy), 1993, 8/5 (335-345)

Isolated cerebral and cerebellar mitochondria produce free radicals when exposed to elevated CA2+ and Na+: implications for neurodegeneration. J Neurochem (UNITED STATES) Aug 1994, 63 (2)

Isoprenoids (coQ10) in aging and neurodegeneration. Neurochem Int (ENGLAND) Jul 1994, 25 (1) p35-8

Therapy for Alzheimer's disease. Symptomatic or neuroprotective? Mol Neurobiol (UNITED STATES) Aug-Dec 1994, 9 (1-3)

The mystery of Alzheimer's disease and its prevention by melatonin. Med Hypotheses (ENGLAND) Oct 1995, 45 (4) p339-40

Advances in the pharmacotherapy of Alzheimer's disease. Eur Arch Psychiatry Clin Neurosci (GERMANY) 1994, 244 (5)

Chrono-neuroendocrinological aspects of physiological aging and senile dementia. Chronobiologia (ITALY) Jan-Jun 1994, 21 (1-2) p121-6

Overview of clinical trials of hydergine in dementia. ARCH. NEUROL. (USA), 1994, 51/8 (787-798)

Combined cholinergic precursor treatment and dihydroergotoxine mesylate in Alzheimer's disease. IRCS MED. SCI. (ENGLAND), 1983, 11/12 (1048-1049)

Hydergine treatment and brain functioning (CNV rebound) in Alzheimer's patients: Preliminary findings. PSYCHOPHARMACOL. BULL. (USA), 1981, 17/3 (202-206)

Single-case study of clinical response to high-dose ergot alkaloid treatment for dementia. Preliminary report. GERONTOLOGY (SWITZERLAND), 1981, 27/1-2 (76-78)

Isoprenoids (coQ10) in aging and neurodegeneration. NEUROCHEM. INT. (United Kingdom), 1994, 25/1 (35-38)

Analyses of energy metabolism and mitochondrial genome in post-mortem brain from patients with Alzheimer's disease. J. NEUROL. (Germany), 1993, 240/6 (377-380)

Muscle biopsy in Alzheimer's disease: Morphological and biochemical findings. CLIN. NEU-ROPATHOL. (Germany), 1991, 10/4 (171-176)

Growth hormone secretion in Alzheimer's disease: Studies with growth hormone- releasing hormone alone and combined with pyridostigmine or arginine. DEMENTIA (Switzerland), 1993, 4/6 (315-320)

Selegiline: A review of its clinical efficacy in Parkinson's disease and its clinical potential in Alzheimer's disease. CNS Drugs (New Zealand), 1995, 4/3 (230-246)

Age-related memory decline and longevity under treatment with selegiline. LIFE SCI. (USA), 1994, 55/25-26

Long-term effects of phosphatidylserine, pyritinol, and cognitive training in Alzheimer's disease. A neuropsychological, EEG, and PET investigation. DEMENTIA (Switzerland), 1994, 5/2 (88-98)

Abnormalities of energy metabolism in Alzheimer's disease studied with PET. ANN. NEW YORK ACAD. SCI. (USA), 1991, 640/- (65-71)

Effects of phosphatidylserine in Alzheimer's disease. USA PSYCHOPHARMACOL. BULL. (USA), 1992, 28/1 (61-66)

Effect of phosphatidylserine on cerebral glucose metabolism in Alzheimer's disease. DEMENTIA (Switzerland), 1990, (197-201)

Decreased methionine adenosyltransferase activity in erythrocytes of patients with dementia disorders. Sweden European Neuropsychopharmacology (Netherlands), 1995, 5/2 (107-114)

Folate, vitamin B12 and cognitive impairment in patients with Alzheimer's disease. ACTA PSYCHIA-TR. SCAND. (Denmark), 1992, 86/4 (301-305)

Alzheimer's Disease: A 'cobalaminergic' hypothesis. MED. HYPOTHESES (United Kingdom), 1992, 37/3 (161-165)

Vitamin B12 and folate concentrations in serum and cerebrospinal fluid of neurological patients with special reference to multiple sclerosis and dementia J. NEUROL. NEUROSURG. PSYCHIATRY (United Kingdom), 1990, 53/11 (951-954)

Vitamin B12 levels in serum and cerebrospinal fluid of people with Alzheimer's disease. ACTA PSY-CHIATR. SCAND. (Denmark), 1990, 82/4 (327-329)

Alzheimers disease/alcohol dementia: Association with zinc deficiency and cerebral vitamin B12 deficiency. J. ORTHOMOL. PSYCHIATRY (CANADA), 1984, 13/2 (97-104)

Carnitine and acetyl-L-carnitine content of human hippocampus and erythrocytes in Alzheimer's disease. Journal of Nutritional and Environmental Medicine (United Kingdom), 1995, 5/1 (35-39)

Advances in the pharmacotherapy of Alzheimer's disease. EUR. ARCH. PSYCHIATRY CLIN. NEU-ROSCI. (Germany), 1994, 244/5 (261-271)

Clinical and neurochemical effects of acetyl-L-carnitine in Alzheimer's disease. NEUROBIOL. AGING (USA), 1995, 16/1 (1-4)

Neuroprotective activity of acetyl-L-carnitine: Studies in vitro. NEUROSCI. RES. (USA), 1994, 37/1 (92-96)

Acetyl-L-carnitine and Alzheimer's disease: Pharmacological beyond the cholinergic sphere. ANN. NEW YORK ACAD. SCI. (USA), 1993, 695/- (324-326)

Acetyl-L-carnitine: A drug able to slow the progress of Alzheimer's disease? ANN. NEW YORK ACAD. SCI. (USA), 1991, 640/- (228-232)

Pharmacokinetics of IV and oral acetyl-L-carnitine in a multiple dose regimen in patients with senile dementia of Alzheimer Type. EUR. J. CLIN. PHARMACOL. (Germany), 1992, 42/1 (89-93)

Double-blind, placebo-controlled study of acetyl-l-carnitine in patients with Alzheimer's disease. CURR. MED. RES. OPIN. (United Kingdom), 1989, 11/10 (638-647)

The pharmacotherapy of Alzheimer's disease based on the cholinergic hypothesis: An update. Neurodegeneration United Kingdom),1995, 4/4 (349-356)

Aniracetam: A new nootropic drug with excellent tolerance for mild to moderate cognitive impairment in elderly people. DRUGS TODAY (Spain), 1994, 30/1 (9-24)

Auditory and visual event-related potentials in patients suffering from Alzheimer's dementia and multiinfarct dementia, before and after treatment with piracetam. FUNCT. NEUROL. (Italy), 1993, 8/5 (335-345)

Amnesia

[Antagonism of piracetam with proline in relation to amnestic effects]. Biull Eksp Biol Med (USSR) Mar 1985, 99 (3) p311-4

[Effect of mental stimulants on electroconvulsive shock-induced retrograde amnesia]. Pharmazie (GERMANY, EAST) Dec 1983, 38 (12) p869-71,

Hypoxia-induced amnesia in one-trial learning and pharmacological protection by piracetam. Psychopharmacologia (GERMANY, WEST) 1972, 25 (1) p32-40

Pre-clinical evaluation of cognition enhancing drugs. Prog Neuropsychopharmacol Biol Psychiatry (ENGLAND) 1989, 13 Suppl pS99-115

Nootropic drugs and brain cholinergic mechanisms. Prog Neuropsychopharmacol Biol Psychiatry (ENGLAND) 1989, 13 Suppl pS77-88

Specificity of piracetam's anti-amnesic activity in three models of amnesia in the mouse. Pharmacol Biochem Behav (UNITED STATES) Mar 1988, 29 (3) p625-9

[Effects of piracetam during prolonged use in an experiment] Effekty piratsetama pri dlitel'nom primenenii v eksperimente. Farmakol Toksikol (USSR) Jul-Aug 1985, 48 (4) p42-6

Amyotrophic Lateral Sclerosis (ALS) (Lou Gehrig's Disease)

Free Radicals Appear to Fuel Lou Gehrig's Disease. Family Practice News, Rockville, MD

In vivo generation of hydroxyl radicals and MPTP-induced dopaminergic toxicity in the basal ganglia. Ann N Y Acad Sci (UNITED STATES) Nov 17, 1994, 738 p25-36

Detection of point mutations in codon 331 of mitochondrial NADH dehydrogenase subunit 2 in Alzheimer's brains. Biochem Biophys Res Commun (UNITED STATES) Jan 15 1992, 182 (1) p238-46

Deprenyl enhances neurite outgrowth in cultured rat spinal ventral horn neurons. J Neurol Sci (NETHERLANDS) Aug 1994, 125 (1) p11-3

Therapeutic trial with N-acetylcysteine in amyotrophic lateral sclerosis. Adv Exp Med Biol (UNITED STATES) 1987, 209 p281-4

Attempted treatment of motor neuron disease with N-acetylcysteine and dithiothreitol. Adv Exp Med Biol (UNITED STATES) 1987, 209 p277-80

Anti-Glutamate Therapy in Amyotrophic Lateral Sclerosis: A Trial Using Lamotrigine. Canadian Journal of Neurological Sciences, 1993; 20:297-301

A Controlled Trial of Riluzole in Amyotrophic Lateral Sclerosis. New England Journal of Medicine, March 3, 1994; 330(9):585-591

Aluminum Deposition in Central Nervous System of Patients with Amyotrophic Lateral Sclerosis From the Kii Peninsula of Japan. Neurotoxicology, 1991; 615-620

Free Radicals and Neuroprotection. By B, J. Wilder, M. D., Professor Emeritus of Neurology University of Florida College of Medicine and Consultant in Neurology Department of Veterans Affairs Medical Center

Anemia-Thrombocytopenia-Leukopenia

Folic acid supplementation improves erythropoietin response. Nephron (SWITZERLAND) 1995, 71 (4) p395-400

Partial amelioration of AZT-induced macrocytic anemia in the mouse by folic acid. Stem Cells (Dayt) (UNITED STATES) Sep 1993, 11 (5) p393-7

Megaloblastic anemia in patients receiving total parenteral nutrition without folic acid or vitamin B12 supplementation. Can Med Assoc J (CANADA) Jul 23 1977, 117 (2) p144-6

Modulation of tumor necrosis factor-alpha (TNF-alpha) toxicity by the pineal hormone melatonin (MLT) in metastatic solid tumor patients. Annals of the New York Academy of Sciences (USA), 1995, 768 (334-336)

[Anemias due to disorder of folate, vitamin B12 and transcobalamin metabolism]. Rev Prat (FRANCE) Jun 1 1993, 43 (11) p1358-63

[Is it necessary to supplement with folic acid patients in chronic dialysis treated with erythropoietin?]. Rev Med Chil (CHILE) Jan 1993, 121 (1) p30-5

Ineffective hematopoiesis in folate-deficient mice. Blood (UNITED STATES) May 1 1992, 79 (9)

References

p2273-80

[Primary prophylaxis against cerebral toxoplasmosis. Efficacy of folinic acid in the prevention of hematologic toxicity of pyrimethamine]. Presse Med (FRANCE) Apr 2 1994, 23 (13) p613-5

Nutritional status of an institutionalized aged population. J Am Coll Nutr (UNITED STATES) 1984, 3 (1) p13-25

[Acquired, vitamin B6-responsive, primary sideroblastic anemia, an enzyme deficiency in heme synthesis]. Schweiz Med Wochenschr (SWITZERLAND) Oct 10 1981, 111 (41) p1533-5

Intakes of vitamins and minerals by pregnant women with selected clinical symptoms. J Am Diet Assoc (UNITED STATES) May 1981, 78 (5) p477-82

[Anemia with hypersideroblastosis during anti-tuberculosis therapy. Cure with vitamin therapy]. Nouv Rev Fr Hematol (FRANCE) Apr 14 1978, 20 (1) p99-110

[Myelopathy and macrocytic anemia associated with a folate deficiency. Cure by folic acid]. Ann Med Interne (Paris) (FRANCE) May 1975, 126 (5) p339-48

[Vitamin B 6 deficiency anemia]. Schweiz Med Wochenschr (SWITZERLAND) Oct 11 1975, 105 (41) p1319-24

Premature infants require additional folate and vitamin B-12 to reduce the severity of the anemia of prematurity. Am J Clin Nutr (UNITED STATES) Dec 1994, 60 (6) p930-5

Apoptosis mediates and thymidine prevents erythroblast destruction in folate deficiency anemia. Proc Natl Acad Sci U S A (UNITED STATES) Apr 26 1994, 91 (9) p4067-71

Acute folate deficiency associated with intravenous nutrition with aminoacid- sorbitol-ethanol: prophylaxis with intravenous folic acid. Br J Haematol (ENGLAND) Dec 1977, 37 (4) p521-6

Interactions between folate and ascorbic acid in the guinea pig. J Nutr (UNITED STATES) Apr 1982, 112 (4) p673-80

Modulation of human lymphoblastoid interferon activity by melatonin in metastatic renal cell carcinoma. A phase II study. Cancer (UNITED STATES) Jun 15 1994, 73 (12) p3015-9

A biological study on the efficacy of low-dose subcutaneous interleukin-2 plus melatonin in the treatment of cancer-related thrombocytopenia. Oncology (SWITZERLAND) Sep-Oct 1995, 52 (5) p360-2

A new class of antihypertensive neutral lipid: 1-alkyl-2-acetyl-sn-glycerols, a precursor of platelet activating factor. BIOCHEM. BIOPHYS. RES. COMMUN. (USA), 1984, 118/1 (344-350)

Metabolism of 1-O-alkyl-2-acetyl-sn-glycerol by washed rabbit platelets: Formation of platelet activating factor. ARCH. BIOCHEM. BIOPHYS. (USA), 1984, 234/1 (318-321)

Conversion of 1-alkyl-2-acetyl-sn-glycerols to platelet activating factor and related phospholipids by rabbit platelets. BIOCHEM. BIOPHYS. RES. COMMUN. (USA), 1984, 124/1 (156-163)

Anti-neoplastic action of peritoneal macrophages after oral admin. of ether analogues of lysophospholipids. EUR. J. CANCER PART A GEN. TOP. 1992, 28/10 (1637-1642)

Anesthesia and Surgery Precautions

Myocardial preservation by therapy with coenzyme Q10 during heart surgery. USA CLIN. INVEST. SUPPL. (Germany), 1993, 71/8 (S 155-S 161)

Effect of CoQ10 on myocardial ischemia/reperfusion injury in the isolated rat heart. Journal of the Japanese Association for Thoracic Surgery (Japan), 1995, 43/4 (466-472)

Free radical reaction products and antioxidant capacity in arterial plasma during coronary artery bypass grafting. J. THORAC. CARDIOVASC. SURG. (USA) 1994, 108/1 (140-147)

Oxygen radicals in cerebral vascular injury. CIRC. R RES. (USA), 1985, 57/4 (508-516)

Postischemic tissue injury by iron-mediated free radical lipid peroxidation. ANN. EMERG. MED. (USA), 1985, 14/8 (804-809)

Oxygen free radical-induced histamine release during intestinal ischemia and reperfusion. EUR. SURG. RES. (Switzerland), 1989, 21/6 (297-304)

Role of iron ions in the genesis of reperfusion injury following successful cardiopulmonary resuscitation: Preliminary data and a biochemical hypothesis. ANN. EMERG. MED. (USA), 1985, 14/8 (777-783)

The biological significance of zinc. ANAESTHESIST (BERL.) (GERMANY, WEST), 1975, 24/8 (329-342)

Cortical pOsub 2 distribution during oligemic hypotension and its pharmacological modifications (Hydergine). SWITZERLAND ARZNEIM.-FORSCH. (GERMANY, WEST), 1978, 28/5 (768-770)

The use of piracetam (Nootrop) in post-anesthetic recovery of elderly patients. (A preliminary study). GREECE ACTA ANAESTHESIOL. HELL. (GREECE), 1981, 15/1-2 (76-80)

Free radical reaction products and antioxidant capacity in arterial plasma during coronary artery bypass grafting. J. THORAC. CARDIOVASC. SURG. (USA), 1994, 108/1 (140-147)

Free radical trapping agents in myocardial protection in cardiac surgery. FRANCE ANN. CARDIOL. ANGEIOL. (FRANCE), 1986, 35/7 BIS (447-452)

Biochemical studies of cerebral ischemia in the rat - Changes in cerebral free amino acids, catecholamines and uric acid. JAPAN BRAIN NERVE (JAPAN), 1986, 38/3 (253-258)

Glutathione status in human blood during surgery. CLIN. CHEM. ENZYMOL. COMMUN. (United Kingdom), 1988, 1/2 (71-76)

Effect of supplemental vitamin A on colon anastomotic healing in rats given preoperative irradiation. AM. J. SURG. (USA), 1987, 153/2 (153-156)

Effect of reduced glutathione on endocrine and renal functions following halothane anesthesia and surgery in man. JPN. J. ANESTHESIOL. (JAPAN), 1982, 31/8 (830-839)

Intraocular irrigating solutions and lens clarity. AMER.J.OPHTHAL. (USA), 1976, 82/4 (594-597)

Intraocular irrigating solutions. Their effect on the corneal endothelium. ARCH.OPHTHAL. (USA), 1975, 93/8 (648-657)

Anxiety and Stress

Endocrine correlates of personality traits: A comparison between emotionally stable and emotionally labile healthy young men. Neuropsychobiology (Switzerland), 1997, 35/4 (205-210)

Tissue changes in glutathione metabolism and lipid peroxidation induced by swimming are partially prevented by melatonin. Pharmacology and Toxicology (Denmark), 1996, 78/5 (308-312)

The role of beta-adrenoceptor blockers in the treatment of psychiatric disorders. CNS Drugs (New Zealand), 1996, 5/2 (115-136)

At least three neurotransmitter systems mediate a stress-induced increase in c-fos mRNA in different rat brain areas. Cellular and Molecular Neurobiology (USA), 1997, 17/2 (157-169)

Calcitonin gene-related peptide is an adipose-tissue neuropeptide with lipolytic actions. Endocrinology and Metabolism (United Kingdom), 1996, 3/4 (235-242)

Adverse CNS-effects of beta-adrenoceptor blockers. Pharmacopsychiatry (Germany), 1996, 29/6 (201-211)

Acute effects of beta blockade and exercise on mood and anxiety. British Journal of Sports Medicine (United Kingdom), 1996, 30/3 (238-242)

Stressor-induced alterations of the splenic plaque-forming cell response: Strain differences and modification by propranolol. Pharmacology Biochemistry and Behavior (USA), 1996, 53/2 (235-241)

Propranolol reduces the anxiety associated with day case surgery. European Journal of Surgery, Acta Chirurgica (Norway), 1996, 162/1 (11-14)

Nutritional management of the metabolically stressed patient. CRIT. CARE NURS. Q. (USA), 1995, 17/4 (79-90)

Propranolol in psychiatry. Therapeutic uses and side effects. Neuropsychobiology (SWITZERLAND) 1986, 15 (1) p20-7

Propranolol in experimentally induced stress. Br J Psychiatry (ENGLAND) Dec 1981, 139 p545-9

Modulation of the immunologic response to acute stress in humans by beta-blockade or benzodiazepines. FASEB J (UNITED STATES) Mar 1996, 10 (4) p517-24

Beta-adrenergic receptors are involved in stress-related behavioral changes. Pharmacol Biochem Behav (UNITED STATES) May 1993, 45 (1) p1-7

The effect of beta blockade on stress-induced cognitive dysfunction in adolescents Clin Pediatr (Phila) (UNITED STATES) Jul 1991, 30 (7) p441-5

Modulation of baseline behavior in rats by putative serotonergic agents in three ethoexperimental paradigms. Behav Neural Biol (UNITED STATES) Nov 1990, 54 (3) p234-53

Effects of propranolol, atenolol, and chlordesmethyldiazepam on response to mental stress in patients with recent myocardial infarction. Clin Cardiol (UNITED STATES) Jun 1987, 10 (6) p293-302

Clinical Trials For Chronic Fatigue and Anxiety. Life Extension Update-February 1996

Nutritional management of the metabolically stressed patient. CRIT. CARE NURS. Q. (USA), 1995, 17/4 (79-90)

Propranolol in psychiatry. Therapeutic uses and side effects. Neuropsychobiology (SWITZERLAND) 1986, 15 (1) p20-7

Propranolol in experimentally induced stress. Br J Psychiatry Dec 1981, 139 p545-9

Modulation of the immunologic response to acute stress in humans by beta- blockade or benzodiazepines. FASEB J (UNITED STATES) Mar 1996, 10 (4) p517-24

Beta-adrenergic receptors are involved in stress-related behavioral changes. Pharmacol Biochem Behav (UNITED STATES) May 1993, 45 (1) p1-7

The effect of beta blockade on stress-induced cognitive dysfunction in adolescents. Clin Pediatr (Phila) (UNITED STATES) Jul 1991, 30 (7) p441-5

Modulation of baseline behavior in rats by putative serotonergic agents in three ethoexperimental paradigms. Behav Neural Biol (UNITED STATES) Nov 1990, 54 (3) p234-53

Effects of propranolol, atenolol, and chlordesmethyldiazepam on response to mental stress in patients with recent myocardial infarction. Clin Cardiol (UNITED STATES) Jun 1987, 10 (6) p293-302

Clinical Trials For Chronic Fatigue and Anxiety. Life Extension Update-February 1996. A study was conducted on 20 patients who had been ill with various forms of chronic fatigue from one-to-three months. Patients were registered and information collected in accordance with the protocol of the European Fatigue Study Group, which includes scales to measure anxiety, depression, muscle fatigue, mental fatigue, sleep disorders, and headache. Four placebo capsules were given to these patients daily during the first two weeks of the study. Then four capsules of garum extract were given daily for the next two weeks of the study. After two weeks on placebo, fatigue symptoms were reduced by an average of 14% and overall symptoms of anxiety, depression, and insomnia were reduced by 4%. After two weeks of taking garum extract, on the other hand, fatigue symptoms were reduced by 51% and overall symptoms by 65%. Two weeks after discontinuing garum extract therapy, fatigue symptoms increased 15% and overall symptoms increased 7%. These results show the broad-spectrum benefits of garum extract for people suffering from chronic stress and fatigue. It is interesting to note that the beneficial effects of garum extract persisted even after the treatment was stopped. Another study involved 40 patients who had been suffering from various forms of chronic fatigue for one-to-three months. Four capsules of garum extract per day was prescribed for two weeks. The results, based on the Fatigue Study Group criteria, showed conclusive average benefit of 50% for the ten functions that most accurately measure fatigue and depression. In a study of 60 patients taking garum extract, only three mild reactions were noted without the necessity of interrupting the treatment. The reactions were: one case of nervous irritation, one case of heartburn, and one case of diarrhea. No emotional tension or insomnia was reported and it was concluded that garum extract is extremely well tolerated and is without contraindications. In a soon to be published study on the treatment of anxiety in college students, garum extract was shown to be safe and effective in reducing anxiety in otherwise healthy subjects. Other studies are showing that, when garum extract reduces anxiety, it results in improved learning, including enhanced EEG (Electroencephalogram) brain wave activity.

Summary: Garum extract benefits 90% of patients with chronic stress and fatigue compared to only 30% of patients on placebo. An analysis of all the human clinical studies of garum extract to date shows overall positive results in the treatment of the symptoms of chronic stress, including fatigue, anxiety and depression.

Additional References:

See Garum. 1 0-volume edition of Dictionnaire Larousse.

Dr. J. BORY, Journees de Biochimie medicale de l'Ouest, Brest, 1981.

Ph. DARCET et al (Ann. Nutr. Alim., 1980, 34 277.901.

G. DURANT, G. PASCAL N. VODOVAR, H. GOUNELLE DE PONTANEL (Med. et Nutr., 1978, vol. XIV, 1 95-204).

GROWFORD and SINCLAIR,1972 (J. Nutrition, 102-1315).

M. HENRY, researcher, Personal contribution.

LAMPTEY and WALTER, 1976 lJ. Nutrition, 106-86).

Professor P METAIS (Cahiers de Nutrition et Dietetique, 1980, vol. XV, n 3, 227

Prostaglandines et physiologic de la reproduction, International INSERM Symposium (Revue francaise des laboratoires-January 1980, n 77 4-5-6)

Arrhythmia (Cardiac)

Fish oil and other nutritional adjuvants for treatment of congestive heart failure. Medical Hypotheses (United Kingdom), 1996, 46/4 (400-406)

Evidence on the participation of the 3',5'-cyclic AMP pathway in the non-genomic action of 1,25-dihy-droxy-vitamin D3 in cardiac muscle. Mol Cell Endocrinol (NETHERLANDS) Dec 1991, 82 (2-3) p229-35

1,25(OH)2 vitamin D3, and retinoic acid antagonize endothelin-stimulated hypertrophy of neonatal rat cardiac myocytes. J Clin Invest Apr 1 1996, 97 (7) p1577-88

[Effect of vitamin E deficiency on the development of cardiac arrhythmias as affected by acute ischemia]. Biull Eksp Biol Med (USSR) Nov 1986, 102 (11) p530-2

Antioxidant protection against adrenaline-induced arrhythmias in rats with chronic heart hypertrophy. Can J Cardiol (CANADA) Mar 1990, 6 (2) p71-4

The antiarrhythmic effects of taurine alone and in combination with magnesium sulfate on ischemia/reperfusion arrhythmia. Chinese Pharmacological Bulletin (China), 1994, 10/5 (358-362)

Prophylactic effects of taurine and diltiazem, alone or combined, on reperfusion arrhythmias in rats. Acta Pharmacologica Sinica (China), 1996, 17/2

The effects of antioxidants on reperfusion dysrhythmias. Ceska a Slovenska Farmacie (Czech Republic), 1995, 44/5 (257-260)

Protective effects of all-trans-retinoic acid against cardiac arrhythmias induced by isoproterenol, lysophosphatidylcholine or ischemia and reperfusion. Journal of Cardiovascular Pharmacology (USA), 1995, 26/6

Effects of dietary supplementation with alpha-tocopherol on myocardial infarct size and ventricular arrhythmias in a dog model of ischemia-reperfusion. J. AM. COLL. CARDIOL. (USA), 1994, 24/6 (1580-1585)

Magnesium flux during and after open heart operations in children. Ann Thorac Surg (UNITED

STATES) Apr 1995, 59 (4) p921-7

Sino-atrial Wenckebach conduction in thyrotoxic periodic paralysis: a case report. Int J Cardiol (IRE-LAND) Jan 6 1995, 47 (3) p285-9

A possible beneficial effect of selenium administration in antiarrhythmic therapy. J Am Coll Nutr (UNITED STATES) Oct 1994, 13 (5) p496-8

Omega-3 fatty acids and prevention of ventricular fibrillation. Prostaglandins Leukot Essent Fatty Acids (SCOTLAND) Feb-Mar 1995, 52

[Effect of anti-arrhythmia drugs on the beta2 receptor-dependent adenyl cyclase system of lymphocytes in patients with cardiac rhythm disorders]. Kardiologiia (USSR) Jul 1989, 29 (7) p25-9

An expanded concept of "insurance" supplementation—broad-spectrum protection from cardiovascular disease. Med Hypotheses (ENGLAND) Oct 1981, 7 (10) p1287-1302

Italian multicenter study on the safety and efficacy of coenzyme Q10 as adjunctive therapy in heart failure (interim analysis). Clin Investig (GERMANY) 1993, 71 (8 Suppl) pS145-9

Isolated diastolic dysfunction of the myocardium and its response to CoQ10 treatment. Clin Investig (GERMANY) 1993, 71 (8 Suppl) pS140-4

Protective effects of propionyl-L-carnitine during ischemia and reperfusion. Cardiovasc Drugs Ther (UNITED STATES) Feb 1991, 5 Suppl 1 p77-83

Consequences of magnesium deficiency on the enhancement of stress reactions; preventive and therapeutic implications (a review). J Am Coll Nutr (UNITED STATES) Oct 1994

Community-based prevention of stroke: nutritional improvement in Japan. Health Rep (CANADA) 1994, 6 (1)

Effect of dietary magnesium supplementation on intralymphocytic free calcium and magnesium in stroke-prone spontaneously hypertensive rats. Clin Exp Hypertens (UNITED STATES) May 1994

Clinical study of cardiac arrhythmias using a 24-hour continuous electrocardiographic recorder (5th report)—antiarrhythmic action of coenzyme Q10 in diabetics. Tohoku J Exp Med (JAPAN) Dec 1983, 141 Suppl p453-63

Usefulness of coenzyme Q10 in clinical cardiology: a long-term study. Mol Aspects Med (ENGLAND) 1994, 15 Suppl

Isolated diastolic dysfunction of the myocardium and its response to CoQ10 treatment. Clin Investig (GERMANY) 1993, 71 (8 Suppl) pS140-4

Effect of coenzyme Q10 on structural alterations in the renal membrane of stroke- prone spontaneously hypertensive rats. Biochem Med Metab Biol (UNITED STATES) Apr 1991

Coenzyme Q10: a new drug for cardiovascular disease. J Clin Pharmacol (UNITED STATES) Jul 1990

[Effects of 2,3-dimethoxy-5-methyl-6-(10'-hydroxydecyl)-1,4-benzoquinone (CV-2619) on adriamycin-induced ECG abnormalities and myocardial energy metabolism in spontaneously hypertensive rats] Nippon Yakurigaku Zasshi (JAPAN) Oct 1982

Bioenergetics in clinical medicine. III. Inhibition of coenzyme Q10-enzymes by clinically used anti-hypertensive drugs. Res Commun Chem Pathol Pharmacol (UNITED STATES) Nov 1975

Bioenergetics in clinical medicine. Studies on coenzyme Q10 and essential hypertension. Res Commun Chem Pathol Pharmacol (UNITED STATES) Jun 1975

[Prevention of cerebrovascular insults] Schweiz Med Wochenschr (SWITZERLAND) Nov 12 1994

[Essential antioxidants in cardiovascular diseases—lessons for Europe] Ther Umsch (SWITZERLAND) Jul 1994

Antioxidant vitamin intake and coronary mortality in a longitudinal population study. Am J Epidemiol (UNITED STATES) Jun 15 1994

Decline in stroke mortality. An epidemiologic perspective. Ann Epidemiol Sep 1993

Can antioxidants prevent ischemic heart disease? J Clin Pharm Ther (ENGLAND) Apr 1993

Antioxidant therapy in the aging process. EXS (SWITZERLAND) 1992, 62

Effect of flosequinan on ischaemia-induced arrhythmias and on ventricular cyclic nucleotide content in the anaesthetized rat. Br J Pharmacol (ENGLAND) Apr 1993, 108 (4) p1111-6

What do the newer inotropic drugs have to offer? CARDIOVASC. DRUGS THER. (USA), 1992, 6/1 (15-18)

Arrhythmogenic effect of forskolin in the isolated perfused rat heart: Influence of nifedipine reduction of external calcium. CLIN. EXP. PHARMACOL. PHYSIOL. (Australia), 1989, 16/10 (751-757)

Hormone secretagogues increase cytosolic calcium by increasing cAMP in corticotropin-secreting cells. PROC. NATL ACAD. SCI. U. S. A. (USA) , 1985, 82/23 (8034-8038)

The genesis of arrhythmias during myocardial ischemia. Dissociation between changes in cyclic adenosine monophosphate and electrical instability in the rat. CIRC. RES. (USA), 1985, 57/5 (668-675) CODEN: CIRUA

Effects of high K on relaxation produced by drugs in the guinea-pig tracheal muscle. RESPIR. PHYSIOL. (NETHERLANDS), 1985, 61/1 (43-55)

Forskolin inhibits ouabain-sensitive ATPase in the medulla of rat kidney. IRCS MED. SCI. (ENGLAND), 1983, 11/11 (957-958)

Arthritis

Treatment of rheumatoid arthritis with blackcurrant seed oil. BR. J. RHEUMATOL. (United Kingdom), 1994, 33/9 (847-852)

Treatment of rheumatoid arthritis with gammalinolenic acid. ANN. INTERN. MED. (USA), 1993, 119/9 (867-873)

Validation of a meta-analysis: The effects of fish oil in rheumatoid arthritis. Journal of Clinical Epidemiology (USA), 1995, 48/11 (1379-1390)

Botanical lipids: Effects on inflammation, immune responses, and rheumatoid arthritis. Seminars in Arthritis and Rheumatism (USA), 1995, 25/2 (87-96)

n-3 Polyunsaturated fatty acids: Update 1995. European Journal of Clinical Investigation (United Kingdom), 1995, 25/9

Marine and botanical lipids as immunomodulatory and therapeutic agents in the treatment of rheumatoid arthritis. Rheumatic Disease Clinics of North America (USA), 1995, 21/3 (759-777)

Attenuation of adjuvant arthritis in rats by treatment with oxygen radical scavengers. IMMUNOL. CELL BIOL. (Australia), 1994, 72/5

Alteration of the cellular fatty acid profile and the production of eicosanoids in human monocytes by gamma-linolenic acid. ARTHRITIS RHEUM. (USA), 1990, 33/10 (1526-1533)

Suppression of acute and chronic inflammation by dietary gamma linolenic acid. J. RHEUMATOL. (Canada), 1989, 16/6 (729-733)

Reactive oxygen species, lipid peroxides and essential fatty acids in patients with rheumatoid arthritis and systemic lupus erythematosus. PROSTAGLANDINS LEUKOTRIENES ESSENT. FATTY ACIDS (United Kingdom), 1991, 43/4

Suppression of acute and chronic inflammation by dietary gamma linolenic acid. J. RHEUMATOL. (Canada), 1989, 16/6 (729-733)

Effects of fish oil supplementation on non-steroidal anti-inflammatory drug requirement in patients with mild rheumatoid arthritis—a double-blind placebo controlled study. Br J Rheumatol (ENGLAND) Nov 1993, 32 (11) p982-9

Association of etretinate and fish oil in psoriasis therapy. Inhibition of hypertriglyceridemia resulting from retinoid therapy after fish oil supplementation. Acta Derm Venereol Suppl (Stockh) (NORWAY) 1994, 186 p151-3

Intravenous infusion of n-3 polyunsaturated fatty acids. Proc Soc Exp Biol Med (UNITED STATES) Jun 1992, 200 (2) p171-3

Effects of dietary fish oil lipids on allergic and inflammatory diseases. Allergy Proc (UNITED STATES) Sep-Oct 1991, 12 (5) p299-303

Omega-3 fatty acids in health and disease and in growth and development. Am J Clin Nutr (UNITED STATES) Sep 1991, 54 (3) p438-63

The effect of dietary fish oil supplement upon the content of dihomo-gammalinolenic acid in human plasma phospholipids. Prostaglandins Leukot Essent Fatty Acids (SCOTLAND) May 1990, 40 (1) p9-12

Summary of the NATO advanced research workshop on dietary omega 3 and omega 6 fatty acids: biological effects and nutritional essentiality. J Nutr (UNITED STATES) Apr 1989, 119 (4) p521-8

Health effects and metabolism of dietary eicosapentaenoic acid. Prog Food Nutr Sci (ENGLAND) 1988, 12 (2) p111-50

[Potential value of eicosapentaenoic acid]. Allerg Immunol (Paris) (FRANCE) Oct 1987, 19 (8 Suppl) p12-3

Collagen antibodies in Ross River virus disease (epidemic polyarthritis). Rheumatol Int (GERMANY, WEST) 1987, 7 (6) p267-9

Effects of dietary supplementation with marine fish oil on leukocyte lipid mediator generation and function in rheumatoid arthritis. Arthritis Rheum (UNITED STATES) Sep 1987, 30 (9) p988-97

Low prevalences of coronary heart disease (CHD), psoriasis, asthma and rheumatoid arthritis in Eskimos: are they caused by high dietary intake of eicosapentaenoic acid (EPA), a genetic variation of essential fatty acid (EFA) metabolism or a combination of both? Med Hypotheses (ENGLAND) Apr 1987, 22 (4) p421-8

Inhibition of elastase enzyme release from human polymorphonuclear leukocytes by N-acetyl-galactosamine and N-acetyl-glucosamine. Clin Exp Rheumatol (ITALY) Jan-Feb 1991, 9 (1) p17-21

Severe rheumatoid arthritis: current options in drug therapy. Geriatrics (UNITED STATES) Dec 1990, 45 (12) p43-8

Terminal N-acetylglucosamine in chronic synovitis. Br J Rheumatol (ENGLAND) Feb 1990, 29 (1) p25-31

Membrane N-acetylglucosamine: expression by cells in rheumatoid synovial fluid, and by pre-cultured monocytes. Br J Exp Pathol (ENGLAND) Oct 1989, 70 (5) p567-77

Serum levels of interleukin-2 receptor and activity of rheumatic diseases characterized by immune system activation. Arthritis Rheum (UNITED STATES) Nov 1988, 31 (11) p1358-64

[Therapy of gonarthrosis using chondroprotective substances. Prospective comparative study of glucosamine sulphate and glycosaminoglycan polysulphate]. Fortschr Med (GERMANY, EAST) Jun 28 1984, 102 (24) p676-82

Oral glucosamine sulphate in the management of arthrosis: report on a multi-centre open investigation in Portugal. Pharmatherapeutica (ENGLAND) 1982, 3 (3) p157-68

Double-blind clinical evaluation of intra-articular glucosamine in outpatients with gonarthrosis. Clin Ther (UNITED STATES) 1981, 3 (5) p336-43

A double-blind placebo controlled trial of Efamol Marine on skin and joint symptoms of psoriatic arthritis. Br J Rheumatol (ENGLAND) Oct 1994, 33 (10) p954-8

Evening primrose oil in patients with rheumatoid arthritis and side-effects of non- steroidal anti-inflammatory drugs. Br J Rheumatol (ENGLAND) Oct 1991, 30 (5) p370-2

Essential fatty acid and prostaglandin metabolism in Sjogren's syndrome, systemic sclerosis and rheumatoid arthritis. Scand J Rheumatol Suppl (SWEDEN) 1986, 61 p242-5

Beneficial effect of eicosapentaenoic and docosahexaenoic acids in the management of systemic lupus erythematosus and its relationship to the cytokine network. Prostaglandins Leukot Essent Fatty Acids (SCOT) Sep 1994,51 (3) p207-13

Fish-oil fatty acid supplementation in active rheumatoid arthritis. A double-blinded, controlled, crossover study. Ann Intern Med (UNITED STATES) Apr 1987, 106 (4) p497-503

Zonal distribution of chondroitin-4-sulphate/dermatan sulphate and chondroitin-6- sulphate in normal and diseased human synovium. Ann Rheum Dis (ENGLAND) Jan 1994, 53 (1) p35-8

Asthma

Alterations in human leukocyte function induced by ingestion of eicosapentaenoic acid. J Clin Immunol (UNITED STATES) Sep 1986, 6 (5) p402-10

The treatment of asthmatic patients using an alpha-adrenergic receptor blocking agent, co-dergocrine mesylate ('Hydergine'). Pharmatherapeutica (ENGLAND) 1980, 2 (5) p330-6

References

Plasma vitamin C (ascorbic acid) levels in asthmatic children. Afr J Med Med Sci (ENGLAND) Sep-Dec 1985, 14 (3-4)

Intravenous magnesium sulfate as an adjunct in the treatment of acute asthma. Chest (UNITED STATES) Jun 1995, 107 (6) p1576-81

[Magnesium in lung diseases]. Tidsskr Nor Laegeforen (NORWAY) Mar 10 1995, 115 (7) p827-8

Asthma, inhaled oxidants, and dietary antioxidants. Am J Clin Nutr (UNITED STATES) Mar 1995, 61 (3 Suppl) p625S-630S

Relaxant effects of forskolin on guinea pig tracheal smooth muscle. LUNG (GERMANY, WEST), 1987, 165/4 (225-237)

Bronchial asthma: Factors which contribute to 'intractable asthma' and approach to new treatments, from the standpoint of the bronchial pathophysiology. JPN. J. THORAC. DIS. (JAPAN), 1985, 23/9 (971-980)

Bronchodilator and antiallergy activity of forskolin. EUR. J. PHARMACOL. (NETHERLANDS), 1985, 111/1 (1-8)

Activation of cAMP-dependent pathways in human airway smooth muscle cells inhibits TNF-alpha-induced ICAM-1 and VCAM-1 expression and T lymphocyte adhesion. J Immunol (UNITED STATES) Mar 1 1995, 154 (5) p2358-65

Consequences of magnesium deficiency on the enhancement of stress reactions; preventive and therapeutic implications (a review). J Am Coll Nutr (UNITED STATES) Oct 1994, 13 (5) p429-46

Rapid infusion of magnesium sulfate obviates need for intubation in status asthmaticus. Am J Emerg Med (UNITED STATES) Mar 1994, 12 (2)

Magnesium sulfate for the treatment of bronchospasm complicating acute bronchitis in a four-months'-pregnant woman. Ann Emerg Med (UNITED STATES) Aug 1993, 22 (8) p1365-7

Acetylcysteine for life-threatening acute bronchial obstruction. ANN. INTERN. MED. (USA), 1978, 88/5 (656)

Effect of the combination of human thioredoxin and L-cysteine on ischemia- reperfusion injury in isolated rat lungs. European Surgical Research (Switzerland), 1995, 27/6 (363-370)

Effects of N-acetyl-L-cysteine on regional blood flow during endotoxic shock. European Surgical Research (Switzerland), 1995, 27/5 (292-300)

A combination of cefuroxime and N-acetyl-cysteine for the treatment of lower respiratory tract infections in children. INT. J. CLIN. PHARMACOL. THER. TOXICOL. (GERMANY, WEST), 1985, 23/5

Irish general practice study of acetylcysteine (Fabrol) in chronic bronchitis. J. INT. MED. RES. (ENGLAND), 1984, 12/2 (96-101)

Regulation of Ca2+-dependent K+-channel activity in tracheal myocytes by phosphorylation. NATURE (United Kingdom), 1989, 341/6238 (152-154)

Effects of N-acetyl-L-cysteine on regional blood flow during endotoxic shock. European Surgical Research (Switzerland), 1995, 27/5 (292-300)

Irish general practice study of acetylcysteine (Fabrol) in chronic bronchitis. J. INT. MED. RES. (ENG-

LAND), 1984, 12/2 (96-101)

Atherosclerosis

Hyperhomocysteinaemia and end stage renal disease. Journal of Nephrology (Italy), 1997, 10/2 (77-84)

Dietary pectin influences fibrin network structure in hypercholesterolaemic subjects. Thrombosis Research (United Kingdom), 1997, 86/3 (183-196)

Possible participation of Fas-mediated apoptosis in the mechanism of atherosclerosis. Gerontology (Switzerland), 1997, 43/SUPPL. 1 (35-42)

Omega3 fatty acids in the prevention-management of cardiovascular disease Simopoulos A.P. Canadian Journal of Physiology and Pharmacology (Canada), 1997, 75/3 (234-239)

Vitamin intake: A possible determinant of plasma homocyst(e)ine among middle-aged adults. Annals of Epidemiology (USA), 1997, 7/4 (285-293)

Dietary soy protein and estrogen replacement therapy improve cardiovascular risk factors and decrease aortic cholesteryl ester content in ovariectomized cynomolgus monkeys. Metabolism: Clinical and Experimental (USA), 1997, 46/6 (698-705)

Augmented Ca2+ in-flux is involved in the mechanism of enhanced proliferation of cultured vascular smooth muscle cells from spontaneously diabetic Goto-Kakizaki rats. Atherosclerosis (Ireland), 1997, 131/2 (167-175)

Atherogenesis and the homocysteine-folate-cobalamin triad: Do we need standardized analyses? Journal of the American College of Nutrition (USA), 1997, 16/3 (258-267)

Regulation of leucocyte-endothelial interactions of special relevance to atherogenesis. Clinical and Experimental Pharmacology and Physiology (Australia), 1997, 24/5 (A33-A35)

Fasting total plasma homocysteine and atherosclerotic peripheral vascular disease. Annals of Vascular Surgery (USA), 1997, 11/3 (217-223)

Estrogen inhibin and proliferation of vascular smooth muscle cells. Atherosclerosis (Ireland), 1997, 130/1 (1-10)

Plasma total homocysteine, B vitamins, and risk of coronary atherosclerosis. Arteriosclerosis, Thrombosis, and Vascular Biology (USA), 1997, 17/5 (989-995)

Correlation between plasma homocyst(e)ine and aortic atherosclerosis. American Heart Journal (USA), 1997, 133/5 (534-540) CODEN: AHJOA

Estrogen reduces proliferation and agonist-induced calcium increase in coronary artery smooth muscle cells. American Journal of Physiology - Heart and Circulatory Physiology (USA), 1997, 272/4 41-4 (H1996-H2003)

Cell cycle effects of nitric oxide on vascular smooth muscle cells. American Journal of Physiology - Heart and Circulatory Physiology (USA), 1997, 272/4 41-4 (H1810-H1818)

Transcriptional and post-transcriptional control of lysyl oxidase expression in vascular smooth muscle cells: Effects of TGF-beta1 and serum deprivation. Journal of Cellular Biochemistry (USA), 1997, 65/3

(395-407)

Effects of dehydroepiandrosterone on proliferation of human aortic smooth muscle cells. Life Sciences (USA), 1997, 60/11 (833-838)

Dietary fish oil: Influence on lesion regression in the porcine model of atherosclerosis. Arteriosclerosis, Thrombosis, and Vascular Biology (USA), 1997, 17/4 (688-694)

Additive hypocholesterolemic effect of psyllium and cholestyramine in the hamster: Influence on fecal sterol and bile acid profiles. Journal of Lipid Research (USA), 1997, 38/3 (491-502)

Calcifying subpopulation of bovine aortic smooth muscle cells is responsive to 17beta-estradiol. Circulation (USA), 1997, 95/7 (1954-1960)

Influence of lifestyle modification on atherosclerotic progression determined by ultrasonographic change in the common carotid intima-media thickness. American Journal of Clinical Nutrition (USA), 1997, 65/4 (1000-1004)

Angiotensin-converting enzyme inhibition prevents arterial nuclear factor-kappaB activation, monocyte chemoattractant protein-1 expression, and macrophage infiltration in a rabbit model of early accelerated atherosclerosis. Circulation (USA), 1997, 95/6 (1532-1541)

Tumor necrosis factor-alpha activates smooth muscle cell migration in culture and is expressed in the balloon-injured rat aorta. Arteriosclerosis, Thrombosis, and Vascular Biology (USA), 1997, 17/3 (490-497)

Vitamin E inhibits low-density lipoprotein-induced adhesion of monocytes to human aortic endothelial cells in vitro. Arteriosclerosis, Thrombosis, and Vascular Biology (USA), 1997, 17/3 (429-436)

Vascular myofibroblasts: Lessons from coronary repair and remodeling. Arteriosclerosis, Thrombosis, and Vascular Biology (USA), 1997, 17/3 (417-422)

Functional CD40 ligand is expressed on human vascular endothelial cells, smooth muscle cells, and macrophages: Implications for CD40-CD40 ligand signaling in atherosclerosis. Proceedings of the National Academy of Sciences of the United States of America (USA), 1997, 94/5 (1931-1936)

Nitric oxide synthase: Role in the genesis of vascular disease. Annual Review of Medicine (USA), 1997, 48/- (489-509)

Endothelial function. General considerations. Drugs (New Zealand), 1997, 53/SUPPL. 1 (1-10)

Hyperhomocyst(e)inemia is associated with impaired endothelium- dependent vasodilation in humans. Circulation (USA), 1997, 95/5 (1119-1121)

The role of folic acid in deficiency states and prevention of disease. Journal of Family Practice (USA), 1997, 44/2 (138-144)

Lipid-lowering trials in the primary and secondary prevention of coronary heart disease: New evidence, implications and outstanding issues. Current Opinion in Lipidology (United Kingdom), 1996, 7/6 (341-355)

Effects of vitamin D on aortic smooth muscle cells in culture. Toxicology in Vitro (United Kingdom), 1996, 10/6 (701-711)

Antagonistic effects of tetrahydropyrans on platelet activating factor-induced DNA synthesis and proliferation of cerebromicrovascular smooth muscle cells. Chinese Journal of Pharmacology and

Toxicology (China), 1996, 10/4 (251-254)

Soy isoflavones enhance coronary vascular reactivity in atherosclerotic female macaques. Fertility and Sterility (USA), 1997, 67/1 (148-154)

Common mutation in methylenetetrahydrofolate reductase: Correlation with homocysteine metabolism and late-onset vascular disease. Circulation (USA), 1996, 94/12 (3074-3078)

Hyperhomocysteinemia confers an independent increased risk of atherosclerosis in end-stage renal disease and is closely linked to plasma folate and pyridoxine concentrations. Circulation (USA), 1996, 94/11 (2743-2748)

Endothelin receptors and atherosclerosis: A potential target for therapeutic intervention. Expert Opinion on Investigational Drugs (United Kingdom), 1996, 5/11 (1495-1508)

Endothelium and atherosclerosis: Monocyte accumulation as a target for therapeutic intervention. Expert Opinion on Investigational Drugs (United Kingdom), 1996, 5/11 (1487-1494)

Upregulation of IGF-I and collagen I mRNA in human atherosclerotic tissue is not accompanied by changes in type 1 IGF receptor or collagen III mRNA: An in situ hybridization study. Coronary Artery Disease (United Kingdom), 1996, 7/8 (569-572)

150-kD oxygen-regulated protein is expressed in human atherosclerotic plaques and allows mononuclear phagocytes to withstand cellular stress on exposure to hypoxia and modified low density lipoprotein. Journal of Clinical Investigation (USA), 1996, 98/8 (1930-1941)

Dietary fats and coronary heart disease. Biomedicine and Pharmacotherapy (France), 1996, 50/6-7 (261-268)

Interferon-inducible protein-10 involves vascular smooth muscle cell migration, proliferation, and inflammatory response. Journal of Biological Chemistry (USA), 1996, 271/39 (24286-24293)

Basic science of abdominal aortic aneurysms: Emerging therapeutic strategies for an unresolved clinical problem. Current Opinion in Cardiology (United Kingdom), 1996, 11/5 (504-518)

Homocystinuria: What about mild hyperhomocysteinaemia? Postgraduate Medical Journal (United Kingdom), 1996, 72/851 (513-518)

Pathogenesis of atherosclerosis. Maturitas (Ireland), 1996, 23/SUPPL. (S47-S49)

Effect of low dose omega-3 fatty acid supplementations on plasmalipids and lipoproteins in patients with coronary sclerosis and dyslipoproteinaemia. Zeitschrift fur Ernahrungswissenschaft (Germany), 1996, 35/2 (191-198)

Antioxidant of the coronary diet and disease. Clinica Cardiovascular (Spain), 1996, 14/2 (29-38)

Gamma imaging of atherosclerotic lesions: The role of antibody affinity in in vivo target localization. Journal of Nuclear Cardiology (USA), 1996, 3/3 (231-241)

Enhanced capacity of n-3 fatty acid-enriched macrophages to oxidize low density lipoprotein mechanisms and effects of antioxidant vitamins. Atherosclerosis (Ireland), 1996, 124/2 (157-169)

Prevention of preatheromatous lesions in sand rats by treatment with a nutritional supplement. Arzneimittel-Forschung/Drug Research (Germany), 1996, 46/6 (610-614)

Dietary methionine imbalance, endothelial cell dysfunction and atherosclerosis. Nutrition Research

(USA), 1996, 16/7 (1251-1266)

Evidence for cultured human vascular smooth muscle cell heterogeneity: Isolation of clonal cells and study of their growth characteristics. Thrombosis and Haemostasis (Germany), 1996, 75/5 (854-858)

Adenosine inhibitory effect on enhanced growth of aortic smooth muscle cells from streptozotocin-induced diabetic rats. British Journal of Pharmacology (United Kingdom), 1996, 118/3 (783-789)

Fish oil supplementation in patients with heterozygous familial hypercholesterolemia. Recenti Progressi in Medicina (Italy), 1996, 87/3 (102-105)

Pathology induced by high vitamin doses. Cahiers de Nutrition et de Dietetique (France), 1996, 31/2 (76-80)

Smooth muscle cell migration and proliferation is enhanced in abdominal aortic aneurysms. Australian and New Zealand Journal of Surgery (Australia), 1996, 66/5 (305-308)

Eicosanoid precursors: Potential factors for atherogenesis in diabetic CAPD patients? Peritoneal Dialysis International (Canada), 1996, 16/SUPPL. 1 (S250-S253)

Increased serum level of total homocysteine in CAPD patients: Despite fish oil therapy. Peritoneal Dialysis International (Canada), 1996, 16/SUPPL. 1(S246-S249)

The central role of calcium in the pathogenesis of cardiovascular disease. Journal of Human Hypertension (United Kingdom), 1996, 10/3 (143-155)

Shosaikoto (Kampo medicine) protects macrophage function from suppression by hypercholesterolemia. Biological and Pharmaceutical Bulletin (Japan), 1996, 19/4 (652-654)

Metabolism of linoleic and alpha-linolenic acids in cultured cardiomyocytes: Effect of different n-6 and n-3 fatty acid supplementation. Molecular and Cellular Biochemistry (USA), 1996, 157/1-2 (217-222)

17beta-estradiol and smooth muscle cell proliferation in aortic cells of male and female rats. Biochemical and Biophysical Research Communications (USA), 1996, 221/1 (8-14)

Homocysteine, folate, and vascular disease. Journal of Myocardial Ischemia (USA), 1996, 8/2 (60-63)

Effect of etofibrate and nicanartine on plasminogen activator inhibitor type-1 production in vitro by cultured vascular cells and on plasma plasminogen activator inhibitor type-1 activity in vivo in rabbits. Current Therapeutic Research - Clinical and Experimental (USA), 1996, 57/3 (192-202)

Phorbol ester inhibits the phosphorylation of the retinoblastoma protein without suppressing cyclin D-associated kinase in vascular smooth muscle cells. Journal of Biological Chemistry (USA), 1996, 271/14 (8345-8351)

Inhibitory effects of NB-818 on migration and proliferation of smooth muscle cells. Japanese Pharmacology and Therapeutics (Japan), 1996, 24/2 (213-217)

A novel cis-acting element is essential for cytokine-mediated transcriptional induction of the serum amyloid A gene in nonhepatic cells. Veterinary Pathobiology Department, University of Missouri US6/4 (1584-1594)

Nutritional interest of flavonoids. Medecine et Nutrition (France), 1996, 32/1 (17-27)

Study of causes underlying the low atherosclerotic response to dietary hypercholesterolemia in a selected strain of rabbits. Atherosclerosis (Ireland), 1996, 121/1 (63-73)

References

Simvastatin releases Ca2+ from a thapsigargin-sensitive pool and inhibits InsP3-dependent Ca2+ mobilization in vascular smooth muscle cells. Journal of Cardiovascular Pharmacology (USA), 1996, 27/3 (383-391)

The effect of reduced glomerular filtration rate on plasma total homocysteine concentration. Scandinavian Journal of Clinical and Laboratory Investigation (Norway), 1996, 56/1 (41-46)

Effects of diet and exercise on qualitative and quantitative measures of LDL and its susceptibility to oxidation. Arteriosclerosis, Thrombosis, and Vascular Biology (USA), 1996, 16/2 (201-207)

Homocysteine: Relation with ischemic vascular diseases. Revue de Medecine Interne (France), 1996, 17/1 (34-45)

Evaluation of hydroxyl radical-scavenging property of garlic. Molecular and Cellular Biochemistry (USA), 1996, 154/1 (55-63)

Effects of interaction of RRR-alpha-tocopheryl acetate and fish oil on low-density-lipoprotein oxidation in postmenopausal women with and without hormone-replacement therapy. American Journal of Clinical Nutrition (USA), 1996, 63/2 (184-193)

Therapeutic actions of garlic constituents. Medicinal Research Reviews (USA), 1996, 16/1 (111-124)

Soybean isoflavones improve cardiovascular risk factors without affecting the reproductive system of peripubertal rhesus monkeys. Journal of Nutrition (USA), 1996, 126/1 (43-50)

Endothelin-1 and angiotensin II act as progression but not competence growth factors in vascular smooth muscle cells. European Journal of Pharmacology (Netherlands), 1996, 295/2-3 (261-269)

Apoptosis of vascular smooth muscle cells induced by in vitro stimulation with interferon-gamma, tumor necrosis factor-alpha, and interleukin-1beta. Arteriosclerosis, Thrombosis, and Vascular Biology (USA), 1996, 16/1 (19-27)

High dose B-vitamin treatment of hyperhomocysteinemia in dialysis patients. Kidney International (USA), 1996, 49/1 (147-152)

Long-term folic acid (but not pyridoxine) supplementation lowers elevated plasma homocysteine level in chronic renal failure. Mineral and Electrolyte Metabolism (Switzerland), 1996, 22/1-3 (106-109)

The mechanism of apolipoprotein B-100 thiol depletion during oxidative modification of low-density lipoprotein. Archives of Biochemistry and Biophysics (USA), 1997, 341/2 (287-294)

Ascorbate and urate are the strongest determinants of plasma antioxidative capacity and serum lipid resistance to oxidation in Finnish men. Atherosclerosis (Ireland), 1997, 130/1 (223-233)

Antioxidants in the prevention of atherosclerosis. Current Opinion in Lipidology (United Kingdom), 1996, 7/6 (374-380)

The carotenoids beta-carotene, canthaxanthin and zeaxanthin inhibit macrophage-mediated LDL oxidation. FEBS Letters (Netherlands), 1997, 401/2-3 (262-266)

Polyunsaturated fatty acids, antioxidants, and cognitive function in very old men. American Journal of Epidemiology (USA), 1997, 145/1 (33-41)

Animal studies on antioxidants. Journal of Cardiovascular Risk (United Kingdom), 1996, 3/4 (358-362)

Alpha-Tocopherol and beta-carotene serum levels in post-menopausal women treated with transdermal estradiol and oral medroxyprogesterone acetate. Hormone and Metabolic Research (Germany), 1996, 28/10 (558-561)

Time-course studies by synchrotron X-ray solution scattering of the structure of human low-density lipoprotein during Cu2+-induced oxidation in relation to changes in lipid composition. Biochemical Journal (United Kingdom), 1996, 319/1 (217-227)

Antioxidant status of hypercholesterolemic patients treated with LDL apheresis. Cardiovascular Drugs and Therapy (USA), 1996, 10/5 (567-571)

Abnormal antioxidant vitamin and carotenoid status in chronic renal failure. QJM - Monthly Journal of the Association of Physicians (United Kingdom), 1996, 89/10 (765-769)

Antioxidants in cardiovascular disease: Randomized trials. Nutrition (USA), 1996, 12/9 (583-588)

Dietary antioxidants and cognitive function in a population-based sample of older persons: The Rotterdam study. American Journal of Epidemiology (USA), 1996, 144/3 (275-280)

Lack of correlation between the alpha-tocopherol content of plasma and LDL, but high correlations for gamma-tocopherol and carotenoids. Journal of Lipid Research (USA), 1996, 37/9 (1936-1946)

Oxidized low density lipoproteins in atherogenesis: Role of dietary modification. Annual Review of Nutrition (USA), 1996, 16/- (51-71)

Effect of dietary supplementation of beta-carotene on human monocyte -macrophage-mediated oxidation of low density lipoprotein. Israel Journal of Medical Sciences (Israel), 1996, 32/6 (473-478)

Increased oxidation resistance of atherogenic plasma lipoproteins at high vitamin E levels in non-vitamin E supplemented men. Atherosclerosis (Ireland), 1996, 124/1 (83-94)

Increased levels of autoantibodies to cardiolipin and oxidised low density lipoprotein are inversely associated with plasma vitamin C status in cigarette smokers. Atherosclerosis (Ireland), 1996, 124/1 (75-81)

Antioxydant vitamins and risk of cardiovascular diseases

The significance of oxidised low-density lipoprotein in atherosclerosis. Ugeskrift for Laeger (Denmark), 1996, 158/19 (2706-2710)

Prevention of atherosclerosis with dietary antioxidants: Fact or fiction? Journal of Nutrition (USA), 1996, 126/4 SUPPL. (1067S-1071S)

Nutritional supplement program halts progression of early coronary atherosclerosis documented by ultrafast computed tomography. Journal of Applied Nutrition (USA), 1996, 48/3 (68-78)

Metal excretion and magnesium retention in patients with intermittent claudication treated with intravenous disodium EDTA. Clinical Chemistry (USA), 1996, 42/12 (1938-1942)

Therapy for acute myocardial infarction. Clinics in Geriatric Medicine (USA), 1996, 12/1 (141-168)

Vitamin E consumption and the risk of coronary disease in women. NEW ENGL. J. MED. (USA), 1993, 328/20 (1444-1449)

The role of free radicals in disease. Australian and New Zealand Journal of Ophthalmology (Australia), 1995, 23/1

References

Coenzyme Q10 and coronary artery disease. CLIN. INVEST. SUPPL. (Germany), 1993, 71/8

Dietary antioxidant vitamins and death from coronary heart disease in postmenopausal women. New England Journal of Medicine (USA), 1996, 334/18

Vitamin E and atherosclerosis: Potential role of vitamin E in the prevention of cardiovascular diseases. Nutrition Clinique et Metabolisme (France), 1996, 10/1 (43-44)

Randomized, controlled trial of antioxidant vitamins and cardioprotective diet on hyperlipidemia, oxidative stress, and development of experimental atherosclerosis: The diet and antioxidant trial on atherosclerosis (DATA). Cardiovascular Drugs and Therapy (USA), 1995, 9/6

Serum levels of vitamin E in relation to cardiovascular diseases. Journal of Clinical Pharmacy and Therapeutics (United Kingdom), 1995, 20/6

Oxidative susceptibility of low density lipoprotein from rabbits fed atherogenic diets containing coconut, palm, or soybean oils. Lipids (USA), 1995, 30/12 (1145-1150)

Coantioxidants make alpha-tocopherol an efficient antioxidant for low- density lipoprotein. American Journal of Clinical Nutrition (USA), 1995, 62/6 SUPPL.

Optimal diet for reducing the risk of arteriosclerosis. Canadian Journal of Cardiology (Canada), 1995, 11/SUPPL. G

Effect of vitamin E, vitamin C and beta-carotene on LDL oxidation and atherosclerosis. Canadian Journal of Cardiology (Canada), 1995, 11/SUPPL. G (97G-103G)

Atherosclerosis: Vitamin E protects coronary arteries. Deutsche Apotheker Zeitung (Germany), 1995, 135/41 (42+44)

Effects on health of dietary supplementation with 100 mg d-alpha-tocopheryl acetate, daily for 6 years. Journal of International Medical Research (United Kingdom), 1995, 23/5

Mechanisms of the cardioprotective effect of a diet enriched with omega-3 polyunsaturated fatty acids. Pathophysiology (Netherlands), 1995, 2/3 (131-140)

Prevention of atherosclerosis: The potential role of antioxidants. Postgraduate Medicine (USA), 1995, 98/1

Vitamin E: Metabolism and role in atherosclerosis. ANN. BIOL. CLIN. (France), 1994, 52/7-8

Vitamin C prevents cigarette smoke-induced leukocyte aggregation and adhesion to endothelium in vivo. PROC. NATL. ACAD. SCI. U. S. A. (USA), 1994, 91/16 (7688-7692)

Homocysteine and coronary atherosclerosis. J Am Coll Cardiol (UNITED STATES) Mar 1 1996, 27 (3) p517-27

Hyperhomocysteinaemia: a role in the accelerated atherogenesis of chronic renal failure? Neth J Med (NETHERLANDS) May 1995, 46 (5) p244-51

Hyperhomocysteinaemia and endothelial dysfunction in young patients with peripheral arterial occlusive disease. Eur J Clin Invest (ENGLAND) Mar 1995, 25 (3) p176-81

Homocysteine and coronary atherosclerosis. J Am Coll Cardiol (UNITED STATES) Mar 1 1996, 27 (3) p517-27

Vitamin nutrition status and homocysteine: an atherogenic risk factor. Nutr Rev (UNITED STATES)

Nov 1994, 52 (11) p383-7

Homocysteine and coronary artery disease. Cleve Clin J Med (UNITED STATES) Nov-Dec 1994, 61 (6) p438-50

Treatment of atherosclerosis and thrombosis with aspirin. Lancet (ENGLAND) Sep 9 1972, 2 (776) p532-4

[Progress in the prevention and treatment of ischemic cerebrovascular diseases with garlic extract] Chung Kuo Chung Hsi I Chieh Ho Tsa Chih (CHINA) Feb 1995, 15 (2) p124-6 (24 Refs.)

Platelets, carotids, and coronaries. Critique on antithrombotic role of antiplatelet agents, exercise, and certain diets. Am J Med (UNITED STATES) Sep 1984, 77 (3) p513-23

Effects of 11-week increases in dietry eicosapentaenoic acid on bleeding time, lipids, and platelet aggregation. Lancet (ENGLAND) Nov 28 1981, 2 (8257) p1190-3

N -3 but not N-6 fatty acids reduce the expression of the combined adhesion and scavenger receptor CD36 in human monocytic cells. Cell Biochem Funct (ENGLAND) Sep 1995, 13 (3) p211-6

Essential fatty acid metabolism in patients with essential hypertension, diabetes mellitus and coronary heart disease. Prostaglandins Leukot Essent Fatty Acids (SCOTLAND) Jun 1995, 52 (6) p387-91

[Changes in fatty acid composition, platelet aggregability and RBC function in elderly subjects with administration of low-dose fish oil concentrate and comparison with younger subjects]. Ronen Igakkai Zasshi (JAPAN) Aug 1994, 31 (8) p596-603

Do fish oils prevent restenosis after coronary angioplasty? Circulation (UNITED STATES) Nov 1994, 90 (5) p2248-57

n-3 fatty acid incorporation into LDL particles renders them more susceptible to oxidation in vitro but not necessarily more atherogenic in vivo. Arterioscler Thromb (UNITED STATES) Jul 1994, 14 (7) p1170-6

Human atherosclerotic plaque contains both oxidized lipids and relatively large amounts of alpha-tocopherol and ascorbate. Arterioscler Thromb Vasc Biol (UNITED STATES) Oct 1995, 15 (10) p1616-24

Attention Deficit Disorder (ADD)

Omega-3 fatty acids in boys with behavior, learning, and health problems. Physiology and Behavior (USA), 1996, 59/4-5 (915-920)

Behavioral effects of dietary neurotransmitter precursors: Basic and clinical aspects. Neuroscience and Biobehavioral Reviews (USA), 1996, 20/2 (313-323)

Coloboma hyperactive mutant mice exhibit regional and transmitter-specific deficits in neurotransmission. Journal of Neurochemistry (USA), 1997, 68/1 (176-186)

Clinical trial of piracetam in patients with myoclonus: Nationwide multiinstitution study in Japan. Movement Disorders (USA), 1996, 11/6 (691-700)

Neurobehavioral aspects of lead neurotoxicity in children. Central European Journal of Public Health (Czech Republic), 1997, 5/2 (65-69)

References

Hair lead levels related to children's classroom attention-deficit behavior. Archives of Environmental Health (USA), 1996, 51/3 (214-220)

Bone lead levels and delinquent behavior. Journal of the American Medical Association (USA), 1996, 275/5 (363-369)

Zinc deficiency in attention-deficit hyperactivity disorder. Biological Psychiatry (USA), 1996, 40/12 (1308-1310)

Iron treatment in children with attention deficit hyperactivity disorder: A preliminary report. Neuropsychobiology (Switzerland), 1997, 35/4 (178-180)

Attention-deficit hyperactivity disorder: Pharmacotherapy and beyond. Postgraduate Medicine (USA), 1997, 101/5 (201+213+222)

Do nutrient supplements and dietary changes affect learning and emotional reactions of children with learning difficulties? A controlled series of 16 cases. Nutr Health (ENGLAND) 1984, 3 (1-2) p69-77

[Effect of supplementary intake of vitamins for 6 months on physical and mental work capacity of children beginning school education at the age of 6 years]. Vopr Pitan (USSR) Jul-Aug 1988

Nutritional therapy for selected inborn errors of metabolism. J Am Coll Nutr (UNITED STATES) 1989, 8 Suppl

Vitamin supplements and purported learning enhancement in mentally retarded children. J Nutr Sci Vitaminol (Tokyo) (JAPAN) Jun 1989

Vitamin B6 in clinical neurology. Ann N Y Acad Sci (UNITED STATES) 1990, 585 p250-60

[Vitamin B12 deficiency due to abnormal eating habits]. Ned Tijdschr Geneeskd (NETHERLANDS) Feb 26 1994

Use and safety of elevated dosages of vitamin E in infants and children. Int J Vitam Nutr Res Suppl (CANADA) 1989, 30 p69-80

Experience over 17 years with antioxidant treatment in Spielmeyer-Sjogren disease. Am J Med Genet Suppl (UNITED STATES) 1988, 5 p265-74

Vitamin E and the nervous system. Crit Rev Neurobiol (UNITED STATES) 1987, 3 (1)

Clinical uses of vitamin E. Acta Vitaminol Enzymol (ITALY) 1985, 7 Suppl p33-43

Neurologic complications of vitamin E deficiency: case report and review of the literature. Bull Clin Neurosci (UNITED STATES) 1985, 50 p53-60

A progressive neurological syndrome associated with an isolated vitamin E deficiency.

Can J Neurol Sci (CANADA) Nov 1984, 11 (4 Suppl) p561-4

[Evaluation of the effectiveness of prophylactic vitamin administration to school children in Moscow]. Vopr Pitan (USSR) May-Jun 1992

The assessment of the vitamin B6 status among Egyptian school children by measuring the urinary cystathionine excretion. Int J Vitam Nutr Res (SWITZERLAND) 1984, 54 (4) p321-7

Dramatic favorable responses of children with learning disabilities or dyslexia and attention deficit disorder to antimotion sickness medications: four case reports. Percept Mot Skills (UNITED STATES) Dec

References

1991, 73 (3 Pt 1) p723-38

New developments in pediatric psychopharmacology. J Dev Behav Pediatr (UNITED STATES) Sep 1983, 4 (3) p202-9

Piracetam in the management of minimal brain dysfunction [letter]. S Afr Med J (SOUTH AFRICA) Aug 7 1976, 50 (34) p1312

Altered dopaminergic function in the prefrontal cortex, nucleus accumbens and caudate-putamen of an animal model of attention-deficit hyperactivity disorder?the spontaneously hypertensive rat. Brain Res (NETHERLANDS) Apr 10 1995, 676 (2) p343-51

Deanol and methylphenidate in minimal brain dysfunction. Clin Pharmacol Ther (UNITED STATES) May 1975, 17 (5) p534-40

Effect of dextroamphetamine and methylphenidate on calcium and magnesium concentration in hyperactive boys. Psychiatry Res (IRELAND) Nov 1994, 54 (2) p199-210

[Deficiency of certain trace elements in children with hyperactivity]. Psychiatr Pol (POLAND) May-Jun 1994, 28 (3) p345-53

[Level of magnesium in blood serum in children from the province of Rzesz?ow]. Wiad Lek (POLAND) Feb 1993, 46 (3-4) p120-2

Gamma-linolenic acid for attention-deficit hyperactivity disorder: placebo-controlled comparison to D-amphetamine. Biol Psychiatry (UNITED STATES) Jan 15 1989, 25 (2) p222-8

Megavitamins and hyperactivity [letter]. Pediatrics (UNITED STATES) Aug 1986, 78 (2) p374-5

Vitamin E and Alzheimer's disease in subjects with Down syndrome. Journal of Mental Deficiency Research, 1988 Dec Vol 32(6) 479-484

Behavioral disorders, learning disabilities and megavitamin therapy. Adolescence 1987 Fal Vol 22(87) 729-738

Macrocytosis and cognitive decline in Down syndrome. British Journal of Psychiatry 1986 Dec Vol 149 797-798

Treatment approaches in Down syndrome: A review. Australia & New Zealand Journal of Developmental Disabilities

A double blind study of vitamin B-sub-6 in Down syndrome infants: I. Clinical and biochemical results. Journal of Mental Deficiency Research 1985 Sep Vol 29(3) 233-240

A double blind study of vitamin B-sub-6 in Down syndrome infants: II. Cortical auditory evoked potentials. Journal of Mental Deficiency Research 1985 Sep Vol 29(3) 241-246

Xylose absorption in Down syndrome. Journal of Mental Deficiency Research 1985 Jun Vol 29(2) 173-177

Nutritional aspects of Down syndrome with special reference to the nervous system. British Journal of Psychiatry 1984 Aug Vol 145 115-120

Children's mental retardation study is attacked: A closer look. International Journal of Biosocial Research 1982 Vol 3(2) 75-86

Effects of nutritional supplementation on IQ and certain other variables associated with Down syndrome. American Journal of Mental Deficiency 1983 Sep Vol 88(2) 214-217

Vitamin A and carotene values of institutionalized mentally retarded subjects with and without Down syndrome. Journal of Mental Deficiency Research 1977 Mar Vol 21(1) 63-74

Sodium-dependent glutamate binding in senile dementia. Neurobiology of Aging 1987 May-Jun Vol 8(3) 219-223

Alzheimer-like neurotransmitter deficits in adult Down syndrome brain tissue. Journal of Neurology, Neurosurgery & Psychiatry 1987 Jun Vol 50(6) 775-778

A report on phosphatidylcholine therapy in a Down Syndrome child. Psychological Reports 1986 Feb Vol 58(1) 207-217

Do nutrient supplements and dietary changes affect learning and emotional reactions of children with learning difficulties? A controlled series of 16 cases. Nutr Health (ENGLAND) 1984, 3 (1-2) p69-77

[Effect of supplementary intake of vitamins for 6 months on physical and mental work capacity of children beginning school education at the age of 6 years]. Vopr Pitan (USSR) Jul-Aug 1988

Nutritional therapy for selected inborn errors of metabolism. J Am Coll Nutr (UNITED STATES) 1989, 8 Suppl

Vitamin supplements and purported learning enhancement in mentally retarded children. J Nutr Sci Vitaminol (Tokyo) (JAPAN) Jun 1989

Vitamin B6 in clinical neurology. Ann N Y Acad Sci (UNITED STATES) 1990, 585 p250-60

[Vitamin B12 deficiency due to abnormal eating habits]. Ned Tijdschr Geneeskd (NETHERLANDS) Feb 26 1994

Use and safety of elevated dosages of vitamin E in infants and children. Int J Vitam Nutr Res Suppl (CANADA) 1989, 30 p69-80

Experience over 17 years with antioxidant treatment in Spielmeyer-Sjogren disease. Am J Med Genet Suppl (UNITED STATES) 1988, 5 p265-74

Vitamin E and the nervous system. Crit Rev Neurobiol (UNITED STATES) 1987, 3 (1)

Clinical uses of vitamin E. Acta Vitaminol Enzymol (ITALY) 1985, 7 Suppl p33-43

Neurologic complications of vitamin E deficiency: case report and review of the literature. Bull Clin Neurosci (UNITED STATES) 1985, 50 p53-60

A progressive neurological syndrome associated with an isolated vitamin E deficiency. Can J Neurol Sci (CANADA) Nov 1984, 11 (4 Suppl) p561-4

[Evaluation of the effectiveness of prophylactic vitamin administration to school children in Moscow]. Vopr Pitan (USSR) May-Jun 1992

The assessment of the vitamin B6 status among Egyptian school children by measuring the urinary cystathionine excretion. Int J Vitam Nutr Res (SWITZERLAND) 1984, 54 (4) p321-7

Dramatic favorable responses of children with learning disabilities or dyslexia and attention deficit disorder to antimotion sickness medications: four case reports. Percept Mot Skills (UNITED STATES) Dec 1991, 73 (3 Pt 1) p723-38

References

New developments in pediatric psychopharmacology. J Dev Behav Pediatr (UNITED STATES) Sep 1983, 4 (3) p202-9

Dramatic favorable responses of children with learning disabilities or dyslexia and attention deficit disorder to antimotion sickness medications: four case reports. Percept Mot Skills (UNITED STATES) Dec 1991, 73 (3 Pt 1) p723-38

Piracetam in the management of minimal brain dysfunction [letter]. S Afr Med J (SOUTH AFRICA) Aug 7 1976, 50 (34) p1312

Altered dopaminergic function in the prefrontal cortex, nucleus accumbens and caudate-putamen of an animal model of attention-deficit hyperactivity disorder—the spontaneously hypertensive rat. Brain Res (NETHERLANDS) Apr 10 1995, 676 (2) p343-51

Deanol and methylphenidate in minimal brain dysfunction. Clin Pharmacol Ther (UNITED STATES) May 1975, 17 (5) p534-40

Effect of dextroamphetamine and methylphenidate on calcium and magnesium concentration in hyperactive boys. Psychiatry Res (IRELAND) Nov 1994, 54 (2) p199-210

[Deficiency of certain trace elements in children with hyperactivity]. Psychiatr Pol (POLAND) May-Jun 1994, 28 (3) p345-53

[Level of magnesium in blood serum in children from the province of Rzesz'ow]. Wiad Lek (POLAND) Feb 1993, 46 (3-4) p120-2

Gamma-linolenic acid for attention-deficit hyperactivity disorder: placebo-controlled comparison to D-amphetamine. Biol Psychiatry (UNITED STATES) Jan 15 1989, 25 (2) p222-8

Megavitamins and hyperactivity [letter]. Pediatrics (UNITED STATES) Aug 1986, 78 (2) p374-5

Vitamin E and Alzheimer's disease in subjects with Down syndrome. Journal of Mental Deficiency Research, 1988 Dec Vol 32(6) 479-484

Behavioral disorders, learning disabilities and megavitamin therapy. Adolescence 1987 Fal Vol 22(87) 729-738

Macrocytosis and cognitive decline in Down syndrome. British Journal of Psychiatry 1986 Dec Vol 149 797-798

Treatment approaches in Down syndrome: A review. Australia & New Zealand Journal of Developmental Disabilities

A double blind study of vitamin B-sub-6 in Down syndrome infants: I. Clinical and biochemical results. Journal of Mental Deficiency Research 1985 Sep Vol 29(3) 233-240

A double blind study of vitamin B-sub-6 in Down syndrome infants: II. Cortical auditory evoked potentials. Journal of Mental Deficiency Research 1985 Sep Vol 29(3) 241-246

Xylose absorption in Down syndrome. Journal of Mental Deficiency Research 1985 Jun Vol 29(2) 173-177

Nutritional aspects of Down syndrome with special reference to the nervous system. British Journal of Psychiatry 1984 Aug Vol 145 115-120

Children's mental retardation study is attacked: A closer look. International Journal of Biosocial

Research 1982 Vol 3(2) 75-86

Effects of nutritional supplementation on IQ and certain other variables associated with Down syndrome. American Journal of Mental Deficiency 1983 Sep Vol 88(2) 214-217

Vitamin A and carotene values of institutionalized mentally retarded subjects with and without Down syndrome. Journal of Mental Deficiency Research 1977 Mar Vol 21(1) 63-74

Sodium-dependent glutamate binding in senile dementia. Neurobiology of Aging 1987 May-Jun Vol 8(3) 219-223

Alzheimer-like neurotransmitter deficits in adult Down syndrome brain tissue. Journal of Neurology, Neurosurgery & Psychiatry 1987 Jun Vol 50(6) 775-778

A report on phosphatidylcholine therapy in a Down Syndrome child. Psychological Reports 1986 Feb Vol 58(1) 207-217

Autoimmune Diseases

Androgen and progesterone levels in females with rheumatoid arthritis. REUMATISMO (Italy), 1994, 46/2 (65-69)

Docosahexaenoic and eicosapentaenoic acids inhibit human lymphoproliferative responses in vitro but not the expression of T cell surface activation markers. Scandinavian Journal of Immunology (United Kingdom), 1996, 43/3

Modulation of antioxidant enzymes and programmed cell death by n-3 fatty acids. Lipids (USA), 1996, 31/3 SUPPL. (S91-S96)

Dietary marine lipids suppress continuous expression of interleukin-1beta gene transcription. Lipids (USA), 1996, 31/3 SUPPL. (S23-S31)

Tissue specific regulation of transforming growth factor beta by omega-3 lipid-rich krill oil in autoimmune murine lupus. Nutrition Research (USA), 1996, 16/3 (489-503)

The effects of dietary lipid manipulation on the production of murine T cell-derived cytokines. Cytokine (United Kingdom), 1995, 7/6 (548-553)

Dietary omega-3 lipids delay the onset and progression of autoimmune lupus nephritis by inhibiting transforming growth factor beta mRNA and protein expression. Journal of Autoimmunity (United Kingdom), 1995, 8/3 (381-393)

Fish oil feeding modulates leukotriene production in murine lupus nephritis. PROSTAGLANDINS (USA), 1994, 48/5 (331-348)

Effects of n-3 and n-6 fatty acids on the activities and expression of hepatic antioxidant enzymes in autoimmune-prone NZBxNZW F1 mice. LIPIDS (USA), 1994, 29/8 (561-568)

Increased TGF-beta and decreased oncogene expression by omega-3 fatty acids in the spleen delays onset of autoimmune disease in B/W mice. J. IMMUNOL. (USA), 1994, 152/12 (5979-5987)

Decreased pro-inflammatory cytokines and increased antioxidant enzyme gene expression by omega-3 lipids in murine lupus nephritis. BIOCHEM. BIOPHYS. RES. COMMUN. (USA), 1994, 200/2 (893-898)

Suppression of autoimmune disease by dietary n-3 fatty acids. J. LIPID RES. (USA), 1993, 34/8 (1435-

1444)

Role of omega-3 fatty acids in health and disease. NUTR. RES. (USA), 1993, 13/SUPPL. 1 (S19-S45)

Omega-3 polyunsaturated fatty acids: A potential new treatment of immune renal disease. MAYO CLIN. PROC. (USA), 1991, 66/10 (1018-1028)

Practicalities of lipids: ICU patient, autoimmune disease, and vascular disease. J. PARENTER. ENTER. NUTR. (USA), 1990, 14/5 SUPPL.

Dietary marine lipids suppress murine autoimmune disease. J. INTERN. MED. SUPPL. (United Kingdom), 1989, 225/731

Depression of humoral responses and phagocytic functions in vivo and in vitro by fish oil and eicosapentanoic acid. CLIN. IMMUNOL. IMMUNOPATHOL. (USA), 1989, 52/2 (257-270)

The type of dietary fat affects the severity of autoimmune disease in NZB/NZW mice. AM. J. PATHOL. (USA), 1987, 127/1 (106-121)

Effects of dietary supplementation on autoimmunity in the MRL/lpr mouse: A preliminary investigation. ANN. RHEUM. DIS. (UK), 1986, 45/12 (1019-1024)

A fish oil diet rich in eicosapentaenoic acid reduces cyclooxygenase metabolites, and suppresses lupus in MRL-lpr mice. J. IMMUNOL. (USA), 1985, 134/3 (1914-1919)

The protective effect of dietary fish oil on murine lupus. PROSTAGLANDINS (USA), 1985, 30/1 (51-75)

Modulation of antioxidant enzymes and programmed cell death by n-3 fatty acids. Lipids (USA), 1996, 31/3 SUPPL. (S91-S96)

Effect of (n-3) polyunsaturated fatty acids on cytokine production and their biologic function. Nutrition (USA), 1996, 12/1 SUPPL. (S8-S14)

Lipid peroxidase and erythrocyte redox system in systemic vasculitides treated with corticoids. Effect of vitamin E administration. Romanian Journal of Internal Medicine (Romania), 1994, 32/4 (283-289)

Free radical tissue damages in the anterior segment of the eye in experimental autoimmune uveitis. Investigative Ophthalmology and Visual Science (USA), 1996, 37/4

Intervention at diagnosis of type I diabetes using either antioxidants or photopheresis. DIABETES METAB. REV. (United Kingdom), 1993, 9/4 (329-336)

Free radical theory of aging: Beneficial effect of antioxidants on the life span of male NZB mice: Role of free radical reactions in the deterioration of the immune system with age and in the pathogenesis of systemic lupus erythematosus. AGE (USA), 1980, 3/3 (64-73)

The connective tissue diseases and the overall influence of gender. Int J of Fertility and Menopausal Studies (USA), 1996, 41/2

Blood dehydroepiandrosterone sulphate (DHEAS) levels in pemphigoid/pemphigus and psoriasis. Clinical and Experimental Rheumatology (Italy), 1995, 13/3

Neuroendocrine-immune system interactions and autoimmunity. Annual Review of Immunology (USA), 1995, 13/- (307-338)

Low serum levels of dehydroepiandrosterone may cause deficient IL-2 production by lymphocytes in patients with systemic lupus erythematosus (SLE). Clinical and Experimental Immunology (United Kingdom), 1995, 99/2

Bacterial Infections

Evaluation of the effect of arginine-enriched amino acid solution on tumor growth. J. PARENTER. ENTER. NUTR. (USA), 1985, 9/4 (428-434)

Activation of mouse macrophages by alkylglycerols, inflammation products of cancerous tissues. Cancer Research, 1988 Nov 1, 48(21):6044-9.

Activation of mouse peritoneal macrophages by lysophospholipids and ether derivatives of neutral lipids and phospholipids. Cancer Research, 1987 Apr 15, 47(8):2008-13.

Activation of macrophages by ether analogues of lysophospholipids. Cancer Immunology, Immunotherapy, 1987, 25(3):185-92

Interactions between alkylglycerols and human neutrophil granulocytes. Scandinavian Journal of Clinical and Laboratory Investigation, 1990 Jun, 50(4):363-70

The effect of antioxidants on bleomycin treatment in in vitro and in vivo genotoxicity assays. Mutation Research - Fundamental and Molecular Mechanisms of Mutagenesis (Netherlands), 1995, 329/1 (37-47)

Inhibitory effect of vitamin C on the mutagenicity and covalent DNA binding of the electrophilic and carcinogenic metabolite, 6-sulfooxymethylbenzo(a)pyrene. CARCINOGENESIS (United Kingdom), 1994, 15/5 (917-920)

Few aspects of bacterial colonies in the stomach during the treatment with acidoinhibitors. BOLL. CHIM. FARM. (Italy), 1992, 131/8 (302-303)

The prevention and management of pressure ulcers. MED. CLIN. NORTH AM. (USA), 1989, 73/6 (1511-1524)

The inhibition of bacterially mediated N-nitrosation by vitamin C: Relevance to the inhibition of endogenous N-nitrosation in the achlorhydric stomach. CARCINOGENESIS (United Kingdom), 1989, 10/2 (397-399)

Partial purification and some properties of an antibacterial compound from Aloe vera. PHYTOTHER. RES. (United Kingdom), 1988, 2/2 (67-69)

Activation of serum complement leads to inhibition of ascorbic acid transport (42530). PROC. SOC. EXP. BIOL. MED. (USA), 1987, 185/2 (153-157)

Effects of vitamins A, C, and E on aflatoxin Bsub 1-induced mutagenesis in Salmonella typhimurium TA-98 and TA-100. TERATOG. CARCINOG. MUTAG. (USA), 1985, 5/1 (29-40)

Effect of vitamin A supplementation on lectin-induced diarrhoea and bacterial translocation in rats. Nutrition Research (USA), 1996, 16/3 (459-465)

Increased translocation of Escherichia coli and development of arthritis in vitamin A- deficient rats. Infection and Immunity (USA), 1995, 63/8 (3062-3068)

Gastrointestinal infections in children. CURR. OPIN. GASTROENTEROL. (United Kingdom), 1994,

10/1 (88-97)

Intestinal malabsorption presenting with night blindness. BR. J. CLIN. PRACT. (United Kingdom), 1993, 47/5 (275-276)

Etiology of acute lower respiratory tract infection in children from Alabang, Metro Manila. REV. INFECT. DIS. (USA), 1990, 12/SUPPL. 8 (S929-S939)

Effect of vitamin A in enteral formulae for burned guinea-pigs. BURNS (United Kingdom), 1990, 16/4 (265-272)

Vitamin A supplementation improves macrophage function and bacterial clearance during experimental salmonella infection. PROC. SOC. EXP. BIOL. MED. (USA), 1989, 191/1 (47-54)

Inhibition by retinoic acid of multiplication of virulent tubercle bacilli in cultured human macrophages. INFECT. IMMUN. (USA), 1989, 57/3 (840-844)

Corneal ulceration, measles, and childhood blindness in Tanzania. BR. J. OPHTHALMOL. (UK), 1987, 71/5 (331-343)

Impact of vitamin A supplementation on childhood mortality. A randomised controlled community trial. LANCET (UK), 1986, 1/8491 (1169-1173)

Effects of vitamins A, C, and E on aflatoxin Bsub 1-induced mutagenesis in Salmonella typhimurium TA-98 and TA-100. TERATOG. CARCINOG. MUTAG. (USA), 1985, 5/1 (29-40)

Impaired blood clearance of bacteria and phagocytic activity in vitamin A-deficient rats (41999). PROC. SOC. EXP. BIOL. MED. (USA), 1985, 178/2 (204-208)

Chronic salmonella septicemia and malabsorption of vitamin A . AM. J. CLIN. NUTR. (USA), 1979, 32/2 (319-324)

Retinol level in patients with psoriasis during treatment with B group vitamins, a bacterial polysaccharide (pyrogenal) and methotrexate (Russian). VESTN.DERM.VENER. (USSR), 1975, 51/1 (55-58)

Essential fatty acids: Biology and their clinical implications. ASIA PAC. J. PHARMACOL. (Singapore), 1991, 6/4 (317-330)

Essential fatty acid deficiency in children. TIJDSCHR. KINDERGENEESKD. (NETHERLANDS), 1981, 49/1 (10-15)

Nitric oxide-dependent killing of Candida albicans by murine peritoneal cells during an experimental infection . FEMS Immunology and Medical Microbiology (Netherlands), 1995, 11/3 (157-162)

Biosynthesis and interaction of endothelium-derived vasoactive mediators. EICOSANOIDS (Germany), 1991, 4/4 (187-202)

Regulation of macrophage physiology by L-arginine: Role of the oxidative L-arginine deiminase pathway. J. IMMUNOL. (USA), 1989, 143/11 (3641-3646)

Comparative evaluation of aloe vera in the management of burn wounds in guinea pigs. PLAST. RECONSTR. SURG. (USA), 1988, 81/3 (386-389)

Effect of topical zinc oxide on bacterial growth and inflammation in full-thickness skin wounds in normal and diabetic rats. Agren MS; Soderberg TA; Reuterving CO; Hallmans G; Tengrup I, Department of Pathology, University of Linkoping, Sweden. Eur J Surg (SWEDEN) Feb 1991, 157 (2) p97-101.

Antimicrobial activity of some commercial extracts of propolis preparedwith different solvents. Phytotherapy Research (United Kingdom), 1996, 10/4 (335-336)

Antibacterial action of a formulation containing propolis of Apis mellifera L. REV. FARM. BIOQUIM. UNIV. SAO PAULO (Brazil), 1994, 30/1 (19-21)

Electron microscopic and microcalorimetric investigations of the possible mechanism of the antibacterial action of a defined propolis provenance. PLANTA MED. (Germany), 1994, 60/3 (222-227)

Synergistic effect of ethanolic extract of propolis and antibiotics on the growth of Staphylococcus aureus. ARZNEIM.-FORSCH. DRUG RES. (Germany), 1993, 43/5 (607-609)

Antibacterial, antifungal, antiamoebic, antiinflammatory and antipyretic studies on propolis bee products. J. ETHNOPHARMACOL. (Ireland), 1991, 35/1 (77-82)

Antibacterial properties of propolis (bee glue). J. R. SOC. MED. (United Kingdom), 1990, 83/3 (159-160)

Biological properties and clinical application of propolis. III. Investigation of the sensitivity of staphylococci isolated from pathological cases to ethanol extract of propolis (EEP). ARZNEIM.-FORSCH. (GERMANY, WEST), 1977, 27/7 (1395)

Biological properties and clinical application of propolis. I. Some physico chemical properties of propolis. ARZNEIMITTEL-FORSCH. (GERMANY, WEST), 1977, 27/4 (889-890)

Balding

United States Patent: [19][11]

Patent Number: 5,352,442

Proctor: [45]

Date of Patent: Oct. 4,1994

Various other U.S. and foreign patents

Further references:

Anderson, Chemical Abstracts, vol. 90, p. 311K (1979).

Ando et al., Chemical Abstracts 93:79872n (1980).

Bazzano et al., Journal of American Academy of Dermatology, vol. 15, pp. 880-883 (1986).

Barry, Pharmacology of the Skin, vol. 1, pp. 121-137 (1987).

Cheng et al., Archives of Dermatological Research, vol. 278, pp. 470-473 (1986).

Cumming. et al., Journal of American Medical Association, vol. 247, pp. 1295-1298 (1982).

Dawber, Dermatologica, vol. 175 suppl. 2, pp. 23-28 (1987).

DeVillez, Archives of Dermatology, vol 121, pp. 197-202, (1985)

Dostert a d., Xenobiotica, vol. 15, No. 10, pp. 799-803 (1985).

Ehman et d., Investigative Radiology, vol. 21, pp. 125-131 (1986).

Feelisch et al., Evr. Journal of Pharmacology, vol. 139, pp. 19-30 (1987).

Feelisch et al., Evr. Journal of Pharmacology, vol. 142, pp. 405-409 (1987).

Fox et al., Annals of the New York Academy of Sciences, vol. 411, pp. 14-19 (1983).

Goffman et al., International Journal of Radiation, Oncology, Biology and Physics, vol. 22, pp. 803-806 (Nov. 4, 1992).

Headington, Current Therapeutic Research, vol. 36, pp. 1098-1105 (1984).

Hearse et al., Circulation Research, vol. 60, pp. 375-383 (1987).

Heschler, Chemical Abstracts, vol. 78, pp. 115-239 (1973). Ignarro et al., Biochemica ct. Biophysica Acta, vol. 631, pp. 221-231 (1980).

J., Soc. Cosmetology Chem., (Italy) vol. 33, pp. 95-96 (Mar./Apr. 1982).

Journal of American Medical Association, vol. 260, No. 20 (1988).

Karlsson et al., Journal of Cyclic Nucleotide and Protein Res., vol. 10, No. 4, pp. 309-315 (1985).

Kvedar, Journal of American Academic Dermatology, vol. 12, pp. 215-225 (1985).

Longevity, vol. 2, No. 3, p. 26 (Jan. 1988).

Lucky, Archives of Dermatology, vol. 121, pp.57-62 (1985). Messina, Current Therapeutic Research vol. 34, pp. 319-324 (1983).

Messina, Current Therapeutic Research, vol. 38, pp. 269-282 (1985).

Mitchell et al., IBC USA Conference, South Natick, Mass: (Jun. 27, 1991).

Mittal et al., Proc. of National Academy of Science USA, vol. 74, No. 10 pp. 4360-4364 (1977).

Bladder Conditions

See references under Urinary Tract Infections.

Breast Cancer

Progress on therapy of breast cancer with vitamin Q10 and the regression of metastases. Biochem Biophys Res Commun (UNITED STATES) Jul 6 1995

Apparent partial remission of breast cancer in 'high risk' patients supplemented with nutritional antioxidants, essential fatty acids and coenzyme Q10. Mol Aspects Med (ENGLAND) 1994, 15 Suppl

Effects of isoprenoids (coQ10) on growth of normal human mammary epithelial cells and breast cancer cells in vitro. Anticancer Res (GREECE) Jan-Feb 1994

Partial and complete regression of breast cancer in patients in relation to dosage of coenzyme Q10. Biochem Biophys Res Commun (UNITED STATES) Mar 30 1994

Modulation of the length of the cell cycle time of MCF-7 human breastcancer cells by melatonin. Life Sci (ENGLAND) 1996, 58 (9)

Melatonin blocks the stimulatory effects of prolactin on human breast cancer cell growth in culture.

References

Br J Cancer (ENGLAND) Dec 1995

Melatonin modulation of estrogen-regulated proteins, growth factors, and proto- oncogenes in human breast cancer. J Pineal Res (DENMARK) Mar 1995

Melatonin inhibition of MCF-7 human breast-cancer cells growth: influence of cell proliferation rate. Cancer Lett (IRELAND) Jul 13 1995

Serial transplants of DMBA-induced mammary tumors in Fischer rats as model system for human breast cancer. IV. Parallel changes of biopterin and melatonin indicate interactions between the pineal gland and cellular immunity in malignancy. Oncology (SWITZERLAND) Jul-Aug 1995

Modulation of cancer endocrine therapy by melatonin: a phase II study of tamoxifen plus melatonin in metastatic breast cancer patients progressing under tamoxifen alone. Br J Cancer (ENGLAND) Apr 1995

Modulation of estrogen receptor mRNA expression by melatonin in MCF-7 human breast cancer cells. Mol Endocrinol (UNITED STATES) Dec 1994

Melatonin modulates growth factor activity in MCF-7 human breast cancer cells. J Pineal Res (DEN-MARK) Aug 1994

Differences between pulsatile or continuous exposure to melatonin on MCF-7 human breast cancer cell proliferation. Cancer Lett (IRELAND) Sep 30 1994

Effects of melatonin on cancer: studies on MCF-7 human breast cancer cells in culture. J Neural Transm Suppl (AUSTRIA) 1986, 21 p433-49

Role of pineal gland in aetiology and treatment of breast cancer. Lancet (ENGLAND) Oct 14 1978

Beta-interferon, retinoids and tamoxifen as maintenance therapy in metastatic breast cancer. A pilot study. Clin Ter (ITALY) Oct 1995

The effects of retinoids on proliferative capacities and macromolecular synthesis in human breast cancer MCF-7 cells. Cancer (UNITED STATES) Nov 15 1980

The anti-proliferative effect of vitamin D3 analogues is not mediated by inhibition of the AP-1 pathway, but may be related to promoter selectivity. Oncogene (ENGLAND) Nov 2 1995

Epidemiology of soy and cancer: perspectives and directions. J Nutr (UNITED STATES) Mar 1995, 125 (3 Suppl)

Effects of tyrosine kinase inhibitors on the proliferation of human breast cancer cell lines and proteins important in the ras signaling pathway. Int J Cancer (UNITED STATES) Jan 17 1996

Selective responsiveness of human breast cancer cells to indole-3-carbinol, a chemopreventive agent. J Natl Cancer Inst (UNITED STATES) Jan 19 1994

Differential stimulatory and inhibitory responses of human MCF-7 breast cancer cells to linoleic acid and conjugated linoleic acid in culture. ANTICANCER RES. (Greece), 1992, 12/6 B

Inhibitory effect of conjugated dienoic derivatives of linoleic acid and beta-carotene on the in vitro growth of human cancer cells. CANCER LETT. (Ireland), 1992, 63/2 (125-133)

Preferential cytotoxicity on tumor cells by caffeic acid phenethyl ester isolated from propolis. EXPE-RIENTIA (Switzerland), 1988, 44/3 (230-232)

Effect of caffeic acid esters on carcinogen-induced mutagenicity and human colon adenocarcinoma cell growth. CHEM.-BIOL. INTERACT. (Ireland), 1992, 84/3 (277-290)

Bursitis

See references under Arthritis.

Cancer Chemotherapy

[Effect of biological membrane stabilizing drugs (coenzyme Q10, dextran sulfate and reduced glutathione) on adriamycin (doxorubicin)-induced toxicity and microsomal lipid peroxidation in mice] Gan To Kagaku Ryoho. 1996 Jan. 23(1). P 93-8

Coenzyme Q10, plasma membrane oxidase and growth control. Mol Aspects Med. 1994. 15 SupplP s1-11

Protective effects of various drugs on adriamycin (doxorubicin)-induced toxicity and microsomal lipid peroxidation in mice and rats. Biol Pharm Bull. 1993 Nov. 16(11). P 1114-7

Tissue concentration of doxorubicin (adriamycin) in mouse pretreated with alpha- tocopherol or coenzyme Q10. Acta Med Okayama. 1991 Jun. 45(3). P 195-9

[Electrocardiogram analysis of adriamycin cardiotoxicity in 160 cases] Chung Hua Chung Liu Tsa Chih. 1991 Jan. 13(1). P 71-3

Adriamycin-Fe3+-induced mitochondrial protein damage with lipid peroxidation. Biol Pharm Bull. 1995 Apr. 18(4). P 514-7

Effect of antioxidants on adriamycin-induced microsomal lipid peroxidation. Biol Trace Elem Res. 1995 Jan-Mar. 47(1-3). P 111-6

Alpha tocopherol improves focal glomerulosclerosis In rats with adriamycin-induced progressive renal failure. Nephron. 1994. 68(3). P 347-52

Adriamycin-induced oxidative stress in rat central nervous system. Biochem Mol Biol Int. 1993 Apr. 29(5). P 807-20

[Cardioprotection in chemo- and radiotherapy for malignant diseases—an echocardiographic pilot study] Schweiz Rundsch Med Prax. 1995 Oct 24. 84(43). P 1220-3

Randomised comparison of fluorouracil, epidoxorubicin and methotrexate (FEMTX) plus supportive care with supportive care alone in patients with non-resectable gastric cancer. Br J Cancer. 1995 Mar. 71(3). P 587-91

Enhancement of the antineoplastic effect of anticarcinogens on benzo[a]pyrene- treated Wistar rats, in relation to their number and biological activity. Cancer Lett. 1994 Jul 29. 82(2). P 153-65

Critical reappraisal of vitamins and trace minerals in nutritional support of cancer patients. Support Care Cancer. 1993 Nov. 1(6). P 295-7

The effects of chemotherapy including cisplatin on vitamin D metabolism. Endocr J. 1993 Dec. 40(6). P 737-42

Vitamin A, a useful biochemical modulator capable of preventing intestinal damage during methotrexate treatment. Pharmacol Toxicol. 1993 Aug. 73(2). P 69-74

Chemotherapy-induced alopecia: new developments South Med J. 1993 May. 86(5). P 489-96

Vitamin E enhances the chemotherapeutic effects of adriamycin on humanprostatic carcinoma cells in vitro. J. UROL. (BALTIMORE) (USA), 1986, 136/2 (529-531)

Hematological aspects of vitamin E, continued. Adriamycin cardiotoxicity amelioration by alpha-tocopherol. AM. J. PEDIATR. HEMATOL. ONCOL. (USA), 1979, 1/2 (151-153)

Treatment of cancer-related thrombocytopenia by low-dose subcutaneous Interleukin- 2 plus the pineal hormone melatonin: A biological phase II study. Journal of Biological Regulators and Homeostatic Agents (Italy), 1995, 9/2 (52-54)

Type 2 Th cells as target of the circadian melatonin signal: Relevance in local immunity. Regional Immunology (USA), 1995, 6/5-6 (350-354)

Hematopoietic rescue via T-cell-dependent, endogenous granulocyte- macrophage colony-stimulating factor induced by the pineal neurohormone melatonin in tumor-bearing mice. CANCER RES. (USA), 1994, 54/9 (2429-2432)

Randomized study with the pineal hormone melatonin versus supportive care alone in advanced non-small cell lung cancer resistant to a first-line chemotherapy containing cisplatin. ONCOLOGY (SWITZERLAND) (Switzerland), 1992, 49/5 (336-339)

Preliminary studies on melatonin in the treatment of myelodysplastic syndromes following cancer chemotherapy. J. PINEAL RES. (Denmark), 1990, 8/4 (347-354)

Melatonin increase as predictor for tumor objective response to chemotherapy in advanced cancer patients. TUMORI (Italy), 1988, 74/3 (339-345)

Cancer Radiation Therapy

Taurine deficiency after intensive chemotherapy and/or radiation. Am J Clin Nutr; 55(3):708-11 1992

Effect of glutaurine and its derivatives and their combinations with radiation protective substances upon irradiated mice. Acta Radiol Oncol Radiat Phys Biol; 20(5):319-324 1981

[Effect of mixed gamma-neutron irradiation on taurine penetration through cellular membranes of rat peripheral blood leukocytes] Res. Inst. Biology and Biophysics, V. V. Kuibyshev Tomsk State Univ., Tomsk, USSR

[Sources of taurine hyperexcretion in irradiated rats] Radiobiologiia; 20(3):455-459 1980

[Taurine and sh-group content in the platelets of irradiated rats] Radiobiologiia; 18(2):271-274

Biological Effects of Alkylglycerolsl. Prog Biochem Pharmacol; 22:48-57 1988, (37 Refs)

Effect of alkoxyglycerols on the frequency of injuries following radiation therapy for carcinoma of the uterine cervix. Acta Obstet Gynecol Scand; 56(4):441-448 1977

In vivo radioprotective activity of Panax ginseng and diethyldithiocarbamate. In Vivo; 7(5):467-70 1993

Inhibition of mutagenesis and transformation by root extracts of panax ginseng in vitro. Planta Med;

57(2):125-8 1991

Restoration of radiation injury by ginseng. Ii. Some properties of the radioprotective substances. J Radiat Res (Tokyo); 22(3):336-343

Restoration of radiation injury by ginseng. I. Responses of x-irradiated mice to ginseng extract. J Radiat Res (Tokyo); 22(3):323-335

[Substances stimulating recovery from radiation injury]. Radioisotopes; 27(11):666-675 1978

Acemannan Immunostimulant in combination with surgery and radiation therapy on spontaneous canine and feline fibrosarcomas. J Am Anim Hosp Assoc; 31(5):439-47 1995

Acemannan-containing wound dressing gel reduces radiation-induced skin reactions in C3H mice. Int J Radiat Oncol Biol Phys; 32(4):1047-52 1995

Cancer Surgery

Interleukin 2 treatment in colorectal cancer: current results and future prospects. Eur J Surg Oncol; 20(6):622-9 1994

Perioperative immunomodulation in cancer surgery. Am J Surg; 167(1):174-9 1994

Immune defects in patients with head and neck cancer. Anticancer Res; 13(6B):2507-19 1993

Effects of alprazolam on cellular immune response to surgical stress in mice. Cancer Lett; 73(2-3):155-60 1993

Morphine attenuates surgery-induced enhancement of metastatic colonization in rats. Pain; 54(1):21-8 1993

Narcotic-induced suppression of natural killer cell activity in ventilated and nonventilated rats. Clin Immunol Immunopathol; 64(2):173-6 1992

The impact of surgery on natural killer cell cytotoxicity and tumor metastasis in rats. Diss Abstr Int [B]; 53(4):1776 1992

Altered lymphocyte subsets and natural killer cells of patients with obstructive jaundice in perioperative period. J Tongji Med Univ; 11(3):145-9 1991

Hierarchical immunosuppression of regional lymph nodes in patients with head and neck squamous cell carcinoma. Otolaryngol Head Neck Surg; 105(4):517-27 1991

Effects of alprazolam on t-cell immunosuppressive response to surgical stress in mice. Cancer Lett; 58(3):183-7 1991

Blood transfusion and survival after laryngectomy for laryngeal carcinoma. J Laryngol Otol; 105(4):293-4 1991

[The effect of surgical intervention on the state of the immune system in brain tumors]. Klin Khir; (12):4-6 1990

[Dynamics of various indicators of immunity in relation to the type of anesthesia during surgical treatment of patients with lung cancer after irradiation]. Vestn Khir Im I I Grek; 145(8):99-102 1990

Mechanism of surgical stress impairment of murine natural killer cell cytotoxicity. Diss Abstr Int [B];

51(6):2809 1990

Highly immunogenic regressor tumor cells can prevent development of postsurgical tumor immunity. Cell Immunol; 119(1):101-13 1989

General concepts in cancer treatment. Surgical Oncology: A European Handbook, p. 121-305, 1989

Effects of low dose perioperative interferon on the surgically induced suppression of antitumour immune responses. Br J Surg; 75(10):976-81 1988

Lymphocyte subsets, natural killer cytotoxicity, and perioperative blood transfusion for elective colorectal cancer surgery. Cancer Detect Prev Suppl; 1:571-6 1987

Effect of surgical stress on murine natural killer cell cytotoxicity. J Immunol; 138(1):171-8 1987

Immune suppression: therapeutic alterations. Principles of Cancer Biotherapy, p. 93-162, 1987

Suppression of natural killer cell activity by surgical stress in cancer patients and the underlying mechanisms. Acta Med Okayama; 40(2):113-9 1986

Surgical stress-mediated suppression of murine natural killer cell cytotoxicity. Cancer Res; 44(9):3888-91 1984

Surgery, trauma and immune suppression. Evolving the mechanism. Ann Surg; 197(4):434-8 1983

Surgical essentials in the care of the elderly cancer patient. Aging; 24:57-61 1983

[Postoperative treatment of malignant brain tumors with acnu and psk-particularly immunological follow-up research]. Gan To Kagaku Ryoho; 9(6):1081-90 1982

Principles of pathology in surgery. Principles of Pathology in Surgery, 453 pp., 1980

Small cell carcinoma of the lung. Ann Thorac Surg; 30(6):602-610 1980

Cancer and immunocompetence. Acta Chir Scand Suppl; (498):146-150 1980

Alteration of lymphocyte function due to anesthesia: in vivo and in vitro suppression of mitogen-induced blastogenesis by sodium pentobarbital. Surgery; 87(5):573-580 1980

A mechanism of suppression of antitumor immunity (lai reactivity) by surgery. Cancer Immunol Immunother; 7(4):263-269 1980

[The state of immune responsiveness in various course of stomach cancer]. Vopr Onkol; 23(4):72-76 1977

Effects of operation on immune response in cancer patients: sequential evaluation of in vitro lymphocyte function. Surgery; 79(1):46-51 1976

[Surgery, hormone therapy, and irradiation in a patient with metastasizing mammary carcinoma]. Fortschr Med; 92(14):615-616 1974

Renal impairment associated with the pre-operative administration of recombinant interleukin-2. Clin Sci (Colch); 87(5):513-8 1994

Cancer Treatment

Practices influencing iron status in university women. Nutrition Research (USA), 1997, 17/1 (9-22)

References

Protease inhibitors and carcinogenesis. Cancer Investigation (USA), 1996, 14/6 (597-608)

Inhibition of epidermal growth factor receptor-associated tyrosine kinase blocks glioblastoma invasion of the brain. Neurosurgery (USA), 1997, 40/1 (141-151)

The fatty acid composition of human gliomas differs from that found in nonmalignant brain tissue. Lipids (USA), 1996, 31/12 (1283-1288)

Microdosimetric evaluation of relative biological effectiveness. International Journal of Radiation Oncology Biology Physics (USA), 1996, 36/3 (689-697)

Whole-grain consumption and chronic disease: Protective mechanisms. Nutrition and Cancer (USA), 1997, 27/1 (14-21)

Effect of oestradiol and insulin on the proliferative pattern and on oestrogen and progesterone receptor contents in MCF-7 cells. Journal of Cancer Research and Clinical Oncology (Germany), 1996, 122/12 (745-749)

Vegetable, fruit, and grain consumption to colorectal adenomatous polyps. American Journal of Epidemiology (USA), 1996, 144/11 (1015-1025)

Improvement by eicosanoids in cancer cachexia induced by LLC-IL6 transplantation. Journal of Cancer Research and Clinical Oncology (Germany), 1996, 122/12 (711-715)

Diet and risk of esophageal cancer by histologic type in a low-risk Group. International Journal of Cancer (USA), 1996, 68/3 (300-304)

The effect of unsaturated fatty acids on membrane composition and signal transduction in HT-29 human colon cancer cells. Cancer Letters (Ireland), 1996, 108/1 (25-33)

Genistein-stimulated adherence of prostate cancer cells is associated with the binding of focal adhesion kinase to beta-1-integrin. Clinical and Experimental Metastasis (United Kingdom), 1996, 14/4 (389-398)

Chemoprevention of mammary cancer by diallyl selenide, a novel organoselenium compound. Anticancer Research (Greece), 1996, 16/5 A (2911-2915)

Tofu and risk of breast cancer in Asian-Americans. Cancer Epidemiology Biomarkers and Prevention (USA), 1996, 5/11(901-906)

Dietary calcium, vitamin D, and the risk of colorectal cancer in Stockholm, Sweden. Cancer Epidemiology Biomarkers and Prevention (USA), 1996, 5/11(897-900)

Effect of omega-3 fatty acids on the progression of metastases after the surgical excision of human breast cancer cell solid tumors growing in nude mice. Clinical Cancer Research (USA), 1996, 2/10 (1751-1756)

Regulation of human colonic cell line proliferation and phenotype by sodium butyrate. Digestive Diseases and Sciences (USA), 1996, 41/10 (1986-1993)

Curcumin inhibits the proliferation and cell cycle progression of human umbilical vein endothelial cell. Cancer Letters (Ireland), 1996, 107/1 (109-115)

Cell cycle arrest and induction of apoptosis in pancreatic cancer cells exposed to eicosapentaenoic acid in vivo. British Journal of Cancer (United Kingdom), 1996, 74/9 (1375-1383)

Effects of dietary conjugated linoleic acid on lymphocyte function and growth of mammary tumors in mice. Anticancer Research (Greece), 1997, 17/2 A (987-993)

Conjugated linoleic acid suppresses the growth of human breast adenocarcinoma cells in SCID mice. Anticancer Research (Greece), 1997, 17/2 A (969-973)

Lymphatic recovery, tissue distribution, and metabolic effects of conjugated lioleic acid in rats. Journal of Nutritional Biochemistry (USA), 1997, 8/1 (38-43)

Proliferative responses of normal human mammary and MCF-7 breast cancer cells to linoleic acid, conjugated linoleic acid and eicosanoid synthesis inhibitors in culture. Anticancer Research (Greece), 1997, 17/1 A (197-203)

Conjugated linoleic acid modulates hepatic lipid composition in mice. Lipids (USA), 1997, 32/2 (199-204)

Dietary conjugated linoleic acid modulation of phorbol ester skin tumor promotion. Nutrition and Cancer (USA), 1996, 26/2 (149-157)

The efficacy of conjugated linoleic acid in mammary cancer prevention is independent of the level or type of fat in the diet. Carcinogenesis (United Kingdom), 1996, 17/5 (1045-1050)

Dietary modifiers of carcinogenesis. Environmental Health Perspectives (USA), 1995, 103/SUPPL. 8 (177-184)

Effects of C18 fatty acid isomers on DNA synthesis in hepatoma and breast cancer cells. Anticancer Research (Greece), 1995, 15/5 B (2017-2021)

Effect of timing and duration of dietary conjugated linoleic acid on mammary cancer prevention. Nutrition and Cancer (USA), 1995, 24/3 (241-247)

Reinvestigation of the antioxidant properties of conjugated linoleic acid. Lipids (USA), 1995, 30/7 (599-605)

Furan fatty acids determined as oxidation products of conjugated octadecadienoic acid. Lipids (USA), 1995, 30/7 (595-598)

The role of phenolics, conjugated linoleic acid, carnosine, and pyrroloquinoline quinone as nonessential dietary antioxidants. Nutrition Reviews (USA), 1995, 53/3 (49-58)

Conjugated linoleic acid is a growth factor for rats as shown by enhanced weight gain and improved feed efficiency. J. NUTR. (USA), 1994, 124/12 (2344-2349)

Conjugated linoleic acid: A powerful anticarcinogen from animal fat sources. CANCER (USA), 1994, 74/3 (1050-1054)

Effect of cheddar cheese consumption on plasma conjugated linoleic acid concentrations in men. NUTR. RES. (USA), 1994, 14/3 (373-386)

Intake of selected micronutrients and the risk of endometrial carcinoma. Cancer (USA), 1996, 77/5 (917-923)

Tea in chemoprevention of cancer: Epidemiologic and experimental studies. International Journal of Oncology (Greece), 1996, 8/2 (221-238)

Genistein suppresses growth stimulatory effect of growth factors in HCE 16/3 cells. Chinese Journal of Oncology (China), 1997, 19/2 (118-122)

Intestinal immunocompetency and/or cancer control. Biotherapy (Japan), 1997, 11/4 (524-525)

Chemoprotection against the formation colon DNA adducts from the food-borne carcinogen 2-amino-1-methyl-6-phenylimidazo(4,5-b)pyridine (PhIP) in the rat. Mutation Research - Fundamental and Molecular Mechanisms of Mutagenesis (Netherlands), 1997, 376/1-2 (115-122)

Effects of protein kinase and phosphatase inhibitors on the growth of human prostatic cancer cells. Medical Science Research (United Kingdom), 1997, 25/5 (353-354)

Estrogenic activity of natural and synthetic estrogens in human breast cancer cells in culture. Environmental Health Perspectives (USA), 1997, 105/SUPPL. 3 (637-645)

Dietary estrogens stimulate human breast cells to enter the cell cycle. Environmental Health Perspectives (USA), 1997, 105/SUPPL. 3 (633-636)

Medical hypothesis: Bifunctional genetic-hormonal pathways to breast cancer. Environmental Health Perspectives (USA), 1997, 105/SUPPL. 3 (571-576)

Natural products and their derivatives as cancer chemopreventive agents. Progress in Drug Research (Switzerland), 1997, 48/- (147-171)

Isolation of isoflavones from soy-based fermentations of the erythromycin-producing bacterium Saccharopolyspora erythraea. Applied Microbiology and Biotechnology (Germany), 1997, 47/4 (398-404)

Migration of highly aggressive MV3 melanoma cells in 3-dimensional collagen lattices results in local matrix reorganization and shedding of alpha2 and beta1 integrins and CD44. Cancer Research (USA), 1997, 57/10 (2061-2070)

Inhibition of growth and induction of differentiation of metastatic melanoma cells in vitro by genistein: Chemosensitivity is regulated by cellular p53. British Journal of Cancer (United Kingdom), 1997, 75/11 (1559-1566)

Phyto-oestrogens and Western diseases. Annals of Medicine (United Kingdom), 1997, 29/2 (95-120)

Preclinical studies of the combination of angiogenic inhibitors with cytotoxic agents. Investigational New Drugs (USA), 1997, 15/1 (39-48)

Curcumin and genistein, plant natural produbreast cancer MCF-7 cells induced by estrogenic pesticides. Biochemical and Biophysical Research Communications (USA), 1997, 233/3 (692-696)

New agents for cancer chemoprevention. Nation996, 63/SUPPL. 26 (1-28)

Glutathione S-transferases of female A/J mouse lung and their induction by anticarcinogenic organosulfides from garlic. Archives of Biochemistry and Biophysics (USA), 1997, 340/2 (279-286)

Metabolic support of the gastrointestinal tract: Potential gut protection during intensive cytotoxic therapy. Cancer (USA), 1997, 79/9 (1794-1803)

Inhibition of malignant cell proliferation by culture media conditioned by cardiac or skeletal muscle. Cell Biology International (United Kingdom), 1997, 21/3 (133-144)

A diet rich in fat and poor in dietary fiber increases the in vitro formation of reactive oxygen species in human feces. Journal of Nutrition (USA), 1997, 127/5 (706-709)

Inhibition of 12-O-tetradecanoylphorbol-13-acetate induced Epstein-Barr virus early antigen activation by natural colorants. Cancer Letters (Ireland), 1997, 115/2 (173-178)

The bovine papillomavirus E6 oncoprotein interacts with paxillin and disrupts the actin cytoskeleton. Proceedings of the National Academy of Sciences of the United States of America (USA), 1997, 94/9 (4412-4417)

Genistein inhibits proliferation and in vitro invasive potential of human prostatic cancer cell lines. Anticancer Research (Greece), 1997, 17/2 A (1199-1204)

Assessment of cyclooxygenase inhibitors using in vitro assay systems. Methods in Cell Science (Netherlands), 1997, 19/1 (25-31)

Activation of gelatinase A (72-kDa type IV collagenase) induced by monensin in normal human fibroblasts. Experimental Cell Research (USA), 1997, 232/2 (322-330)

Selective modulation of cell adhesion molecules on lymphocytes by bromelain protease 5. Pathobiology (Switzerland), 1996, 64/6 (339-346)

Overview of the epidemiology of colorectal cancer. Diseases of the Colon and Rectum (USA), 1997, 40/4 (483-493)

Suppression of nitric oxide production in lipopolysaccharide-stimulated macrophage cells by omega3 polyunsaturated fatty acids. Japanese Journal of Cancer Research (Japan), 1997, 88/3 (234-237)

The effect of nutritional intervention on immune functions and other biomarkers in high cancer risk individuals

Adenocarcinomas of the esophagus and gastric cardia: The role of diet. Nutrition and Cancer (USA), 1997, 27/3 (298-309)

Effects of high- and low-risk diets on gut microflora-associated biomarkers of colon cancer in human flora-associated rats. Nutrition and Cancer (USA), 1997, 27/3 (250-255)

Eating to beat breast cancer: Potential role for soy supplements. Annals of Oncology (Netherlands), 1997, 8/3 (223-225)

Position of the American Dietetic Association: Phytochemicals and functional foods. Journal of Nutraceuticals, Functional and Medical Foods (USA), 1997, 1/1 (33-45)

Angiogenesis as a target for tumor treatment. Oncology (Switzerland), 1997, 54/3 (177-184)

Identification of compounds with preferential inhibitory activity against low-Nm23-expressing human breast carcinoma and melanoma cell lines. Nature Medicine (USA), 1997, 3/4 (395-401)

Activation of mitogenic signaling by endothelin 1 in ovarian carcinoma cells. Cancer Research (USA), 1997, 57/7 (1306-1311)

Modulation of apoptosis by sulindac, curcumin, phenylethyl-3- methylcaffeate, and 6-phenylhexyl isothiocyanate: Apoptotic index as a biomarker in colon cancer chemoprevention and promotion. Cancer Research (USA), 1997, 57/7 (1301-1305)

Reduction of urinary mutagen excretion in rats fed garlic. Cancer Letters (Ireland), 1997, 114/1-2 (185-186)

Meat, starch and non-starch polysaccharides, are epidemiological and experimental findings consistent with acquired genetic alterations in sporadic colorectal cancer? Cancer Letters (Ireland), 1997, 114/1-2 (25-34)

Induction of human adenocarcinoma cell differentiation by the phytoestrogen genistein is independent of its antiestrogenic function. International Journal of Oncology (Greece), 1997, 10/4 (753-757)

Metabolism of the chemoprotective agent diallyl sulfide to glutathione conjugates in rats. Chemical Research in Toxicology (USA), 1997, 10/3 (318-327)

Incorporation of long-chain n-3 fatty acids in tissues and enhanced bone marrow cellularity with docosahexaenoic acid feeding in post-weanling Fischer 344 rats. Lipids (USA), 1997, 32/3 (293-302)

Differential effects of polyunsaturated fatty acids on chemosensitivity of NIH3T3 cells and its transformants. International Journal of Cancer (USA), 1997, 70/3 (357-361)

The new dietary fats in health and disease. Journal of the American Dietetic Association (USA), 1997, 97/3 (280-286)

Inhibition of proliferation of estrogen receptor-positive MCF-7 human breast cancer cells by flavonoids in the presence and absence of excess estrogen. Cancer Letters (Ireland), 1997, 112/2 (127-133)

S-allylmercaptocysteine inhibits cell proliferation and reduces the viability of erythroleukemia, breast, and prostate cancer cell lines. Nutrition and Cancer (USA), 1997, 27/2 (186-191)

Inhibition of N-methyl-N-nitrosourea-induced mammary tumors in rats by the soybean isoflavones Anticancer Research (Greece), 1996, 16/6 A (3293-3298)

Experimental approaches to therapy and prophylaxis for heat stress and heatstroke. Wilderness and Environmental Medicine (USA), 1996, 7/4 (312-334)

Genistein-induced apoptosis of prostate cancer cells is preceded by a specific decrease in focal adhesion kinase activity. Molecular Pharmacology (USA), 1997, 51/2 (193-200)

Male rats fed methyl- and folate-deficient diets with or without niacin develop hepatic carcinomas associated with decreased tissue NAD concentrations and altered poly(ADP-ribose) polymerase activity. Journal of Nutrition (USA), 1997, 127/1 (30-36)

Nutritional and lifestyle habits and water-fiber interaction in colorectal adenoma etiology. Cancer Epidemiology Biomarkers and Prevention (USA), 1997, 6/2 (79-85)

Prevention of mammary preneoplastic transformation by naturally-occurring tumor inhibitors. Cancer Letters (Ireland), 1997, 111/1-2 (141-147)

Nitric oxide scavenging by curcuminoids. Journal of Pharmacy and Pharmacology (United Kingdom), 1997, 49/1 (105-107)

Antiproliferative potency of structurally distinct dietary flavonoids on human colon cancer cells. Cancer Letters (Ireland), 1996, 110/1-2 (41-48)

Dietary fat and colon cancer: Modulating effect of types and amount of dietary fat on ras-p21 function during promotion and progression stages

Short-chain fructo-oligosaccharides reduce the occurrence of colon tumors and develop gut-associated lymphoid tissue in Min mice. Cancer Research (USA), 1997, 57/2 (225-228)

Usage and users of natural remedies in a middle-aged population: Demographic and psychosocial characteristics. Results from the Malmo Diet and Cancer Study. Pharmacoepidemiology and Drug Safety (United Kingdom), 1996, 5/5 (303-314)

T-cell adjuvants. Int J Immunopharmacol; 16(9):703-10 1994

Therapy of secondary t-cell immunodeficiencies with biological substances and drugs. Med Oncol Tumor Pharmacother; 6(1):11-7 1989

Immunological effects of isoprinosine as a pulse immunotherapy in melanoma and arc patients. Cancer Detect Prev Suppl; 1:457-62 1987

Isoprinosine as an immunopotentiator in an animal model of human osteosarcoma. Int J Immunopharmacol; 3(4):383-389 1981

Immune effects of preoperative immunotherapy with high-dose subcutaneous interleukin-2 versus neuroimmunotherapy with low-dose interleukin-2 plus the neurohormone melatonin in gastrointestinal tract tumor patients. J Biol Regul Homeost Agents; 9(1):31-3 1995

The immunoneuroendocrine role of melatonin. J Pineal Res; 14(1):1-10 1993

Endocrine and immune effects of melatonin therapy in metastatic cancer patients. Eur J Cancer Clin Oncol; 25(5):789-95 1989

Potential of tyrosine kinase receptors as therapeutic targets in cancer. Cancer Therapy in the Twenty-First Century, Vol 1, p.49-81, 1994.

In vitro inhibition of proliferation of MDA-MB-435 human breast cancer cells by combinations of tocotrienols and flavonoids (Meeting abstract). FASEB J; 9(4):A868 1995

Effects of tyrosine kinase inhibitors on the proliferation of human breast cancer cell lines and proteins important in the ras signaling pathway. Int J Cancer; 65(2):186-91 1996

Reversal of multidrug resistance in vivo by dietary administration of the phytochemical indole-3-carbinol. Cancer Res; 56(3):574-81 1996

Differential sensitivity of human prostatic cancer cell lines to the effects of protein kinase and phosphatase inhibitors. Cancer Lett; 98(1):103-10 1995

Growth regulation of the human papillary thyroid cancer cell line by protein tyrosine kinase and cAMP-dependent protein kinase. Endocr J; 41(4):399-407 1994

The effects of different combinations of flavonoids on the proliferation of MDA-MB-435 human breast cancer cells (Meeting abstract). Proc Annu Meet Am Assoc Cancer Res; 36:A3538 1995

Preferential requirement for protein tyrosine phosphatase activity in the 12-O- tetradecanoylphorbol-13-acetate-induced differentiation of human colon cancer cells. Biochem Pharmacol; 50(8):1217-22 1995

Bioactive organosulfur phytochemicals in Brassica oleracea vegetables—a review. Food Chem Toxicol; 33(6):537-43 1995

[Growth and invasion of differentiated thyroid gland carcinoma: importance of signal transduction]. Langenbecks Arch Chir; 380(2):96-101 1995

Nerve growth factor stimulates clonal growth of human lung cancer cell lines and a human glioblastoma cell line expressing high-affinity nerve growth factor binding sites involving tyrosine kinase signaling. Cancer Res; 55(10):2212-9 1995

Evaluation of the biochemical targets of genistein in tumor cells. J Nutr; 125(3 Suppl):784S-789S 1995

In vitro hormonal effects of soybean isoflavones. J Nutr; 125(3 Suppl):751S-756S 1995

Resistance of melanoma cell lines to interferons correlates with reduction of IFN- induced tyrosine phosphorylation. Induction of the anti-viral state by IFN is prevented by tyrosine kinase inhibitors. J Immunol; 154(5):2248-56 1995

Biotherapy of B-cell precursor leukemia by targeting genistein to CD19-associated tyrosine kinases. Science; 267(5199):886-91 1995

Genistein inhibits the growth of prostate cancer cells. What is the mechanism? Proc Annu Meet Am Assoc Cancer Res; 36:A2310 1995

Growth-inhibitory effects of the natural phyto-oestrogen genistein in MCF-7 human breast cancer cells. Eur J Cancer; 30A(11):1675-82 1994

Natural flavonoids and lignans are potent cytostatic agents against human leukemic HL-60 cells. Life Sci; 55(13):1061-9 1994

The natural tyrosine kinase inhibitor genistein produces cell cycle arrest and apoptosis in Jurkat T-leukemia cells. Leuk Res; 18(6):431-9 1994

Selective responsiveness of human breast cancer cells to indole-3-carbinol, a chemopreventive agent. J Natl Cancer Inst; 86(2):126-31 1994

Genistein is an effective stimulator of sex hormone-binding globulin production in hepatocarcinoma human liver cancer cells and suppresses proliferation of these cells in culture. Steroids; 58(7):301-4 1993

Lycopene is a more potent inhibitor of human cancer cell proliferation than either alpha-carotene or beta-carotene. Nutr Cancer; 24(3):257-66 1995

Inhibitory effect of 220-oxa-1,25-dihydroxyvitamin D3 on the proliferation of pancreatic cancer cell lines. Gastroenterology; 110(5):1605-13 1996

Antiproliferative responses to two human colon cancer cell lines to vitamin D3 are differently modified by 9-cis-retinoic acid. Cancer Res; 56(3):623-32 1996

Vitamin D: a modulator of cell proliferation and differentiation. J Steroid Biochem Mol Biol; 37(6):873-6 1990

Preferential cytotoxicity on tumor cells by caffeic acid phenethyl ester isolated from propolis. EXPERIENTIA (Switzerland), 1988, 44/3 (230-232)

Effect of caffeic acid esters on carcinogen-induced mutagenicity and human colon adenocarcinoma cell growth. CHEM.-BIOL. INTERACT. (Ireland), 1992, 84/3 (277-290)

Candida (Fungal, Yeast) Infections

[Fecal microflora in healthy young people]. Zh Mikrobiol Epidemiol Immunobiol (USSR) Feb 1983, (2) p36-40

Biotherapeutic agents. A neglected modality for the treatment and prevention of selected intestinal and vaginal infections. JAMA (UNITED STATES) Mar 20 1996, 275 (11) p870-6

Influence of lactobacilli on the adhesion of Staphylococcus aureus and Candida albicans to fibers and epithelial cells. J Ind Microbiol (ENGLAND) Sep 1995, 15 (3) p248-53

Effect of Lactobacillus acidophilus on antibiotic-associated gastrointestinal morbidity: a prospective randomized trial. J Otolaryngol (CANADA) Aug 1995, 24 (4) p230-3

Inhibition of Candida albicans by Lactobacillus acidophilus: evidence for the involvement of a peroxidase system. Microbios (ENGLAND) 1994, 80 (323) p125-33

Ingestion of yogurt containing Lactobacillus acidophilus as prophylaxis for candidal vaginitis [see comments]. Ann Intern Med (UNITED STATES) Mar 1 1992, 116 (5) p353-7

Evidence for the involvement of thiocyanate in the inhibition of Candida albicans by Lactobacillus acidophilus. Microbios (ENGLAND) 1990, 62 (250) p37-46

Viricidal effects of Lactobacillus and yeast fermentation. Appl Environ Microbiol (UNITED STATES) Aug 1983, 46 (2) p452-8

Inhibition of Candida albicans by Lactobacillus acidophilus. J Dairy Sci (UNITED STATES) May 1980, 63 (5) p830-2

Thrush bowel infection: existence, incidence, prevention and treatment, particularly by a Lactobacillus acidophilus preparation. Curr Med Drugs (ENGLAND) Dec 1967, 8 (4) p3-11

[Candida infection of the female genitalia. Complaints and clinical findings] Candidainfektion des weiblichen dGenitales. Beschwerden und Befund. Med Klin (GERMANY, WEST) Jan 31 1969, 64 (5) p203-6

Dietary supplement of neosugar alters the fecal flora and decreases activities of some reductive enzymes in human subjects. Am J Clin Nutr (UNITED STATES) May 1996, 63 (5) p709-16

In vitro fructooligosaccharide utilization and inhibition of Salmonella spp. by selected bacteria. Poult Sci (UNITED STATES) Sep 1995, 74 (9) p1418-25

Dietary fructooligosaccharide, xylooligosaccharide and gum arabic have variable effects on cecal and colonic microbiota and epithelial cell proliferation in mice and rats. J Nutr (UNITED STATES) Oct 1995, 125 (10) p2604-9

A comparison of susceptibility to five antifungal agents of yeast cultures from burn patients. Burns (ENGLAND) May 1995, 21 (3) p167-70

[A trial of the use of diflucan (fluconazole) in patients with vaginal candidiasis]. Antibiot Khimioter. 1993 Dec. 38(12). P 39-41

[Fluconazole—a new antifungal agent]. Tidsskr Nor Laegeforen. 1992 Jun 10. 112(15). P 1961-3

[Endogenous candida endophthalmitis: a new therapy]. Klin Monatsbl Augenheilkd. 1991 Dec. 199(6). P 446-9

Perspective Evaluation of Candida Antigen Detection Test For Invasive Candidiasis and Immunocompromised Adult Patients With Cancer. The American Journal of Medicine, December 1989;87(621-627)

Pathogenesis of Candidiasis: Immunosuppression By Cell Wall Mannan Catabolites, Archives of Surgery, November 1989; 124:1290-1294

Ingestion of Yogurt Containing Lactobacillus Acidophilus as Prophylaxis for Candidal Vaginitis. Annals of Internal Medicine, March 1, 1992;116(5):353-357

Garlic: A Review of Its Relationship to Malignant Disease. Preventive Medicine, May 1990;19(3):346-361

Anticandidal and Anticarcinogenic Potentials For Garlic. International Clinical Nutrition Review, October 1990;10(4):423-429.

Vaginal Flora and Urinary Tract Infections. Current Opinion in Infectious Disease, 1991;4:37-41

Regulation of The Immune Response to Candida Albicans by Monocyte and Progesterone. American Journal of Obstetrics and Gynecology, 1991;164:1351-4

Hydrogen Peroxide-Producing Organisms Toxic To Vaginal Bacteria. Infectious Disease News, August 8, 1991;5

The Vaginal Ecosystem. Mardh, Per-Anders, M.D., American Journal of Obstetrics and Gynecology, October 1991;165(4): Part II:1163-1168.

Ingestion of Yogurt Containing Lactobacillus Acidophilus as Prophylaxis for Candidal Vaginitis. Annals of Internal Medicine, March 1, 1992;116(5);353-357

Catabolic Wasting

Feeding conjugated linoleic acid to animals partially overcomes catabolic responses due to endotoxin injection. Biochem Biophys Res Commun (UNITED STATES) Feb 15 1994, 198

Inhibition of lipolysis and muscle protein degradation by EPA in cancer cachexia. Nutrition (USA), 1996, 12/1 SUPPL. (S31-S33)

The effect of polyunsaturated fatty acids on the progress of cachexia in patients with pancreatic cancer. Nutrition (USA), 1996, 12/1 SUPPL. (S27-S30)

Comparison of the effectiveness of eicosapentaenoic acid administered as either the free acid or ethyl ester as an anticachectic and antitumour agent. PROSTAGLANDINS LEUKOTRIENES ESSENT. FATTY ACIDS (United Kingdom), 1994, 51/2 (141-145)

Kinetics of the inhibition of tumour growth in mice by eicosapentaenoic acid-reversal by linoleic acid. BIOCHEM. PHARMACOL. (United Kingdom), 1993, 45/11 (2189-2194)

Anticachectic and antitumor effect of eicosapentaenoic acid and its effect on protein turnover. CANCER RES. (USA), 1991, 51/22 (6089-6093)

Muscle wasting and dedifferentiation induced by oxidative stress in a murine model of cachexia is prevented by inhibitors of nitric oxide synthesis and antioxidants. EMBO Journal (United Kingdom), 1996, 15/8 (1753-1765)

Modulation of immune function and weight loss by L-arginine in obstructive jaundice in the rat. BR. J. SURG. (United Kingdom), 1994, 81/8 (1199-1201)

Effects of L-carnitine on serum triglyceride and cytokine levels in rat models of cachexia and septic shock. British Journal of Cancer (United Kingdom), 1995, 72/5

L-carnitine deficiency in AIDS patients. AIDS (United Kingdom), 1992, 6/2 (203-205)

The enzymatic activities of branched-chain amino acid catabolism in tumour-bearing rats. CANCER LETT. (Ireland), 1992, 61/3 (239-242)

Branched chain amino acids as the protein component of parenteral nutrition in cancer cachexia. BR. J. SURG. (United Kingdom), 1989, 76/2 (149-153)

Zinc in different tissues: Relation to age and local concentrations in cachexia, liver cirrhosis and long-term intensive care. INFUSIONSTHER. KLIN. ERNAHR. (SWITZERLAND), 1979, 6/4 (225-229)

The role of serum protein in congestive heart failure. Nutritional support in organ failure: proceedings of the International Symposium, 1990, -/- (45- 52)

Clinical rise of a combination containing phosphocreatinine as adjuvant to physiokinesiotherapy. RIABILITAZIONE (ITALY), 1976, 9/2 (51-62)

Myopathy and HIV infection. Current Opinion in Rheumatology (USA), 1995, 7/6 (497-502)

Effects of L-carnitine on serum triglyceride and cytokine levels in rat models of cachexia and septic shock. British Journal of Cancer (United Kingdom), 1995, 72/5

Cataract

Stereospecific effects of R-lipoic acid on buthionine sulfoximine-induced cataract formation in newborn rats. Biochem Biophys Res Commun (UNITED STATES) Apr 16 1996, 221 (2) p422-9

Alpha-Lipoic acid as a biological antioxidant. Free Radic Biol Med (UNITED STATES) Aug 1995, 19 (2) p 227-50

Alpha-lipoic acid supplementation prevents symptoms of vitamin E deficiency. Biochem Biophys Res Commun (UNITED STATES) Oct 14 1994

A review of the evidence supporting melatonin's role as an antioxidant. J Pineal Res (DENMARK) Jan 1995, 18 (1) p1-11

Glutathione deficiency decreases tissue ascorbate levels in newborn rats: ascorbate spares glutathione and protects against oxidative damage. Proc Natl Acad Sci U S A (UNITED STATES) Jun 1 1991, 88 (11) p4656-60

51Cr release and oxidative stress in the lens. Lens Eye Toxic Res (UNITED STATES) 1989, 6 (1-2) p183-202

Free radical tissue damage: protective role of antioxidant nutrients. FASEB J (UNITED STATES) Dec 1987, 1 (6) p441-5

Oxidative damage and defense. Am J Clin Nutr (US) Jun 1996, 63 (6) p985S-990S

[Antioxidative vitamins and cataracts in the elderly]. Z Ernahrungswiss (GERMANY) Sep 1995, 34 (3) p167-76

Alpha-lipoic acid prevents buthionine sulfoximine-induced cataract formation in newborn rats. Free Radic Biol Med (UNITED STATES) Apr 1995, 18 (4) p823-9

Prevention of cataracts by nutritional and metabolic antioxidants. Crit Rev Food Sci Nutr (UNITED STATES) 1995, 35 (1-2) p111-29

Free radicals, exercise, and antioxidant supplementation. Int J Sport Nutr (UNITED STATES) Sep 1994, 4 (3) p205-20, Comment in Int J Sport Nutr 1994 Sep;4(3):203-4

The use of vitamin supplements and the risk of cataract among US male physicians. Am J Public Health (UNITED STATES) May 1994, 84 (5) p788-92

Modelling cortical cataractogenesis VII: Effects of vitamin E treatment on galactose- induced cataracts. Exp Eye Res (ENGLAND) Feb 1985, 40 (2) p213-22

Modeling cortical cataractogenesis. V. Steroid cataracts induced by solumedrol partially prevented by vitamin E in vitro. Exp Eye Res (ENGLAND) Jul 1983, 37 (1) p65-76

Antioxidant vitamins in cataract prevention. Z Ernahrungswiss (GERMANY, WEST) Mar 1989, 28 (1) p56-75

Biochemical and morphological changes in the lenses of selenium and/or vitamin E deficient rats. Biomed Environ Sci (UNITED STATES) Jun 1994, 7 (2) p109-15

Biochemical changes and cataract formation in lenses from rats receiving multiple, low doses of sodium selenite. Exp Eye Res (ENGLAND) Nov 1992, 55 (5) p671-8

Defense system of the lens against oxidative damage: effect of oxidative challenge on cataract formation in glutathione peroxidase deficient-acatalasemic mice. Exp Eye Res (ENGLAND) Oct 1980, 31 (4) p425-33 (no abstract)

Intraocular irrigating solutions and lens clarity. AMER.J.OPHTHAL. (USA), 1976, 82/4 (594-597)

Intraocular irrigating solutions. Their effect on the corneal endothelium. ARCH.OPHTHAL. (USA), 1975, 93/8 (648-657)

Cerebral Vascular Disease

The effect of hypertension on cerebral atherosclerosis in the cynomolgus monkey. STROKE (USA), 1993, 24/8 (1218-1227)

The case for intravenous magnesium treatment of arterial disease in general practice: Review of 34 years of experience. J. NUTR. MED. (United Kingdom), 1994, 4/2 (169-177)

Neuropsychiatric complications of cardiac surgery. J. CARDIOTHORAC. VASC. ANESTH. (USA), 1994, 8/1 SUPPL. 1 (13-18)

Effects of the dipyridamol-dihydroergotoxine (Hydergine) methane sulphonate associations on pOsub 2 and its incidence in brain tissue. GEN. PHARMACOL. (ENGLAND), 1983, 14/6 (579-583)

The protective effects of dietary fish oil on focal cerebral infarction. PROSTAGLANDINS MED. (USA), 1979, 3/5 (257-268)

What causes infarction in ischemic brain? NEUROLOGY (USA), 1983, 33/2 (222-233)

Effects of antihypertensive drugs on blood velocity: implications for prevention of cerebral vascular disease. CANAD.J.NEUROL.SCI. (CANADA), 1977, 4/2 (93-97)

Oxygen radicals in cerebral vascular injury. CIRC. R RES. (USA), 1985, 57/4 (508-516)

Postischemic tissue injury by iron-mediated free radical lipid peroxidation. USA ANN. EMERG. MED. (USA), 1985, 14/8 (804-809)

Role of iron ions in the genesis of reperfusion injury following successful cardiopulmonary resuscitation: Preliminary data and a biochemical hypothesis. ANN. EMERG. MED. (USA), 1985, 14/8 (777-783)

Cortical pOsub 2 distribution during oligemic hypotension and its pharmacological modifications (Hydergine). SWITZERLAND ARZNEIM.-FORSCH. (GERMANY, WEST), 1978, 28/5 (768-770)

The use of piracetam (Nootropil) in post-anesthetic recovery of elderly patients. (A preliminary study). GREECE ACTA ANAESTHESIOL. HELL. (GREECE), 1981, 15/1-2 (76-80)

Free radical reaction products and antioxidant capacity in arterial plasma during coronary artery bypass grafting. J. THORAC. CARDIOVASC. SURG. (USA), 1994, 108/1 (140-147)

Biochemical studies of cerebral ischemia in the rat - Changes in cerebral free amino acids, catecholamines and uric acid. JAPAN BRAIN NERVE (JAPAN), 1986, 38/3 (253-258)

Free radicals scavenging action and anti-enzyme activities of procyanidines from Vitis vinifera. A mechanism for their capillary protective action. Arzneimittelforschung (GERMANY) May 1994, 44 (5) p592-601

Prevention of postischemic cardiac injury by the orally active iron chelator 1,2- dimethyl-3-hydroxy-4-pyridone (L1) and the antioxidant (+)-cyanidanol-3. CIRCULATION (USA), 1989, 80/1 (158-164)

Iron-load increases the susceptibility of rat hearts to oxygen reperfusion damage. Protection by the antioxidant (+)-cyanidanol-3 and deferoxamine. CIRCULATION (USA), 1988, 78/2 (442-449)

Cholesterol Reduction

Clinical trials with gugulipid. A new hypolipidaemic agent. J Assoc Physicians India (INDIA) May 1989, 37 (5) p323-8

Hypolipidemic and antioxidant effects of Commiphora mukul as an adjunct to dietary therapy in patients with hypercholesterolemia. Cardiovasc Drugs Ther (UNITED STATES) Aug 1994, 8 (4) p659-64

Beneficial effects of Allium sativum (garlic), Allium cepa and Commiphora mukul on experimental hyperlipidemia and atherosclerosis—a comparative evaluation. J Postgrad Med (INDIA) Jul 1991, 37 (3) p132-5

Curcumin, a major component of food spice turmeric (Curcuma longa) inhibits aggregation and alters eicosanoid metabolism in human blood platelets. Prostaglandins Leukotrienes and Essential Fatty Acids (United Kingdom), 1995, 52/4 (223- 227)

Influence of capsaicin, eugenol, curcumin and ferulic acid on sucrose-induced hypertriglyceridemia in rats. NUTR. REP. INT. (USA), 1988, 38/3 (571-581)

Inhibitory effect of curcumin, an anti-inflammatory agent, on vascular smooth muscle cell proliferation. EUR. J. PHARMACOL. (Netherlands), 1992, 221/2-3 (381-384)

Polyphenols as cancer chemopreventive agents. J Cell Biochem Suppl (UNITED STATES) 1995, 22 p169-80

Anti-tumour and antioxidant activity of natural curcuminoids. Cancer Lett (IRELAND) Jul 20 1995, 94 (1) p79-83

Phospholipid epitopes for mouse antibodies against bromelain-treated mouse erythrocytes. Immunology (ENGLAND) Sep 1987, 62 (1) p11-6

The effect of spices on cholesterol 7 alpha-hydroxylase activity and on serum and hepatic cholesterol levels in the rat. Int J Vitam Nutr Res (SWITZERLAND) 1991, 61 (4) p364-9

Effect of gugulipid on bioavailability of diltiazem and propranolol. J Assoc Physicians India (INDIA) Jun 1994, 42 (6) p454-5

Clinical trials with gugulipid. A new hypolipidaemic agent. J Assoc Physicians India (INDIA) May 1989, 37 (5) p323-8

Biological effects of isoflavones in young women: Importance of the chemical composition of soy-abean products. British Journal of Nutrition (United Kingdom), 1995, 74/4 (587-601)

Overview of proposed mechanisms for the hypocholesterolemic effect of soy. Journal of Nutrition (USA), 1995, 125/3 SUPPL. (606S-611S)

Biological effects of a diet of soy protein rich in isoflavones on the menstrual cycle of premenopausal women. AM. J. CLIN. NUTR. (USA), 1994, 60/3 (333-340)

A review of the clinical effects of phytoestrogens. Obstetrics and Gynecology (USA), 1996, 87/5 II SUPPL. (897-904)

Nutritional interest of flavonoids. Medecine et Nutrition (France), 1996, 32/1 (17-27)

Inhibition of protein tyrosine kinase alters the effect of serum basic protein I on triacylglycerols and cholesterol differently in normal and hyperapoB fibroblasts. Arteriosclerosis, Thrombosis, and Vascular Biology (USA), 1995, 15/8 (1195-1203)

Influence of dietary curcumin and cholesterol on the progression of experimentally induced diabetes in albino rat. Molecular and Cellular Biochemistry (USA), 1995, 152/1 (13-21)

Effect of retinol deficiency and curcumin or turmeric feeding on brain Na+-K+ adenosine triphos-phatase activity. MOL. CELL. BIOCHEM. (USA), 1994, 137/2 (101-107)

Bioactive substances in food: Identification and potential uses. CAN. J. PHYSIOL. PHARMACOL. (Canada), 1994, 72/4 (423-434)

Mechanism of antiinflammatory actions of curcumine and boswellic acids. J. ETHNOPHARMACOL. (Ireland), 1993, 38/2-3 (113-119)

Influence of dietary spices on adrenal steroidogenesis in rats. NUTR. RES. (USA), 1993, 13/4 (435-444)

Differential effects of dietary lipids and curcumin on kidney microsomal fatty acids and Na+, K+ - ATPase activity in rat. NUTR. RES. (USA), 1992, 12/7 (893-904)

Chronic Fatigue Syndrome

Isolated diastolic dysfunction of the myocardium and its response to CoQ10 treatment. Clin Investig (GERMANY) 1993, 71 (8 Suppl) pS140-4

Analysis of dietary intake and selected nutrient concentrations in patients with chronic fatigue syndrome. J Am Diet Assoc (UNITED STATES) Apr 1996, 96 (4) p383-6

[Chronic fatigue syndrome]. Nippon Naika Gakkai Zasshi (JAPAN) Sep 10 1993, 82 (9) p1571-6

Electron-microscopic investigation of muscle mitochondria in chronic fatigue syndrome. Neuropsychobiology (SWITZERLAND) 1995, 32 (4) p175-81

Serum levels of carnitine in chronic fatigue syndrome: clinical correlates. Neuropsychobiology (SWITZERLAND) 1995, 32 (3) p132-8

Acylcarnitine deficiency in chronic fatigue syndrome. Clin Infect Dis (UNITED STATES) Jan 1994, 18 Suppl 1 pS62-7

Cirrhosis

See references under Liver (Cirrhosis)

Common Cold

Problems and prospects of developing effective therapy for common cold viruses. Trends in Microbiology (United Kingdom), 1997, 5/2 (58-63)

Vitamin C intake and susceptibility to the common cold. British Journal of Nutrition (United Kingdom), 1997, 77/1 (59-72)

Vitamin C supplementation and common cold symptoms: Problems with inaccurate reviews. Nutrition (USA), 1996, 12/11-12 (804-809):

Vitamin C, the placebo effect, and the common cold: A case study of how preconceptions influence the analysis of results. Journal of Clinical Epidemiology (USA), 1996, 49/10 (1079-1085,1087)

Vitamin C and common cold incidence: A review of studies with subjects under heavy physical stress. International Journal of Sports Medicine (Germany), 1996, 17/5 (379-383)

Herbal immuno-stimulants. Zeitschrift fur Phytotherapie (Germany), 1996, 17/2 (79-95)

Epidemiology, pathogenesis, and treatment of the common cold. Annals of Allergy, Asthma and Immunology (USA), 1997, 78/6 (531-540)

Zinc lozenges for the common cold (4). Journal of Family Practice (USA), 1997, 44/6 (526)

Zinc lozenges reduce the duration of common cold symptoms. Nutrition Reviews (USA), 1997, 55/3 (82-85):

The age-associated decline in immune function of healthy individuals is not related to changes in plasma concentrations of beta-carotene, retinol, alpha-tocopherol or zinc. Mechanisms of Ageing and Development (Ireland), 1997, 94/1-3 (55-69)

Zinc gluconate lozenges for treating the common cold (1) (multiple letters). Annals of Internal

References

Medicine (USA), 1997, 126/9 (738-739)

Zinc for the common cold. Medical Letter on Drugs and Therapeutics (USA), 1997, 39/993 (9-10)

The common cold. Primary Care - Clinics in Office Practice (USA), 1996, 23/4 (657-675)

How does zinc modify the common cold? Clinical observations and implications regarding mechanisms of action. Medical Hypotheses (United Kingdom), 1996, 46/3 (295-302)

Zinc for treating the common cold: review of all clinical trials since 1984. Altern Ther Health Med (UNITED STATES) Nov 1996, 2 (6) p63-72

Zinc gluconate lozenges for treating the common cold. A randomized, double-blind, placebo-controlled study [see comments]. Ann Intern Med (UNITED STATES) Jul 15 1996, 125 (2) p81-8, Comment in Ann Intern Med 1996 Jul 15;125(2):142-4

Social ties and susceptibility to the common cold. JAMA (UNITED STATES) Jun 25 1997, 277 (24) p1940-4

In vivo anti-influenza virus activity of a zinc finger peptide. Antimicrob Agents Chemother (UNITED STATES) Mar 1997, 41 (3) p687-92

Common (but not always considered) viral infections of the lower respiratory tract. Pediatr Ann (UNITED STATES) Oct 1996, 25 (10) p577-84

Vitamin C and the common cold: a retrospective analysis of Chalmers' review. J Am Coll Nutr (UNITED STATES) Apr 1995

Interrelation of vitamin C, infection, haemostatic factors, and cardiovascular disease. BMJ (ENGLAND) Jun 17 1995, 310 (6994) p1559-63

Does vitamin C alleviate the symptoms of the common cold?--a review of current evidence. Scand J Infect Dis (SWEDEN) 1994, 26 (1) p1-6

Recommended dietary allowance: support from recent research. J Nutr Sci Vitaminol (Tokyo) (JAPAN) 1992, Spec No p173-6

Vitamin C and the common cold. Br J Nutr (ENGLAND) Jan 1992, 67 (1) p3-16

Vitamin C and the common cold: using identical twins as controls. Med J Aust (AUSTRALIA) Oct 17 1981, 2 (8) p411-2

The effects of ascorbic acid and flavonoids on the occurrence of symptoms normally associated with the common cold. Am J Clin Nutr (UNITED STATES) Aug 1979, 32 (8) p1686-90

Winter illness and vitamin C: the effect of relatively low doses. Can Med Assoc J (CANADA) Apr 5 1975, 112 (7) p823-6

Acetylcysteine: a drug with an interesting past and a fascinating future. Respiration (SWITZERLAND) 1986, 50 Suppl 1 p26-30

[Effect of Astragalus membranaceus on Ca2+ influx and coxsackie virus B3 RNA replication in cultured neonatal rat heart cells]. Chung Kuo Chung Hsi I Chieh Ho Tsa Chih (CHINA) Aug 1995

The inhibitory effect of astragalus membranaceus on coxsackie B-3 virus RNA replication. Chin Med Sci J (CHINA) Sep 1995, 10 (3) p146-50

References

[The effect of astragalus polysaccharides (APS) on cell mediated immunity (CMI) in burned mice]. Chung Hua Cheng Hsing Shao Shang Wai Ko Tsa Chih (CHINA) Mar 1994

Immunomodulating Chinese herbal medicines. Mem Inst Oswaldo Cruz (BRAZIL) 1991, 86 Suppl 2 p159-64

[The effect of vitamin A and Astragalus on the splenic T lymphocyte-CFU of burned mice]. Chung Hua Cheng Hsing Shao Shang Wai Ko Tsa Chih (CHINA) Jun 1989

Nutritional antioxidants and the modulation of inflammation: theory and practice. New Horiz (UNITED STATES) May 1994

Evaluation of zinc complexes on the replication of rhinovirus 2 in vitro. Res Commun Chem Pathol Pharmacol (UNITED STATES) Dec 1989

Zinc gluconate and the common cold: a controlled clinical study. J Int Med Res (ENGLAND) Jun 1992, 20 (3) p234-46

Prophylaxis and treatment of rhinovirus colds with zinc gluconate lozenges. J Antimicrob Chemother (ENGLAND) Dec 1987

Reduction in duration of common colds by zinc gluconate lozenges in a double-blind study. Antimicrob Agents Chemother (UNITED STATES) Jan 1984, 25 (1) p20-4

Antivirals for the chemoprophylaxis and treatment of influenza. Semin Respir Infect (UNITED STATES) Mar 1992

Utilization of pulse oximetry for the study of the inhibitory effects of antiviral agents on influenza virus in mice. Antimicrob Agents Chemother (UNITED STATES) Feb 1992

Further studies with short duration ribavirin aerosol for the treatment of influenza virus infection in mice and respiratory syncytial virus infection in cotton rats. Antiviral Res (NETHERLANDS) Jan 1992

High dose-short duration ribavirin aerosol treatment--a review. Bull Int Union Tuberc Lung Dis (FRANCE) Jun-Sep 1991

Viral pneumonia. Infect Dis Clin North Am (UNITED STATES) Sep 1991

Aerosol and intraperitoneal administration of ribavirin and ribavirin triacetate: pharmacokinetics and protection of mice against intracerebral infection with influenza A/WSN virus. Antimicrob Agents Chemother (UNITED STATES) Jul 1991

Antiviral drug therapy. Am Fam Physician (UNITED STATES) Jan 1991

Molecular mechanisms of action of ribavirin. Rev Infect Dis (UNITED STATES) Nov-Dec 1990

New acquisitions in the chemotherapy of viral infections. Verh K Acad Geneeskd Belg (BELGIUM) 1990

Comparison of oral and aerosol ribavirin regimens in the high risk elderly. J Clin Pharmacol (UNITED STATES) Dec 1989

Comparative activities of several nucleoside analogs against influenza A, B, and C viruses in vitro. Antimicrob Agents Chemother (UNITED STATES) Jun 1988

Antiviral drugs for common respiratory diseases. What's here, what's to come. Postgrad Med (UNITED STATES) Feb 1 1988, 83 (2) p136-9, 142-3, 146-8

Oral ribavirin treatment of influenza A and B. Antimicrob Agents Chemother (UNITED STATES) Aug 1987

Clinical review of ribavirin. Infect Control (UNITED STATES) May 1987, 8 (5) p215-8

Clinical use of antiviral drugs. Drug Intell Clin Pharm (UNITED STATES) May 1987

Protection of mice from lethal influenza virus infection with high dose-short duration ribavirin aerosol. Antimicrob Agents Chemother (UNITED STATES) Dec 1986, 30 (6) p942-4

Ribavirin: a clinical overview. Eur J Epidemiol (ITALY) Mar 1986

Effect of ribavirin triphosphate on primer generation and elongation during influenza virus transcription in vitro. Antiviral Res (NETHERLANDS) Feb 1985, 5 (1) p39-48

Ribavirin. Drug Intell Clin Pharm (UNITED STATES) Feb 1984

[Immunomodulating activity of ethanol-water extracts of the roots of Echinacea gloriosa L., Echinacea angustifolia DC. and Rudbeckia speciosa Wenderoth tested on the immune system in C57BL6 inbred mice]. Cesk Farm (CZECH REPUBLIC) Aug 1993

Application of purified polysaccharides from cell cultures of the plant Echinacea purpurea to mice mediates protection against systemic infections with Listeria monocytogenes and Candida albicans. Int J Immunopharmacol (ENGLAND) 1991, 13 (1)

Macrophage activation by the polysaccharide arabinogalactan isolated from plant cell cultures of Echinacea purpurea. J Natl Cancer Inst (UNITED STATES) May 3 1989

Macrophage activation and induction of macrophage cytotoxicity by purified polysaccharide fractions from the plant Echinacea purpurea. Infect Immun (UNITED STATES) Dec 1984

Combined antiviral and antimediator treatment of rhinovirus colds. J Infect Dis (UNITED STATES) Oct 1992, 166 (4)

[Common cold: diagnostic steps? Antibiotics?]. Ther Umsch (SWITZERLAND) Apr 1992, 49 (4)

Alpha 2-interferon for the common cold. Ann Pharmacother (UNITED STATES) Mar 1992, 26 (3) (no abstract)

Managing viral upper respiratory infections. Aust Fam Physician (AUSTRALIA) May 1991, 20 (5)

Immunological barriers in the nose and paranasal sinuses. Acta Otolaryngol (Stockh) (SWEDEN) May-Jun 1987, 103

Interferon for the treatment of infections. Annu Rev Med (UNITED STATES) 1987, 38 p51-9

Effect of Astragalus membranaceus on electrophysiological activities of acute experimental coxsackie B-3 viral myocarditis in mice CHIN. MED. SCI. J. (China), 1993, 8/4 (203-206)

Efficacy and safety of the standardized ginseng extract G 115 for potentiating vaccination against common cold and/or influenza syndrome Drugs under Experimental and Clinical Research (Switzerland), 1996, 22/2 65-72)

An emerging green pharmacy: Modern plant medicines and health. Laboratory Medicine (USA), 1996, 27/3 (170-176)

Immunity in myocardiac hypertrophy rat and effect of total saponins of panax ginseng in vivo and in vitro. Chinese Pharmacological Bulletin (China), 1996, 12/1 (84-86)

Treatment of experimental coxsackie B-3 viral myocarditis with astragalus membranaceus in mice. CHIN. MED. J. (CHINA) (China), 1990, 103/1 (14-18)

Effect of Astragalus membranaceus injecta on coxsackie b-2 virus infected rat beating heart cell culture. CHIN. MED. J. (PEKING) (CHINA), 1987, 100/7 (595-602)

SAMBUCOL(TM) INHIBITED SEVERAL STRAINS OF INFLUENZA VIRUS AND REDUCED SYMPTOMS DURING AN OUTBREAK OF INFLUENZA B PANAMA. Weizmann Institute of Science 2-15-94

THE EFFECT OF SAMBUCOL(TM) on HIV INFECTION IN VITRO. Congress of Microbiology 2-6-95

Vitamin C and the common cold: a retrospective analysis of Chalmers' review. J Am Coll Nutr (UNITED STATES) Apr 1995

Interrelation of vitamin C, infection, haemostatic factors, and cardiovascular disease. BMJ (ENGLAND) Jun 17 1995, 310 (6994) p1559-63

Does vitamin C alleviate the symptoms of the common cold?—a review of current evidence. Scand J Infect Dis (SWEDEN) 1994, 26 (1) p1-6

Recommended dietary allowance: support from recent research. J Nutr Sci Vitaminol (Tokyo) (JAPAN) 1992, Spec No p173-6

Vitamin C and the common cold. Br J Nutr (ENGLAND) Jan 1992, 67 (1) p3-16

Vitamin C and the common cold: using identical twins as controls. Med J Aust (AUSTRALIA) Oct 17 1981, 2 (8) p411-2

The effects of ascorbic acid and flavonoids on the occurrence of symptoms normally associated with the common cold. Am J Clin Nutr (UNITED STATES) Aug 1979, 32 (8) p1686-90

Winter illness and vitamin C: the effect of relatively low doses. Can Med Assoc J (CANADA) Apr 5 1975, 112 (7) p823-6

Acetylcysteine: a drug with an interesting past and a fascinating future. Respiration (SWITZERLAND) 1986, 50 Suppl 1 p26-30

[Effect of Astragalus membranaceus on Ca2+ influx and coxsackie virus B3 RNA replication in cultured neonatal rat heart cells]. Chung Kuo Chung Hsi I Chieh Ho Tsa Chih (CHINA) Aug 1995

The inhibitory effect of astragalus membranaceus on coxsackie B-3 virus RNA replication. Chin Med Sci J (CHINA) Sep 1995, 10 (3) p146-50

[The effect of astragalus polysaccharides (APS) on cell mediated immunity (CMI) in burned mice]. Chung Hua Cheng Hsing Shao Shang Wai Ko Tsa Chih (CHINA) Mar 1994

Immunomodulating Chinese herbal medicines. Mem Inst Oswaldo Cruz (BRAZIL) 1991, 86 Suppl 2 p159-64

[The effect of vitamin A and Astragalus on the splenic T lymphocyte-CFU of burned mice]. Chung Hua Cheng Hsing Shao Shang Wai Ko Tsa Chih (CHINA) Jun 1989

Nutritional antioxidants and the modulation of inflammation: theory and practice. New Horiz (UNITED STATES) May 1994

References

Evaluation of zinc complexes on the replication of rhinovirus 2 in vitro. Res Commun Chem Pathol Pharmacol (UNITED STATES) Dec 1989

Zinc gluconate and the common cold: a controlled clinical study. J Int Med Res (ENGLAND) Jun 1992, 20 (3) p234-46

Prophylaxis and treatment of rhinovirus colds with zinc gluconate lozenges. J Antimicrob Chemother (ENGLAND) Dec 1987

Reduction in duration of common colds by zinc gluconate lozenges in a double-blind study. Antimicrob Agents Chemother (UNITED STATES) Jan 1984, 25 (1) p20-4

Antivirals for the chemoprophylaxis and treatment of influenza. Semin Respir Infect (UNITED STATES) Mar 1992

Utilization of pulse oximetry for the study of the inhibitory effects of antiviral agents on influenza virus in mice. Antimicrob Agents Chemother (UNITED STATES) Feb 1992

Further studies with short duration ribavirin aerosol for the treatment of influenza virus infection in mice and respiratory syncytial virus infection in cotton rats. Antiviral Res (NETHERLANDS) Jan 1992

High dose-short duration ribavirin aerosol treatment—a review. Bull Int Union Tuberc Lung Dis (FRANCE) Jun-Sep 1991

Viral pneumonia. Infect Dis Clin North Am (UNITED STATES) Sep 1991

Aerosol and intraperitoneal administration of ribavirin and ribavirin triacetate: pharmacokinetics and protection of mice against intracerebral infection with influenza A/WSN virus. Antimicrob Agents Chemother (UNITED STATES) Jul 1991

Antiviral drug therapy. Am Fam Physician (UNITED STATES) Jan 1991

Molecular mechanisms of action of ribavirin. Rev Infect Dis (UNITED STATES) Nov-Dec 1990

New acquisitions in the chemotherapy of viral infections. Verh K Acad Geneeskd Belg (BELGIUM) 1990

Comparison of oral and aerosol ribavirin regimens in the high risk elderly. J Clin Pharmacol (UNITED STATES) Dec 1989

Comparative activities of several nucleoside analogs against influenza A, B, and C viruses in vitro. Antimicrob Agents Chemother (UNITED STATES) Jun 1988

Antiviral drugs for common respiratory diseases. What's here, what's to come. Postgrad Med (UNITED STATES) Feb 1 1988, 83 (2) p136-9, 142-3, 146-8

Oral ribavirin treatment of influenza A and B. Antimicrob Agents Chemother (UNITED STATES) Aug 1987

Clinical review of ribavirin. Infect Control (UNITED STATES) May 1987, 8 (5) p215-8

Clinical use of antiviral drugs. Drug Intell Clin Pharm (UNITED STATES) May 1987

Protection of mice from lethal influenza virus infection with high dose-short duration ribavirin aerosol. Antimicrob Agents Chemother (UNITED STATES) Dec 1986, 30 (6) p942-4

Ribavirin: a clinical overview. Eur J Epidemiol (ITALY) Mar 1986

References

Effect of ribavirin triphosphate on primer generation and elongation during influenza virus transcription in vitro. Antiviral Res (NETHERLANDS) Feb 1985, 5 (1) p39-48

Ribavirin. Drug Intell Clin Pharm (UNITED STATES) Feb 1984

[Immunomodulating activity of ethanol-water extracts of the roots of Echinacea gloriosa L., Echinacea angustifolia DC. and Rudbeckia speciosa Wenderoth tested on the immune system in C57BL6 inbred mice]. Cesk Farm (CZECH REPUBLIC) Aug 1993

Application of purified polysaccharides from cell cultures of the plant Echinacea purpurea to mice mediates protection against systemic infections with Listeria monocytogenes and Candida albicans. Int J Immunopharmacol (ENGLAND) 1991, 13 (1)

Macrophage activation by the polysaccharide arabinogalactan isolated from plant cell cultures of Echinacea purpurea. J Natl Cancer Inst (UNITED STATES) May 3 1989

Macrophage activation and induction of macrophage cytotoxicity by purified polysaccharide fractions from the plant Echinacea purpurea. Infect Immun (UNITED STATES) Dec 1984

Combined antiviral and antimediator treatment of rhinovirus colds. J Infect Dis (UNITED STATES) Oct 1992, 166 (4)

[Common cold: diagnostic steps? Antibiotics?]. Ther Umsch (SWITZERLAND) Apr 1992, 49 (4)

Alpha 2-interferon for the common cold. Ann Pharmacother (UNITED STATES) Mar 1992, 26 (3) (no abstract)

Managing viral upper respiratory infections. Aust Fam Physician (AUSTRALIA) May 1991, 20 (5)

Immunological barriers in the nose and paranasal sinuses. Acta Otolaryngol (Stockh) (SWEDEN) May-Jun 1987, 103

Interferon for the treatment of infections. Annu Rev Med (UNITED STATES) 1987, 38 p51-9

Effect of Astragalus membranaceus on electrophysiological activities of acute experimental coxsackie B-3 viral myocarditis in mice.CHIN. MED. SCI. J. (China), 1993, 8/4 (203-206)

Efficacy and safety of the standardized ginseng extract G 115 for potentiating vaccination against common cold and/or influenza syndrome. Drugs under Experimental and Clinical Research (Switzerland), 1996, 22/2 65-72)

An emerging green pharmacy: Modern plant medicines and health. Gruber J.W.; DerMarderosian A. Laboratory Medicine (USA), 1996, 27/3 (170-176)

Immunity in myocardiac hypertrophy rat and effect of total saponins of panax ginseng in vivo and in vitro. Chinese Pharmacological Bulletin (China), 1996, 12/1 (84-86)

Treatment of experimental coxsackie B-3 viral myocarditis with astragalus membranaceus in mice. CHIN. MED. J. (CHINA) (China), 1990, 103/1 (14-18)

Effect of Astragalus membranaceus injecta on coxsackie b-2 virus infected rat beating heart cell culture.CHIN. MED. J. (PEKING) (CHINA), 1987, 100/7 (595-602)

Sambucol Inhibited Several Strains of Influenza Virus And Reduced Symptoms During an Outbreak of Influenza B Panama.Weizmann Institute of Science 2-15-94

The Effect of Sambucol on HIV Infection in Vitro. Congress of Microbiology 2-6-95

Congestive Heart Failure/Cardiomyopathy

The clinical and hemodynamic effects of Coenzyme Q10 in congestive cardiomyopathy. American Journal of Therapeutics (USA), 1997, 4/2-3 (66-72)

Fish oil and other nutritional adjuvants for treatment of congestive heart failure. Medical Hypotheses (United Kingdom), 1996, 46/4 (400-406)

The use of oral magnesium in mild-to-moderate congestive heart failure. Congestive Heart Failure (USA), 1997, 3/2 (21-24)

Guidelines on treatment of hypertension in the elderly, 1995 -A tentative plan for comprehensive research projects on aging and health. Japanese Journal of Geriatrics (Japan), 1996, 33/12 (945-974)

Predictors of sudden death and death from pump failure in congestive heart failure are different. Analysis of 24 h Holter monitoring, clinical variables, blood chemistry, exericise test and radionuclide angiography. International Journal of Cardiology (Ireland), 1997, 58/2 (151-162)

Magnesium supplementation in patients with congestive heart failure. Journal of the American College of Nutrition (USA), 1997, 16/1 (22-31)

How best to determine magnesium requirement: Need to consider cardiotherapeutic drugs that affect its retention. Journal of the American College of Nutrition (USA), 1997, 16/1 (4-6)

Magnesium: A critical appreciation. Zeitschrift fur Kardiologie (Germany), 1996, 85/SUPPL. 6 (147-151)

Sarcoplasmic reticular Ca2+ pump ATPase activity in congestive myocardial infarction. Canadian Journal of Cardiology (Canada), 1996, 12/10 (1065-1073)

Significance of magnesium in congestive heart failure. American Heart Journal (USA), 1996, 132/3 (664-671)

The rationale of magnesium as alternative therapy for patients with acute myocardial infarction without thrombolytic therapy. American Heart Journal (USA), 1996, 132/2 II (483-486)

Mortality risk and patterns of practice in 4606 acute care patients with congestive heart failure: The relative importance of age, sex, and medical therapy. Archives of Internal Medicine (USA), 1996, 156/15 (1669-1673)

The study of renal magnesium handling in chronic congestive heart failure. Sapporo Medical Journal (Japan), 1996, 65/1 (23-32)

Management of acute myocardial infarction in the elderly. Drugs and Aging (New Zealand), 1996, 8/5 (358-377)

Supraventricular tachycardia after coronary artery bypass grafting surgery and fluid and electrolyte variables. Heart and Lung: Journal of Acute and Critical Care (USA), 1996, 25/1 (31-36)

Growth hormone in end-stage heart failure (multiple letters) (6). Lancet (United Kingdom), 1997, 349/9068 (1841-1843)

Haemodynamic effects of intravenous growth hormone in congestive heart failure (1). Lancet (United Kingdom), 1997, 349/9058 (1067-1068)

Skeletal muscle metabolism in experimental heart failure. Journal of Molecular and Cellular

Cardiology (United Kingdom), 1996, 28/11 (2263-2273)

Hydralazine prevents nitroglycerin tolerance by inhibiting activation of a membrane-bound NADH oxidase: A new action for an old drug. Journal of Clinical Investigation (USA), 1996, 98/6 (1465-1470)

Edema and principles of diuretic use. Medical Clinics of North America (USA), 1997, 81/3 (689-704)

Alterations in ATP-sensitive potassium channel sensitivity to ATP in failing human hearts. American Journal of Physiology - Heart and Circulatory Physiology (USA), 1997, 272/4 41-4 (H1656-H1665)

Effective water clearance and tonicity balance: The excretion of water revisited. Clinical and Investigative Medicine (Canada), 1997, 20/1 (16-24)

Hypertension update. Survey of Ophthalmology (USA), 1996, 41/1 (79-89)

Does aspirin cause acute or chronic renal failure in experimental animals and in humans? American Journal of Kidney Diseases (USA), 1996, 28/1 SUPPL. (S24-S29)

Elevated myocardial interstitial norepinephrine concentration contributes to the regulation of $Na+,K+$-ATPase in heart failure. European Journal of Pharmacology (Netherlands), 1996, 309/3 (235-241)

[Magnesium: current studies--critical evaluation--consequences]. Z Kardiol (GERMANY) 1996, 85 Suppl 6 p147-51

Nonsustained polymorphous ventricular tachycardia during amiodarone therapy for atrial fibrillation complicating cardiomyopathy. Management with intravenous magnesium sulfate. Chest (UNITED STATES) May 1997, 111 (5) p1454-7

Magnesium deficiency-related changes in lipid peroxidation and collagen metabolism in vivo in rat heart. Int J Biochem Cell Biol (ENGLAND) Jan 1997, 29 (1) p129-34

[Value of magnesium in acute myocardial infarct]. Z Kardiol (GERMANY) 1996, 85 Suppl 6 p129-34

NADH-coenzyme Q reductase (complex I) deficiency: heterogeneity in phenotype and biochemical findings. J Inherit Metab Dis (NETHERLANDS) 1996, 19 (5) p675-86

Familial cardiomyopathy with cataracts and lactic acidosis: a defect in complex I (NADH-dehydrogenase) of the mitochondria respiratory chain. Pediatr Res (UNITED STATES) Mar 1996, 39 (3) p513-21

Comparison of calcium-current in isolated atrial myocytes from failing and nonfailing human hearts. Mol Cell Biochem (NETHERLANDS) Apr 12-26 1996, 157 (1-2) p157-62

Mitochondrial complex I deficiency leads to increased production of superoxide radicals and induction of superoxide dismutase. J Clin Invest (UNITED STATES) Jul 15 1996, 98 (2) p345-51

A preliminary study of growth hormone in the treatment of dilated cardiomyopathy. N Engl J Med (UNITED STATES) Mar 28 1996, 334 (13) p809-14 Comment in N Engl J Med 1996 Mar 28;334(13):856-7; Comment in: N Engl J Med 1996 Aug 29;335(9):672; discussion 673-4; Comment in: N Engl J Med 1996 Aug 29;335(9):672-3; discussion 673-4

Effect of protection and repair of injury of mitochondrial membrane-phospholipid on prognosis in patients with dilated cardiomyopathy. Blood Press Suppl (NORWAY) 1996, 3 p53-5

[Therapeutic effects of coenzyme Q10 on dilated cardiomyopathy: assessment by 123I-BMIPP myocardial single photon emission computed tomography (SPECT): a multicenter trial in Osaka

University Medical School Group]. Kaku Igaku (JAPAN) Jan 1996, 33 (1) p27-32

The effects of calcium channel blockers on blood fluidity. J Cardiovasc Pharmacol (UNITED STATES) 1990, 16 Suppl 6 pS40-4

Increased whole blood and plasma viscosity in patients with angina pectoris and 'normal' coronary arteries. ACTA MED. SCAND. (Sweden), 1988, 224/2 (109-114)

Can lifestyle changes reverse coronary heart disease? LANCET (United Kingdom), 1990, 336/8708 (129-133)

The natural history of atherosclerosis: An ecologic perspective. ATHEROSCLEROSIS (Ireland), 1990, 82/1-2 (157-164)

Concordant dyslipidemia, hypertension and early coronary disease in Utah families. KLIN. WOCHEN-SCHR. (Germany, Federal Republic of), 1990, 68/SUPPL. 20 (53-59)

Correction: Mediterranean alpha-linolenic acid rich diet in secondary prevention of coronary heart disease (Lancet (1994) June 11 (1454). Lancet (United Kingdom), 1995, 345/8951 (738)

Mediterranean alpha-linolenic acid-rich diet in secondary prevention of coronary heart disease. LANCET (United Kingdom), 1994, 343/8911 (1454-1459)

Effect of antioxidant-rich foods on plasma ascorbic acid, cardiac enzyme, and lipid peroxide levels in patients hospitalized with acute myocardial infarction. Journal of the American Dietetic Association (USA), 1995, 95/7 (775-780)

Dietary supplementation with orange and carrot juice in cigarette smokers lowers oxidation products in copper-oxidized low-density lipoproteins. Journal of the American Dietetic Association (USA), 1995, 95/6 (671-675)

Women, hormones and blood pressure. Canadian Journal of Cardiology (Canada), 1996, 12/6 SUPPL. D (9D-12D)

Protective effect of fruits and vegetables on development of stroke in men. Journal of the American Medical Association (USA), 1995, 273/14 (1113-1117)

The effect of caffeine on ventricular ectopic activity in patients with malignant ventricular arrhythmia. ARCH. INTERN. MED. (USA), 1989, 149/3 (637-639)

Coffee, cocktails and coronary candidates. N. ENGL. J. MED. (USA), 1977, 297/8 (443-444)

Concentrations of magnesium, calcium, potassium, and sodium in human heart muscle after acute myocardial infarction. Clin Chem (UNITED STATES) Nov 1980, 26 (12) p1662-5

[Therapeutic efficacy of pantothenic acid preparations in ischemic heart disease patients]. Vopr Pitan (USSR) Mar-Apr 1987, (2) p15-7

Antifibrillatory effect of tetrahydroberberine. Chung Kuo Yao Li Hsueh Pao (CHINA) Jul 1993, 14 (4) p301-5

Effects of tetrahydroberberine on ischemic and reperfused myocardium in rats. Chung Kuo Yao Li Hsueh Pao (CHINA) Mar 1993, 14 (2) p130-3

[Ventricular tachyarrhythmias treated with berberine]. Chung Hua Hsin Hsueh Kuan Ping Tsa Chih (CHINA) Jun 1990, 18 (3) p155-6, 190

[Effects of berberine on ischemic ventricular arrhythmia]. Chung Hua Hsin Hsueh Kuan Ping Tsa Chih (CHINA) Oct 1989, 17 (5) p300-1, 319

[Protective effects of berberine on spontaneous ventricular fibrillation in dogs after myocardial infarction]. Chung Kuo Yao Li Hsueh Pao (CHINA) Jul 1989, 10 (4) p320-4

Protective effects of berberine and phentolamine on myocardial reoxygenation damage. Chin Med Sci J (ENGLAND) Dec 1992, 7 (4) p221-5

Beneficial effects of berberine on hemodynamics during acute ischemic left ventricular failure in dogs. Chin Med J (Engl) (CHINA) Dec 1992, 105 (12) p1014-9

[The role and mechanism of berberine on coronary arteries]. Chung Hua Hsin Hsueh Kuan Ping Tsa Chih (CHINA) Aug 1990, 18 (4) p231-4, 254-5

Effect of tincture of Crataegus on the LDL-receptor activity of hepatic plasma membrane of rats fed an atherogenic diet. Atherosclerosis (IRELAND) Jun 1996, 123 (1-2) p235-41

Effect of a hawthorn extract on contraction and energy turnover of isolated rat cardiomyocytes. Arzneimittelforschung (GERMANY) Nov 1995, 45 (11) p1157-61

[Crataegus Special Extract WS 1442. Assessment of objective effectiveness in patients with heart failure (NYHA II)]. Fortschr Med (GERMANY) Aug 30 1996, 114 (24) p291-6

[Crataegus Special Extract WS 1442 in NYHA II heart failure. A placebo controlled randomized double-blind study]. Fortschr Med (GERMANY) Jul 20 1993, 111 (20-21) p352-4

Abnormal membrane concentrations of 20 and 22-carbon essential fatty acids: a common link between risk factors and coronary and peripheral vascular disease? Prostaglandins Leukot Essent Fatty Acids (SCOTLAND) Dec 1995, 53 (6) p385-96

Differential changes in left and right ventricular adenylyl cyclase activities in congestive heart failure. American Journal of Physiology - Heart and Circulatory Physiology (USA), 1997, 272/2 41-2 (H884-H893)

Chronic opiate-receptor inhibition in experimental congestive heart failure in dogs. American Journal of Physiology - Heart and Circulatory Physiology (USA), 1997, 272/1 41-1 (H478-H484)

beta-adrenoceptor mediated signal transduction in congestive heart failure in cardiomyopathic (UM-X7.1) hamsters. Molecular and Cellular Biochemistry (USA), 1996, 157/1-2 (191-196)

Pharmacology and inotropic potential of FORSKOLIN in the human heart. J Clin Invest (UNITED STATES) Jul 1984, 74 (1) p212-23

[Effects of FORSKOLIN on canine congestive heart failure]. Nippon Yakurigaku Zasshi (JAPAN) Nov 1986, 88 (5) p389-94

Italian multicenter study on the safety and efficacy of COENZYME Q10 as adjunctive therapy in heart failure. Mol Aspects Med (ENGLAND) 1994, 15 Suppl ps287-94

[Coenzyme Q10 (ubiquinone) in the treatment of heart failure. Are any positive effects documented?]. Tidsskr Nor Laegeforen (NORWAY) Mar 20 1994, 114 (8) p939-42

Italian multicenter study on the safety and efficacy of COENZYME Q10 as adjunctive therapy in heart failure (interim analysis). The CoQ10 Drug Surveillance Investigators. Clin Investig (GERMANY) 1993, 71 (8 Suppl) pS145-9

Isolated diastolic dysfunction of the myocardium and its response to CoQ10 treatment. Clin Investig (GERMANY) 1993, 71 (8 Suppl) pS140-4

Effect of COENZYME Q10 therapy in patients with congestive heart failure: a long-term multicenter randomized study. Clin Investig (GERMANY) 1993, 71 (8 Suppl) pS134-6

Role of metabolic therapy in cardiovascular disease. Clin Investig (GERMANY) 1993, 71 (8 Suppl) pS124-8

Usefulness of TAURINE in chronic congestive heart failure and its prospective application. Jpn Circ J (JAPAN) Jan 1992, 56 (1) p95-9

Co-enzyme Q10: a new drug for cardiovascular disease. J Clin Pharmacol (UNITED STATES) Jul 1990, 30 (7) p596-608

COENZYME Q10: a new drug for myocardial ischemia? Med Clin North Am (UNITED STATES) Jan 1988, 72 (1) p243-58

Cardiac performance and COENZYME Q10 in thyroid disorders. Endocrinol Jpn (JAPAN) Dec 1984, 31 (6) p755-61

A clinical study of the effect of COENZYME Q on congestive heart failure. Jpn Heart J (JAPAN) Jan 1976, 17 (1) p32-42

[MAGNESIUM in cardiology]. Schweiz Rundsch Med Prax (SWITZERLAND) May 2 1995, 84 (18) p526-32

MAGNESIUM therapy in acute myocardial infarction when patients are not candidates for thrombolytic therapy. J Cardiol (UNITED STATES) Feb 15 1995, 75 (5) p321-3

[Oral MAGNESIUM supplementation to patients receivingdiuretics -- normalization of MAGNESIUM, POTASSIUM and sodium, and POTASSIUM pumps in the skeletal muscles]. Ugeskr Laeger (DENMARK) Jul 4 1994, 156 (27) p4007-10, 4013

Effects of intravenous MAGNESIUM sulfate on arrhythmias in patients with congestive heart failure. Am Heart J (UNITED STATES) Jun 1993, 125 (6) p1645-50

MAGNESIUM-POTASSIUM interactions in cardiac arrhythmia. Examples of ionic medicine. Magnes Trace Elem (SWITZERLAND) 92 1991, 10 (2-4) p193-204

Clinical clues to MAGNESIUM deficiency. Isr J Med Sci (ISRAEL) Dec 1987, 23 (12) p1238-41

Platelet TAURINE in patients with arterial hypertension, myocardial failure or infarction. Acta Med Scand Suppl (SWEDEN) 1980, 642 p79-84

Physiological and experimental regulation of TAURINE content in the heart. Fed Proc (UNITED STATES) Jul 1980, 39 (9) p2685-90

A relation between myocardial TAURINE contest and pulmonary wedge pressure in dogs with heart failure. Physiol Chem Phys (UNITED STATES) 1977, 9 (3) p259-63

Adrenergic stimulation of TAURINE transport by the heart. Science (UNITED STATES) Oct 28 1977, 198 (4315) p409-11

Effects of L-CARNITINE administration on left ventricular remodeling after acute anterior myocardial infarction. J Am Coll Cardiol (UNITED STATES) Aug 1995, 26 (2) p380-7

The myocardial distribution and plasma concentration of CARNITINE in patients with mitral valve disease. Surg Today (JAPAN) 1994, 24 (4) p313-7

Myocardial CARNITINE metabolism in congestive heart failure induced by incessant tachycardia. Basic Res Cardiol (GERMANY) Jul-Aug 1993, 88 (4) 362-70

[The clinical and hemodynamic effects of propionyl-L-CARNITINE in the treatment of congestive heart failure]. Clin Ter (ITALY) Nov 1992, 141 (11) p379-84

L-CARNITINE treatment for congestive heart failure--experimental and clinical study. Jpn Circ J (JAPAN) Jan 1992, 56 (1) p86-94

The therapeutic potential of CARNITINE in cardiovascular disorders. Clin Ther (UNITED STATES) Jan-Feb 1991, 13 (1) p2-21; discussion 1

[Dilated cardiomyopathy due to primary CARNITINE deficiency] Cardiomiopatia dilatativa da deficit primitivo di carnitina. Squarcia Pediatr Med Chir (ITALY) Mar-Apr 1986, 8 (2) p157-61

Characterization of inwardly rectifying K+ channel in human cardiac myocytes. Alterations in channel behavior in myocytes isolated from patients with idiopathic dilated cardiomyopathy. Circulation (UNITED STATES) Jul 15 1995, 92 (2) p164-74

Impaired forearm vasodilation to hyperosmolal stimuli in patients with congestive heart failure secondary to idiopathic dilated cardiomyopathy or to ischemic cardiomyopathy. Am J Cardiol (UNITED STATES) Nov 15 1992, 70 (15) p1315-9

Usefulness of coenzyme Q10 in clinical cardiology: a long-term study. Mol Aspects Med (ENGLAND) 1994, 15 Suppl

Bioenergetics in clinical medicine. Studies on coenzyme Q10 and essential hypertension. Res Commun Chem Pathol Pharmacol (UNITED STATES) Jun 1975

Can antioxidants prevent ischemic heart disease? J Clin Pharm Ther (ENGLAND) Apr 1993

Antioxidant therapy in the aging process. EXS (SWITZERLAND) 1992, 62

Pharmacology and inotropic potential of FORSKOLIN in the human heart. J Clin Invest (UNITED STATES) Jul 1984, 74 (1) p212-23

[Effects of FORSKOLIN on canine congestive heart failure]. Nippon Yakurigaku Zasshi (JAPAN) Nov 1986, 88 (5) p389-94

Italian multicenter study on the safety and efficacy of COENZYME Q10 as adjunctive therapy in heart failure. CoQ10 Drug Surveillance Investigators. Mol Aspects Med (ENGLAND) 1994, 15 Suppl ps287-94

[Coenzyme Q10 (ubiquinone) in the treatment of heart failure. Are any positive effects documented?]. Tidsskr Nor Laegeforen (NORWAY) Mar 20 1994, 114 (8) p939-42

Italian multicenter study on the safety and efficacy of COENZYME Q10 as adjunctive therapy in heart failure (interim analysis). The CoQ10 Drug Surveillance Investigators. Clin Investig (GERMANY) 1993, 71 (8 Suppl) pS145-9

Isolated diastolic dysfunction of the myocardium and its response to CoQ10 treatment. Clin Investig (GERMANY) 1993, 71 (8 Suppl) pS140-4

References

Effect of coenzyme Q10 therapy in patients with congestive heart failure: a long-term multicenter randomized study. Clin Investig (GERMANY) 1993, 71 (8 Suppl) pS134-6

Role of metabolic therapy in cardiovascular disease. Clin Investig (GERMANY) 1993, 71 (8 Suppl) pS124-8

Usefulness of TAURINE in chronic congestive heart failure and its prospective application. Jpn Circ J (JAPAN) Jan 1992, 56 (1) p95-9

Coenzyme Q10: a new drug for cardiovascular disease. J Clin Pharmacol (UNITED STATES) Jul 1990, 30 (7) p596-608

Coenzyme Q10: a new drug for myocardial ischemia? Med Clin North Am (UNITED STATES) Jan 1988, 72 (1) p243-58

Cardiac performance and coenzyme Q10 in thyroid disorders. Endocrinol Jpn (JAPAN) Dec 1984, 31 (6) p755-61

A clinical study of the effect of COENZYME Q on congestive heart failure. Jpn Heart J (JAPAN) Jan 1976, 17 (1) p32-42

[MAGNESIUM in cardiology]. Schweiz Rundsch Med Prax (SWITZERLAND) May 2 1995, 84 (18) p526-32

MAGNESIUM therapy in acute myocardial infarction when patients are not candidates for thrombolytic therapy. J Cardiol (UNITED STATES) Feb 15 1995, 75 (5) p321-3

[Oral MAGNESIUM supplementation to patients receivingdiuretics — normalization of MAGNESIUM, POTASSIUM and sodium, and POTASSIUM pumps in the skeletal muscles]. Ugeskr Laeger (DENMARK) Jul 4 1994, 156 (27) p4007-10, 4013

Effects of intravenous MAGNESIUM sulfate on arrhythmias in patients with congestive heart failure. Am Heart J (UNITED STATES) Jun 1993, 125 (6) p1645-50

MAGNESIUM-POTASSIUM interactions in cardiac arrhythmia. Examples of ionic medicine. Magnes Trace Elem (SWITZERLAND) 92 1991, 10 (2-4) p193-204

Clinical clues to MAGNESIUM deficiency. Isr J Med Sci (ISRAEL) Dec 1987, 23 (12) p1238-41

Platelet TAURINE in patients with arterial hypertension, myocardial failure or infarction. Acta Med Scand Suppl (SWEDEN) 1980, 642 p79-84

Physiological and experimental regulation of TAURINE content in the heart. Fed Proc (UNITED STATES) Jul 1980, 39 (9) p2685-90

A relation between myocardial TAURINE contest and pulmonary wedge pressure in dogs with heart failure. Physiol Chem Phys (UNITED STATES) 1977, 9 (3) p259-63

Adrenergic stimulation of TAURINE transport by the heart. Science (UNITED STATES) Oct 28 1977, 198 (4315) p409-11

Effects of L-CARNITINE administration on left ventricular remodeling after acute anterior myocardial infarction. J Am Coll Cardiol (UNITED STATES) Aug 1995, 26 (2) p380-7

The myocardial distribution and plasma concentration of CARNITINE in patients with mitral valve disease. Surg Today (JAPAN) 1994, 24 (4) p313-7

Myocardial CARNITINE metabolism in congestive heart failure induced by incessant tachycardia. Basic Res Cardiol (GERMANY) Jul-Aug 1993, 88 (4) p362-70

[The clinical and hemodynamic effects of propionyl-L-CARNITINE in the treatment of congestive heart failure]. Clin Ter (ITALY) Nov 1992, 141 (11) p379-84

L-CARNITINE treatment for congestive heart failure—experimental and clinical study. Jpn Circ J (JAPAN) Jan 1992, 56 (1) p86-94

The therapeutic potential of CARNITINE in cardiovascular disorders. Clin Ther (UNITED STATES) Jan-Feb 1991, 13 (1) p2-21; discussion 1

[Dilated cardiomyopathy due to primary CARNITINE deficiency] Cardiomiopatia dilatativa da deficit primitivo di carnitina. Squarcia. Pediatr Med Chir (ITALY) Mar-Apr 1986, 8 (2) p157-61

Characterization of inwardly rectifying K+ channel in human cardiac myocytes. Alterations in channel behavior in myocytes isolated from patients with idiopathic dilated cardiomyopathy. Circulation (UNITED STATES) Jul 15 1995, 92 (2) p164-74

Impaired forearm vasodilation to hyperosmolal stimuli in patients with congestive heart failure secondary to idiopathic dilated cardiomyopathy or to ischemic cardiomyopathy. Am J Cardiol (UNITED STATES) Nov 15 1992, 70 (15) p1315-9

Usefulness of coenzyme Q10 in clinical cardiology: a long-term study. Mol Aspects Med (ENGLAND) 1994, 15 Suppl

Co-enzyme Q10: a new drug for cardiovascular disease. J Clin Pharmacol (UNITED STATES) Jul 1990

Bioenergetics in clinical medicine. Studies on coenzyme Q10 and essential hypertension. Res Commun Chem Pathol Pharmacol (UNITED STATES) Jun 1975

Can antioxidants prevent ischemic heart disease? J Clin Pharm Ther (ENGLAND) Apr 1993

Antioxidant therapy in the aging process. EXS (SWITZERLAND) 1992, 62

Constipation

[Intake of dietary fiber and other nutrients by children with and without functional chronic constipation]. Arq Gastroenterol (BRAZIL) Apr-Jun 1996, 33 (2) p93-101

The treatment of chronic constipation in adults. A systematic review. J Gen Intern Med (UNITED STATES) Jan 1997, 12 (1) p15-24

Health help. Fluid + fiber = frequency. Home Care Provid (UNITED STATES) Jan-Feb 1996, 1 (1) p30

Fecal incontinence in children. Am Fam Physician (UNITED STATES) May 1 1997, 55 (6) p2229-38

Chronic constipation--is the work-up worth the cost? Dis Colon Rectum (UNITED STATES) Mar 1997, 40 (3) p280-6

Changing bowel hygiene practice successfully: a program to reduce laxative use in a chronic care hospital. Geriatr Nurs (UNITED STATES) Jan-Feb 1997, 18 (1) p12-7

[A clinical study of the use of a combination of glucomannan with lactulose in the constipation of pregnancy]. Minerva Ginecol (ITALY) Dec 1996, 48 (12) p577-82

Clinical response to dietary fiber treatment of chronic constipation. Am J Gastroenterol (UNITED STATES) Jan 1997, 92 (1) p95-8

Lack of influence of intestinal transit on oxidative status in premenopausal women. Eur J Clin Nutr (ENGLAND) Aug 1996, 50 (8) p565-8

Dietary fiber and laxation in postop orthopedic patients. Clin Nurs Res (UNITED STATES) Nov 1996, 5 (4) p428-40

[The relationship between intake of dietary fiber and chronic constipation in children]. Ned Tijdschr Geneeskd (NETHERLANDS) Oct 12 1996, 140 (41) p2036-9

Assessment of the effect of increased dietary fibre intake on bowel function in patients with spinal cord injury. Spinal Cord (ENGLAND) May 1996, 34 (5) p277-83

Chronic idiopathic constipation: pathophysiology and treatment. J Clin Gastroenterol (UNITED STATES) Apr 1996, 22 (3) p190-6

Pediatric constipation. Gastroenterol Nurs (UNITED STATES) May-Jun 1996, 19 (3) p88-95

Constipation and fecal incontinence in the elderly population. Mayo Clin Proc (UNITED STATES) Jan 1996, 71 (1) p81-92

Therapeutic availability of iron administered orally as the ferrous gluconate together with magnesium-L-aspartate hydrochloride. Arzneimittelforschung (GERMANY) Mar 1996, 46 (3) p302-6

The osmotic and intrinsic mechanisms of the pharmacological laxative action of oral high doses of magnesium sulphate. Importance of the release of digestive polypeptides and nitric oxide. Magnes Res (ENGLAND) Jun 1996, 9 (2) p133-8

Small bowel obstruction caused by a medication bezoar: report of a case. Surg Today (JAPAN) 1996, 26 (1) p68-70

Challenges in the treatment of colonic motility disorders. American Journal of Health-System Pharmacy (USA), 1996, 53/22 SUPPL. (S17-S26)

Acute hypermagnesemia after laxative use. Annals of Emergency Medicine (USA), 1996, 28/5 (552-555)

The connection between dietary fibre intake and chronic constipation in children. Nederlands Tijdschrift voor Geneeskunde (Netherlands), 1996, 140/41 (2036-2039)

Constipation in children. American Family Physician (USA), 1996, 54/2 (611-630)

Products for indigestion. Pharmaceutical Journal (United Kingdom), 1996, 256/6892 (678-682)

Antacids drugs: Multiple but too often unknown pharmacological properties. Journal de Pharmacie Clinique (France), 1996, 15/1 (41-51)

Treatment of retentive encopresis with diet modification and scheduled toileting vs. mineral oil and rewards for toileting: A clinical decision. Ambulatory Child Health (United Kingdom), 1996, 1/3 (214-222)

Comparison of the effects of magnesium hydroxide and a bulk laxative on lipids, carbohydrates, vitamins A and E, and minerals in geriatric hospital patients in the treatment of constipation. J Int Med Res (ENGLAND) Sep-Oct 1989, 17 (5) p442-54

[Magnesium: current concepts of its physiopathology, clinical aspects and therapy]. Acta Vitaminol Enzymol (ITALY) 1982, 4 (1-2) p87-97

[Treatment of constipation with vitamin B5 or dexpanthenol]. Med Chir Dig (FRANCE) 1979, 8 (7) p671-4

Endogenous nitric oxide modulates morphine-induced constipation. Biochem Biophys Res Commun (UNITED STATES) Dec 16 1991, 181 (2) p889-93

Effectiveness of bran supplement on the bowel management of elderly rehabilitation patients. J Gerontol Nurs (UNITED STATES) Oct 1995, 21 (10) p21-30

Mechanisms of constipation in older persons and effects of fiber compared with placebo. J Am Geriatr Soc (UNITED STATES) Jun 1995, 43 (6)

Comparison of the effects of magnesium hydroxide and a bulk laxative on lipids, carbohydrates, vitamins A and E, and minerals in geriatric hospital patients in the treatment of constipation. J Int Med Res (ENGLAND) Sep-Oct 1989, 17 (5) p442-54

[Magnesium: current concepts of its physiopathology, clinical aspects and therapy]. Acta Vitaminol Enzymol (ITALY) 1982, 4 (1-2) p87-97

[Treatment of constipation with vitamin B5 or dexpanthenol] Med Chir Dig (FRANCE) 1979, 8 (7) p671-4

Endogenous nitric oxide modulates morphine-induced constipation. Biochem Biophys Res Commun (UNITED STATES) Dec 16 1991, 181 (2) p889-93

Effectiveness of bran supplement on the bowel management of elderly rehabilitation patients. J Gerontol Nurs (UNITED STATES) Oct 1995, 21 (10) p21-30

Mechanisms of constipation in older persons and effects of fiber compared with placebo. J Am Geriatr Soc (UNITED STATES) Jun 1995, 43 (6)

Deafness

See references under Hearing Loss.

Depression

Natural product formulations available in europe for psychotropic indications. Psychopharmacology Bulletin (USA), 1995, 31/4 (745-751)

Antidepressive effectiveness of a highly dosed hypericum extract. Munchener Medizinische Wochenschrift (Germany), 1996, 138/3 (35-39)

St. John's Wort in the treatment of depression. Johanniskraut zur antidepressiven therapie. Fortschritte der Medizin (Germany), 1995, 113/25 (32-33)

Hypericum perforatum. Fitoterapia (Italy), 1995, 66/1 (43-68)

Psychomotoric performance improvement: Antidepressant therapy with St John's wort. THERA-PIEWOCHE (Germany), 1995, 45/2 (106+108+110+112)

Hypericum in the treatment of seasonal affective disorders. J. GERIATR. PSYCHIATRY NEUROL. (Canada), 1994, 7/SUPPL. 1 (S29-S33)

Effectiveness and tolerance of the hypericum extract LI 160 compared to maprotiline: A multicenter double-blind study. J. GERIATR. PSYCHIATRY NEUROL. (Canada), 1994, 7/SUPPL. 1 (S24-S28)

Effectiveness and tolerance of the hypericum extract LI 160 in comparison with imipramine: Randomized double-blind study with 135 outpatients. J. GERIATR. PSYCHIATRY NEUROL. (Canada), 1994, 7/SUPPL. 1 (S19-S23)

Multicenter double-blind study examining the antidepressant effectiveness of the hypericum extract LI 160. J. GERIATR. PSYCHIATRY NEUROL. (Canada), 1994, 7/SUPPL. 1 (S15-S18)

Hypericum treatment of mild depressions with somatic symptoms. J. GERIATR. PSYCHIATRY NEU-ROL. (Canada), 1994, 7/SUPPL. 1 (S12-S14)

St. Johns' wort: A prescription from nature against depressions. Johanniskraut: ein rezept der natur gegen depressionen. THERAPIEWOCHE (Germany), 1994, 44/14 (808+811-815)

Psychopharmacological therapy after acquired brain damage. MUNCH. MED. WOCHENSCHR. (Germany), 1994, 136/4 (51-55)

Extract of St. John's wort in the treatment of depression - Attention and reaction remain unimpaired. FORTSCHR. MED. (Germany), 1993, 111/19 (37-40)

Investigations of the antidepressive effects of St. Johns Wort. PZ WISS. (Germany), 1993, 138/2 (50-54)

Experimental animal studies of the psychotropic activity of a Hypericum extract. ARZNEIM.-FORSCH./DRUG RES. (GERMANY, WEST), 1987, 37/1 (10-13)

Plasma tryptophan and five other amino acids in depressed and normal subjects. Archives of General Psychiatry 38(6):642-646, 1981

Trace amine deficit in depressive illness: the phenylalanine connexion. Acta Psychiatrica Scandinavica 61(Suppl. 280):29-39, 1980

Phenylalanine levels in endogenous psychoses. Psychiatrie, Neurologie und Medizinische Psychologie 32(10):631-633, 1980

Evaluation of the relative potency of individual competing amino acids to tryptophan transport in endogenously depressed patients. Psychiatry Research 3(2):141-150, 1980

Amino acids in mental illness. Biological psychiatry today. Vol. B Amsterdam, Elsevier/North Holland, 1979, p1581-4

Lithium prevention of amphetamine-induced 'manic' excitement and of reserpine- induced 'depression' in mice: possible role of 2-phenylethylamine. Psychopharmacology (Berlin) 59(3):259-262, 1978

Depression, pregnancy and phenylalanine. Neuropisiquiatria (Buenos Aires) 8(1):60-64, 1977

Theoretical and therapeutic potential of indoleamine precursors in affective disorders. Neuropsychobiology (Basel) 3(4):199-233, 1977

Phenylethylamine and glucose in true depression. Journal of Orthomolecular Psychiatry (Regina) 5(3):199-202, 1976

Therapeutic action of D-phenylalanine in Parkinson's disease. Arzneimittel-Forschung (Aulendorf) 26(4):577-579, 1976

Effects of D-phenylalanine on clinical picture and phenethylaminuria in depression. Biological Psychiatry 10(2):235-239, 1975

Phenylalanine for endogenous depression. Journal of Orthomolecular Psychiatry (Regina) 3(2):80-81, 1974

Rapidity of onset of the antidepressant effect of parenteral S-adenosyl-L-methionine. Psychiatry Research (Ireland), 1995, 56/3

The clinical potential of ademetionine (S-adenosylmethionine) in neurological disorders. DRUGS (New Zealand), 1994, 48/2 (137-152)

Primary fibromyalgia is responsive to S-adenosyl-L-methionine. CURR. THER. RES. CLIN. EXP. (USA), 1994, 55/7

S-adenosyl-L-methionine in Sjogren's syndrome and fibromyalgia. CURR. THER. RES. CLIN. EXP. (USA), 1994, 55/6

Effects of S-adenosyl-L-methionine on cognitive and vigilance functions in the elderly. CURR. THER. RES. CLIN. EXP. (USA), 1994, 55/6

Results of treatment with s-adenosyl-l-methionine in patients with major depression and internal illnesses. CURR. THER. RES. CLIN. EXP. (USA), 1994, 55/6

S-adenosyl-l-methionine (SAM) as antidepressant: Meta-analysis of clinical studies. ACTA NEUROL. SCAND. SUPPL. (Denmark), 1994, 89/154

S-adenosyl-L-methionine in the treatment of major depression complicating chronic alcoholism. CURR. THER. RES. CLIN. EXP. (USA), 1994, 55/1

Clinical evaluation of S-adenosyl-L-methionine versus transcutaneous electrical nerve stimulation in primary fibromyalgia. CURR. THER. RES. CLIN. EXP. (USA), 1993, 53/2

Double blind, placebo-controlled study of S-adenosyl-L-methionine in depressed postmenopausal women. PSYCHOTHER. PSYCHOSOM. (Switzerland), 1993, 59/1

S-Adenosyl-methionine (SAM) as antidepressant. NEW TRENDS CLIN. NEUROPHARMACOL. (Italy), 1992, 6/1-4

Efficacy of S-adenosyl-L-methionine in speeding the onset of action of imipramine. PSYCHIATRY RES. (Ireland), 1992, 44/3

Oral S-adenosyl-L-methionine in depression. CURR. THER. RES. CLIN. EXP. (USA), 1992, 52/3

Neuroendocrine effects of S-adenosyl-(L)-methionine, a novel putative antidepressant. J. PSYCHIATR. RES. (United Kingdom), 1990, 24/2

The antidepressant potential of oral S-adenosyl-l-methionine. ACTA PSYCHIATR. SCAND. (Denmark), 1990, 81/5

S-Adenosyl-L-methionine. A review of its pharmacological properties and therapeutic potential in liver dysfunction and affective disorders in relation to its physiological role in cell metabolism. DRUGS (New Zealand), 1989, 38/3

Antidepressants: A Comparative review of the clinical pharmacology and therapeutic use of the 'newer' versus the 'older' drugs. DRUGS (New Zealand), 1989, 37/5 (713-738)

Neuropharmacology of S-adenosyl-L-methionine. AM. J. MED. (USA), 1987, 83/5 A (95-103)

Vitamins in psychiatry. Do they have a role?. DRUGS (AUSTRALIA), 1985, 30/1

S-adenosyl-L-methionine (SAM) in clinical practice: Preliminary report on 75

minor depressives. CURR. THER. RES., CLIN. EXP. (USA), 1985, 37/4

S-Adenosyl-L-Methionine (SAM) treatment in psychogeriatry: a controlled clinical trial in depressed patients. G.GERONTOL. (ITALY), 1977, 25/3

A methyl donor, adenosylmethionine, in depression. FOLIA NEUROPSYCHIAT.(LECCE) (ITALY), 1973, 16/4

Therapeutic effects and mechanism of action of S adenosyl l methionine in depressive syndromes. MINERVA MED. (ITALY), 1973, 64/29 (1515-1529)

S-Adenosyl-methionine (SAM) as antidepressant. NEW TRENDS CLIN. NEUROPHARMACOL. (Italy), 1992, 6/1-4

Antidepressants: A Comparative review of the clinical pharmacology and therapeutic use of the 'newer' versus the 'older' drugs. DRUGS (New Zealand), 1989, 37/5 (713-738)

Monitoring S-adenosyl-methionine blood levels and antidepressant effect. ACTA NEUROL. (ITALY), 1980, 35/6 (488-495)

Long-term high dose treatment of depression with St John's wort extract. TW Neurologie Psychiatrie (Germany), 1995, 9/4 (220-221)

Effective phytotherapy for depressive patients. Effiziente phytotherapie fur depressive. Munchener Medizinische Wochenschrift (Germany), 1996, 138/7 (58)

St John's wort - An effective alternative with almost no side-effects for the treatment of depression. Depressionen: johanniskraut - die effektive und nebenwirkungsarme alternative. Zeitschrift fur Allgemeinmedizin (Germany), 1996, 72/1 (63)

Hypericum perforatum (Saint Johns wort) in the treatment of depression. THERAPIEWOCHE (Germany), 1993, 43/17 (962)

Good results with Hypericum perforatum in the treatment of depressions. FORTSCHR. MED. (Germany), 1993, 111/8 (57-58)

The efficacy of hypericum extract is double-blind verified. PRAX. MAG. MED. (Germany), 1993, -/4 (46)

Medicinal plants improve the results of brain performance test. FORTSCHR. MED. (Germany), 1993, 111/6 (50)

The efficacy of Hypericum extract in the treatment of depression. MUNCH. MED. WOCHENSCHR. (Germany), 1993, 135/8 (65)

Phytotherapeutic antidepressive agent with few side-effects. FORTSCHR. MED. (Germany), 1993, 111/3 (54+56)

Depression - To brighten up the mind with Saint-John's-Wort. TW NEUROL. PSYCHIATR. (Germany), 1992, 6/12 (793-794)

Saint Johns wort in the treatment of depressions. THERAPIEWOCHE (Germany), 1992, 42/51-52 (3074-3075)

Saint Johns wort (Hypericum perforatum extract) in the treatment of depressions. FORTSCHR. MED. (Germany), 1992, 110/31 (68-69)

Herbal medicine in depressions? PHARM. ZTG. (Germany), 1992, 137/41 (78-79)

Identification of selective MAO-type-A inhibitors in Hypericum perforatum. PHARMACOPSYCHIATRY (Germany, Federal Republic of), 1989, 22/5 (194)

Diabetes Type I (Juvenile Diabetes)

Oral alpha lipoic acid preparation proves good bioavailability in diabetic polyneuropathy. Therapiewoche (Germany), 1995, 45/23 (1367-1370)

Lipoic acid improves nerve blood flow, reduces oxidative stress, and improves distal nerve conduction in experimental diabetic neuropathy. Diabetes Care (USA), 1995, 18/8 (1160-1167)

Thioctic (lipoic) acid: A therapeutic metal-chelating antioxidant? Biochemical Pharmacology (United Kingdom), 1995, 50/1 (123-126)

Diabetic polyneuropathy. Most effective measure: Keep blood sugar close to normal from the start. Munchener Medizinische Wochenschrift (Germany), 1995, 137/6

Primary preventive and secondary interventionary effects of acetyl-L-carnitine on diabetic neuropathy in the bio-breeding Worcester rat. Journal of Clinical Investigation (USA), 1996, 97/8 (1900-1907)

Effects of acetyl- and proprionyl-L-carnitine on peripheral nerve function and vascular supply in experimental diabetes. Metabolism: Clinical and Experimental (USA), 1995, 44/9

Acetyl-L-carnitine corrects the altered peripheral nerve function of experimental diabetes. Metabolism: Clinical and Experimental (USA), 1995, 44/5

Diabetic neuropathy in the rat: 1. Alcar augments the reduced levels and axoplasmic transport of substance P. J. NEUROSCI. RES. (USA), 1995, 40/3 (414-419)

Hypothesis: the role of vitamin C in diabetic angiopathy. PERSPECT.BIOL.MED. (USA), 1974, 17/2 (210-217)

Treatment of symptomatic diabetic peripheral neuropathy with the anti-oxidant alpha- lipoic acid. A 3-week multicentre randomized controlled trial (ALADIN Study). Diabetologia (Germany), 1995, 38/12 (1425-1433)

Alternative therapeutic principles in the prevention of microvascular and Neuropathic complications. Diabetes Research and Clinical Practice (Ireland), 1995, 28/SUPPL.

Effects of aminoguanidine on rat pancreatic islets in culture and on the pancreatic islet blood flow of anaesthetized rats. Biochemical Pharmacology (USA), 1996, 51/12 (1711-1717)

Aminoguanidine prevents the decreased myocardial compliance produced by streptozotocin-induced diabetes mellitus in rats. Circulation (USA), 1996, 93/10 (1905-1912)

Slowing of peripheral motor nerve conduction was ameliorated by aminoguanidine in streptozocin-induced diabetic rats. European Journal of Endocrinology (Norway), 1996, 134/4 (467-473)

Thiamine pyrophosphate and pyridoxamine inhibit the formation of antigenic advanced glycation end-products: Comparison with aminoguanidine. Biochemical and Biophysical Research Communications (USA), 1996, 220/1

Advanced glycosylation end products in diabetic renal and vascular disease. American Journal of Kidney Diseases (USA), 1995, 26/6 (875-888)

Aminoguanidine treatment inhibits the development of experimental diabetic retinopathy. PROC. NATL ACAD. SCI. U. S. A. (USA), 1991, 88/24 (11555-11558)

Aminoguanidine effects on nerve blood flow, vascular permeability, electrophysiology, and oxygen free radicals. PROC. NATL ACAD. SCI. U. S. A. (USA), 1991, 88/14 (6107-6111)

Diabetes Type II (Adult Onset Diabetes)

Acetyl-L-carnitine effects on nerve conduction and glycemic regulation in experimental diabetes. Endocrine Research (USA), 1997, 23/1-2 (27-36)

Age-related decreases in chromium levels in 51,665 hair, sweat, and serum samples from 40,872 patients - Implications for the prevention of cardiovascular disease and type II diabetes mellitus. Metabolism: Clinical and Experimental (USA), 1997, 46/5 (469-473)

Lipoic acid (thioctic acid): Antioxidant properties and their clinical implications. Diabetes und Stoffwechsel (Germany), 1996, 5/3 SUPPL. (98-101)

Effect of lipoic acid (thioctic acid) on peripheral nerve of experimental diabetic neuropathy. USA Diabetes und Stoffwechsel (Germany), 1996, 5/3 SUPPL. (94-97)

Lipoic acid alpha-potential modulator of insulin sensitivity in patients with non-insulin-dependent diabetes mellitus. Diabetes und Stoffwechsel (Germany), 1996, 5/3 SUPPL. (64-70)

Lipoic acid acutely ameliorates insulin sensitivity in obese subjects with type 2 diabetes. Diabetes und Stoffwechsel (Germany), 1996, 5/3 SUPPL. (59-63)

Treatment of symptomatic diabetic peripheral neuropathy with alpha-lipoic acid. A 3-week multicentre randomized controlled trial (ALADIN Study). Diabetes und Stoffwechsel (Germany), 1996, 5/3 SUPPL. (102-110)

Effect of lipoic acid (thioctic acid) on glucose homeostasis and muscle glucose transporters in diabetic rats. Diabetes und Stoffwechsel (Germany), 1996, 5/3 SUPPL. (50-54)

Altered 14C-deoxyglucose incorporation in rat brain following treatment with alpha-lipoic acid (thioctic acid). Clinical implications for diabetic neuropathy and neurodegenerative disorders. Diabetes und Stoffwechsel (Germany), 1996, 5/3 SUPPL. (31-35)

Studies on the bioavailability of alpha lipoic acid in type I and type II diabetics with diabetic neuropathy. Diabetes und Stoffwechsel (Germany), 1996, 5/3 SUPPL. (23-26)

On the pharmacokinetics of alpha-lipoic acid in patients with diabetic polyneuropathy. Diabetes und Stoffwechsel (Germany), 1996, 5/3 SUPPL. (17-22)

Chromium oligopeptide activates insulin receptor tyrosine kinase activity. Biochemistry (USA), 1997, 36/15 (4382-4385)

Effect of chromium nicotinic acid supplementation on selected cardiovascular disease risk factors. Biological Trace Element Research (USA), 1996, 55/3 (297-305)

Modulation of cellular reducing equivalent homeostasis by alpha-lipoic acid. Mechanisms and implications for diabetes and ischemic injury. Biochemical Pharmacology (USA), 1997, 53/3 (393-399)

Endothelial dysfunction: Clinical implications. Progress in Cardiovascular Diseases (USA), 1997, 39/4 (287-324)

Effects of treatment with the antioxidant alpha-lipoic acid on cardiac autonomic neuropathy in NIDDM patients: A 4-month randomized controlled multicenter trial (DEKAN study). Diabetes Care (USA), 1997, 20/3 (369-373)

alpha-Lipoic acid corrects neuropeptide deficits in diabetic rats via induction of trophic support. Neuroscience Letters (Ireland), 1997, 222/3 (191-194)

Chromium picolinate supplementation improves cardiac metabolism, but not myosin isoenzyme distribution in the diabetic heart. Journal of Nutritional Biochemistry (USA), 1996, 7/11 (617-622)

Dehydroepiandrosterone and diseases of aging. Drugs and Aging (New Zealand), 1996, 9/4 (274-291)

Sex hormones and DHEA-SO4 in relation to ischemic heart disease mortality in diabetic subjects: The Wisconsin Epidemiologic Study of Diabetic Retinopathy. Diabetes Care (USA), 1996, 19/10 (1045-1050)

The effects of acetyl-L-carnitine and sorbinil on peripheral nerve structure, chemistry, and function in experimental diabetes. Metabolism: Clinical and Experimental (USA), 1996, 45/7 (902-907)

Acetyl-L-carnitine deficiency as a cause of altered nerve myo-inositol content, Na,K-ATPase activity, and motor conduction velocity in the streptozotocin-diabetic rat. Metabolism: Clinical and Experimental (USA), 1996, 45/7 (865-872)

Unrecognized pandemic subclinical diabetes of the affluent nations: Causes, cost and prevention. Journal of Orthomolecular Medicine (Canada), 1996, 11/2 (95-99)

Evidence of a relationship between childhood-onset type I diabetes and low groundwater concentration of zinc. Diabetes Care (USA), 1996, 19/8 (873-875)

Improved pallesthetic sensitivity of pudendal nerve in impotent diabetic patients treated with acetyl-L-carnitine. Acta Urologica Italica (Italy), 1996, 10/3 (185-187)

Primary preventive and secondary interventionary effects of acetyl-L- carnitine on diabetic neuropathy in the bio-breeding Worcester rat. Journal of Clinical Investigation (USA), 1996, 97/8 (1900-1907)

Vitamin and mineral deficiencies which may predispose to glucose intolerance of pregnancy. Journal of the American College of Nutrition (USA), 1996, 15/1 (14-20)

Antioxidant status in patients with uncomplicated insulin-dependent and non-insulin-dependent diabetes mellitus. European Journal of Clinical Investigation (United Kingdom), 1997, 27/6 (484-490)

Nutrient intake and food use in an Ojibwa-Cree community in Northern Ontario assessed by 24h dietary recall. Nutrition Research (USA), 1997, 17/4 (603-618)

Effect of vitamin C supplementation on hepatic cytochrome P450 mixed-function oxidase activity in streptozotocin-diabetic rats. Toxicology Letters (Ireland), 1996, 89/3 (249-256)

The effect of dietary treatment on lipid peroxidation and antioxidant status in newly diagnosed noninsulin dependent diabetes. Free Radical Biology and Medicine (USA), 1996, 21/5 (719-726)

Vitamin B6 alleviates the vascular complications of insulin-treated STZ-induced diabetic rats. Nutritional Sciences Journal (Taiwan), 1996, 21/3 (235-248)

Total vitamin C, ascorbic acid, and dehydroascorbic acid concentrations in plasma of critically ill patients. American Journal of Clinical Nutrition (USA), 1996, 63/5 (760-765)

Clinical study of vitamin influence in diabetes mellitus. Journal of the Medical Society of Toho University (Japan), 1996, 42/6 (577-581)

Vitamins and metals: Potential dangers for the human being. Schweizerische Medizinische Wochenschrift (Switzerland), 1996, 126/15 (607-611)

Leukocyte lipid peroxidation, superoxide dismutase, glutathione peroxidase and serum and leukocyte vitamin C levels of patients with type II diabetes mellitus. Clinica Chimica Acta (Netherlands), 1996, 244/2 (221-227)

Erythrocyte and plasma antioxidant activity in type I diabetes mellitus. Presse Medicale (France), 1996, 25/5 (188-192)

Vitamin C improves endothelium-dependent vasodilation in patients with non-insulin-dependent diabetes mellitus. Journal of Clinical Investigation (USA), 1996, 97/1 (22-28)

Effects of aspirin or basic amino acids on collagen cross-links and complications in NIDDM. Diabetes Care (UNITED STATES) May 1997, 20 (5) p832-5

Acute and chronic response to vanadium following two methods of streptozotocin-diabetes induction. Can J Physiol Pharmacol (CANADA) Feb 1997, 75 (2) p83-90

[Comparison of metabolism of water-soluble vitamins in healthy children and in children with insulin-dependent diabetes mellitus depending upon the level of vitamins in the diet]. Vopr Med Khim (RUSSIA) Apr-Jun 1996, 42 (2) p153-8

Spice constituents scavenging free radicals and inhibiting pentosidine formation in a model system. Biosci Biotechnol Biochem (JAPAN) Feb 1997, 61 (2) p263-6

L-Arginine reduces lipid peroxidation in patients with diabetes mellitus. Free Radic Biol Med (UNITED STATES) 1997, 22 (1-2) p355-7

Short-term oral administration of L-arginine reverses defective endothelium-dependent relaxation and cGMP generation in diabetes. Eur J Pharmacol (NETHERLANDS) Dec 19 1996, 317 (2-3) p317-20

A diet enriched in protein accelerates diabetes manifestation in NOD mice. Acta Diabetol (GERMANY) Sep 1996, 33 (3) p236-40

Metformin improves hemodynamic and rheological responses to L-arginine in NIDDM patients. Diabetes Care (UNITED STATES) Sep 1996, 19 (9) p934-9

References

Impairment of coronary blood flow regulation by endothelium-derived nitric oxide in dogs with alloxan-induced diabetes. J Cardiovasc Pharmacol (UNITED STATES) Jul 1996, 28 (1) p60-7

Involvement of the L-arginine-nitric oxide pathway in hyperglycaemia-induced coronary artery dysfunction of isolated guinea pig hearts. Eur J Clin Invest (ENGLAND) Aug 1996, 26 (8) p707-12

Deficient nitric oxide responsible for reduced nerve blood flow in diabetic rats: effects of L-NAME, L-arginine, sodium nitroprusside and evening primrose oil. Br J Pharmacol (ENGLAND) May 1996, 118 (1) p186-90

Interactions between essential fatty acid, prostanoid, polyol pathway and nitric oxide mechanisms in the neurovascular deficit of diabetic rats. Diabetologia (GERMANY) Feb 1996, 39 (2) p172-82

Effects of vanadyl sulfate on carbohydrate and lipid metabolism in patients with non-insulin-dependent diabetes mellitus. Metabolism (UNITED STATES) Sep 1996, 45 (9) p1130-5

Contraction and relaxation of aortas from diabetic rats: effects of chronic anti-oxidant and aminoguanidine treatments. Naunyn Schmiedebergs Arch Pharmacol (GERMANY) Apr 1996, 353 (5) p584-91

[Erythrocyte and plasma antioxidant activity in diabetes mellitus type I]. Activite anti-oxydante erythrocytaire et plasmatique dans le diabete de type I. Presse Med (FRANCE) Feb 10 1996, 25 (5) p188-92

Hyperglycemia-induced latent scurvy and atherosclerosis: the scorbutic-metaplasia hypothesis. Med Hypotheses (ENGLAND) Feb 1996, 46 (2) p119-29

Oral vanadyl sulfate improves insulin sensitivity in NIDDM but not in obese nondiabetic subjects. Diabetes (UNITED STATES) May 1996, 45 (5) p659-66

Homologous physiological effects of phenformin and chromium picolinate. Med Hypotheses (ENGLAND) Oct 1993, 41 (4) p316-24

[The effect of chromium picolinate on the liver levels of trace elements] Efecto del picolinato de cromo en los niveles hepaticos de algunos elementos traza. Nutr Hosp (SPAIN) Nov-Dec 1995, 10 (6) p373-6

Anabolic effects of insulin on bone suggest a role for chromium picolinate in preservation of bone density. Med Hypotheses (ENGLAND) Sep 1995, 45 (3) p241-6

Longevity effect of chromium picolinate--'rejuvenation' of hypothalamic function? Med Hypotheses(ENGLAND) Oct 1994, 43 (4) p253-65

Thiamine pyrophosphate and pyridoxamine inhibit the formation of antigenic advanced glycation endproducts: comparison with aminoguanidine. Biochem Biophys Res Commun (UNITED STATES) Mar 7 1996, 220 (1) p113-9

Loss of glucose-induced insulin secretion and GLUT2 expression in transplanted beta-cells. Diabetes (UNITED STATES) Jan 1995, 44 (1) p75-9

Case report: amelioration of insulin resistance in diabetes with dehydroepiandrosterone. Am J Med Sci (UNITED STATES) Nov 1993, 306 (5) p320-4

Therapeutic effects of dehydroepiandrosterone metabolites in diabetes mutant mice (C57BL/KsJ-db/db). Endocrinology (UNITED STATES) Jul 1984, 115 (1) p239-43

The endocrine pancreas in pyridoxine deficient rats. Med (JAPAN) Jul 1981, 134 (3) p331-6

Vitamin B6 metabolism and diabetes. Biochem Med Metab Biol (UNITED STATES) Jun 1994, 52 (1) p10-7

A deficiency of vitamin B6 is a plausible molecular basis of the retinopathy of patients with diabetes mellitus. Biochem Biophys Res Commun (UNITED STATES) Aug 30 1991, 179 (1) p615-9

Erythrocyte O2 transport and metabolism and effects of vitamin B6 therapy in type II diabetes mellitus. Diabetes (UNITED STATES) Jul 1989, 38 (7) p881-6

Diabetes and adrenal disease. Baillieres Clin Endocrinol Metab (ENGLAND) Oct 1992, 6 (4) p829-47

[Preventive treatment of diabetic microangiopathy: blocking the pathogenic mechanisms]. Diabete Metab (FRANCE) 1994, 20 (2 Pt 2) p219-28

Alternative therapeutic principles in the prevention of microvascular and neuropathic complications. Diabetes Res Clin Pract (IRELAND) Aug 1995, 28 Suppl pS201-7

Enhancement of glucose disposal in patients with type 2 diabetes by alpha-lipoic acid. Arzneimittelforschung (GERMANY) Aug 1995, 45 (8) p872-4

Inhibition with N-acetylcysteine of enhanced production of tumor necrosis factor in streptozotocin-induced diabetic rats. Clin Immunol Immunopathol (UNITED STATES) Jun 1994, 71 (3) p333-7

Effects of acetyl- and proprionyl-L-carnitine on peripheral nerve function and vascular supply in experimental diabetes. Metabolism (UNITED STATES) Sep 1995, 44 (9) p1209-14

Acetyl-L-carnitine for symptomatic diabetic neuropathy [letter]. Diabetologia (GERMANY) Jan 1995, 38 (1) p123

Peptide alterations in autonomic diabetic neuropathy prevented by acetyl-L-carnitine. Int J Clin Pharmacol Res (SWITZERLAND) 1992, 12 (5-6) p225-30

Prevention of cardiovascular and renal pathology of aging by the advanced glycation inhibitor aminoguanidine. Proc Natl Acad Sci U S A (UNITED STATES) Apr 30 1996, 93 (9) p3902-7

Prevention of long-term complications of non-insulin-dependent diabetes mellitus. Clin Invest Med (CANADA) Aug 1995, 18 (4) p332-9

Secondary intervention with aminoguanidine retards the progression of diabetic retinopathy in the rat model. Diabetologia (GERMANY) Jun 1995, 38 (6) p656-60

Prevention of glomerular basement membrane thickening by aminoguanidine in experimental diabetes mellitus. Metabolism (UNITED STATES) Oct 1991, 40 (10) p1016-9

Can metformin reduce insulin resistance in polycystic ovary syndrome? Fertil Steril (UNITED STATES) May 1996, 65 (5) p946-9

Effects of diet and metformin administration on sex hormone-binding globulin, androgens, and insulin in hirsute and obese women. J Clin Endocrinol Metab (UNITED STATES) Jul 1995, 80 (7) p2057-62

[The value of metformin in therapy of type 2 diabetes: effect on insulin resistance, diabetic control and cardiovascular risk factors]. Wien Klin Wochenschr (AUSTRIA) 1994, 106 (24) p793-802

Oral vanadyl sulfate improves hepatic and peripheral insulin sensitivity in patients with non-insulin-dependent diabetes mellitus. J Clin Invest (UNITED STATES) Jun 1995, 95 (6) p2501-9

References

Toxicity studies on one-year treatment of non-diabetic and streptozotocin-diabetic rats with vanadyl sulphate. Pharmacol Toxicol (DENMARK) Nov 1994, 75 (5) p265-73

Antidiabetic action of vanadyl in rats independent of in vivo insulin-receptor kinase activity. Diabetes (UNITED STATES) Apr 1991, 40 (4) p492-8

Homologous physiological effects of phenformin and chromium picolinate. Med Hypotheses (ENGLAND) Oct 1993, 41 (4) p316-24

[The effect of chromium picolinate on the liver levels of trace elements] Efecto del picolinato de cromo en los niveles hepaticos de algunos elementos traza. Nutr Hosp (SPAIN) Nov-Dec 1995, 10 (6) p373-6

Anabolic effects of insulin on bone suggest a role for chromium picolinate in preservation of bone density. Med Hypotheses (ENGLAND) Sep 1995, 45 (3) p241-6

Longevity effect of chromium picolinate—'rejuvenation' of hypothalamic function? Med Hypotheses(ENGLAND) Oct 1994, 43 (4) p253-65

Thiamine pyrophosphate and pyridoxamine inhibit the formation of antigenic advanced glycation end-products: comparison with aminoguanidine. Biochem Biophys Res Commun (UNITED STATES) Mar 7 1996, 220 (1) p113-9

Loss of glucose-induced insulin secretion and GLUT2 expression in transplanted beta- cells. Diabetes (UNITED STATES) Jan 1995, 44 (1) p75-9

Case report: amelioration of insulin resistance in diabetes with dehydroepiandrosterone. Am J Med Sci (UNITED STATES) Nov 1993, 306 (5) p320-4

Therapeutic effects of dehydroepiandrosterone metabolites in diabetes mutant mice (C57BL/KsJ-db/db). Endocrinology (UNITED STATES) Jul 1984, 115 (1) p239-43

The endocrine pancreas in pyridoxine deficient rats. Med (JAPAN) Jul 1981, 134 (3) p331-6

Vitamin B6 metabolism and diabetes. Biochem Med Metab Biol (UNITED STATES) Jun 1994, 52 (1) p10-7

A deficiency of vitamin B6 is a plausible molecular basis of the retinopathy of patients with diabetes mellitus. Biochem Biophys Res Commun (UNITED STATES) Aug 30 1991, 179 (1) p615-9

Erythrocyte O2 transport and metabolism and effects of vitamin B6 therapy in type II diabetes mellitus. Diabetes (UNITED STATES) Jul 1989, 38 (7) p881-6

Diabetes and adrenal disease. Baillieres Clin Endocrinol Metab (ENGLAND) Oct 1992, 6 (4) p829-47

[Preventive treatment of diabetic microangiopathy: blocking the pathogenic mechanisms] Diabete Metab (FRANCE) 1994, 20 (2 Pt 2) p219-28

Alternative therapeutic principles in the prevention of microvascular and neuropathic complications. Diabetes Res Clin Pract (IRELAND) Aug 1995, 28 Suppl pS201-7

Enhancement of glucose disposal in patients with type 2 diabetes by alpha-lipoic acid. Arzneimittelforschung (GERMANY) Aug 1995, 45 (8) p872-4

Inhibition with N-acetylcysteine of enhanced production of tumor necrosis factor in streptozotocin-induced diabetic rats. Clin Immunol Immunopathol (UNITED STATES) Jun 1994, 71 (3) p333-7

Effects of acetyl- and proprionyl-L-carnitine on peripheral nerve function and vascular supply in experimental diabetes. Metabolism (UNITED STATES) Sep 1995, 44 (9) p1209-14

Acetyl-L-carnitine for symptomatic diabetic neuropathy [letter] Diabetologia (GERMANY) Jan 1995, 38 (1) p123

Peptide alterations in autonomic diabetic neuropathy prevented by acetyl-L-carnitine. Int J Clin Pharmacol Res (SWITZERLAND) 1992, 12 (5-6) p225-30

Prevention of cardiovascular and renal pathology of aging by the advanced glycation inhibitor aminoguanidine. Proc Natl Acad Sci U S A (UNITED STATES) Apr 30 1996, 93 (9) p3902-7

Prevention of long-term complications of non-insulin-dependent diabetes mellitus. Clin Invest Med (CANADA) Aug 1995, 18 (4) p332-9

Secondary intervention with aminoguanidine retards the progression of diabetic retinopathy in the rat model. Diabetologia (GERMANY) Jun 1995, 38 (6) p656-60

Prevention of glomerular basement membrane thickening by aminoguanidine in experimental diabetes mellitus. Metabolism (UNITED STATES) Oct 1991, 40 (10) p1016-9

Can metformin reduce insulin resistance in polycystic ovary syndrome? Fertil Steril (UNITED STATES) May 1996, 65 (5) p946-9

Effects of diet and metformin administration on sex hormone-binding globulin, androgens, and insulin in hirsute and obese women. J Clin Endocrinol Metab (UNITED STATES) Jul 1995, 80 (7) p2057-62

[The value of metformin in therapy of type 2 diabetes: effect on insulin resistance, diabetic control and cardiovascular risk factors] Wien Klin Wochenschr (AUSTRIA) 1994, 106 (24) p793-802

Oral vanadyl sulfate improves insulin sensitivity in NIDDM but not in obese nondiabetic subjects. Diabetes (UNITED STATES) May 1996, 45 (5) p659-66

Oral vanadyl sulfate improves hepatic and peripheral insulin sensitivity in patients with non-insulin-dependent diabetes mellitus. J Clin Invest (UNITED STATES) Jun 1995, 95 (6) p2501-9

Toxicity studies on one-year treatment of non-diabetic and streptozotocin-diabetic rats with vanadyl sulphate. Pharmacol Toxicol (DENMARK) Nov 1994, 75 (5) p265-73

Antidiabetic action of vanadyl in rats independent of in vivo insulin-receptor kinase activity. Diabetes (UNITED STATES) Apr 1991, 40 (4) p492-8

Digestive Disorders

Digestive processes in the human colon. Nutrition (USA), 1995, 11/1 (37-45)

The ileum and carbohydrate-mediated feedback regulation of postprandial pancreaticobiliary secretion in normal humans.PANCREAS (USA), 1991, 6/5 (495-505)

Factors influencing carbohydrate digestion: Acute and long-term consequences.DIABETES NUTR. METAB. CLIN. EXP. (Italy), 1990, 3/3 (251-258): Two distinct adaptive responses in the synthesis of exocrine pancreatic enzymes to inverse changes in protein and carbohydrate in the diet. AM. J. PHYSIOL. (USA), 1984, 10/6 (G611-G616)

Carbohydrate absorption.MED.CLIN.N.AMER. (USA), 1974, 58/6 (1387-1395)

Dietary carbohydrates. Their indications and contraindications in clinical medicine.PRACTITIONER (ENGLAND), 1974, 212/1270 (448-453)

An analysis on fat digestion in the upper small intestine after intragastric infusion of a test meal in patients with exocrine pancreatic insufficiency.Japanese Journal of Gastroenterology (Japan), 1995, 92/8 (1169-1177)

Pancreatic triglyceride lipase and colipase: Insights into dietary fat digestion.GASTROENTEROLOGY (USA), 1994, 107/5 (1524-1536)

Role of nonpancreatic lipolytic activity in exocrine pancreatic insufficiency.GASTROENTEROLOGY (USA), 1987, 92/1 (125-129)

Rat lingual lipase: Effect of proteases, bile, and pH on enzyme stability Roberts I.M. AM. J. PHYSIOL. (USA), 1985, 12/4 (G496-G500)

Fat digestion by lingual lipase: Mechanism of lipolysis in the stomach and upper small intestine. PEDI-ATR. RES. (USA), 1984, 18/5 (402-409)

Fat digestion in the stomach: Stability of lingual lipase in the gastric environment.PEDIATR. RES. (USA), 1984, 18/3 (248-254)

Colipase and lipase secretion in childhood-onset pancreatic insufficiency. Delineation of patients with steatorrhea secondary to relative colipase deficiency.GASTROENTEROLOGY (USA), 1984, 86/1 (1-7)

New results about the role of lipase, colipase and bile acids in the fat digestion.DTSCH. Z. VERDAU.-STOFFWECHSELKR. (GERMANY, EAST), 1980, 40/6 (246-252)

Lipases, bile salts and fat digestion: New insights. ITAL. J. GASTROENTEROL. (ITALY), 1980, 12/2 (140-145)

Congenital pancreatic lipase deficiency. J. PEDIATR. (USA), 1980, 96/3I (412-416)

Controlled, double-blind multicenter trial of alyophilized total pancreas preparation against placebo in functional digestive disorders. FRANCE MED. CHIR. DIG. (FRANCE), 1987, 16/2 (137-141)

Down Syndrome

Vitamin E and Alzheimer's disease in subjects with Down syndrome. Journal of Mental Deficiency Research 1988 Dec Vol 32(6) 479-484

Behavioral disorders, learning disabilities and megavitamin therapy. Adolescence 1987 Fal Vol 22(87) 729-738

Macrocytosis and cognitive decline in Down syndrome. British Journal of Psychiatry 1986 Dec Vol 149 797-798

Treatment approaches in Down syndrome: A review. Australia & New Zealand Journal of Developmental Disabilities

A double blind study of vitamin B-sub-6 in Down syndrome infants: I. Clinical and biochemical results. Journal of Mental Deficiency Research 1985 Sep Vol 29(3) 233-240

A double blind study of vitamin B-sub-6 in Down syndrome infants: II. Cortical auditory evoked potentials. Journal of Mental Deficiency Research 1985 Sep Vol 29(3) 241-246

Xylose absorption in Down syndrome. Journal of Mental Deficiency Research 1985 Jun Vol 29(2) 173-177

Nutritional aspects of Down syndrome with special reference to the nervous system. British Journal of Psychiatry 1984 Aug Vol 145 115-120

Children's mental retardation study is attacked: A closer look. International Journal of Biosocial Research 1982 Vol 3(2) 75-86

Effects of nutritional supplementation on IQ and certain other variables associated with Down syndrome. American Journal of Mental Deficiency 1983 Sep Vol 88(2) 214-217

Vitamin A and carotene values of institutionalized mentally retarded subjects with and without Down syndrome. Journal of Mental Deficiency Research 1977 Mar Vol 21(1) 63-74

Sodium-dependent glutamate binding in senile dementia. Neurobiology of Aging 1987 May-Jun Vol 8(3) 219-223

Alzheimer-like neurotransmitter deficits in adult Down syndrome brain tissue. Journal of Neurology, Neurosurgery & Psychiatry 1987 Jun Vol 50(6) 775-778

A report on phosphatidylcholine therapy in a Down Syndrome child. Psychological Reports 1986 Feb Vol 58(1) 207-217

Emphysema And Chronic Obstructive Pulmonary Disease

Muscle and serum magnesium in pulmonary intensive care unit patients. Crit Care Med (UNITED STATES) Aug 1988, 16 (8) p751-60

Fluid and electrolyte considerations in diuretic therapy for hypertensive patients with chronic obstructive pulmonary disease. Arch Intern Med (UNITED STATES) Jan 1986, 146 (1) p129-33

Safety and effectiveness of ticarcillin plus clavulanate potassium in treatment of lower respiratory tract infections. Am J Med (UNITED STATES) Nov 29 1985, 79 (5B) p78-80

Frequently nebulized beta-agonists for asthma: effects on serum electrolytes. Ann Emerg Med (UNITED STATES) Nov 1992, 21 (11) p1337-42

Effect of nebulized albuterol on serum potassium and cardiac rhythm in patients with asthma or chronic obstructive pulmonary disease. Pharmacotherapy (UNITED STATES) Nov-Dec 1994, 14 (6) p729-33

The intrabronchial microbial flora in chronic bronchitis patients: a target for N-acetylcysteine therapy? Eur Respir J (DENMARK) Jan 1994, 7 (1) p94-101

[The influence of n-acetylcysteine on chemiluminescence of granulocytes in peripheral blood of patients with chronic bronchitis] Pneumonol Alergol Pol (POLAND) 1993, 61 (11-12)

Effects of coenzyme Q10 administration on pulmonary function and exercise performance in patients with chronic lung diseases. Clin Investig (GERMANY) 1993, 71 (8 Suppl) pS162-6

Protection by N-acetylcysteine of the histopathological and cytogenetical damage produced by exposure of rats to cigarette smoke. Cancer Lett (NETHERLANDS) Jun 15 1992, 64 (2) p123-31

Investigation of the protective effects of the antioxidants ascorbate, cysteine, and dapsone on the phagocyte-mediated oxidative inactivation of human alpha-1-protease inhibitor in vitro. Am Rev Respir Dis (UNITED STATES) Nov 1985, 132 (5) p1049-54

The role of dornase alfa (PULMOZYME) in the treatment of cystic fibrosis. Annals of Pharmacotherapy (USA), 1996, 30/6 (656-661)

Inhalation therapy with recombinant human deoxyribonuclease I Gonda I (PULMOZYME). Advanced Drug Delivery Reviews (Netherlands), 1996, 19/1 (37-46)

Aerosolized dornase alpha (rhDNase-PULMOZYME)) in cystic fibrosis. Journal of Clinical Pharmacy and Therapeutics (United Kingdom), 1995, 20/6

New pharmacologic approaches: rhDNase. Revue de Pneumologie Clinique (France), 1995, 51/3 (193-200)

Taurine and serine supplementation modulates the metabolic response to tumor necrosis factor alpha in rats fed a low protein diet. J. NUTR. (USA), 1992, 122/7 (1369-1375)

L-Carnitine and its role in medicine: A current consideration of its pharmacokinetics, its role in fatty acid metabolism and its use in ischaemic cardiac disease and primary and secondary L-carnitine deficiencies. Epitheorese Klinikes Farmakologias kai Farmakokinetikes (Greece), 1996, 14/1 (11-64)

Esophageal Reflux (Heartburn)

Prevention of esophageal cancer: the nutrition intervention trials in Linxian, China. Linxian Nutrition Intervention Trials Study Group. Cancer Res. 1994 Apr 1. 54(7 Suppl). P 2029s-2031s

Effects of vitamin/mineral supplementation on the proliferation of esophageal squamous epithelium in Linxian, China. Cancer Epidemiol Biomarkers Prev. 1994 Apr-May. 3(3). P 277-9

[Preliminary report on the results of nutrition prevention trials of cancer and other common diseases among residents in Linxian, China] Chung Hua Chung Liu Tsa Chih. 1993 May. 15(3). P 165-81

Chemoprevention of oral leukoplakia and chronic esophagitis in an area of high incidence of oral and esophageal cancer. Ann Epidemiol. 1993 May. 3(3). P 225-34

[Clinical aspects, diagnosis and treatment of esophageal spasm] Grud Serdechnososudistaia Khir. 1991 Jun. (6). P 57-60

Association of esophageal cytological abnormalities with vitamin and lipotrope deficiencies in populations at risk for esophageal cancer. ANTICANCER RES. (Greece), 1988, 8/4 (711-716)

The effect of gamma-linolenic acid on clinical status, red cell fatty acid composition and membrane microviscosity in infants with atopic dermatitis. SO:Drugs Exp Clin Res. 1994. 20(2). P 77-84

Fatty acid compositions of plasma lipids in atopic dermatitis/asthma patients. SO:Arerugi. 1994 Jan. 43(1). P 37-43

Possible immunologic involvement of antioxidants in cancer prevention. Am J Clin Nutr. 1995 Dec. 62(6 Suppl). P 1477S-1482S

Estrogen Replacement Therapy

Dietary soy protein and estrogen replacement therapy improve cardiovascular risk factors and decrease aortic cholesteryl ester content in ovariectomized cynomolgus monkeys. Metabolism: Clinical and Experimental (USA), 1997, 46/6 (698-705)

Daidzein sulfoconjugates are potent inhibitors of sterol sulfatase (EC 3.1.6.2). Biochemical and Biophysical Research Communications (USA), 1997, 233/3 (579-583)

Adrenal puberty or adrenarche. Andrologie (France), 1997, 7/2 (165-186)

Urinary steroids at time of surgery in postmenopausal women with breast cancer. Breast Cancer Research and Treatment (USA), 1997, 44/1 (83-89)

Relation of serum levels of testosterone and dehydroepiandrosterone sulfate to risk of breast cancer in postmenopausal women. American Journal of Epidemiology (USA), 1997, 145/11 (1030-1038)

Role of glucose-6-phosphate dehydrogenase inhibition in the antiproliferative effects of dehydroepiandrosterone on human breast cancer cells. British Journal of Cancer (United Kingdom), 1997, 75/4 (589-592)

Effects of soya consumption for one month on steroid hormones in premenopausal women: Implications for breast cancer risk reduction. Cancer Epidemiology Biomarkers and Prevention (USA), 1996, 5/1 (63-70)

Chemoprevention by dietary dehydroepiandrosterone against promotion/progressi on phase of radiation-induced mammary tumorigenesis in rats. Journal of Steroid Biochemistry and Molecular Biology (United Kingdom), 1995, 54/1-2 (47-53)

Epidemiology of soy and cancer: Perspectives and directions. Journal of Nutrition (USA), 1995, 125/3 SUPPL. (709S-712S)

Prevention by dehydroepiandrosterone of the development of mammary carcinoma induced by 7,12-dimethylbenz(a)anthracene (DMBA) in the rat. BREAST CANCER RES. TREAT. (USA), 1994, 29/2 (203-217)

Serum sex hormone levels after menopause and subsequent breast cancer. Journal of the National Cancer Institute (USA), 1996, 88/5 (291-296)

Relationship of serum dehydroepiandrosterone (DHEA), DHEA sulfate, and 5-androstene-3beta,17beta-diol to risk of breast cancer in postmenopausal women. Cancer Epidemiology Biomarkers and Prevention (USA), 1997, 6/3 (177-181)

Effects of oestrogen and progesterone on age-related changes in arteries of postmenopausal women. Clin Exp Pharmacol Physiol (AUSTRALIA) Jun 1997, 24 (6) p457-9

Hormone replacement therapy in postmenopausal women: urinary N-telopeptide of type I collagen monitors therapeutic effect and predicts response of bone mineral density. Am J Med (UNITED STATES) Jan 1997, 102 (1) p29-37

Estrogen inhibits cuff-induced intimal thickening of rat femoral artery: effects on migration and proliferation of vascular smooth muscle cells. Atherosclerosis (IRELAND) Apr 1997, 130 (1-2) p1-10

Ovarian aging and hormone replacement therapy. Hormonal levels, symptoms, and attitudes of African-American and white women. J Gen Intern Med (UNITED STATES) Apr 1997, 12 (4) p230-6

References

In vivo estrogen regulation of epidermal growth factor receptor in human endometrium. J Clin Endocrinol Metab (UNITED STATES) May 1997, 82 (5) p1467-71

The perimenopausal hot flash: epidemiology, physiology, and treatment. Nurse Pract (UNITED STATES) Mar 1997, 22 (3) p55-6, 61-6

Effects of hormone replacement modalities on low density lipoprotein composition and distribution in ovariectomized cynomolgus monkeys. Atherosclerosis (IRELAND) Apr 5 1996, 121 (2) p217-29

Cause-specific mortality in women receiving hormone replacement therapy. Epidemiology (UNITED STATES) Jan 1997, 8 (1) p59-65

Hormone replacement therapy increases trabecular and cortical bone density in osteoporotic women. Medicina (B Aires) (ARGENTINA) 1996, 56 (3) p247-51

DHEA: a hormone with multiple effects. Curr Opin Obstet Gynecol (UNITED STATES) Oct 1996, 8 (5) p351-4

Mammographic changes in women on hormonal replacement therapy. Maturitas (IRELAND) Aug 1996, 25 (1) p51-7

Androgen replacement therapy in women: myths and realities. Int J Fertil Menopausal Stud (UNITED STATES) Jul-Aug 1996, 41 (4) p412-22

Sequential addition of low dose of medrogestone or medroxyprogesterone acetate to transdermal estradiol: a pilot study on their influence on the endometrium. Eur J Obstet Gynecol Reprod Biol (IRELAND) Sep 1996, 68 (1-2) p137-41

Hormone replacement therapy: clinical benefits and side-effects. Maturitas (IRELAND) May 1996, 23 Suppl pS31-6

Progestins. Maturitas (IRELAND) May 1996, 23 Suppl pS13-8

Evidence for primary and secondary prevention of coronary artery disease in women taking oestrogen replacement therapy. Eur Heart J (ENGLAND) Aug 1996, 17 Suppl D p9-14

Practical aspects of preventing and managing athersclerotic disease in post-menopausal women. Eur Heart J (ENGLAND) Aug 1996, 17 Suppl D p32-7

Hormone replacement therapy is associated with improved arterial physiology in healthy post-menopausal women. Clin Endocrinol (Oxf) (ENGLAND) Oct 1996, 45 (4) p435-41

An examination of the effect of combined cyclical hormone replacement therapy on lipoprotein(a) and other lipoproteins. Atherosclerosis (IRELAND) Jan 26 1996, 119 (2) p215-22

Effects of estrogens and progestogens on the renin-aldosterone system and blood pressure. Steroids (UNITED STATES) Apr 1996, 61 (4) p166-71

Effects of progestogens on haemostasis. Maturitas (IRELAND) May 1996, 24 (1-2) p1-19

Effects of hormone therapy on bone mineral density: results from the postmenopausal estrogen/progestin interventions (PEPI) trial. The Writing Group for the PEPI JAMA (UNITED STATES) Nov 6 1996, 276 (17) p1389-96

Transdermal estrogen replacement therapy in normal perimenopausal women: effects on pituitary-ovarian function. Gynecol Endocrinol (ENGLAND) Feb 1996, 10 (1) p49-53

The effects of androgens and other sex hormones on serum lipoproteins. Lijec Vjesn (CROATIA) Mar 1996, 118 Suppl 1 p33-7

Hormonal and environmental factors affecting cell proliferation and neoplasia in the mammary gland. Prog Clin Biol Res (UNITED STATES) 1996, 394 p211-53

The menopause and hormone replacement therapy: lipids, lipoproteins, coagulation and fibrinolytic factors. Maturitas (IRELAND) Mar 1996, 23 (2) p209-16

Hormonal therapy and genital tract cancer. Curr Opin Obstet Gynecol (UNITED STATES) Feb 1996, 8 (1) p38-41

Health consequences of short- and long-term postmenopausal hormone therapy. Clin Chem (UNITED STATES) Aug 1996, 42 (8 Pt 2) p1342-4

Current concepts in postmenopausal hormone replacement therapy. J Fam Pract (UNITED STATES) Jul 1996, 43 (1) p69-75

Regulation of estrogen/progestogen receptors in the endometrium. Int J Fertil Menopausal Stud (UNITED STATES) Jan-Feb 1996, 41 (1)p16-21

Hormone replacement therapy and breast cancer risk. Arch Fam Med (UNITED STATES) Jun 1996, 5 (6) p341-8

Hormone replacement therapy, hormone levels, and lipoprotein cholesterol concentrations in elderly women. Am J Obstet Gynecol (UNITED STATES) Mar 1996, 174 (3) p897-902

Hormone replacement therapy as treatment of breast cancer--a phase II study of Org OD 14 (tibilone). Br J Cancer (ENGLAND) May 1996, 73 (9) p1086-8

Postmenopausal hormone therapy and breast cancer. Obstet Gynecol (UNITED STATES) Feb 1996, 87 (2 Suppl)

Future aspects of hormone-replacement therapy. Acta Chirurgica Austriaca (Austria), 1996, 28/5 (282-284)

Neuroendocrine aspects of the menopause and hormone replacement therapy. Journal of Cardiovascular Pharmacology (USA), 1996, 28/SUPPL. 5 (S58-S60)

Hormone therapy and phytoestrogens. Journal of Clinical Pharmacy and Therapeutics (United Kingdom), 1996, 21/2 (101-111)

The effects of hormone replacement therapy on plasma vitamin E levels in post-menopausal women. European Journal of Obstetrics Gynecology and Reproductive Biology (Ireland), 1996, 66/2 (151-154)

Effects of hormonal therapies and dietary soy phytoestrogens on vaginal cytology in surgically post-menopausal macaques. Fertility and Sterility (USA), 1996, 65/5 (1031-1035)

Dietary and behavioral determinants of menopause. Clinical Consultations in Obstetrics and Gynecology (USA), 1996, 8/1 (21-26)

A review of the clinical effects of phytoestrogens. Obstetrics and Gynecology (USA), 1996, 87/5 II SUPPL. (897-904)

Molecular effects of genistein on estrogen receptor mediated pathways. Carcinogenesis (United Kingdom), 1996, 17/2 (271-275)

Rationale for the use of genistein-containing soy matrices in chemoprevention trials for breast and prostate cancer. Journal of Cellular Biochemistry (USA), 1995, 58/SUPPL. 22

Dietary flour supplementation decreases post-menopausal hot flushes: Effect of soy and wheat. Maturitas (Ireland), 1995, 21/3 (189-195)

Soy and experimental cancer: Animal studies. Journal of Nutrition (USA), 1995, 125/3 SUPPL.

Aromatase in bone cell: Association with osteoporosis in postmenopausal women. Journal of Steroid Biochemistry and Molecular Biology (United Kingdom), 1995, 53/1-6 (165-174)

Estrogen replacement therapy and fatal ovarian cancer. Am J Epidemiol (UNITED STATES) May 1 1995

Inhibition of breast cancer cell growth by combined treatment with vitamin D3 analogues and tamoxifen. Cancer Res (UNITED STATES) Nov 1 1994, 54 (21) p5711-7

Melatonin modulation of estrogen-regulated proteins, growth factors, and proto-oncogenes in human breast cancer. J Pineal Res (DENMARK) Mar 1995

Melatonin inhibition of MCF-7 human breast-cancer cells growth: influence of cell proliferation rate. Cancer Lett (IRELAND) Jul 13 1995

Modulation of cancer endocrine therapy by melatonin: a phase II study of tamoxifen plus melatonin in metastatic breast cancer patients progressing under tamoxifen alone. Br J Cancer (ENGLAND) Apr 1995

Modulation of estrogen receptor mRNA expression by melatonin in MCF-7 human breast cancer cells. Mol Endocrinol (UNITED STATES) Dec 1994

Melatonin modulates growth factor activity in MCF-7 human breast cancer cells. J Pineal Res (DENMARK) Aug 1994

Role of pineal gland in aetiology and treatment of breast cancer. Lancet (ENGLAND) Oct 14 1978

3beta-hydroxysteroid dehydrogenase/isomerase and aromatase activity in primary cultures of developing zebra finch telencephalon: Dehydroepiandrosterone as substrate for synthesis of androstenedione and estrogens. General and Comparative Endocrinology (USA), 1996, 102/3 (342-350)

Abnormal production of androgens in women with breast cancer. ANTICANCER RES. (Greece), 1994, 14/5 B (2113-2117)

Endogenous sex hormones: Impact on lipids, lipoproteins, and insulin. AM. J. MED. (USA), 1995, 98/1 A (40S-47S)

Dehydroepiandrosterone antiestrogenic action through androgen receptor in MCF-7 human breast cancer cell line. ANTICANCER RES. (Greece), 1993, 13/6 A (2267-2272)

Effect of flax seed ingestion on the menstrual cycle. J. CLIN. ENDOCRINOL. METAB. (USA), 1993, 77/5 (1215-1219)

Estrogen and nerve growth factor-related systems in brain. Effects on basal forebrain cholinergic neurons and implications for learning and memory processes and aging. ANN. NEW YORK ACAD. SCI. (USA), 1994, 743/- (165-199)

Postmenopausal estrogen replacement: A long-term cohort study. AM. J. MED. (USA), 1994, 97/1

(66-77)

Impact of the menopause on the epidemiology and risk factors of coronary artery heart disease in women. EXP. GERONTOL. (USA), 1994, 29/3-4 (357-375)

Hormone therapy and endometrium cancer. REPROD. HUM. HORM. (France), 1994, 7/4 (137-139)

Progestin replacement in the menopause: Effects on the endometrium and serum lipids. CURR. OPIN. OBSTET. GYNECOL. (USA), 1994, 6/3 (284-292)

Effects of hormone replacement therapy on lipoprotein(a) and lipids in postmenopausal women. ARTERIOSCLER. THROMB. (USA), 1994, 14/2 (275-281)

A review of the clinical effects of phytoestrogens. Obstetrics and Gynecology (USA), 1996, 87/5 II SUPPL. (897-904)

Molecular effects of genistein on estrogen receptor mediated pathways. Carcinogenesis (United Kingdom), 1996, 17/2 (271-275)

Rationale for the use of genistein-containing soy matrices in chemoprevention trials for breast and prostate cancer. Journal of Cellular Biochemistry (USA), 1995, 58/SUPPL. 22

Dietary flour supplementation decreases post-menopausal hot flushes: Effect of soy and wheat. Maturitas (Ireland), 1995, 21/3 (189-195)

Soy and experimental cancer: Animal studies. Journal of Nutrition (USA), 1995, 125/3 SUPPL.

Aromatase in bone cell: Association with osteoporosis in postmenopausal women. Journal of Steroid Biochemistry and Molecular Biology (United Kingdom), 1995, 53/1-6 (165-174)

Estrogen replacement therapy and fatal ovarian cancer. Am J Epidemiol (UNITED STATES) May 1 1995

Inhibition of breast cancer cell growth by combined treatment with vitamin D3 analogues and tamoxifen. Cancer Res (UNITED STATES) Nov 1 1994, 54 (21) p5711-7

Melatonin modulation of estrogen-regulated proteins, growth factors, and proto-oncogenes in human breast cancer. J Pineal Res (DENMARK) Mar 1995

Melatonin inhibition of MCF-7 human breast-cancer cells growth: influence of cell proliferation rate. Cancer Lett (IRELAND) Jul 13 1995

Modulation of cancer endocrine therapy by melatonin: a phase II study of tamoxifen plus melatonin in metastatic breast cancer patients progressing under tamoxifen alone. Br J Cancer (ENGLAND) Apr 1995

Modulation of estrogen receptor mRNA expression by melatonin in MCF-7 human breast cancer cells. Mol Endocrinol (UNITED STATES) Dec 1994

Melatonin modulates growth factor activity in MCF-7 human breast cancer cells. J Pineal Res (DENMARK) Aug 1994

Role of pineal gland in aetiology and treatment of breast cancer. Lancet (ENGLAND) Oct 14 1978

3beta-hydroxysteroid dehydrogenase/isomerase and aromatase activity in primary cultures of developing zebra finch telencephalon: Dehydroepiandrosterone as substrate for synthesis of androstenedione and estrogens. General and Comparative Endocrinology (USA), 1996, 102/3 (342- 350)

Aromatase in bone cell: Association with osteoporosis in postmenopausal women. Journal of Steroid Biochemistry and Molecular Biology (United Kingdom), 1995, 53/1-6 (165-174)

Abnormal production of androgens in women with breast cancer. ANTICANCER RES. (Greece), 1994, 14/5 B (2113-2117)

Endogenous sex hormones: Impact on lipids, lipoproteins, and insulin. AM. J. MED. (USA), 1995, 98/1 A (40S-47S)

Dehydroepiandrosterone antiestrogenic action through androgen receptor in MCF-7 human breast cancer cell line. ANTICANCER RES. (Greece), 1993, 13/6 A (2267-2272)

Effect of flax seed ingestion on the menstrual cycle. J. CLIN. ENDOCRINOL. METAB. (USA), 1993, 77/5 (1215-1219)

Transdermal estrogen replacement therapy in normal perimenopausal women: Effects on pituitary-ovarian function. Gynecological Endocrinology (United Kingdom), 1996, 10/1 (49-53)

Hormone replacement therapy, hormone levels, and lipoprotein cholesterol concentrations in elderly women. American Journal of Obstetrics and Gynecology (USA), 1996, 174/3

Estrogen and nerve growth factor-related systems in brain. Effects on basal forebrain cholinergic neurons and implications for learning and memory processes and aging. ANN. NEW YORK ACAD. SCI. (USA), 1994, 743/- (165-199)

Postmenopausal estrogen replacement: A long-term cohort study. AM. J. MED. (USA), 1994, 97/1 (66-77)

Impact of the menopause on the epidemiology and risk factors of coronary artery heart disease in women. EXP. GERONTOL. (USA), 1994, 29/3-4 (357-375)

Hormone therapy and endometrium cancer. REPROD. HUM. HORM. (France), 1994, 7/4 (137-139)

Progestin replacement in the menopause: Effects on the endometrium and serum lipids. CURR. OPIN. OBSTET. GYNECOL. (USA), 1994, 6/3 (284-292)

Effects of hormone replacement therapy on lipoprotein(a) and lipids in postmenopausal women. ARTERIOSCLER. THROMB. (USA), 1994, 14/2 (275-281)

Fibrinogen and Cardiovascular Disease

Dietary (n-3) fatty acids increase superoxide dismutase activity and decrease thromboxane production in the rat heart. Nutrition Research (USA), 1997, 17/1 (163-175)

Effects of n-3 fatty acids and fenofibrate on lipid and hemorrheological parameters in familial dysbetalipoproteinemia and familial hypertriglyceridemia. Metabolism: Clinical and Experimental (USA), 1996, 45/10 (1305-1311)

Repeated fasting and refeeding with 20:5, n-3 Eicosapentaenoic Acid (EPA): A novel approach for rapid fatty acid exchanges and its effect on blood pressure, plasma lipids and hemostasis. Journal of Human Hypertension (United Kingdom), 1996, 10/SUPPL. 3 (S135-S139)

Acute phase response and plasma carotenoid concentrations in older women: Findings from the nun study. Nutrition (USA), 1996, 12/7-8 (475-478)

References

Epidemiology of coagulation factors, inhibitors and activation markers: The Third Glasgow MONICA Survey. II. Relationships to cardiovascular risk factors and prevalent cardiovascular disease. Br J Haematol (ENGLAND) Jun 1997, 97 (4) p785-97

A long-term study on the effect of spontaneous consumption of reduced fat products as part of a normal diet on indicators of health. Int J Food Sci Nutr (ENGLAND) Jan 1997, 48 (1) p19-29

Acute phase response and plasma carotenoid concentrations in older women: findings from the nun study. Nutrition (UNITED STATES) Jul-Aug 1996, 12 (7-8) p475-8

Cadmium and atherosclerosis in the rabbit: reduced atherogenesis by superseding of iron? Food Chem Toxicol (ENGLAND) Jul 1996, 34 (7) p611-21

Vitamin intake: A possible determinant of plasma homocyst(e)ine among middle-aged adults Annals of Epidemiology (USA), 1997, 7/4 (285-293)

Vitamin C blocks inflammatory platelet-activating factor mimetics created by cigarette smoking Journal of Clinical Investigation (USA), 1997, 99/10 (2358-2364)

V677 mutation of methylenetetrahydrofolate reductase and cardiovascular disease in Canadian Inuit (5). Lancet (United Kingdom), 1997, 349/9060 (1221-1222)

Dietary vitamin C, beta-carotene and 30-year risk of stroke: Results from the western electric study. Neuroepidemiology (Switzerland), 1997, 16/2 (69-77)

Beta-carotene, vitamin C, and vitamin E: The protective micronutrients. Nutrition Reviews (USA), 1996, 54/11 II (S109-S114)

Alpha-2 adrenoceptor subtype causing nitric oxide-mediated vascular relaxation in rats. Journal of Pharmacology and Experimental Therapeutics (USA), 1996, 278/3 (1235-1243)

Vitamin C and cardiovascular disease: A systematic review. Journal of Cardiovascular Risk (United Kingdom), 1996, 3/6 (513-521)

Position of the American Dietetic Association: Phytochemicals and functional foods. Journal of Nutraceuticals, Functional and Medical Foods (USA), 1997, 1/1 (33-45)

The effect of hormone replacement therapy on vitamin E status in postmenopausal women. Maturitas (Ireland), 1997, 26/2 (121-124)

Vitamin E inhibits low-density lipoprotein-induced adhesion of monocytes to human aortic endothelial cells in vitro. Arteriosclerosis, Thrombosis, and Vascular Biology (USA), 1997, 17/3 (429-436)

Endothelial dysfunction: Clinical implications. Progress in Cardiovascular Diseases (USA), 1997, 39/4 (287-324)

Interactions between dietary fat, fish, and fish oils and their effects on platelet function in men at risk of cardiovascular disease. Arteriosclerosis, Thrombosis, and Vascular Biology (USA), 1997, 17/2 (279-286)

The role of folic acid in deficiency states and prevention of disease. Journal of Family Practice (USA), 1997, 44/2 (138-144)

Use of antioxidant vitamins in the cardiovascular disease. A review of epidemiological study and clinical trials. Giornale Italiano di Farmacia Clinica (Italy), 1996, 10/3 (155-162)

Intake of dietary fiber and risk of coronary heart disease in a cohort of Finnish men: The Alpha-Tocopherol, Beta-Carotene Cancer Prevention Study. Circulation (USA), 1996, 94/11 (2720-2727)

alpha-Tocopherol inhibits aggregation of human platelets by a protein kinase C-dependent mechanism. Circulation (USA), 1996, 94/10 (2434-2440)

Dietary and physiological studies involving magnesium homeostasis in the heart. Annals of the New York Academy of Sciences (USA), 1996, 793/- (473-478)

Prevention of neural tube defects. CNS Drugs (New Zealand), 1996, 6/5 (399-412)

Neurally mediated cardiac effects of forskolin in conscious dogs. American Journal of Physiology - Heart and Circulatory Physiology (USA), 1996, 271/4 40-4 (H1473-H1482)

Will an increased dietary folate intake reduce the incidence of cardiovascular disease? Nutrition Reviews (USA), 1996, 54/7 (213-216)

Genetic polymorphism of methylenetetrahydrofolate reductase and myocardial infarction: A case-control study Circulation (USA), 1996, 94/8 (1812-1814)

The effect of dietary treatment on lipid peroxidation and antioxidant status in newly diagnosed noninsulin dependent diabetes. Free Radical Biology and Medicine (USA), 1996, 21/5 (719-726)

Antioxidant properties of ethanolic and aqueous extracts of green tea compared to black tea. Biochemical Society Transactions (United Kingdom), 1996, 24/3 (390S)

Nutrition and women's health. Current Problems in Obstetrics, Gynecology and Fertility (USA), 1996, 19/4 (112-166)

Smoking, plasma antioxidants and essential fatty acids before and after nutratherapy. Canadian Journal of Cardiology (Canada), 1996, 12/7 (665-670)

Relation of total homocysteine and lipid levels in children to premature cardiovascular death in male relatives. Pediatric Research (USA), 1996, 40/1 (47-52)

Reduction of plasma peroxide levels by oral antioxidants. Medical Science Research (United Kingdom), 1996, 24/5 (357-359)

Changes in atherosclerotic aorta of rabbit fed with high cholesterol diet: The effect of vitamin E. Klinik Gelisim (Turkey), 1996, 9/2 (4063-4068)

In vitro effects of a flavonoid-rich extract on LDL oxidation. Atherosclerosis (Ireland), 1996, 123/1-2 (83-91)

Folate status is the major determinant of fasting total plasma homocysteine levels in maintenance dialysis patients. Atherosclerosis (Ireland), 1996, 123/1-2 (193-202)

Dietary antioxidant vitamins and death from coronary heart disease in postmenopausal women. New England Journal of Medicine (USA), 1996, 334/18 (1156-1162)

The cardiovascular protective role of docosahexaenoic acid. European Journal of Pharmacology (Netherlands), 1996, 300/1-2 (83-89)

Vitamins as homocysteine-lowering agents. Journal of Nutrition (USA), 1996, 126/4 SUPPL. (1276S-1280S)

The effect of modest vitamin E supplementation on lipid peroxidation products and other cardiovascular risk factors in diabetic patients. Lipids (USA), 1996, 31/3 SUPPL. (S87-S90)

Plasma ascorbic acid concentrations in the Republic of Karelia, Russia and in North Karelia, Finland. European Journal of Clinical Nutrition (United Kingdom), 1996, 50/2 (115-120)

Vegetable, fruit, and cereal fiber intake and risk of coronary heart disease among men. Journal of the American Medical Association (USA), 1996, 275/6 (447-451)

Homocysteine: Relation with ischemic vascular diseases. Revue de Medecine Interne (France), 1996, 17/1 (34-45)

Effects of various fatty acids alone or combined with vitamin E on cell growth and fibrinogen concentration in the medium of HepG2 cells. Thromb Res (UNITED STATES) Oct 1 1995, 80 (1) p75-83

[The role of platelets in the protective effect of a combination of vitamins A, E, C and P in thrombinemia] Gematol Transfuziol (RUSSIA) Sep-Oct 1995, 40 (5) p9-11

[Improvement of hemorheology with ginkgo biloba extract. Decreasing a cardiovascular risk factor] Fortschr Med (GERMANY) May 10 1992, 110 (13) p247-50

On the pharmacology of bromelain: an update with special regard to animal studies on dose-dependent effects. Planta Med (GERMANY, WEST) Jun 1990, 56 (3) p249-53

Effects of various fatty acids alone or combined with vitamin E on cell growth and fibrinogen concentration in the medium of HepG2 cells. Thromb Res (UNITED STATES) Oct 1 1995, 80 (1) p75-83

Protein/platelet interaction with an artificial surface: effect of vitamins and platelet inhibitors. Thromb Res (UNITED STATES) Jan 1 1986, 41 (1) p9-22

[Preventive effects of green tea extract on lipid abnormalities in serum, liver and aorta of mice fed a atherogenic diet] Nippon Yakurigaku Zasshi (JAPAN) Jun 1991, 97 (6) p329-37

Relationship between plasma essential fatty acids and smoking, serum lipids, blood pressure and haemostatic and rheological factors. Prostaglandins Leukot Essent Fatty Acids (SCOTLAND) Aug 1994, 51 (2) p101-8

Omega-3 fatty acids in health and disease and in growth and development Am J Clin Nutr (UNITED STATES) Sep 1991, 54 (3) p438-63

Fibromyalgia

Sleep disturbances, fibromyalgia and primary Sjogren's syndrome. Clin Exp Rheumatol (ITALY) Jan-Feb 1997, 15 (1) p71-4

Effects of experimental muscle pain on muscle activity and co-ordination during static and dynamic motor function. Electroencephalogr Clin Neurophysiol (IRELAND) Apr 1997, 105 (2) p156-64

Trigger points and tender points: one and the same? Does injection treatment help? Rheum Dis Clin North Am (UNITED STATES) May 1996, 22 (2) p305-22

Fibromyalgia and migraine, two faces of the same mechanism. Serotonin as the common clue for pathogenesis and therapy. Adv Exp Med Biol (UNITED STATES) 1996, 398 p373-9

Self-reported illness and health status among Gulf War veterans. A population-based study. The Iowa Persian Gulf Study Group. JAMA (UNITED STATES) Jan 15 1997, 277 (3) p238-45

[Fibromyalgia in dentistry]. J Can Dent Assoc (CANADA) Nov 1996, 62 (11) p874-6, 879-80

Fibromyalgia, depression, and alcoholism: a family history study. J Rheumatol (CANADA) Jan 1996, 23 (1) p149-54

Chronic regional muscular pain in women with precise manipulation work. A study of pain characteristics, muscle function, and impact on daily activities. Scand J Rheumatol (NORWAY) 1996, 25 (4) p213-23

The management of treatment-resistant depression in disorders on the interface of psychiatry and medicine. Fibromyalgia, chronic fatigue syndrome, migraine, irritable bowel syndrome, atypical facial pain, and premenstrual dysphoric disorder. Psychiatr Clin North Am (UNITED STATES) Jun 1996, 19 (2) p351-69

Profile of patients with chemical injury and sensitivity. Environmental Health Perspectives (USA), 1997, 105/SUPPL. 2 (417-436)

The relationship between fibromyalgia and interstitial cystitis. Journal of Psychiatric Research (United Kingdom), 1997, 31/1 (125-131)

Pressure and heat pain thresholds and tolerances in patients with fibromyalgia. Journal of Musculoskeletal Pain (USA), 1997, 5/2 (43-53)

Measuring change in fibromyalgic pain: The relevance of pain distribution. Journal of Musculoskeletal Pain (USA), 1997, 5/2 (29-41)

Thyroid status of 38 fibromyalgia patients: Implications for the etiology of fibromyalgia. Clinical Bulletin of Myofascial Therapy (USA), 1997, 2/1 (47-64)

A prospective long-term study of fibromyalgia syndrome. Arthritis and Rheumatism (USA), 1996, 39/4 (682-685)

Oral S-adenosylmethionine in primary fibromyalgia?Double-blind clinical evaluation. Scand J Rheumatol (SWEDEN) 1991, 20 (4) p294-302

Cerebrospinal fluid S-adenosylmethionine in depression and dementia: effects of treatment with parenteral and oral S-adenosylmethionine. J Neurol Neurosurg Psychiatry (ENGLAND) Dec 1990, 53 (12) p1096-8

The antidepressant potential of oral S-adenosyl-l-methionine. Acta Psychiatr Scand (DENMARK) May 1990, 81 (5) p432-6

Oral S-adenosylmethionine in depression: a randomized, double-blind, placebo-controlled trial. Am J Psychiatry (UNITED STATES) May 1990, 147 (5) p591-5

Disability and impairment in fibromyalgia syndrome: Possible pathogenesis and etiology. Critical Reviews in Physical and Rehabilitation Medicine (USA), 1995, 7/3 (189-232)

Primary fibromyalgia is responsive to S-adenosyl-L-methionine. CURR. THER. RES. CLIN. EXP. (USA), 1994, 55/7 (797-806)

S-adenosyl-L-methionine in Sjogren's syndrome and fibromyalgia. CURR. THER. RES. CLIN. EXP. (USA), 1994, 55/6 (699-706)

Clinical evaluation of S-adenosyl-L-methionine versus transcutaneous electrical nerve stimulation in primary fibromyalgia. CURR. THER. RES. CLIN. EXP. (USA), 1993, 53/2 (222-229)

Evaluation of S-adenosylmethionine in primary fibromyalgia. A double-blind crossover study. AM. J. MED. (USA), 1987, 83/5 A (107-110)

S-adenosylmethionine blood levels in major depression: Changes with drug treatment. ACTA NEU-ROL. SCAND. SUPPL. (Denmark), 1994, 89/154 (15-18)

Psychological distress during puerperium: A novel therapeutic approach using S-adenosylmethionine. CURR. THER. RES. CLIN. EXP. (USA), 1993, 53/6 (707-716)

Double blind, placebo-controlled study of S-adenosyl-L-methionine in depressed postmenopausal women. PSYCHOTHER. PSYCHOSOM. (Switzerland), 1993, 59/1 (34-40)

S-adenosylmethionine treatment of depression: A controlled clinical trial. AM. J. PSYCHIATRY (USA), 1988, 145/9 (1110-1114)

Treatment of depression in rheumatoid arthritic patients. A comparison of S-adenosylmethionine (Samyr) and placebo in a double-blind study. CLIN. TRIALS J. (UK), 1987, 24/4 (305-310)

Monitoring S-adenosyl-methionine blood levels and antidepressant effect. ACTA NEUROL. (ITALY), 1980, 35/6 (488-495)

Evaluation of S-adenosylmethionine (SAMe) effectiveness on depression. CURR. THER. RES., CLIN. EXP. (USA), 1980, 27/6II (908-918)

Oral S-adenosylmethionine in primary fibromyalgia—Double-blind clinical evaluation. Scand J Rheumatol (SWEDEN) 1991, 20 (4) p294-302,

Cerebrospinal fluid S-adenosylmethionine in depression and dementia: effects of treatment with par-enteral and oral S-adenosylmethionine. J Neurol Neurosurg Psychiatry (ENGLAND) Dec 1990, 53 (12) p1096-8

The antidepressant potential of oral S-adenosyl-l-methionine. Acta Psychiatr Scand (DENMARK) May 1990, 81 (5) p432-6,

Oral S-adenosylmethionine in depression: a randomized, double-blind, placebo- controlled trial. Am J Psychiatry (UNITED STATES) May 1990, 147 (5) p591-5,

Disability and impairment in fibromyalgia syndrome: Possible pathogenesis and etiology. Critical Reviews in Physical and Rehabilitation Medicine (USA), 1995, 7/3 (189-232)

Primary fibromyalgia is responsive to S-adenosyl-L-methionine. CURR. THER. RES. CLIN. EXP. (USA), 1994, 55/7 (797-806)

S-adenosyl-L-methionine in Sjogren's syndrome and fibromyalgia. CURR. THER. RES. CLIN. EXP. (USA), 1994, 55/6 (699-706)

Clinical evaluation of S-adenosyl-L-methionine versus transcutaneous electrical nerve stimulation in primary fibromyalgia. CURR. THER. RES. CLIN. EXP. (USA), 1993, 53/2 (222-229)

Oral S-adenosylmethionine in primary fibromyalgia. Double-blind clinical evaluation. SCAND. J. RHEUMATOL. (Sweden), 1991, 20/4 (294-302)

Evaluation of S-adenosylmethionine in primary fibromyalgia. A double-blind crossover study. AM. J. MED. (USA), 1987, 83/5 A (107-110)

S-adenosylmethionine blood levels in major depression: Changes with drug treatment. ACTA NEU-

ROL. SCAND. SUPPL. (Denmark), 1994, 89/154 (15-18)

Psychological distress during puerperium: A novel therapeutic approach using S-adenosylmethionine. CURR. THER. RES. CLIN. EXP. (USA), 1993, 53/6 (707-716)

Double blind, placebo-controlled study of S-adenosyl-L-methionine in depressed postmenopausal women. PSYCHOTHER. PSYCHOSOM. (Switzerland), 1993, 59/1 (34-40)

S-adenosylmethionine treatment of depression: A controlled clinical trial. AM. J. PSYCHIATRY (USA), 1988, 145/9 (1110-1114)

Treatment of depression in rheumatoid arthritic patients. A comparison of S-adenosylmethionine (Samyr) and placebo in a double-blind study. CLIN. TRIALS J. (UK), 1987, 24/4 (305-310)

Monitoring S-adenosyl-methionine blood levels and antidepressant effect. ACTA NEUROL. (ITALY), 1980, 35/6 (488-495)

Evaluation of S-adenosylmethionine (SAM) effectiveness on depression. CURR. THER. RES., CLIN. EXP. (USA), 1980, 27/6II (908-918)

Flu-Influenza Virus

The value of the dehydroepiandrosterone-annexed vitamin C infusion treatment in the clinical control of chronic fatigue syndrome (CFS). II. Characterization of CFS patients with special reference to their response to a new vitamin C infusion treatment. In Vivo (GREECE) Nov-Dec 1996, 10 (6) p585-96

Inhibitory effects of recombinant manganese superoxide dismutase on influenza virus infections in mice. Antimicrob Agents Chemother (UNITED STATES) Nov 1996, 40 (11) p2626-31

Influenza. More than mom and chicken soup. J Fla Med Assoc (UNITED STATES) Jan 1996, 83 (1) p19-22

[Drugs active against respiratory viruses]. Rev Prat (FRANCE) Mar 15 1997, 47 (6) p646-51

Oxidant stress responses in influenza virus pneumonia: Gene expression and transcription factor activation. American Journal of Physiology - Lung Cellular and Molecular Physiology (USA), 1996, 271/3 15-3 (L383-L391)

Antiviral activity of influenza virus M1 zinc finger peptides. Journal of Virology (USA), 1996, 70/12 (8639-8644)

Viral and atypical pneumonias. Primary Care - Clinics in Office Practice (USA), 1996, 23/4 (837-848)

In vivo anti-influenza virus activity of a zinc finger peptide. Antimicrobial Agents and Chemotherapy (USA), 1997, 41/3 (687-692)

Efficacy and safety of aerosolized ribavirin in young children hospitalized with influenza: a double-blind, multicenter, placebo-controlled trial. J Pediatr (UNITED STATES) Jul 1994

Antivirals for the chemoprophylaxis and treatment of influenza. Semin Respir Infect (UNITED STATES) Mar 1992

Utilization of pulse oximetry for the study of the inhibitory effects of antiviral agents on influenza virus in mice. Antimicrob Agents Chemother (UNITED STATES) Feb 1992

References

Further studies with short duration ribavirin aerosol for the treatment of influenza virus infection in mice and respiratory syncytial virus infection in cotton rats. Antiviral Res (NETHERLANDS) Jan 1992

High dose-short duration ribavirin aerosol treatment--a review. Bull Int Union Tuberc Lung Dis (FRANCE) Jun-Sep 1991

Molecular mechanisms of action of ribavirin. Rev Infect Dis (UNITED STATES) Nov-Dec 1990

Ribavirin aerosol treatment of influenza. Infect Dis Clin North Am (UNITED STATES) Jun 1987

Comparative activities of several nucleoside analogs against influenza A,B, and C viruses in vitro. Antimicrob Agents Chemother (UNITED STATES) Jun 1988

Ribavirin aerosol in the elderly. Chest (UNITED STATES) Jun 1988

Favorable outcome after treatment with amantadine and ribavirin in a pregnancy complicated by influenza pneumonia. A case report. Department of Obstetrics and Gynecology, Baylor College of Medicine, Houston, TX 77030

Oral ribavirin treatment of influenza A and B. Antimicrob Agents Chemother (UNITED STATES) Aug 1987

Ribavirin: a clinical overview. Eur J Epidemiol (ITALY) Mar 1986

Ribavirin small-particle aerosol treatment of infections caused by influenza virus strains A/Victoria/7/83 (H1N1) and B/Texas/1/84. Antimicrob Agents Chemother (UNITED STATES) Mar 1985

Effect of ribavirin triphosphate on primer generation and elongation during influenza virus transcription in vitro. Antiviral Res (NETHERLANDS) Feb 1985, 5 (1) p39-48

Ribavirin aerosol treatment of influenza B virus infection. Trans Assoc Am Physicians (UNITED STATES) 1983, 96

Treatment of influenza A (H1N1) virus infection with ribavirin aerosol. Antimicrob Agents Chemother (UNITED STATES) Aug 1984

Immune modulating properties of root extracts of different Echinacea species Zeitschrift fur Phytotherapie (Germany), 1995, 16/3 (157-162+165-166)

Echinacea PHARM. J. (United Kingdom), 1994, 253/6806 (342-343)

Echinacea combinations; efficacy and acceptability in 'flu' and nasopharyngeal inflammations. DTSCH. APOTH.-ZTG (GERMANY, WEST), 1987, 127/16 (853-854)

Papilloma virus infections of the skin. Universitats-Hautklinik, D-7800 Freinburg i. Breisgau GERMANY, WEST

Direct characterization of caffeoyl esters with antihyaluronidase activity in crude extracts from Echinacea angustifolia roots by fast atom bombardment tandem mass spectrometry. FARMACO (Italy), 1993, 48/10 (1447-1461)

Anti-inflammatory activity of Echinacea angustifolia fractions separated on the basis of molecular weight. PHARMACOL. RES. COMMUN. (United Kingdom), 1988, 20/SUPPL. 5 (87-90)

In vitro activity of Mercurius cyanatus against relevant pathogenic bacteria isolates. Arzneimittel-Forschung/Drug Research (Germany), 1995, 45/9 (1018-1020)

Mechanisms of propolis water extract antiherpetic activity. II. Activity of propolis water extract lectines. REV. ROUM. VIROL. (Romania), 1993, 44/1-2 (49-54)

Comparison of the anti-herpes simplex virus activities of propolis and 3- methyl-but-2-enyl caffeate. J. NAT. PROD. LLOYDIA (USA), 1994, 57/5 (644-647)

Synergistic effect of flavones and flavonols against herpes simplex virus type 1 in cell culture. Comparison with the antiviral activity of propolis. J. NAT. PROD. LLOYDIA (USA), 1992, 55/12 (1732-1740)

Recent advances in the chemotherapy of herpes virus infections. REV. ROUM. MED. (RUMANIA), 1981, 32/1 (57-77)

Anti-influenza virus effect of some propolis constituents and their analogues (esters of substituted cinnamic acids). J. NAT. PROD. LLOYDIA (USA), 1992, 55/3 (294-297)

The effect of an aqueous propolis extract, of rutin and of a rutin-quercetin mixture on experimental influenza virus infection in mice. REV. ROUM. MED. (RUMANIA), 1981, 32/3 (213-215)

Gingivitis

Vitamin C, oral scurvy and periodontal disease. S Afr Med J (SOUTH AFRICA) May 26 1984, 65 (21)

[Anticalculus dentifrices. A new era in preventive dentistry?] Ned Tijdschr Tandheelkd (NETHER-LANDS) Dec 1989, 96 (12)

Effect of tea polyphenols on glucan synthesis by glucosyltransferase from Streptococcus mutans. Chem Pharm Bull (Tokyo) (JAPAN) Mar 1990, 38 (3)

Green Tea to Prevent Dental Cares. Chung Hua Kou Chiang Hsueh Tsa Chih (CHINA) Jul 1993, 28 (4) p197-9 54

[Management of gingival inflammation with active ingredients in toothpaste] Dtsch Zahnarztl Z (GERMANY, WEST) Jun 1975, 30 (6) p382-4

Evidence for enhanced treatment of periodontal disease by therapy with coenzyme Q. Int J Vitam Nutr Res (SWITZERLAND) Apr 1973, 43 (4) p537-48

Zinc in etiology of periodontal disease. Med Hypotheses (ENGLAND) Mar Stomatological Clinic, Medical 1993, 40 (3) p182-5

Diabetes and periodontal diseases. Possible role of vitamin c deficiency: an hypothesis. J Periodontol (UNITED STATES) May 1981, 52 (5) p251-4

Relationship of mineral status and intake to periodontal disease. Am J Clin Nutr (UNITED STATES) Jul 1976, 29 (7)

Comparative In Vitro Activity of Sanguinarine Against Oral. ANTIMICROBIAL AGENTS AND CHEMOTHEROPY, Apr. 1985, p. 663-65 Vol. 27, No. 4

MICs of sanguinarine were determined for 52 oral reference strains and 129 fresh isolates from human dental plaque. Sanguinarine was found to completely inhibit the growth of 98% of the isolates at a concentration of 16,ug/ml.

Zinc And Sanguinaria. J Periodontol 60(2):91-5, 1989)

Supplementation or local application may reduce gingival exudate from inflamed and infected gums - which suggests improved tissue health. (Folate mouthwash appears to to be more effective than oral folate.) J Clin Periodonlol 14(6):315-9, 1987)

Effects on established gingivitis in periodontal patients. J Clin Periodontol 11:619-28, 1984).

Effects of extended systemic and topical folate supplementation on gingivitis of pregnancy. J Clin periodontal 9(3):27580, 1982).

Effects of topical and systemic folic acid supplementation on gingivitis in pregnancy. J Clin Periodontol 7(5):402-14, 1980).

The effect of topical application of folic acid on gingival health. J Oral Med 33(1):20-22,1978).

The effect of folic acid on gingival health. J periodontol 47(11):667-8, 1976).

Glaucoma

Neurotransmitters and intraocular pressure. FUNDAM. CLIN. PHARMACOL. (France), 1988, 2/4 (305-325)

HP 663: A novel compound for the treatment of glaucoma. DRUG DEV. RES. (USA), 1988, 12/3-4 (197-209)

Intraocular pressure effects of multiple doses of drugs applied to glaucomatous monkey eyes. ARCH. OPHTHALMOL. (USA), 1987, 105/2 (249-252)

Laser-induced glaucoma in rabbits. EXP. EYE RES. (UK), 1986, 43/6 (885-894)

Regulation of aqueous flow by the adenylate cyclase receptor complex in the ciliary epithelium. AM. J. OPHTHALMOL. (USA), 1985, 100/1 (194-198)

Forskolin suppresses sympathetic neuron function and causes ocular hypotension. CURR. EYE RES. (ENGLAND), 1985, 4/2 (87-96)

Forskolin lowers intraocular pressure by reducing aqueous inflow. INVEST. OPHTHALMOL. VISUAL SCI. (USA), 1984, 25/3 (268-276)

Indomethacin and epinephrine effects on outflow facility and cyclic adenosine monophosphate formation in monkeys. Investigative Ophthalmology and Visual Science (USA), 1996, 37/7 (1348-1359)

Hair Loss

See references under Balding

Hearing Loss

[The influence on sound damages by an extract of ginkgo biloba]. Arch Otorhinolaryngol (UNITED STATES) Jul 8, 1975, 209 (3) p203-15

[Hydergine in pathology of the inner ear]. An Otorrinolaringol Ibero Am (SPAIN) 1990, 17 (1) p85-98

[Ginkgo extract EGb 761 (tenobin)/HAES versus naftidrofuryl A randomized study of therapy of sudden deafness]. Laryngorhinootologie (GERMANY) Mar 1994, 73 (3) p149-52

[Therapeutic trial in acute cochlear deafness. A comparative study of Ginkgo biloba extract and nicergoline]. Presse Med (FRANCE) Sep 25 1986, 15 (31) p1559-61

[The influence on sound damages by an extract of ginkgo biloba]. Arch Otorhinolaryngol (UNITED STATES) Jul 8 1975, 209 (3) p203-15

Results of combined low-power laser therapy and extracts of Ginkgo biloba in cases of sensorineural hearing loss and tinnitus. Adv Otorhinolaryngol (SWITZERLAND) 1995, 49 p101-4

Trial of an extract of Ginkgo biloba (EGB) for tinnitus and hearing loss [letter]. Clin Otolaryngol (ENGLAND) Dec 1988, 13 (6) p501-2

[Hydergine in pathology of the inner ear] An Otorrinolaringol Ibero Am (SPAIN) 1990, 17 (1) p85-98

[Ginkgo extract EGb 761 (tenobin)/HAES versus naftidrofuryl A randomized study of therapy of sudden deafness] Laryngorhinootologie (GERMANY) Mar 1994, 73 (3) p149-52,

[Therapeutic trial in acute cochlear deafness. A comparative study of Ginkgo biloba extract and nicergoline] Presse Med (FRANCE) Sep 25 1986, 15 (31) p1559-61,

[The influence on sound damages by an extract of ginkgo biloba] Arch Otorhinolaryngol (UNITED STATES) Jul 8 1975, 209 (3) p203-15

Results of combined low-power laser therapy and extracts of Ginkgo biloba in cases of sensorineural hearing loss and tinnitus. Adv Otorhinolaryngol (SWITZERLAND) 1995, 49 p101-4

Trial of an extract of Ginkgo biloba (EGB) for tinnitus and hearing loss [letter]. Clin Otolaryngol (ENGLAND) Dec 1988, 13 (6) p501-2,

Hemochromatosis

Biological markers of oxidative stress induced by ethanol and iron overload in rat. Int J Occup Med Environ Health (POLAND) 1994, 7 (4) p355-63

Antioxidant status and lipid peroxidation in hereditary haemochromatosis. Free Radic Biol Med (UNITED STATES) Mar 1994, 16 (3)

Iron storage, lipid peroxidation and glutathione turnover in chronic anti-HCV positive hepatitis. J Hepatol (DENMARK) Apr 1995, 22 (4) p449-56

Induction of oxidative single- and double-strand breaks in DNA by ferric citrate. Free Radic Biol Med (UNITED STATES) Aug 1993

A unique rodent model for both the cardiotoxic and hepatotoxic effects of prolonged iron overload. Lab Invest (UNITED STATES) Aug 1993, 69 (2) p217-22

Biochemical and biophysical investigations of the ferrocene-iron-loaded rat. An animal model of primary haemochromatosis. Eur J Biochem (GERMANY) Dec 5 1991, 202 (2) p405-10

Antioxidant and iron-chelating activities of the flavonoids catechin, quercetin and diosmetin on iron-loaded rat hepatocyte cultures. BIOCHEM. PHARMACOL. (United Kingdom), 1993

Iron absorption and phenolic compounds: Importance of different phenolic structures. EUROP. J.

References

CLIN. NUTR. (United Kingdom), 1989

Inhibition of the tobacco-specific nitrosamine-induced lung tumorigenesis by compounds derived from cruciferous vegetables and green tea. ANN. NEW YORK ACAD. SCI. (USA), 1993, 686

The effects of caffeic acid and its related catechols on hydroxyl radical formation by 3- hydroxyanthranilic acid, ferric chloride, and hydrogen peroxide. ARCH. BIOCHEM. BIOPHYS. (USA), 1990, 276/1

A novel antioxidant flavonoid (IdB 1031) affecting molecular mechanisms of cellular activation. FREE RADIC. BIOL. MED. (USA), 1994, 16/5 (547-553)

Prevention of postischemic cardiac injury by the orally active iron chelator 1,2- dimethyl-3-hydroxy-4-pyridone (L1) and the antioxidant (+)-cyanidanol-3. CIRCULATION (USA), 1989, 80/1 (158-164)

Hepatotoxicity of menadione predominates in oxygen-rich zones of the liver lobule. J. PHARMACOL. EXP. THER. (USA), 1989, 248/3 (1317-1322)

Iron-load increases the susceptibility of rat hearts to oxygen reperfusion damage. Protection by the antioxidant (+)-cyanidanol-3 and deferoxamine. CIRCULATION (USA), 1988, 78/2 (442-449)

Hepatocyte injury resulting from the inhibition of mitochondrial respiration at low oxygen concentrations involves reductive stress and oxygen activation. Chemico-Biological Interactions (Ireland), 1995, 98/1 (27-44)

Modulating hypoxia-induced hepatocyte injury by affecting intracellular redox state. Biochimica et Biophysica Acta - Molecular Cell Research (Netherlands), 1995, 1269/2 (153-161)

Protection of rat myocardial phospholipid against peroxidative injury through superoxide-(xanthine oxidase)-dependent, iron-promoted fenton chemistry by the male contraceptive gossypol. BIOCHEM. PHARMACOL. (United Kingdom), 1988, 37/17 (3335-3342)

Protective effect of tea polyphenol on rat myocardial injury induced by isoproterenol. Chinese Traditional and Herbal Drugs (China)(Apr) 1995

Effect of the interaction of tannins with coexisting substances. Part 2. reduction of heavy metal ions and solubilization of precipitates. Journal of the Pharmaceutical Society of Japan (Japan), V102, (8), 1982

Free radicals scavenging action and anti-enzyme activities of procyanidines from Vitis vinifera. A mechanism for their capillary protective action. Arzneimittelforschung (GERMANY) May 1994, 44 (5) p592-601

The inhibitory action of chlorogenic acid on the intestinal iron absorption in rats. Acta Physiol Pharmacol Ther Latinoam (ARGENTINA) 1992, 42 (3)

Inhibition of tobacco-specific nitrosamine-induced lung tumorigenesis by compounds derived from cruciferous vegetables and green tea. Ann N Y Acad Sci (UNITED STATES) May 28 1993, 686

Ascorbic acid prevents the dose-dependent inhibitory effects of polyphenols and phytates on non-heme-iron absorption. Am J Clin Nutr (UNITED STATES) Feb 1991, 53 (2)

Phytic acid. A natural antioxidant. J Biol Chem (UNITED STATES) Aug 25 1987, 262 (24)

[Effect of polyphenols of coffee pulp on iron absorption]. Arch Latinoam Nutr (VENEZUELA) Jun 1985, 35 (2)

Factors affecting the absorption of iron from cereals. Br J Nutr (ENGLAND) Jan 1984, 51 (1) p37-46

The effect of red and white wines on nonheme-iron absorption in humans. Am J Clin Nutr (UNITED STATES) Apr 1995

Prevention of iron deficiency. Baillieres Clin Haematol (ENGLAND) Dec 1994, 7 (4)

Iron absorption and phenolic compounds: importance of different phenolic structures. Eur J Clin Nutr (ENGLAND) Aug 1989, 43 (8) p547-57

Hepatitis B

[Markers of chronic hepatitis B in children after completion of therapywith isoprinosine] Pol Tyg Lek (POLAND) Mar 15-29 1993, 48 (11-13) p263-4

[Course of chronic virus hepatitis B in children and attempts at modifying its treatment] Pol Tyg Lek (POLAND) Mar 15-29 1993, 48 (11-13) p258-60

Isoprinosine in the treatment of chronic active hepatitis type B. Scand J Infect Dis (SWEDEN) 1990, 22 (6) p645-8

[Evaluation of the treatment of chronic active hepatitis (HBsAg+) with isoprinosine. II. Immunological studies] Pol Tyg Lek (POLAND) Apr 16-30 1990, 45 (16-18) p347-51

In vitro studies on the effect of certain natural products against hepatitis B virus. Indian J Med Res (INDIA) Apr 1990, 92 p133-8

Effects of glycyrrhizin on hepatitis B surface antigen: a biochemical and morphological study. J Hepatol (DENMARK) Oct 1994, 21 (4) p601-9

Glycyrrhizin withdrawal followed by human lymphoblastoid interferon in the treatment of chronic hepatitis B. Gastroenterol Jpn (JAPAN) Dec 1991, 26 (6) p742-6

Combination therapy of glycyrrhizin withdrawal and human fibroblast Interferon for chronic hepatitis B. Clin Ther (UNITED STATES) 1989, 11 (1) p161-9

Alpha-interferon combined with immunomodulation in the treatment of chronic hepatitis B. J Gastroenterol Hepatol (AUSTRALIA) 1991, 6 Suppl 1 p13-4

Improvement of liver fibrosis in chronic hepatitis C patients treated with natural interferon alpha. J Hepatol (DENMARK) Feb 1995, 22 (2) p135-42

Diagnosis and treatment of the major hepatotropic viruses. Am J Med Sci (UNITED STATES) Oct 1993, 306 (4) p248-61

Treatment of chronic viral hepatitis.J Antimicrob Chemother (ENGLAND) Jul 1993, 32 Suppl A p107-20

[Mechanisms of the effect of interferon (IFN) therapy in patients with type B and C chronic hepatitis] Hokkaido Igaku Zasshi (JAPAN) May 1993, 68 (3) p297-309

A pilot study of ribavirin therapy for recurrent hepatitis C virus infection after liver transplantation. Transplantation (UNITED STATES) May 27 1996, 61 (10) p1483-8

Ribavirin as therapy for chronic hepatitis C. A randomized, double- blind, placebo-controlled trial. Ann

Intern Med (UNITED STATES) Dec 15 1995, 123 (12) p897-903

Treatment with ribavirin+alpha interferon in HCV chronic active hepatitis non-responders to interferon alone: preliminary results. J Chemother (ITALY) Feb 1995, 7 (1) p58-61

Combined treatment with interferon alpha-2b and ribavirin for chronic hepatitis C in patients with a previous non-response or non-sustained response to interferon alone. J Med Virol (UNITED STATES) May 1995, 46 (1) p43-7

Increase in hepatic iron stores following prolonged therapy with ribavirin in patients with chronic hepatitis C. J Hepatol (DENMARK) Dec 1994, 21 (6) p1109-12

Therapy for chronic hepatitis C. Gastroenterol Clin North Am (UNITED STATES) Sep 1994, 23 (3) p603- 13

Treatment of chronic viral hepatitis. Baillieres Clin Gastroenterol (ENGLAND) Jun 1994, 8 (2) p233-53

Elevated serum iron predicts poor response to interferon treatment in patients with chronic HCV infection. Dig Dis Sci (UNITED STATES) Nov 1995, 40 (11) p2431-3

Distribution of iron in the liver predicts the response of chronic hepatitis C infection to interferon therapy [published erratum appears in Am J Clin Pathol 1995 Aug;104(2):232] Am J Clin Pathol (UNITED STATES) Apr 1995, 103 (4) p419-24

Increased serum iron and iron saturation without liver iron accumulation distinguish chronic hepatitis C from other chronic liver diseases. Dig Dis Sci (UNITED STATES) Dec 1994, 39 (12) p2656-9

Response related factors in recombinant interferon alfa-2b treatment of chronic hepatitis C. Gut (ENGLAND) 1993, 34 (2 Suppl) pS139-40

Measurements of iron status in patients with chronic hepatitis [see comments] Gastroenterology (UNITED STATES) Jun 1992, 102 (6) p2108-13

[Effect of green tea on iron absorption in elderly patients with iron deficiency anemia] Nippon Ronen Igakkai Zasshi (JAPAN) Sep 1990, 27 (5) p555-8

[Current knowledge in the treatment of chronic hepatitis C] Acquisitions recentes dans le traitement de l'hepatite C chronique. Rev Med Liege (BELGIUM) Dec 1995, 50 (12) p501-4

Hepatitis C

Ribavirin as therapy for chronic hepatitis C. A randomized, double- blind, placebo-controlled trial. Ann Intern Med (UNITED STATES) Dec 15 1995, 123 (12) p897-903

Treatment with ribavirin+alpha interferon in HCV chronic active hepatitis non-responders to interferon alone: preliminary results. J Chemother (ITALY) Feb 1995, 7 (1) p58-61

Combined treatment with interferon alpha-2b and ribavirin for chronic hepatitis C in patients with a previous non-response or non-sustained response to interferon alone. J Med Virol (UNITED STATES) May 1995, 46 (1) p43-7

[Evaluation of the treatment of chronic active hepatitis (HBsAg+) with isoprinosine. II. Immunological studies] Pol Tyg Lek (POLAND) Apr 16-30 1990, 45 (16-18) p347-51

In vitro studies on the effect of certain natural products against hepatitis B virus. Indian J Med Res (INDIA) Apr 1990, 92 p133-8

Effects of glycyrrhizin on hepatitis B surface antigen: a biochemical and morphological study. (DENMARK) Oct 1994, 21 (4) p601-9

Glycyrrhizin withdrawal followed by human lymphoblastoid interferon in the treatment of chronic hepatitis B. Gastroenterol Jpn (JAPAN) Dec 1991, 26 (6) p742-6

Combination therapy of glycyrrhizin withdrawal and human fibroblast interferon for chronic hepatitis B. Clin Ther (UNITED STATES) 1989, 11 (1) p161-9

Alpha-interferon combined with immunomodulation in the treatment of chronic hepatitis B. J Gastroenterol Hepatol (AUSTRALIA) 1991, 6 Suppl 1 p13-4

Improvement of liver fibrosis in chronic hepatitis C patients treated with natural interferon alpha. J Hepatol (DENMARK) Feb 1995, 22 (2) p135-42

Diagnosis and treatment of the major hepatotropic viruses. Am J Med Sci (UNITED STATES) Oct 1993, 306 (4) p248-61

Treatment of chronic viral hepatitis. J Antimicrob Chemother (ENGLAND) Jul 1993, 32 Suppl A p107-20

[Mechanisms of the effect of interferon (IFN) therapy in patients with type B and C chronic hepatitis] Hokkaido Igaku Zasshi (JAPAN) May 1993, 68 (3) p297-309

A pilot study of ribavirin therapy for recurrent hepatitis C virus infection after liver transplantation. Transplantation (UNITED STATES) May 27 1996, 61 (10) p1483-8

Therapy for chronic hepatitis C. Gastroenterol Clin North Am (UNITED STATES) Sep 1994, 23 (3) p603-13

Treatment of chronic viral hepatitis. Baillieres Clin Gastroenterol (ENGLAND) Jun 1994, 8 (2) p233-53

Elevated serum iron predicts poor response to interferon treatment in patients with chronic HCV infection. Dig Dis Sci (UNITED STATES) Nov 1995, 40 (11) p2431- 3

Distribution of iron in the liver predicts the response of chronic hepatitis C infection to interferon therapy [published erratum appears in Am J Clin Pathol 1995 Aug;104(2):232] Am J Clin Pathol (UNITED STATES) Apr 1995, 103 (4) p419-24

Increased serum iron and iron saturation without liver iron accumulation distinguish chronic hepatitis C from other chronic liver diseases. Dig Dis Sci (UNITED STATES) Dec 1994, 39 (12) p2656- 9

Response related factors in recombinant interferon alfa-2b treatment of chronic hepatitis C. Gut (ENGLAND) 1993, 34 (2 Suppl) pS139-40

Measurements of iron status in patients with chronic hepatitis. Gastroenterology (UNITED STATES) Jun 1992, 102 (6) p2108-13

[Markers of chronic hepatitis B in children after completion of therapy with isoprinosine] Pol Tyg Lek (POLAND) Mar 15-29 1993, 48 (11-13) p263-4

[Course of chronic virus hepatitis B in children and attempts at modifying its treatment] Pol Tyg Lek

(POLAND) Mar 15-29 1993, 48 (11-13) p258-60

Isoprinosine in the treatment of chronic active hepatitis type B. Scand J Infect Dis (SWEDEN) 1990, 22 (6) p645-8

Antioxidant and iron-chelating activities of the flavonoids catechin, quercetin and diosmetin on iron-loaded rat hepatocyte cultures. BIOCHEM. PHARMACOL. (United Kingdom), 1993

Iron absorption and phenolic compounds: Importance of different phenolic structures. EUROP. J. CLIN. NUTR. (United Kingdom), 1989

Inhibition of the tobacco-specific nitrosamine-induced lung tumorigenesis by compounds derived from cruciferous vegetables and green tea. ANN. NEW YORK ACAD. SCI. (USA), 1993, 686

The effects of caffeic acid and its related catechols on hydroxyl radical formation by 3-hydroxyanthranilic acid, ferric chloride, and hydrogen peroxide. ARCH. BIOCHEM. BIOPHYS. (USA), 1990, 276/1

A novel antioxidant flavonoid (IdB 1031) affecting molecular mechanisms of cellular activation. FREE RADIC. BIOL. MED. (USA), 1994, 16/5 (547-553)

Prevention of postischemic cardiac injury by the orally active iron chelator 1,2-dimethyl-3-hydroxy-4-pyridone (L1) and the antioxidant (+)-cyanidanol-3. CIRCULATION (USA), 1989, 80/1 (158-164)

Hepatotoxicity of menadione predominates in oxygen-rich zones of the liver lobule. J. PHARMACOL. EXP. THER. (USA), 1989, 248/3 (1317-1322)

HIV Infection (AIDS)
(Opportunistic Infections)

Selenium and HIV in Pediatrics. J. NUTR. IMMUNOL. (USA), 1994, 3/1 (41-49)

N-Acetylcysteine enhances T cell functions and T cell growth in culture. INT. IMMUNOL. (United Kingdom), 1993, 5/1 (97-101

Cysteine and glutathione deficiency in HIV-infected patients. The basis for treatment with N-acetylcysteine. AIDS-FORSCHUNG (Germany), 1992, 7/4 (197-199)

N-acetylcysteine (NAC) enhances interleukin-2 but suppresses interleukin-4 secretion from normal and HIV+ CD4+ T-cells. Cell Mol Biol (Noisy-le-grand) (FRANCE) 1995, 41 Suppl 1 pS35-40

N-acetylcysteine enhances antibody-dependent cellular cytotoxicity in neutrophils and mononuclear cells from healthy adults and human immunodeficiency virus-infected patients. J Infect Dis (UNITED STATES) Dec 1995, 172 (6) p1492-502

Glutathione precursor and antioxidant activities of N-acetylcysteine and oxothiazolidine carboxylate compared in in vitro studies of HIV replication. AIDS Res Hum Retroviruses (UNITED STATES) Aug 1994, 10 (8) p961-7

Role for oxygen radicals in self-sustained HIV-1 replication in monocyte-derived macrophages: enhanced HIV-1 replication by N-acetyl-L-cysteine. J Leukoc Biol (UNITED STATES) Dec 1994, 56 (6) p702- 7

Effects of glutathione precursors on human immunodeficiency virus replication. Chem Biol Interact (IRELAND) Jun 1994, 91 (2-3) p217-24

Effect of glutathione depletion and oral N-acetyl-cysteine treatment on CD4+ and CD8+ cells. FASEB J (UNITED STATES) Apr 1 1994, 8 (6) p448-51

N-acetylcysteine enhances T cell functions and T cell growth in culture. Int Immunol (ENGLAND) Jan 1993, 5 (1) p97-101

Comparative study of the anti-HIV activities of ascorbate and thiol- containing reducing agents in chronically HIV-infected cells. Am J Clin Nutr (UNITED STATES) Dec 1991, 54 (6 Suppl) p1231S-1235S

Role for oxygen radicals in self-sustained HIV-1 replication in monocyte-derived macrophages: Enhanced HIV-1 replication by N-acetyl-L-cysteine. J. LEUKOCYTE BIOL. (USA), 1994, 56/6 (702-707)

Effects of glutathione precursors on human immunodeficiency virus replication. CHEM.-BIOL. INTERACT. (Ireland), 1994, 91/2-3 (217- 224)

Antioxidant status and lipid peroxidation in patients infected with HIV. CHEM.-BIOL. INTERACT. (Ireland), 1994, 91/2-3 (165- 180)

N-acetylcysteine inhibits latent HIV expression in chronically infected cells. AIDS RES. HUM. RETRO-VIRUSES (USA), 1991, 7/6 (563- 567)

Selenium mediated inhibition of transcription factor NF-kappaB and HIV-1 LTR promoter activity. Archives of Toxicology (Germany), 1996, 70/5 (277- 283)

Release of nitric oxide from astroglial cells: A key mechanism in neuroimmune disorders. Advances in Neuroimmunology (United Kingdom), 1995, 5/4 (421-430)

Carnitine depletion in peripheral blood mononuclear cells from patients with AIDS: Effect of oral L-carnitine. AIDS (United Kingdom), 1994, 8/5 (655-660)

High dose L-carnitine improves immunologic and metabolic parameters in AIDS patients. IMMUNOPHARMACOL. IMMUNOTOXICOL. (USA), 1993, 15/1 (1-12)

Stress, Immunity and Ageing. A role for acetyl-L-carnitine: proceedings of the workshop. ICS844. Universita degli Studi dell'Aquila degli Abruzzi, L'Aquila Italy

Vitamin B-12 abnormalities in HIV-infected patients. EUR. J. HAEMATOL. (Denmark), 1991, 47/1 (60-64)

HIV-infected patients with vitamin B-12 deficiency and autoantibodies to intrinsic factor: Disease pathogenesis and therapy. AIDS PATIENT CARE (USA), 1991, 5/3 (125-128)

One-year follow-up on the safety and efficacy of isoprinosine for human immunodeficiency virus infection. J. INTERN. MED. (United Kingdom), 1992, 231/6 (607- 615)

Immunotherapy of human immunodeficiency virus infection. TRENDS PHARMACOL. SCI. (United Kingdom), 1991, 12/3 (107-111)

The efficacy of inosine pranobex in preventing the acquired immunodeficiency syndrome in patients with human immunodeficiency virus infection. NEW ENGL. J. MED. (USA), 1990, 322/25 (1757-1763)

The activities of coenzyme Q10 and vitamin B6 for immune responses. BIOCHEM. BIOPHYS. RES. COMMUN. (USA), 1993, 193/1 (88-92)

Coenzyme Q10 increases T4/T8 ratios of lymphocytes in ordinary subjects and relevance to patients having the AIDS related complex. BIOCHEM. BIOPHYS. RES. COMMUN. (USA), 1991, 176/2 (786-791)

Biochemical deficiencies of coenzyme Q10 in HIV-infection and exploratory treatment. BIOCHEM. BIOPHYS. RES. COMMUN. (USA), 1988, 153/2 (888-896)

Coenzyme Q10 increases T4/T8 ratios of lymphocytes in ordinary subjects and relevance to patients having the AIDS related complex. BIOCHEM. BIOPHYS. RES. COMMUN. (USA), 1991, 176/2 (786-791)

Relationship between sex steroid hormone levels and CD4 lymphocytes in HIV infected men. Experimental and Clinical Endocrinology and Diabetes (Germany),1996,104

Inhibition of 3'azido-3'deoxythymidine-resistant HIV-1 infection by dehydroepiandrosterone in vitro. BIOCHEM. BIOPHYS. RES. COMMUN. (USA), 1994, 201/3 (1424-1432)

Inhibition of HIV-1 latency reactivation by dehydroepiandrosterone (DHEA) and an analog of DHEA. AIDS RES. HUM. RETROVIRUSES (USA), 1993, 9/8 (747- 754)

Evidence for changes in adrenal and testicular steroids during HIV infection. J. ACQUIRED IMMUNE DEFIC. SYNDR. (USA), 1992, 5/8 (841-846)

Dehydroepiandrosterone as predictor for progression to AIDS in asymptomatic human immunodeficiency virus-infected men. J. INFECT. DIS. (USA), 1992, 165/3 (413-418)

Decreased serum dehydroepiandrosterone is associated with an increased progression of human immunodeficiency virus infection in men with CD4 cell counts of 200-499. J. INFECT. DIS. (USA), 1991, 164/5 (864-868)

Hypertension (High Blood Pressure)

Summary of the NATO advanced research workshop on dietary omega 3 and omega 6 fatty acids: biological effects and nutritional essentiality. J Nutr (UNITED STATES) Apr 1989, 119 (4) p521-8

Simopoulos AP. J Nutr (UNITED STATES) Apr 1989, 119 (4) p521-8

Vasodilating agents and platelet function: intracellular free calcium concentration, cyclic nucleotides, and shape-change response. J Cardiovasc Pharmacol (UNITED STATES) 1986, 8 Suppl 8 pS102-6

L-arginine restores dilator responses of the basilar artery to acetylcholine during chronic hypertension. Hypertension (UNITED STATES) Apr 1996, 27 (4) p893-6

Prospective study of nutritional factors, blood pressure, and hypertension among US women. Hypertension (UNITED STATES) May 1996, 27 (5) p1065-72

Association of macronutrients and energy intake with hypertension. J Am Coll Nutr (UNITED STATES) Feb 1996, 15 (1) p21-35

Relations between magnesium, calcium, and plasma renin activity in black and white hypertensive patients. Miner Electrolyte Metab (SWITZERLAND) 1995, 21 (6) p417-22

Effect of renal perfusion pressure on excretion of calcium, magnesium, and phosphate in the rat. Clin Exp Hypertens (UNITED STATES) Nov 1995, 17 (8) p1269-85

Potassium depletion and salt-sensitive hypertension in Dahl rats: effect on calcium, magnesium, and phosphate excretions. Clin Exp Hypertens (UNITED STATES) Aug 1995, 17 (6) p989-1008

Dietary L-arginine attenuates blood pressure in mineralocorticoid-salt hypertensive rats. Clin Exp Hypertens (UNITED STATES) Oct 1995, 17 (7) p1009-24

Associations between blood pressure and dietary intake and urinary excretion of electrolytes in a Chinese population. J Hypertens (ENGLAND) Jan 1995, 13 (1) p49-56

Concentration of free intracellular magnesium in the myocardium of spontaneously hypertensive rats treated chronically with calcium antagonist or angiotensin converting enzyme inhibitor. Arch Mal Coeur Vaiss (FRANCE) Aug 1994, 87 (8) p1041-5

Nonpharmacologic treatment of hypertension. Curr Opin Nephrol Hypertens (UNITED STATES) Oct 1992, 1 (1) p85-90

Micronutrient effects on blood pressure regulation. Nutr Rev (UNITED STATES) Nov 1994, 52 (11) p367-75

Role of magnesium and calcium in alcohol-induced hypertension and strokes as probed by in vivo television microscopy, digital image microscopy, optical spectroscopy, 31P-NMR, spectroscopy and a unique magnesium ion-selective electrode. Alcohol Clin Exp Res (UNITED STATES) Oct 1994, 18 (5) p1057-68

Consequences of magnesium deficiency on the enhancement of stress reactions; preventive and therapeutic implications (a review). J Am Coll Nutr (UNITED STATES) Oct 1994, 13 (5) p429-46

Dietary management of blood pressure. J Assoc Acad Minor Phys (UNITED STATES) 1994, 5 (4) p147-51

Community-based prevention of stroke: nutritional improvement in Japan. Health Rep (CANADA) 1994, 6 (1) p181-8

Effect of dietary magnesium supplementation on intralymphocytic free calcium and magnesium in stroke-prone spontaneously hypertensive rats. Clin Exp Hypertens (UNITED STATES) May 1994, 16 (3) p317-26

Impact of increasing calcium in the diet on nutrient consumption, plasma lipids, and lipoproteins in humans. Am J Clin Nutr (UNITED STATES) Apr 1994, 59 (4) p900-7

Electrolytes and hypertension: results from recent studies. Am J Med Sci (UNITED STATES) Feb 1994, 307 Suppl 1 pS17-20

Calcium antagonists in pregnancy as an antihypertensive and tocolytic agent. Wien Med Wochenschr (AUSTRIA) 1993, 143 (19-20) p519-21

Augmentation of the renal tubular dopaminergic activity by oral calcium supplementation in patients with essential hypertension. Am J Hypertens (UNITED STATES) Nov 1993, 6 (11 Pt 1) p933-7

Nutrition and diseases of women: cardiovascular disorders. J Am Coll Nutr (UNITED STATES) Aug 1993, 12 (4) p417-25

The pathogenesis of eclampsia: the 'magnesium ischaemia' hypothesis. Med Hypotheses (ENGLAND) Apr 1993, 40 (4) p250-6

Longitudinal changes during the development of hypertension in rats fed excess chloride and sodium. Proc Soc Exp Biol Med (UNITED STATES) Jul 1993, 203 (3) p377-85

Salivary electrolytes in treated hypertensives at low or normal sodium diet. Clin Exp Hypertens (UNIT-

ED STATES) Mar 1993, 15 (2) p245-56

Can guava fruit intake decrease blood pressure and blood lipids? J Hum Hypertens (ENGLAND) Feb 1993, 7 (1) p33-8

Preventive nutrition: disease-specific dietary interventions for older adults. Geriatrics (UNITED STATES) Nov 1992, 47 (11) p39-40, 45-9

Intracellular Mg2+, Ca2+, Na2+ and K+ in platelets and erythrocytes of essential hypertension patients: relation to blood pressure. Clin Exp Hypertens [A] (UNITED STATES) 1992, 14 (6) p1189-209

A prospective study of nutritional factors and hypertension among US men. Circulation (UNITED STATES) Nov 1992, 86 (5) p1475-84

The effects of nonpharmacologic interventions on blood pressure of persons with high normal levels. Results of the Trials of Hypertension Prevention, Phase I [published erratum appears in JAMA 1992 May 6;267(17):2330]. JAMA (UNITED STATES) Mar 4 1992, 267 (9) p1213-20

Overview: studies on spontaneous hypertension-development from animal models toward man. Clin Exp Hypertens [A] (UNITED STATES) 1991, 13 (5) p631-44

Electrolytes in the epidemiology, pathophysiology, and treatment of hypertension. Prim Care (UNITED STATES) Sep 1991, 18 (3) p545-57

Effect of migration on blood pressure: the Yi People Study. Epidemiology (UNITED STATES) Mar 1991, 2 (2) p88-97

Minerals and blood pressure. Ann Med (FINLAND) Aug 1991, 23 (3) p299-305

Renal function of cations excretion in children predisposed to essential hypertension. Chung Hua Yu Fang I Hsueh Tsa Chih (CHINA) May 1991, 25 (3) p152-4

Nutrition and blood pressure among elderly men and women (Dutch Nutrition Surveillance System). J Am Coll Nutr (UNITED STATES) Apr 1991, 10 (2) p149-55

The effect of Ca and Mg supplementation and the role of the opioidergic system on the development of DOCA-salt hypertension. Am J Hypertens (UNITED STATES) Jan 1991, 4 (1 Pt 1) p72-5

Cellular mechanisms in hypertension and therapeutic implications in blacks. Cardiovasc Drugs Ther (UNITED STATES) Mar 1990, 4 Suppl 2 p317-9

Experimental intervention of hypertension and cardiovascular diseases. Clin Exp Hypertens [A] (UNITED STATES) 1990, 12 (5) p939-52

Attenuated vasodilator responses to Mg2+ in young patients with borderline hypertension. Circulation (UNITED STATES) Aug 1990, 82 (2) p384-93

Dietary modulators of blood pressure in hypertension. Eur J Clin Nutr (ENGLAND) Apr 1990, 44 (4) p319-27

Daily intake of macro and trace elements in the diet. 4. Sodium, potassium, calcium, and magnesium. Ann Ig (ITALY) Sep-Oct 1989, 1 (5) p923-42

Fish oils modulate blood pressure and vascular contractility in the rat and vascular contractility in the primate. Blood Press (NORWAY) May 1995, 4 (3) p177-86

Vasorelaxant properties of n-3 polyunsaturated fatty acids in aortas from spontaneously hypertensive and normotensive rats. J Cardiovasc Risk (ENGLAND) Jun 1994, 1 (1) p75-80

Effects of fish oil, nifedipine and their combination on blood pressure and lipids in primary hypertension. J Hum Hypertens (ENGLAND) Feb 1993, 7 (1) p25-32

Effects of a combination of evening primrose oil (gamma linolenic acid) and fish oil (eicosapentaenoic + docahexaenoic acid) versus magnesium, and versus placebo in preventing pre-eclampsia. Women Health (UNITED STATES) 1992, 19 (2-3) p117-31

Microbial infection or trauma at cardiovascular representation area of medulla oblongata as some of the possible causes of hypertension or hypotension. Acupunct Electrother Res (UNITED STATES) 1988, 13 (2-3) p131-45

Garlic (Allium sativum)--a potent medicinal plant. Fortschr Med (GERMANY) Jul 20 1995, 113 (20-21) p311-5

A meta-analysis of the effect of garlic on blood pressure. J Hypertens (ENGLAND) Apr 1994, 12 (4) p463-8

Patient preferences for novel therapy: an N-of-1 trial of garlic in the treatment for hypertension. J Gen Intern Med (UNITED STATES) Nov 1993, 8 (11) p619-21

Can garlic lower blood pressure? A pilot study. Pharmacotherapy (UNITED STATES) Jul-Aug 1993, 13 (4) p406-7

Hypertension and hyperlipidaemia: garlic helps in mild cases. Br J Clin Pract Symp Suppl (ENGLAND) Aug 1990, 69 p3-6

Antithrombotic activity of garlic: its inhibition of the synthesis of thromboxane-B2 during infusion of arachidonic acid and collagen in rabbits. Prostaglandins Leukot Essent Fatty Acids (SCOTLAND) Oct 1990, 41 (2) p95-9

Garlic (Allium sativum) and onion (Allium cepa): a review of their relationship to cardiovascular disease. Prev Med (UNITED STATES) Sep 1987, 16 (5) p670-85

Bulgarian traditional medicine: a source of ideas for phytopharmacological investigations. J Ethnopharmacol (SWITZERLAND) Feb 1986, 15 (2) p121-32

Garlic as a natural agent for the treatment of hypertension: a preliminary report. Cytobios (ENGLAND) 1982, 34 (135-36) p145-52

Plants and hypotensive, antiatheromatous and coronarodilatating action. Am J Chin Med (UNITED STATES) Autumn 1979, 7 (3) p197-236

Treatment of essential hypertension with coenzyme Q10. Mol Aspects Med (ENGLAND) 1994, 15 Suppl pS265-72

Coenzyme Q10 in essential hypertension. Mol Aspects Med (ENGLAND) 1994, 15 Suppl ps257-63

Usefulness of coenzyme Q10 in clinical cardiology: a long-term study. Mol Aspects Med (ENGLAND) 1994, 15 Suppl ps165-75

Influence of coenzyme Q-10 on the hypotensive effects of enalapril and nitrendipine in spontaneously hypertensive rats. Pol J Pharmacol (POLAND) Sep-Oct 1994, 46 (5) p457-61

Isolated diastolic dysfunction of the myocardium and its response to CoQ10 treatment. Clin Investig

References

(GERMANY) 1993, 71 (8 Suppl) pS140-4

Muscle fibre types, ubiquinone content and exercise capacity in hypertension and effort angina. Ann Med (FINLAND) Aug 1991, 23 (3) p339-44

Effect of coenzyme Q10 on structural alterations in the renal membrane of stroke-prone spontaneously hypertensive rats. Biochem Med Metab Biol (UNITED STATES) Apr 1991, 45 (2) p216-26

Co-enzyme Q10: a new drug for cardiovascular disease. J Clin Pharmacol (UNITED STATES) Jul 1990, 30 (7) p596-608

Coenzyme Q10: a new drug for myocardial ischemia? Med Clin North Am (UNITED STATES) Jan 1988, 72 (1) p243-58

Clinical study of cardiac arrhythmias using a 24-hour continuous electrocardiographic recorder (5th report)--antiarrhythmic action of coenzyme Q10 in diabetics. Tohoku J Exp Med (JAPAN) Dec 1983, 141 Suppl p453-63

Bioenergetics in clinical medicine. XVI. Reduction of hypertension in patients by therapy with coenzyme Q10. Res Commun Chem Pathol Pharmacol (UNITED STATES) Jan 1981, 31 (1) p129-40

Prospects for nutritional control of hypertension. Med Hypotheses (ENGLAND) Mar 1981, 7 (3) p271-83

Bioenergetics in clinical medicine XV. Inhibition of coenzyme Q10-enzymes by clinically used adrenergic blockers of beta-receptors. Res Commun Chem Pathol Pharmacol (UNITED STATES) May 1977, 17 (1) p157-64

Bioenergetics in clinical medicine. VIII. Adminstration of coenzyme Q10 to patients with essential hypertension. Res Commun Chem Pathol Pharmacol (UNITED STATES) Aug 1976, 14 (4) p721-7

Bioenergetics in clinical medicine. III. Inhibition of coenzyme Q10-enzymes by clinically used antihypertensive drugs. Res Commun Chem Pathol Pharmacol (UNITED STATES) Nov 1975, 12 (3) p533-40

Bioenergetics in clinical medicine. Studies on coenzyme Q10 and essential hypertension. Res Commun Chem Pathol Pharmacol (UNITED STATES) Jun 1975, 11 (2) p273-88

Antioxidant status in controlled and uncontrolled hypertension and its relationship to endothelial damage. J Hum Hypertens (ENGLAND) Nov 1994, 8 (11) p843-9

The role of antioxidants in the prevention of cardiovascular diseases. Bratisl Lek Listy (SLOVAKIA) May 1994, 95 (5) p199-211

Prevention of cerebrovascular insults. Schweiz Med Wochenschr (SWITZERLAND) Nov 12 1994, 124 (45) p1995-2004

A double-blind, placebo-controlled parallel trial of vitamin C treatment in elderly patients with hypertension. Gerontology (SWITZERLAND) 1994, 40 (5) p268-72

Essential antioxidants in cardiovascular diseases--lessons for Europe. Ther Umsch (SWITZERLAND) Jul 1994, 51 (7) p475-82

Antioxidant vitamin intake and coronary mortality in a longitudinal population study. Am J Epidemiol (UNITED STATES) Jun 15 1994, 139 (12) p1180-9

References

The decline in stroke mortality. An epidemiologic perspective. Ann Epidemiol (UNITED STATES) Sep 1993, 3 (5) p571-5

Can anti-oxidants prevent ischaemic heart disease? J Clin Pharm Ther (ENGLAND) Apr 1993, 18 (2) p85-95

Antioxidant therapy in the aging process. EXS (SWITZERLAND) 1992, 62 p428-37

Anthropometry, lipid- and vitamin status of 215 health-conscious Thai elderly. Int J Vitam Nutr Res (SWITZERLAND) 1991, 61 (3) p215-23

Anti-oxidants show an anti-hypertensive effect in diabetic and hypertensive subjects. Clin Sci (Colch) (ENGLAND) Dec 1991, 81 (6) p739-42

Calcium intake: covariates and confounders. Am J Clin Nutr (UNITED STATES) Mar 1991, 53 (3) p741-4

Factors associated with age-related macular degeneration. An analysis of data from the first National Health and Nutrition Examination Survey. Am J Epidemiol (UNITED STATES) Oct 1988, 128 (4) p700-10

Vitamin C deficiency and low linolenate intake associated with elevated blood pressure J Hypertens Suppl (ENGLAND) Dec 1987, 5 (5) pS521-4

Relationship of magnesium intake and other dietary factors to blood pressure: the Honolulu heart study. Am J Clin Nutr (UNITED STATES) Feb 1987, 45 (2) p469-75

Pathogenetic factors of aging macular degeneration. Ophthalmology (UNITED STATES) May 1985, 92 (5) p628-35

Nutrition and the elderly: a general overview. J Am Coll Nutr (UNITED STATES) 1984, 3 (4) p341-50

Blood pressure and nutrient intake in the United States. Science (UNITED STATES) Jun 29 1984, 224 (4656) p1392-8

Nitric oxide and the regulation of blood pressure in the hypertension-prone and hypertension-resistant Sabra rat. Hypertension (UNITED STATES) Sep 1996, 28 (3) p367-71

Serum calcium, magnesium, copper and zinc and risk of cardiovascular death. Eur J Clin Nutr (ENGLAND) Jul 1996, 50 (7) p431-7

Vascular effects of metformin. Possible mechanisms for its antihypertensive action in the spontaneously hypertensive rat. Am J Hypertens (UNITED STATES) Jun 1996, 9 (6) p570-6

Plasma ubiquinol-10 is decreased in patients with hyperlipidaemia. Atherosclerosis (Ireland), 1997, 129/1 (119-126)

Role of exogenous L-arginine in hepatic ischemia-reperfusion injury. Journal of Surgical Research (USA), 1997, 69/2 (429-434)

Effects of taurine and guanidinoethane sulfonate on toxicity of the pyrrolizidine alkaloid monocrotaline. Biochemical Pharmacology (USA), 1996, 51/3 (321-329)

The Inuit diet. Fatty acids and antioxidants, their role in ischemic heart disease, and exposure to organochlorines and heavy metals. An international study. Arctic Med Res (FINLAND) 1996, 55 Suppl 1 p20-4

References

Renal denervation prevents intraglomerular platelet aggregation and glomerular injury induced by chronic inhibition of nitric oxide synthesis. Nephron (SWITZERLAND) 1996, 73 (1) p34-40

Enhanced vasodilation to acetylcholine in athletes is associated with lower plasma cholesterol. Am J Physiol (UNITED STATES) Jun 1996, 270 (6 Pt 2) pH2008-13

Central depressor action of nitric oxide is deficient in genetic hypertension. Am J Hypertens (UNITED STATES) Mar 1996, 9 (3) p237-41

Cigarette smoking potentiates endothelial dysfunction of forearm resistance vessels in patients with hypercholesterolemia. Role of oxidized LDL. Circulation (UNITED STATES) Apr 1 1996, 93 (7) p1346-53

Effect of salt intake and inhibitor dose on arterial hypertension and renal injury induced by chronic nitric oxide blockade. Hypertension (UNITED STATES) May 1996, 27 (5) p1165-72

Role of nitric oxide in the maintenance of resting cerebral blood flow during chronic hypertension. Life Sci (ENGLAND) 1996, 58 (15) p1231-8

Angiotensin II-mediated hypertension in the rat increases vascular superoxide production via membrane NADH/NADPH oxidase activation. Contribution to alterations of vasomotor tone. J Clin Invest (UNITED STATES) Apr 15 1996, 97 (8) p1916-23

Endothelial function in deoxycorticosterone-NaCl hypertension: effect of calcium supplementation. Circulation (UNITED STATES) Mar 1 1996, 93 (5) p1000-8

Can the kidney prevent cardiovascular diseases? Clin Exp Hypertens (UNITED STATES) Apr-May 1996, 18 (3-4) p501-11

Vitamin C status and blood pressure. J Hypertens (ENGLAND) Apr 1996, 14 (4) p503-8

[Evaluation of selected parameters of zinc metabolism in patients with primary hypertension]. Pol Arch Med Wewn (POLAND) Mar 1996, 95 (3) p198-204

Acute sympathoinhibitory actions of metformin in spontaneously hypertensive rats. Hypertension (UNITED STATES) Mar 1996, 27 (3 Pt 2) p619-25

[Overview--suppression effect of essential trace elements on arteriosclerotic development and it's mechanism]. Nippon Rinsho (JAPAN) Jan 1996, 54 (1) p59-66

L-arginine prevents corticotropin-induced increases in blood pressure in the rat. Hypertension (UNITED STATES) Feb 1996, 27 (2) p184-9

Improvement of cardiac output and liver blood flow and reduction of pulmonary vascular resistance by intravenous infusion of L-arginine during the early reperfusion period in pig liver transplantation. Transplantation (UNITED STATES) May 15 1997, 63 (9) p1225-33

Hypertension, diabetes mellitus, and insulin resistance: the role of intracellular magnesium. Am J Hypertens (UNITED STATES) Mar 1997, 10 (3) p346-55

Prevention of preeclampsia with calcium supplementation and its relation with the L-arginine:nitric oxide pathway. Braz J Med Biol Res (BRAZIL) Jun 1996, 29 (6) p731-41

[Guidelines on treatment of hypertension in the elderly, 1995--a tentative plan for comprehensive research projects on aging and health-- Members of the Research Group for "Guidelines on Treatment of Hypertension in the Elderly", Comprehensive Research Projects on Aging and Health, the Ministry of

Health and Welfare of Japan]. Nippon Ronen Igakkai Zasshi (JAPAN) Dec 1996, 33 (12) p945-75

Treatment of essential hypertension with coenzyme Q10. Mol Aspects Med (ENGLAND) 1994, 15 Suppl

Coenzyme Q10 in essential hypertension. Mol Aspects Med (ENGLAND) 1994, 15 Suppl

Usefulness of coenzyme Q10 in clinical cardiology: a long-term study. Mol Aspects Med (ENGLAND) 1994, 15 Suppl

Influence of coenzyme Q-10 on the hypotensive effects of enalapril and nitrendipine in spontaneously hypertensive rats. Pol J Pharmacol (POLAND) Sep-Oct 1994, 46 (5) p457- 61

Isolated diastolic dysfunction of the myocardium and its response to CoQ10 treatment. Clin Investig (GERMANY) 1993, 71 (8 Suppl)

Effect of coenzyme Q10 on structural alterations in the renal membrane of stroke-prone spontaneously hypertensive rats. Biochem Med Metab Biol (UNITED STATES) Apr 1991

Coenzyme Q10: a new drug for cardiovascular disease. J Clin Pharmacol (UNITED STATES) Jul 1990

Coenzyme Q10: a new drug for myocardial ischemia? Med Clin North Am (UNITED STATES) Jan 1988

Bioenergetics in clinical medicine. XVI. Reduction of hypertension in patients by therapy with coenzyme Q10. Res Commun Chem Pathol Pharmacol (UNITED STATES) Jan 1981

Bioenergetics in clinical medicine. VIII. Adminstration of coenzyme Q10 to patients with essential hypertension. Res Commun Chem Pathol Pharmacol (UNITED STATES) Aug 1976

Bioenergetics in clinical medicine. III. Inhibition of coenzyme Q10- enzymes by clinically used antihypertensive drugs. Res Commun Chem Pathol Pharmacol (UNITED STATES) Nov 1975

Bioenergetics in clinical medicine. Studies on coenzyme Q10 and essential hypertension. Res Commun Chem Pathol Pharmacol (UNITED STATES) Jun 1975

[Garlic (Allium sativum)—a potent medicinal plant] Fortschr Med (GERMANY) Jul 20 1995

A meta-analysis of the effect of garlic on blood pressure. J Hypertens (ENGLAND) Apr 1994

Patient preferences for novel therapy: an N-of-1 trial of garlic in the treatment for hypertension. J Gen Intern Med (UNITED STATES) Nov 1993

Can garlic lower blood pressure? A pilot study. Pharmacotherapy (UNITED STATES) Jul-Aug 1993

Hypertension and hyperlipidaemia: garlic helps in mild cases. Br J Clin Pract Symp Suppl (ENGLAND) Aug 1990

Defective renal adenylate cyclase response to prostaglandin E2 in spontaneously hypertensive rats. J Hypertens (ENGLAND) Apr 1985, 3 (2)

Renal response to L-arginine in salt-sensitive patients with essential hypertension. Hypertension (UNITED STATES) Mar 1996

L-arginine restores dilator responses of the basilar artery to acetylcholine during chronic hypertension. Hypertension (UNITED STATES) Apr 1996

Vitamin C deficiency and low linolenate intake associated with elevated blood pressure: the Kuopio

Ischaemic Heart Disease Risk Factor Study. J Hypertens Suppl (ENGLAND) Dec 1987

Regulation of blood pressure by nitroxidergic nerve. J Diabetes Complications (UNITED STATES) Oct-Dec 1995

[Endothelial function and arterial hypertension] Ann Ital Med Int (ITALY) Oct 1995, 10 Suppl

Contrasting effect of antihypertensive treatment on the renal response to L-arginine. Hypertension (UNITED STATES) Dec 1995

Prospective study of nutritional factors, blood pressure, and hypertension among US women. Hypertension (UNITED STATES) May 1996

[Overview—suppression effect of essential trace elements on arteriosclerotic development and it's mechanism] Nippon Rinsho (JAPAN) Jan 1996

[Interrelationship between dietary intake of minerals and prevalence of hypertension] Vopr Pitan (RUSSIA) 1995, (6)

Potassium depletion and salt-sensitive hypertension in Dahl rats: effect on calcium, magnesium, and phosphate excretions. Clin Exp Hypertens (UNITED STATES) Aug 1995

Consequences of magnesium deficiency on the enhancement of stress reactions; preventive and therapeutic implications (a review). J Am Coll Nutr (UNITED STATES) Oct 1994

Relationship of magnesium intake and other dietary factors to blood pressure: the Honolulu heart study. Am J Clin Nutr (UNITED STATES) Feb 1987

[Role of electrolytes in the development and maintenance of hypertension] Nippon Naibunpi Gakkai Zasshi (JAPAN) May 20 1994

Effect of dietary magnesium supplementation on intralymphocytic free calcium and magnesium in stroke-prone spontaneously hypertensive rats. Clin Exp Hypertens (UNITED STATES) May 1994

Vasorelaxant properties of n-3 polyunsaturated fatty acids in aortas from spontaneously hypertensive and normotensive rats. J Cardiovasc Risk (ENGLAND) Jun 1994

Effects of a combination of evening primrose oil (gamma linolenic acid) and fish oil (eicosapentaenoic + docahexaenoic acid) versus magnesium, and versus placebo in preventing pre-eclampsia. Women Health (UNITED STATES) 1992, 19 (2-3)

Antithrombotic activity of garlic: its inhibition of the synthesis of thromboxane-B2 during infusion of arachidonic acid and collagen in rabbits. Prostaglandins Leukot Essent Fatty Acids (SCOTLAND) Oct 1990

Bulgarian traditional medicine: a source of ideas for phytopharmacological investigations. J Ethnopharmacol (SWITZERLAND) Feb 1986

Garlic as a natural agent for the treatment of hypertension: a preliminary report. Cytobios (ENGLAND) 1982, 34 (135-36)

The decline in stroke mortality. An epidemiologic perspective. Ann Epidemiol (UNITED STATES) Sep 1993

Antioxidant therapy in the aging process. EXS (SWITZERLAND) 1992, 62

Antioxidants show an anti-hypertensive effect in diabetic and hypertensive subjects. Clin Sci (Colch)

(ENGLAND) Dec 1991

[Relation between vitamin C consumption and risk of ischemic heart disease] Vopr Pitan (USSR) Nov-Dec 1983

Blood pressure and nutrient intake in the United States. Science (UNITED STATES) Jun 29 1984

Hypoglycemia

Preventing Hypoglycemia. Anti-Aging News, January 1982 Vo.2, No. 1 pg 6-7

Glutathione protects against hypoxic/hypoglycemic decreases in 2- deoxyglucose uptake and presynaptic spikes in hippocampal slices. Eur J Pharmacol (NETHERLANDS) Jan 24 1995, 273 (1-2) p191-5

Glutathione protects against hypoxic/hypoglycemic decreases in 2- deoxyglucose uptake and presynaptic spikes in hippocampal slices. Eur J Pharmacol (NETHERLANDS) Jan 24 1995, 273 (1-2) p191-5

Immune Enhancement

Isoprinosine In The Treatment Of Genital Warts. Cancer Detect Prev; 12(1-6):497-501 1988

Summary of the NATO advanced research workshop on dietary omega 3 and omega 6 fatty acids: biological effects and nutritional essentiality. J Nutr (UNITED STATES) Apr 1989, 119 (4) p521-8

Carnitine in human immunodeficiency virus type 1 infection/acquired immune deficiency syndrome. J Child Neurol (UNITED STATES) Nov 1995, 10 Suppl 2 pS40-4

Utilization of intracellular acylcarnitine pools by mononuclear phagocytes. Biochim Biophys Acta (NETHERLANDS) Nov 11 1994, 1201 (2) p321-7

Carnitine depletion in peripheral blood mononuclear cells from patients with AIDS: effect of oral L-carnitine. AIDS (UNITED STATES) May 1994, 8 (5) p655-60

Nutritional factors in the pathogenesis and therapy of respiratory insufficiency in neuromuscular diseases. Monaldi Arch Chest Dis (ITALY) Aug 1993, 48 (4) p327-30

Sudden infant death syndrome (SIDS): oxygen utilization and energy production. Med Hypotheses (ENGLAND) Jun 1993, 40 (6) p364-6

High dose L-carnitine improves immunologic and metabolic parameters in AIDS patients. Immunopharmacol Immunotoxicol (UNITED STATES) Jan 1993, 15 (1) p1-12

Effects of acetyl-L-carnitine oral administration on lymphocyte antibacterial activity and TNF-alpha levels in patients with active pulmonary tuberculosis. A randomized double blind versus placebo study. Immunopharmacol Immunotoxicol (UNITED STATES) 1991, 13 (1-2) p135-46

Immunological parameters in aging: studies on natural immunomodulatory and immunoprotective substances. Int J Clin Pharmacol Res (SWITZERLAND) 1990, 10 (1-2) p53-7

Carnitine deficiency with cardiomyopathy presenting as neonatal hydrops: successful response to carnitine therapy. J Inherit Metab Dis (NETHERLANDS) 1990, 13 (1) p69-75

Medium-chain triglycerides--useful energy carriers in parenteral nutrition Wien Klin Wochenschr (AUS-TRIA) Apr 14 1989, 101 (8) p300-3

Rationales for micronutrient supplementation in diabetes. Med Hypotheses (ENGLAND) Feb 1984, 13 (2) p139-51

Recent knowledge concerning the biochemistry and significance of ascorbic acid. Z Gesamte Inn Med (GERMANY, EAST) Jan 15 1984, 39 (2) p21-7

Reversibility by L-carnitine of immunosuppression induced by an emulsion of soya bean oil, glycerol and egg lecithin. Arzneimittelforschung (GERMANY, WEST) 1982, 32 (11) p1485-8

Vitamins and immunity: II. Influence of L-carnitine on the immune system. Acta Vitaminol Enzymol (ITALY) 1982, 4 (1-2) p135-40

Suppression of tumor growth and enhancement of immune status with high levels of dietary vitamin B6 in BALB/c mice. J Natl Cancer Inst (UNITED STATES) May 1987, 78 (5) p951-9

Ontogenetic analysis of immune amplification by thymus-derived cells in chickens. Exp Hematol (DENMARK) Sep 1981, 9 (8) p856-64

The activities of coenzyme Q10 and vitamin B6 for immune responses. Biochem Biophys Res Commun (UNITED STATES) May 28 1993, 193 (1) p88-92

Food uses and health effects of corn oil. J Am Coll Nutr (UNITED STATES) Oct 1990, 9 (5) p438-70

A modified determination of coenzyme Q10 in human blood and CoQ10 blood levels in diverse patients with allergies. Biofactors (ENGLAND) Dec 1988, 1 (4) p303-6

Biochemical deficiencies of coenzyme Q10 in HIV-infection and exploratory treatment. Biochem Biophys Res Commun (UNITED STATES) Jun 16 1988, 153 (2) p888-96

Research on coenzyme Q10 in clinical medicine and in immunomodulation. Drugs Exp Clin Res (SWITZERLAND) 1985, 11 (8) p539-45

The polypeptide composition of the mitochondrial NADH: ubiquinone reductase complex from several mammalian species. Biochem J (ENGLAND) Sep 15 1985, 230 (3) p739-46

An analysis of the polypeptide composition of bovine heart mitochondrial NADH-ubiquinone oxidoreductase by two-dimensional polyacrylamide-gel electrophoresis. Biochem J (ENGLAND) Aug 1 1979, 181 (2) p435-43

Immunological senescence in mice and its reversal by coenzyme Q10. Mech Ageing Dev (SWITZER-LAND) Mar 1978, 7 (3) p189-97

Melatonin reduces the severity of dextran-induced colitis in mice. J Pineal Res (DENMARK) Aug 1995, 19 (1) p31-9

Melatonin affects proopiomelanocortin gene expression in the immune organs of the rat. Eur J Endocrinol (NORWAY) Dec 1995, 133 (6) p754-60

Immune effects of preoperative immunotherapy with high-dose subcutaneous interleukin-2 versus neuroimmunotherapy with low-dose interleukin-2 plus the neurohormone melatonin in gastrointestinal tract tumor patients. J Biol Regul Homeost Agents (ITALY) Jan-Mar 1995, 9 (1) p31-3

Serial transplants of DMBA-induced mammary tumors in Fischer rats as model system for human breast cancer. IV. Parallel changes of biopterin and melatonin indicate interactions between the pineal gland and cellular immunity in malignancy. Oncology (SWITZERLAND) Jul-Aug 1995, 52 (4) p278-83

Inhibitory effect of melatonin on production of IFN gamma or TNF alpha in peripheral blood mononuclear cells of some blood donors. J Pineal Res (DENMARK) Nov 1994, 17 (4) p164-9

Specific binding of 2-[125I]iodomelatonin by rat splenocytes: characterization and its role on regulation of cyclic AMP production. J Neuroimmunol (NETHERLANDS) Mar 1995, 57 (1-2) p171-8

Pineal-opioid system interactions in the control of immunoinflammatory responses. Ann N Y Acad Sci (UNITED STATES) Nov 25 1994, 741 p191-6

Evidence for a direct action of melatonin on the immune system. Biol Signals (SWITZERLAND) Mar-Apr 1994, 3 (2) p107-17

The immuno-reconstituting effect of melatonin or pineal grafting and its relation to zinc pool in aging mice. J Neuroimmunol (NETHERLANDS) Sep 1994, 53 (2) p189-201

Multiple sclerosis: the role of puberty and the pineal gland in its pathogenesis. Int J Neurosci (ENGLAND) Feb 1993, 68 (3-4) p209-25

Modulation of human lymphoblastoid interferon activity by melatonin in metastatic renal cell carcinoma. A phase II study. Cancer (UNITED STATES) Jun 15 1994, 73 (12) p3015-9

Modulation of 2[125I]iodomelatonin binding sites in the guinea pig spleen by melatonin injection is dependent on the dose and period but not the time. Life Sci (ENGLAND) 1994, 54 (19) p1441-8

Binding of [125I]-labelled iodomelatonin in the duck thymus. Biol Signals (SWITZERLAND) Sep-Oct 1992, 1 (5) p250-6

Characteristics of 2-[125I]iodomelatonin binding sites in the pigeon spleen and modulation of binding by guanine nucleotides. J Pineal Res (DENMARK) May 1993, 14 (4) p169-77

Pinealectomy ameliorates collagen II-induced arthritis in mice. Clin Exp Immunol (ENGLAND) Jun 1993, 92 (3) p432-6

The immunoneuroendocrine role of melatonin. J Pineal Res (DENMARK) Jan 1993, 14 (1) p1-10

2[125I]iodomelatonin binding sites in spleens of guinea pigs. Life Sci (ENGLAND) 1992, 50 (22) p1719-26

Melatonin: a chronobiotic with anti-aging properties? Med Hypotheses (ENGLAND) Apr 1991, 34 (4) p300-9

Effect of dose and time of melatonin injections on the diurnal rhythm of immunity in chicken. J Pineal Res (DENMARK) Jan 1991, 10 (1) p30-5

The pineal neurohormone melatonin stimulates activated CD4+, Thy-1+ cells to release opioid agonist(s) with immunoenhancing and anti-stress properties. J Neuroimmunol (NETHERLANDS) Jul 1990, 28 (2) p167-76

Alterations of pineal gland and of T lymphocyte subsets in metastatic cancer patients: preliminary results. J Biol Regul Homeost Agents (UNITED STATES) Oct-Dec 1989, 3 (4) p181-3

Endocrine and immune effects of melatonin therapy in metastatic cancer patients. Eur J Cancer Clin Oncol (ENGLAND) May 1989, 25 (5) p789-95

References

Replacement of DHEA in aging men and women. Potential remedial effects. Ann N Y Acad Sci (UNITED STATES) Dec 29 1995, 774 p128-42

Dehydroepiandrosterone (DHEA) treatment reverses the impaired immune response of old mice to influenza vaccination and protects from influenza infection. Vaccine (ENGLAND) 1995, 13 (15) p1445-8

Dehydroepiandrosterone modulation of lipopolysaccharide-stimulated monocyte cytotoxicity. J Immunol (UNITED STATES) Jan 1 1996, 156 (1) p328-35

Dehydroepiandrosterone modulates the spontaneous and IL-6 stimulated fibrinogen production of human hepatoma cells. Acta Microbiol Immunol Hung (HUNGARY) 1995, 42 (2) p229-33

Administration of dehydroepiandrosterone reverses the immune suppression induced by high dose antigen in mice. Immunol Invest (UNITED STATES) May 1995, 24 (4) p583-93

Effects of dehydroepiandrosterone in immunosuppressed adult mice infected with Cryptosporidium parvum. J Parasitol (UNITED STATES) Jun 1995, 81 (3) p429-33

Relationship between dehydroepiandrosterone and calcitonin gene-related peptide in the mouse thymus. Am J Physiol (UNITED STATES) Jan 1995, 268 (1 Pt 1) pE168-73

Dehydroepiandrosterone functions as more than an antiglucocorticoid in preserving immunocompetence after thermal injury. Endocrinology (UNITED STATES) Feb 1995, 136 (2) p393-401

Pregnenolone and dehydroepiandrosterone as precursors of native 7-hydroxylated metabolites which increase the immune response in mice. J Steroid Biochem Mol Biol (ENGLAND) Jul 1994, 50 (1-2) p91-100

In vitro potentiation of lymphocyte activation by dehydroepiandrosterone, androstenediol, and androstenetriol. J Immunol (UNITED STATES) Aug 15 1994, 153 (4) p1544-52

Immune senescence and adrenal steroids: immune dysregulation and the action of dehydroepiandrosterone (DHEA) in old animals. Eur J Clin Pharmacol (GERMANY) 1993, 45 Suppl 1 pS21-3; discussion S43-4

Effects of dehydroepiandrosterone in immunosuppressed rats infected with Cryptosporidium parvum. J Parasitol (UNITED STATES) Jun 1993, 79 (3) p364-70

Dehydroepiandrosterone protects mice inoculated with West Nile virus and exposed to cold stress. J Med Virol (UNITED STATES) Nov 1992, 38 (3) p159-66

The relationship of serum DHEA-S and cortisol levels to measures of immune function in human immunodeficiency virus-related illness. Am J Med Sci (UNITED STATES) Feb 1993, 305 (2) p79-83

Mobilization of cutaneous immunity for systemic protection against infections. Ann N Y Acad Sci (UNITED STATES) Apr 15 1992, 650 p363-6

Dehydroepiandrosterone-induced reduction of Cryptosporidium parvum infections in aged Syrian golden hamsters. J Parasitol (UNITED STATES) Jun 1992, 78 (3) p554-7

Dehydroepiandrosterone enhances IL2 production and cytotoxic effector function of human T cells. Clin Immunol Immunopathol (UNITED STATES) Nov 1991, 61 (2 Pt 1) p202-11

Protection from glucocorticoid induced thymic involution by dehydroepiandrosterone. Life Sci (ENGLAND) 1990, 46 (22) p1627-31

Regulation of murine lymphokine production in vivo. II. Dehydroepiandrosterone is a natural enhancer of interleukin 2 synthesis by helper T cells. Eur J Immunol (GERMANY, WEST) Apr 1990, 20 (4) p793-802

Biomarks in secondary osteoporosis. Clin Rheumatol (BELGIUM) Jun 1989, 8 Suppl 2 p89-94

Protection against acute lethal viral infections with the native steroid dehydroepiandrosterone (DHEA). J Med Virol (UNITED STATES) Nov 1988, 26 (3) p301-14

Food intake reduction and immunologic alterations in mice fed dehydroepiandrosterone. Exp Gerontol (ENGLAND) 1984, 19 (5) p297-304

Steroid induction of gonadotropin surges in the immature rat. I. Priming effects of androgens. Endocrinology (UNITED STATES) Nov 1978, 103 (5) p1822-8

Effect of thyroxine and chicken growth hormone on immune function in autoimmune thyroiditis (obese) strain chicks. Proc Soc Exp Biol Med (UNITED STATES) Jan 1992, 199 (1) p114-22

Binding and functional effects of thyroid stimulating hormone on human immune cells. J Clin Immunol (UNITED STATES) Jul 1990, 10 (4) p204-10

The in vitro effect of a thymic polypeptidic extract on the function of T-cells and macrophages. Endocrinologie (ROMANIA) Apr-Jun 1987, 25 (2) p83-9

Effect of immunization on functional state of thyroid gland and thyroxine binding in rat organs. Biull Eksp Biol Med (USSR) Feb 1982, 93 (2) p46-8

Thyroid function and triiodothyronine and thyroxine kinetics in rabbits immunized with thyroid hormones. Acta Endocrinol (Copenh) (DENMARK) Feb 1975, 78 (2) p276-88

Effect of isoprinosine on lymphocyte proliferation and natural killer cell activity following thermal injury. Immunopharmacol Immunotoxicol (UNITED STATES) 1989, 11 (4) p631-44

Immunopharmacology of the immunotherapy of cancer, infection, and autoimmunity. Fundam Clin Pharmacol (FRANCE) 1987, 1 (4) p283-96

Immunorestoration in children with recurrent respiratory infections treated with isoprinosine. Int J Immunopharmacol (ENGLAND) 1987, 9 (8) p947-9

A randomized double-blind study of inosiplex (isoprinosine) therapy in patients with alopecia totalis. J Am Acad Dermatol (UNITED STATES) May 1987, 16 (5 Pt 1) p977-83

Isoprinosine abolishes the blocking factor-mediated inhibition of lymphocyte responses to Epstein-Barr virus antigens and phytohemagglutinin. Int J Immunopharmacol (ENGLAND) 1986, 8 (1) p101-6

Isoprinosine as an immunopotentiator in an animal model of human osteosarcoma. Int J Immunopharmacol (ENGLAND) 1981, 3 (4) p383-9

Determination of the antiinfectious activity of RU 41740 (Biostim) as an example of an immunomodulator. Adv Exp Med Biol (UNITED STATES) 1992, 319 p165-74

Effect of an immunostimulatory substance of Klebsiella pneumoniae on inflammatory responses of human granulocytes, basophils and platelets. Arzneimittelforschung (GERMANY) Aug 1991, 41 (8) p815-20

Determination of the anti-infective action of an immunomodulator. Biostim as an example. Allerg

Immunol (Paris) (FRANCE) Apr 1991, 23 (4) p145-52

The effect of Biostim (RU-41740) on the expression of cytokine mRNAs in murine peritoneal macrophages in vitro. Toxicol Lett (NETHERLANDS) Oct 1990, 53 (3) p327-37

Immunotolerance of RU 41740. Presse Med (FRANCE) Jul 27 1988, 17 (28) p1458-60

Clinical immunopharmacology of RU 41740. Presse Med (FRANCE) Jul 27 1988, 17 (28) p1438-40

Effect of an immunomodulator, RU 41740, on experimental infections. Presse Med (FRANCE) Jul 27 1988, 17 (28) p1430-2

The effect of the immunomodulator RU 41,740 (biostim) on the specific and nonspecific immuno-suppression induced by thermal injury or protein deprivation. Arch Surg (UNITED STATES) Feb 1988, 123 (2) p207-11

The effect of RU 41.740, an immune modulating compound, in the prevention of acute exacerbations in patients with chronic bronchitis. Eur J Respir Dis (DENMARK) Oct 1986, 69 (4) p235-41

Activation of murine B lymphocytes by RU 41740, a glycoprotein extract from Klebsiella pneumoniae. C R Acad Sci III (FRANCE) 1984, 298 (6) p135-8

Influence of RU 41.740, a glycoprotein extract from Klebsiella pneumoniae, on the murine immune system. I. T-independent polyclonal B cell activation. J Immunol (UNITED STATES) Feb 1984, 132 (2) p616-21

Vitamins and immunity: II. Influence of L-carnitine on the immune system. Acta Vitaminol Enzymol (ITALY) 1982, 4 (1-2)

Suppression of tumor growth and enhancement of immune status with high levels of dietary vitamin B6 in BALB/c mice. J Natl Cancer Inst (UNITED STATES) May 1987

The activities of coenzyme Q10 and vitamin B6 for immune responses. Biochem Biophys Res Commun (UNITED STATES) May 28 1993, 193 (1)

Research on coenzyme Q10 in clinical medicine and in immunomodulation. Drugs Exp Clin Res (SWITZERLAND) 1985, 11 (8) p539-45

Immunoenhancing effect of flavonoid compounds on lymphocyte proliferation and immunoglobulin synthesis. Int J Immunopharmacol (ENGLAND) 1984, 6 (3) p205-15

Immunological senescence in mice and its reversal by coenzyme Q10. Mech Ageing Dev (SWITZER-LAND) Mar 1978, 7 (3)

Immune effects of preoperative immunotherapy with high-dose subcutaneous interleukin-2 versus neuroimmunotherapy with low-dose interleukin-2 plus the neurohormone melatonin in gastrointestinal tract tumor patients. J Biol Regul Homeost Agents (ITALY) Jan-Mar 1995, 9 (1) p31-3

Pineal-opioid system interactions in the control of immunoinflammatory responses. Ann N Y Acad Sci (UNITED STATES) Nov 25 1994

Evidence for a direct action of melatonin on the immune system. Biol Signals (SWITZERLAND) Mar-Apr 1994

The immuno-reconstituting effect of melatonin or pineal grafting and its relation to zinc pool in aging mice. Neuroimmunol (NETHERLANDS) Sep 1994

The immunoneuroendocrine role of melatonin. J Pineal Res (DENMARK) Jan 1993, 14 (1) p1-10

The pineal neurohormone melatonin stimulates activated CD4+, Thy-1+ cells to release opioid agonist(s) with immunoenhancing and anti-stress properties. J Neuroimmunol (NETHERLANDS) Jul 1990, 28 (2)

Endocrine and immune effects of melatonin therapy in metastatic cancer patients. Eur J Cancer Clin Oncol (ENGLAND) May 1989

Dehydroepiandrosterone (DHEA) treatment reverses the impaired immune response of old mice to influenza vaccination and protects from influenza infection. Vaccine (ENGLAND) 1995, 13 (15) p1445-8

Dehydroepiandrosterone modulation of lipopolysaccharide-stimulated monocyte cytotoxicity. J Immunol (UNITED STATES) Jan 1 1996, 156 (1)

Administration of dehydroepiandrosterone reverses the immune suppression induced by high dose antigen in mice. Immunol Invest (UNITED STATES) May 1995

Pregnenolone and dehydroepiandrosterone as precursors of native 7-hydroxylated metabolites which increase the immune response in mice. J Steroid Biochem Mol Biol (ENGLAND) Jul 1994

The relationship of serum DHEA-S and cortisol levels to measures of immune function in human immunodeficiency virus-related illness. Am J Med Sci (UNITED STATES) Feb 1993

Dehydroepiandrosterone enhances IL2 production and cytotoxic effector function of human T cells. Clin Immunol Immunopathol (UNITED STATES) Nov 1991

Protection from glucocorticoid induced thymic involution by dehydroepiandrosterone. Life Sci (ENGLAND) 1990, 46 (22)

Immune development in young-adult C.RF-hyt mice is affected by congenital and maternal hypothyroidism. Proc Soc Exp Biol Med (UNITED STATES) Oct 1993

Binding and functional effects of thyroid stimulating hormone on human immune cells. J Clin Immunol (UNITED STATES) Jul 1990

Immunorestoration in children with recurrent respiratory infections treated with isoprinosine. Int J Immunopharmacol (ENGLAND) 1987, 9 (8)

Isoprinosine abolishes the blocking factor-mediated inhibition of lymphocyte responses to Epstein-Barr virus antigens and phytohemagglutinin. Int J Immunopharmacol (ENGLAND) 1986, 8 (1)

Isoprinosine as an immunopotentiator in an animal model of human osteosarcoma. Int J Immunopharmacol (ENGLAND) 1981, 3 (4)

The effect of Biostim (RU-41740) on the expression of cytokine mRNAs in murine peritoneal macrophages in vitro. Toxicol Lett (NETHERLANDS) Oct 1990

Isoprinosine (INOSINE PRANOBEX BAN, INPX) in the treatment of Aids and other acquired immunodeficiencies of importance. Cancer Detect Prev Suppl; 1:597-609 1987

Immunological effects of Isoprinosine as a pulse immunotherapy in melanoma and ARC patients in melanoma and ARC patients. Cancer Detect Prev Suppl; 1:457-62 1987

A modified determination of coenzyme Q10 in human blood and CoQ10 blood levels in diverse patients with allergies. Biofactors (ENGLAND) Dec 1988, 1 (4)

Carnitine in human immunodeficiency virus type 1 infection/acquired immune deficiency syndrome. J Child Neurol (UNITED STATES) Nov 1995, 10 Suppl

Oxidative damage and mitochondrial decay in aging. Proc Natl Acad Sci U S A (UNITED STATES) Nov 8 1994

Carnitine depletion in peripheral blood mononuclear cells from patients with AIDS: effect of oral L-carnitine. AIDS (UNITED STATES) May 1994, 8 (5) p655-60

Immunological parameters in aging: studies on natural immunomodulatory and immunoprotective substances. Int J Clin Pharmacol Res (SWITZERLAND) 1990, 10 (1- 2)

Insomnia

Melatonin replacement therapy of elderly insomniacs. Sleep (USA), 1995, 18/7 (598-603)

Improvement of sleep equality in elderly people by controlled-release melatonin. Lancet (United Kingdom), 1995, 346/8974 (541-544)

Sleep-inducing effects of low doses of melatonin ingested in the evening. Clinical Pharmacology and Therapeutics (USA), 1995, 57/5 (552-558)

Light, melatonin and the sleep-wake cycle. J. PSYCHIATRY NEUROSCI. (Canada), 1994, 19/5 (345-353)

Melatonin rhythms in night shift workers. SLEEP (USA), 1992, 15/5 (434-441)

Effect of melatonin replacement on serum hormone rhythms in a patient lacking endogenous melatonin. BRAIN RES. BULL. (USA), 1991, 27/2 (181-185)

Melatonin administration in insomnia. NEUROPSYCHOPHARMACOLOGY (USA), 1990, 3/1 (19-23)

Melatonin replacement therapy of elderly insomniacs. Sleep (UNITED STATES) Sep 1995, 18 (7) p598-603

Melatonin replacement corrects sleep disturbances in a child with pineal tumor. Neurology (USA), 1996, 46/1 (261-263)

Use of melatonin in circadian rhythm disorders and following phase shifts. Acta Neurobiologiae Experimentalis (Poland), 1996, 56/1 (359-362)

Treatment of delayed sleep phase syndrome. General Hospital Psychiatry (USA), 1995, 17/5 (335-345)

Nutritional factors in the etiology of the premenstrual tension syndromes. J Reprod Med (UNITED STATES) Jul 1983, 28 (7) p446-64

Effects of intravenously administered vitamin B12 on sleep in the rat. Physiol Behav (UNITED STATES) Jun 1995, 57 (6) p1019-24

Treatment of persistent sleep-wake schedule disorders in adolescents with methylcobalamin (vitamin B12). Sleep (UNITED STATES) Oct 1991, 14 (5) p414-8

Treatment of persistent sleep-wake schedule disorders in adolescents with methylcobalamin (vitamin B12). Sleep (UNITED STATES) Oct 1991, 14 (5) p414-8,

Vitamin B12 treatment for sleep-wake rhythm disorders. Sleep (UNITED STATES) Feb 1990, 13 (1) p15-23

[Folate and the nervous system (author's transl)] Folates et systeme nerveux. Sem Hop (FRANCE) Sep 18-25 1979, 55 (31-32) p1383-7

The effects of nicotinamide upon sleep in humans. Biol Psychiatry (UNITED STATES) Feb 1977, 12 (1) p139-43

Jet Lag

A double-blind trial of MELATONIN as a treatment for jet lag in international cabin crew. Biol Psychiatry (UNITED STATES) Apr 1 1993

MELATONIN and jet lag: confirmatory result using a simplified protocol. Biol Psychiatry (UNITED STATES) Oct 15 1992, 32 (8) p705-11

Role of biological clock in human pathology] Presse Med (FRANCE) Jun 17 1995, 24 (22) p1041-6

Melatonin marks circadian phase position and resets the endogenous circadian pacemaker in humans. Ciba Found Symp (NETHERLANDS) 1995, 183 p303-17; discussion 317-21

The role of pineal gland in circadian rhythms regulation. Bratisl Lek Listy (SLOVAKIA) Jul 1994, 95 (7) p295- 303

Light, melatonin and the sleep-wake cycle. J Psychiatry Neurosci (CANADA) Nov 1994, 19 (5) p345-53

Circadian rhythms, jet lag, and chronobiotics: an overview. Chronobiol Int (UNITED STATES) Aug 1994, 11 (4) p253-65

[Chronobiological sleep disorders and their treatment possibilities] Ther Umsch (SWITZERLAND) Oct 1993, 50 (10) p704-8

Chronopharmacological actions of the pineal gland. Drug Metabol Drug Interact (ENGLAND) 1990, 8 (3-4) p189-201

Some effects of MELATONIN and the control of its secretion in humans. Ciba Found Symp (NETHER-LANDS) 1985, 117 p266-83

Kidney Disease

Kidney stone clinic: Ten years of experience. Nederlands Tijschrift voor de Klinische Chemie (Netherlands), 1996, 21/1

Magnesium in the physiopathology and treatment of renal calcium stones. PRESSE MED. (FRANCE), 1987, 16/1 (25-27)

Urinary factors of kidney stone formation in patients with Crohn's disease. KLIN. WOCHENSCHR. (Germany, Federal Republic of), 1988, 66/3 (87-91)

Renal stone formation in patients with inflammatory bowel disease. SCANNING MICROSC. (USA), 1993, 7/1 (371-380)

Calcium and calcium magnesium carbonate specimens submitted as urinary tract stones. J. UROL. (USA), 1993, 149/2 (244-249)

Etiology and treatment of urolithiasis. AM. J. KIDNEY DIS. (USA), 1991, 18/6 (624-637)

Pathogenesis of nephrolithiasis post-partial ileal bypass surgery: Case-control study. KIDNEY INT. (USA), 1991, 39/6 (1249-1254)

The effect of glucose intake on urine saturation with calcium oxalate, calcium phosphate, uric acid and sodium urate. INT. UROL. NEPHROL. (Netherlands), 1988, 20/6

Magnesium metabolism in health and disease. DIS. MON. (USA), 1988, 34/4 (166-218)

Prophylaxis of recurring urinary stones: hard or soft mineral water. MINERVA MED. (Italy), 1987, 78/24 (1823-1829)

Urothelial injury to the rabbit bladder from various alkaline and acidic solutions used to dissolve kidney stones. J. UROL. (BALTIMORE) (USA), 1986, 136/1 (181-183)

Kidney stones, magnesium and spa treatment. PRESSE THERM. CLIM. (FRANCE), 1983, 120/1 (33-35)

Learning Disorders

Refer to references under Attention Deficit Disorder (ADD), or Age Associated Mental Impairment (Brain Aging).

Leukemia-Lymphoma
(And Hodgkin's Disease)

Thrombotic complications in acute promyelocytic leukemia during all-trans-retinoic acid therapy. Acta Haematol (SWITZERLAND) 1997, 97 (4) p228-30

Secondary cytogenetic changes in acute promyelocytic leukemia--prognostic importance in patients treated with chemotherapy alone and association with the intron 3 breakpoint of the PML gene: a Cancer and Leukemia Group B study. J Clin Oncol (UNITED STATES) May 1997, 15 (5) p1786-95

Thrombosis in patients with acute promyelocytic leukemia treated with and without all-trans retinoic acid. Leuk Lymphoma (SWITZERLAND) Feb 1996, 20 (5-6) p435-9

The in vitro effects of all-trans-retinoic acid and hematopoietic growth factors on the clonal growth and self-renewal of blast stem cells in acute promyelocytic leukemia. Leuk Res (ENGLAND) Apr 1997, 21 (4) p285-94

All-trans retinoic acid in hematological malignancies, an update. GER (GruppoEmatologico Retinoidi). Haematologica (ITALY) Jan-Feb 1997, 82 (1) p106-21

Molecular genetics of acute leukaemia. Lancet (ENGLAND) Jan 18 1997, 349 (9046) p196-200

All-trans retinoic acid (Tretinoin). Gan To Kagaku Ryoho (JAPAN) Apr 1997, 24 (6) p741-6

A case of acute eosinophilic granulocytic leukemia with PML-RAR alpha fusion gene expression and response to all-trans retinoic acid. Leukemia (ENGLAND) Apr 1997, 11 (4) p609-11

Effects of receptor class- and subtype-selective retinoids and an apoptosis-inducing retinoid on the adherent growth of the NIH:OVCAR-3 ovarian cancer cell line in culture. Cancer Lett (IRELAND) May 1 1997, 115 (1) p1-7

All-trans retinoic acid (ATRA) in the treatment of acute promyelocytic leukemia (APL). Hematol Oncol (ENGLAND) Sep 1996, 14 (3) p147-54

Inhibition of proliferation by retinoic acid on adult T cell leukemia cells. Nihon Rinsho Meneki Gakkai Kaishi (JAPAN) Oct 1996, 19 (5) p477-87

Curcumin, an antioxidant and anti-tumor promoter, induces apoptosis in human leukemia cells. Biochim Biophys Acta (NETHERLANDS) Nov 15 1996, 1317 (2) p95-100

All-trans and 9-cis retinoic acid enhance 1,25-dihydroxyvitamin D3-induced monocytic differentiation of U937 cells. Leuk Res (ENGLAND) Aug 1996, 20 (8) p665-76

Experience in administration low dose all-trans retinoic acid for a child with acute promyelocytic leukemia. Rinsho Ketsueki (JAPAN) Feb 1996, 37 (2) p129-33

Down-regulation of bcl-2 in AML blasts by all-trans retinoic acid and its relationship to CD34 antigen expression. Br J Haematol (ENGLAND) Sep 2 1996, 94 (4) p671-5

Induction therapy with all-trans retinoic acid for acute promyelocytic leukemia: a clinical study of 10 cases, including a fatal [correction of fetal] case with thromboembolism. Intern Med (JAPAN) Jan 1996, 35 (1) p10-4

Effect of the protein tyrosine kinase inhibitor genistein on normal and leukaemic haemopoietic progenitor cells. Br J Haematol (ENGLAND) Jun 1 1996, 93 (3) p551-7

Differentiating therapy in acute myeloid leukemia. Leukemia (ENGLAND) Jun 1996, 10 Suppl 2 ps33-8

Expression of Retinoid X Receptor alpha is increased upon monocytic cell differentiation. Biochem Biophys Res Commun (UNITED STATES) Mar 18 1996, 220 (2) p315-22

In vivo and in vitro characterization of the B1 and B2 zinc-binding domains from the acute promyelocytic leukemia protooncoprotein PML. Proc Natl Acad Sci U S A (UNITED STATES) Feb 20 1996, 93 (4) p1601-6

All-trans retinoic acid combined with interferon-alpha effectively inhibits granulocyte-macrophage colony formation in chronic myeloid leukemia. Leuk Res (ENGLAND) Mar 1996, 20 (3) p243-8

Expression of the p53 tumor suppressor gene induces differentiation and promotes induction of differentiation by 1,25-dihydroxycholecalciferol in leukemic U-937 cells. Blood (UNITED STATES) Feb 1 1996, 87 (3) p1064-74

Retinoids and carcinogenesis. Biotherapy (Japan), 1997, 11/4 (512-517)

Combination of a potent 20-epi-vitamin D3 analogue (KH 1060) with 9- cis-retinoic acid irreversibly inhibits clonal growth, decreases bcl-2 expression, and induces apoptosis in HL-60 leukemic cells. Cancer Research (USA), 1996, 56/15 (3570-3576)

Monocytic differentiation modulates apoptotic response to cytotoxic anti-Fas antibody and tumor necrosis factor alpha in human monoblast U937 cells. Journal of Leukocyte Biology (USA), 1996, 60/6 (778-783)

References

Myeloma cell growth arrest, apoptosis, and interleukin-6 receptor modulation induced by EB1089, a vitamin D3 derivative, alone or in association with dexamethasone. Blood (USA), 1996, 88/12 (4659-4666)

Mutation in the ligand-binding domain of the retinoic acid receptor alpha in HL-60 leukemic cells resistant to retinoic acid and with increased sensitivity to vitamin D3 analogs. Leukemia Research (United Kingdom), 1996, 20/9 (761-769)

Selection of myeloid progenitors lacking BCR/ABL mRNA in chronic myelogenous leukemia patients after in vitro treatment with the tyrosine kinase inhibitor genistein. Blood (USA), 1996, 88/8 (3091-3100)

Influence of dietary components on occurrence of and mortality due to neoplasms in male F344 rats. Aging - Clinical and Experimental Research (Italy), 1996, 8/4 (254-262)

The activities of tyrosine protein kinase and phosphotyrosine protein phosphatase by two differentiation inducers in HL-60 cells. Chinese Journal of Clinical Oncology (China), 1996, 23/2 (84-88)

Retinoids in cancer treatment. J Clin Pharmacol. 1992 Oct. 32(10). P 868-88

Induction of differentiation and enhancement of vincristine sensitivity of human erythroleukemia HEL cells by vesnarinone, a positive inotropic agent. Exp Hematol. 1996 Jan. 24(1). P 37-42

1,25-dihydroxyvitamin D3 primes acute promyelocytic cells for TPA-induced monocytic differentiation through both PKC and tyrosine phosphorylation cascades. Exp Cell Res. 1996 Jan 10. 222(1). P 61-9

Probing the pathobiology of response to all-trans retinoic acid in cute promyelocytic leukemia: premature chromosome condensation/fluorescence in situ hybridization analysis. Blood. 1996 Jan 1. 87(1). P 218-26

Acute renal failure associated with the retinoic acid syndrome in acute promyelocytic leukemia. Am J Kidney Dis. 1996 Jan. 27(1). P 134-7

[Synthesis of retinoids with a modified polar group and their antitumor activity. Report I]. Bioorg Khim. 1995 Dec. 21(12). P 941-9

Induction of differentiation in murine erythroleukemia cells by 1 alpha,25-dihydroxy vitamin D3. Cancer Lett. 1995 Apr 14. 90(2). P 225-30

Synergistic differentiation of U937 cells by all-trans retinoic acid and 1 alpha, 25-dihydroxyvitamin D3 is associated with the expression of retinoid X receptor alpha. Biochem Biophys Res Commun. 1994 Aug 30. 203(1). P 272-80

1,25(OH)2-16ene-vitamin D3 is a potent antileukemic agent with low potential to cause hypercalcemia. Leuk Res (1994 Jun) 18(6):453-63

Genistein enhances the ICAM-mediated adhesion by inducing the expression of ICAM-1 and its counter-receptors. Biochem Biophys Res Commun (1994 Aug 30) 203(1):443-9

Induction of differentiation and dna breakage in human hl-60 and k-562 leukemia cells by genistein. Proc Annu Meet Am Assoc Cancer Res (1990) 31:A2605

Tretinoin. A review of its pharmacodynamic and pharmacokinetic properties and use in the management of acute promyelocytic leukaemia. Drugs. 1995 Nov. 50(5). P 897-923

[Treatment of acute promyelocytic leukemia with trans-retinoic acid. Experience of the Santa Maria Hospital, Medical School of Lisbon]. Acta Med Port. 1994 Dec. 7(12). P 717-24

Vitamin A preserves the cytotoxic activity of adriamycin while counteracting its peroxidative effects in human leukemic cells in vitro. Biochem Mol Biol Int. 1994 Sep. 34(2). P 329-35

In vitro all-trans retinoic acid (ATRA) sensitivity and cellular retinoic acid binding protein (CRABP) levels in relapse leukemic cells after remission induction by ATRA in acute promyelocytic leukemia. Leukemia. 1994 Jun. 8(6). P 914-7

Mechanisms of protection of hematopoietic stem cells from irradiation. Leuk Lymphoma. 1994 Mar. 13(1-2). P 27-32

Treatment of mucositis with vitamin E during administration of neutropenic antineoplastic agents. Ann Med Interne (Paris). 1994. 145(6). P 405-8

Effects of sodium ascorbate (vitamin C) and 2-methyl-1,4-naphthoquinone (vitamin K3) treatment on human tumor cell growth in vitro. II. Synergism with combined chemotherapy action. Anticancer Res. 1993 Jan-Feb. 13(1). P 103-6

[Remission of acute promyelocytic leukemia after all-trans-retinoic acid]. Harefuah. 1992 Dec 1. 123(11). P 445-8, 507

Abnormal vitamin B6 status in childhood leukemia. Cancer. 1990 Dec 1. 66(11). P 2421-8

Retinoids in cancer treatment. J Clin Pharmacol. 1992 Oct. 32(10). P 868-88

Induction of differentiation and enhancement of vincristine sensitivity of human erythroleukemia HEL cells by vesnarinone, a positive inotropic agent. Exp Hematol. 1996 Jan. 24(1). P 37-42

1,25-dihydroxyvitamin D3 primes acute promyelocytic cells for TPA- induced monocytic differentiation through both PKC and tyrosine phosphorylation cascades. Exp Cell Res. 1996 Jan 10. 222(1). P 61-9

Probing the pathobiology of response to all-trans retinoic acid in cute promyelocytic leukemia: premature chromosome condensation/fluorescence in situ hybridization analysis. Blood. 1996 Jan 1. 87(1). P 218-26

Acute renal failure associated with the retinoic acid syndrome in acute promyelocytic leukemia. Am J Kidney Dis. 1996 Jan. 27(1). P 134-7

[Synthesis of retinoids with a modified polar group and their antitumor activity. Report I] Bioorg Khim. 1995 Dec. 21(12). P 941-9

Induction of differentiation in murine erythroleukemia cells by 1 alpha,25-dihydroxy vitamin D3. Cancer Lett. 1995 Apr 14. 90(2). P 225-30

Synergistic differentiation of U937 cells by all-trans retinoic acid and 1 alpha, 25-dihydroxyvitamin D3 is associated with the expression of retinoid X receptor alpha. Biochem Biophys Res Commun. 1994 Aug 30. 203(1). P 272-80

1,25(OH)2-16ene-vitamin D3 is a potent antileukemic agent with low potential to cause hypercalcemia. Leuk Res (1994 Jun) 18(6):453-63

Genistein enhances the ICAM-mediated adhesion by inducing the expression of ICAM-1 and its counter-receptors. Biochem Biophys Res Commun (1994 Aug 30) 203(1):443-9

Induction of differentiation and dna breakage in human hl-60 and k- 562 leukemia cells by genistein. Proc Annu Meet Am Assoc Cancer Res (1990) 31:A2605

Tretinoin. A review of its pharmacodynamic and pharmacokinetic properties and use in the management of acute promyelocytic leukaemia. Drugs. 1995 Nov. 50(5). P 897-923

[Treatment of acute promyelocytic leukemia with trans-retinoic acid. Experience of the Santa Maria Hospital, Medical School of Lisbon] Acta Med Port. 1994 Dec. 7(12). P 717-24

Vitamin A preserves the cytotoxic activity of adriamycin while counteracting its peroxidative effects in human leukemic cells in vitro. Biochem Mol Biol Int. 1994 Sep. 34(2). P 329-35

In vitro all-trans retinoic acid (ATRA) sensitivity and cellular retinoic acid binding protein (CRABP) levels in relapse leukemic cells after remission induction by ATRA in acute promyelocytic leukemia. Leukemia. 1994 Jun. 8(6). P 914-7

Mechanisms of protection of hematopoietic stem cells from irradiation. Leuk Lymphoma. 1994 Mar. 13(1-2). P 27-32

In vitro all-trans retinoic acid (ATRA) sensitivity and cellular retinoic acid binding protein (CRABP) levels in relapse leukemic cells after remission induction by ATRA in acute promyelocytic leukemia. Leukemia. 1994. 8 Suppl 2P S16-9

Treatment of mucositis with vitamin E during administration of neutropenic antineoplastic agents. Ann Med Interne (Paris). 1994. 145(6). P 405-8

Effects of sodium ascorbate (vitamin C) and 2-methyl-1,4- naphthoquinone (vitamin K3) treatment on human tumor cell growth in vitro. II. Synergism with combined chemotherapy action. Anticancer Res. 1993 Jan-Feb. 13(1). P 103-6

[Remission of acute promyelocytic leukemia after all-trans-retinoic acid] Harefuah. 1992 Dec 1. 123(11). P 445-8, 507

Abnormal vitamin B6 status in childhood leukemia. Cancer. 1990 Dec 1. 66(11). P 2421-8

Liver (Cirrhosis)

Anemias in Thai patients with cirrhosis. International Journal of Hematology (Ireland), 1997, 65/4 (365-373)

Therapeutic efficacy of L-ornithine-L-aspartate infusions in patients with cirrhosis and hepatic encephalopathy: Results of a placebo-controlled, double-blind study. Hepatology (USA), 1997, 25/6 (1351-1360)

The use of methotrexate, colchicine, and other immunomodulatory drugs in the treatment of primary biliary cirrhosis. Seminars in Liver Disease (USA), 1997, 17/2 (129-136)

Inhibition by green tea extract of diethylnitrosamine-initiated but not choline-deficient, L-amino acid-defined diet-associated development of putative preneoplastic, glutathione S-transferase placental form-positive lesions in rat liver. Japanese Journal of Cancer Research (Japan), 1997, 88/4 (356-362)

Chronic alcoholism in the absence of Wernicke-Korsakoff syndrome and cirrhosis does not result in the loss of serotonergic neurons from the median raphe nucleus. Metabolic Brain Disease (USA), 1996, 11/3 (217-228)

Iron in liver diseases other than hemochromatosis. Seminars in Liver Disease (USA), 1996, 16/1 (65-82)

Antioxidant defenses in metal-induced liver damage. Seminars in Liver Disease (USA), 1996, 16/1 (39-46)

Vitamins and metals: Potential dangers for the human being. Schweizerische Medizinische Wochenschrift (Switzerland), 1996, 126/15 (607-611)

Effects of hepatic stimulator substance, herbal medicine, selenium/vitamin E, and ciprofloxacin on cirrhosis in the rat. Gastroenterology (USA), 1996, 110/4 (1150-1155)

Hepatic encephalopathy. Pathogenesis and therapy. Infezioni in Medicina (Italy), 1997, 5/1 (14-19)

Long-term (12 months) treatment with an anti-oxidant drug (silymarin) is effective on hyperinsulinemia, exogenous insulin need and malondialdehyde levels in cirrhotic diabetic patients. Journal of Hepatology (Denmark), 1997, 26/4 (871-879)

Comparative effects of colchicine and silymarin on CCl4-chronic liver damage in rats. Archives of Medical Research (Mexico), 1997, 28/1 (11-17)

Properties and medical use of flavonolignans (Silymarin) from Silybum marianum. Phytotherapy Research (United Kingdom), 1996, 10/SUPPL. 1 (S25-S26)

Phytotherapy in Germany: Its role in self-medication and in medical prescribing. Natural Medicines (Japan), 1996, 50/4 (259-264)

Reliable phytotherapy in chronic liver diseases. Therapiewoche (Germany), 1996, 46/17 (916+918-919)

Oral supplementation with branched-chain amino acids improves transthyretin turnover in rats with carbon tetrachloride-induced liver cirrhosis. Journal of Nutrition (USA), 1996, 126/5 (1412-1420)

Inhibition by acetylsalicylic acid, a cyclo-oxygenase inhibitor, and p-bromophenacylbromide, a phospholipase A2 inhibitor, of both cirrhosis and enzyme-altered nodules caused by a choline-deficient, L-amino acid-defined diet in rats. Carcinogenesis (United Kingdom), 1996, 17/3 (467-475)

Overview of randomized clinical trials of oral branched-chain amino acid treatment in chronic hepatic encephalopathy Journal of Parenteral and Enteral Nutrition (USA), 1996, 20/2 (159-164)

Leucine metabolism in rats with cirrhosis. J Hepatol (DENMARK) Feb 1996, 24 (2) p209-16

Renal and pressor effects of aminoguanidine in cirrhotic rats with ascites. J Am Soc Nephrol (UNITED STATES) Dec 1996, 7 (12) p2694-9

Nutrient-induced thermogenesis and protein-sparing effect by rapid infusion of a branched chain-enriched amino acid solution to cirrhotic patients. J Med (UNITED STATES) 1996, 27 (3-4) p176-82

Serum amino acid changes in rats with thioacetamide-induced liver cirrhosis. Toxicology (IRELAND) Jan 8 1996, 106 (1-3) p197-206

Vitamin A concentration in the liver decreases with age in patients with cystic fibrosis. J Pediatr Gastroenterol Nutr (UNITED STATES) Mar 1997, 24 (3) p264-70

The prolyl 4-hydroxylase inhibitor HOE 077 prevents activation of Ito cells, reducing procollagen gene expression in rat liver fibrosis induced by choline-deficient L-amino acid-defined diet. Hepatology (UNITED STATES) Apr 1996, 23 (4) p755-63

Glutathione kinetics in normal man and in patients with liver cirrhosis. J Hepatol (DENMARK) Mar

References

1997, 26 (3) p606-13

Proton magnetic resonance spectroscopy of the brain in symptomatic and asymptomatic patients with liver cirrhosis Gastroenterology (UNITED STATES) May 1997, 112 (5) p1610-6

Effect of branched chain amino acid infusions on body protein metabolism in cirrhosis of liver. Gut (1986 Nov) 27 Suppl 1:96-102

Severe recurrent hepatic encephalopathy that responded to oral branched chain amino acids. American Journal of Gastroenterology (USA), 1996, 91/6 (1266-1268)

[Branched-chain amino acids in the treatment of latent porto-systemic encephalopathy. A placebo-controlled double-blind cross-over study]. Z Ernahrungswiss. 1986 Mar. 25(1). P 9-28

A prospective, randomized, double-blind, controlled trial. J Parenter Enteral Nutr. 1985 May-Jun. 9(3). P 288- 95

Prevention of CCL4-induced liver cirrhosis by silymarin. Fundam Clin Pharmacol (1989) 3(3):183-91

Free radicals in tissue damage in liver diseases and therapeutic approach. Tokai J Exp Clin Med (1986) 11 Suppl:121-34

Serum neutral amino acid concentrations in cirrhotic patients with impaired carbohydrate metabolism. Acta Med Okayama. 1983 Aug. 37(4). P 381-4

Is intravenous administration of branched chain amino acids effective in the treatment of hepatic encephalopathy? A multicenter study. Hepatology. 1983 Jul-Aug. 3(4). P 475-80

Branched-chain amino acid-enriched elemental diet in patients with cirrhosis of the liver. A double blind crossover trial. Gastroenterol. 1983 Nov. 21(11). P 644-50

Effect of euglycemic insulin infusion on plasma levels of branched- chain amino acids in cirrhosis. Hepatology. 1983 Mar-Apr. 3(2). P 184-7

Effect of glucose and/or branched chain amino acid infusion on plasma amino acid imbalance in chronic liver failure. J Parenter Enteral Nutr. 1981 Sep-Oct. 5(5). P 414-9

A comparison of the effects of intravenous infusion of individual branched-chain amino acids on blood amino acid levels in man. Clin Sci (Colch). 1981 Jan. 60(1). P 95-100

[Pathogenesis of hepatic encephalopathy (author's transl)] Leber Magen Darm. 1977 Aug. 7(4). P 241-54

Clearance rate of plasma branched-chain amino acids correlates significantly with blood ammonia level in patients with liver cirrhosis. International Hepatology Communications (Ireland), 1995, 3/2 (91-96)

Nutritional treatment of liver cirrhosis with branched chain amino acids. (BCAA) Nutritional support in organ failure: proceedings of the International Symposium, 1990

Branched-chain amino acids - A highly effective substrate of parenteral nutrition for critically ill children with Reye's syndrome. CLIN. NUTR. (USA), 1987, 6/2 (101-104)

Ammonia detoxification by accelerated oxidation of branched chain amino acids in brains of acute hepatic failure rats. BIOCHEM. MED. METAB. BIOL. (USA), 1986, 35/3 (367- 375)

Branched chain amino acids in the treatment of latent portosystemic encephalopathy. A double-blind placebo-controlled crossover study. GASTROENTEROLOGY (USA), 1985, 88/4 (887-895)

L-leucine prevent ammonia-induced changes in glutamate receptors in the brain and in visual evoked potentials in the rabbit. J. PARENTER. ENTER. NUTR. (USA), 1984, 8/6 (700-704)

Effects of amino acid infusions on liver regeneration after partial hepatectomy in the rat. J. PARENTER. ENTER. NUTR. (USA), 1986, 10/1 (17-20)

A comparison of the effects of intravenous infusion of individual branched-chain amino acids on blood amino acid levels in man. Clin Sci (ENGLAND) Jan 1981, 60 (1) p95-100

The role of insulin and glucagon in the plasma aminoacid imbalance of chronic hepatic encephalopathy. Z Gastroenterol (GERMANY, WEST) Jul 1979, 17 (7) p469-76

Drug metabolism in cirrhosis. Selective changes in cytochrome P-450 isozymes in the choline-deficient rat model. Biochem Pharmacol (ENGLAND) Jun 1 1986, 35 (11) p1817-24

Action of curcumin on the cytochrome P450-system catalyzing the activation of aflatoxin B1. Chem Biol Interact (IRELAND) Mar 8 1996, 100 (1) p41-51

Inhibition of lipid peroxidation and cholesterol levels in mice by curcumin. Indian J Physiol Pharmacol (INDIA) Oct 1992, 36 (4) p239-43

Induction of glutathione S-transferase activity by curcumin in mice. Arzneimittelforschung (GERMANY) Jul 1992, 42 (7) p962-4

Effect of polyene phosphatidylcholine (Essentiale forte, cps.) in the treatment of steatosis of the liver, focused on the ultrasonographic finding - Preliminary investigation. CAS. LEK. CESK. (Czech Republic), 1994, 133/12 (366- 369)

Relationship between liver cirrhosis death rate and nutritional factors in 38 countries. INT. J. EPIDEMIOL. (United Kingdom), 1988, 17/2 (414-418)

Vitamin B6 status in cirrhotic patients in relation to apoenzyme of serum alanine aminotransferase. CLIN. BIOCHEM. (Canada), 1988, 21/6 (367-370)

Vitamin B6 concentrations in patients with chronic liver disease and hepatocellular carcinoma. BR. MED. J. (UK), 1986, 293/6540 (175)

Choline and human nutrition. ANNU. REV. NUTR. (USA), 1994, 14/- (269-296)

Prostaglandin E2 production by hepatic macrophages and peripheral monocytes in liver cirrhosis patients. LIFE SCI. (USA), 1993, 53/4 (323-331)

Biochemistry of pharmacology of S-adenosyl-L-methionine and rationale for its use in liver disease. DRUGS (New Zealand), 1990, 40/SUPPL. 3 (98-110)

Choline may be an essential nutrient in malnourished patients with cirrhosis. GASTROENTEROLOGY (USA), 1989, 97/6 (1514-1520)

Use of polyunsaturated phosphatidyl choline in HBsAg negative chronic active hepatitis: Results of prospective double-blind controlled trial. LIVER (DENMARK), 1982, 2/2 (77-81)

Acetyl-L-carnitine increases cytochrome oxidase subunit I mRNA content in hypothyroid rat liver. FEBS LETT. (Netherlands), 1990, 277/1-2 (191-193)

S-Adenosyl-L-methionine. A review of its pharmacological properties and therapeutic potential in liver dysfunction and affective disorders in relation to its physiological role in cell metabolism. DRUGS (New Zealand), 1989, 38/3

Lupus

Refer to references under Autoimmune Diseases.

Macular Degeneration (Dry)

Treatment of senile macular degeneration with Ginkgo biloba extract. A preliminary double-blind, drug versus placebo study. PRESSE MED. (FRANCE), 1986, 15/31 (1556-1558)

Hydergine—a new promise in neuro-retinal disorders. AFRO-ASIAN J. OPHTHALMOL. (India), 1989, 8/1

Inhibition of glutathione reductase by flavonoids. A structure-activity study. BIOCHEM. PHARMACOL. (United Kingdom), 1992, 44/8

Flavonoids, a class of natural products of high pharmacological potency. BIOCHEM. PHARMACOL. (ENGLAND), 1983, 32/7

Results with anthocyanosides from Vaccinium myrtillus equivalent to 25% of anthocyanidines in the treatment of haemorrhagic diathesis due to defective primary haemostasis. GAZZ. MED. ITAL. (ITALY), 1981, 140/10 (445-449)

Studies on vaccinium myrtillus anthocyanosides. I. Vasoprotective and antiinflammatory activity. ARZNEIMITTEL-FORSCH. (GERMANY, WEST), 1976, 26/5

Atrophic macular degeneration. Rate of spread of geographic atrophy and visual loss. OPHTHAL-MOLOGY (USA), 1989, 96/10

Study of aging macular degeneration in China. JPN. J. OPHTHALMOL. (JAPAN), 1987, 31/3

Subretinal neovascularization in senile macular degeneration. AM. J. OPHTHALMOL. (USA), 1984, 97/2

Delayed macular choriocapillary circulation in age related macular. International Ophthalmology (Netherlands), 1995, 19/1

Cystoid macular degeneration in experimental branch retinal vein occlusion. OPHTHALMOLOGY (USA), 1988, 95/10

The clinical picture of retinal thrombosis. KLIN. MONATSBL. AUGENHEILKD. (GERMANY, WEST), 1977, 170/2

Results of fluorescence angiography of the posterior pole of the eye. BER.DTSCH.OPHTHAL.GESELLSCH. (GERMANY, WEST), 1975, vol 73

The evoked cortical potential in macular degeneration. J.AMER.GERIAT.SOC. (USA), 1974, 22/12

The development of neovascularization of senile disciform macular degeneration. AMER.J.OPHTHAL. (USA), 1973, 76/1

Macular Degeneration (Wet)

Dietary carotenoids, vitamins A, C, and E, and advanced age-related macular degeneration. Eye Disease Case-Control Study Group. JAMA (UNITED STATES) Nov 9 1994

Evidence by in vivo and in vitro studies that binding of pycnogenols to elastin affects its rate of degradation by elastases. BIOCHEM. PHARMACOL. (ENGLAND), 1984

Studies on the mechanism of early onset macular degeneration in cynomolgus monkeys. II. Suppression of metallothionein synthesis in the retina in oxidative stress. Experimental Eye Research (United Kingdom), 1996, 62/4 (399-408)

Antioxidant enzymes of the human retina: Effect of age on enzyme activity of macula and periphery. Current Eye Research (United Kingdom), 1996, 15/3 (273-278)

Low glutathione reductase and peroxidase activity in age-related macular degeneration. BR. J. OPHTHALMOL. (United Kingdom), 1994, 78/10 (791-794)

Antioxidant enzymes in RBCs as a biological index of age related macular degeneration. ACTA OPHTHALMOL. (Denmark), 1993, 71/2 (214-218)

Oxidative effects of laser photocoagulation. FREE RADIC. BIOL. MED. (USA), 1991, 11/3 (327-330)

Antioxidant status and neovascular age-related macular degeneration. ARCH. OPHTHALMOL. (USA), 1993, 111/1 (104-109)

Nutrition in the elderly. ANN. INTERN. MED. (USA), 1988, 109/11 (890-904)

Meningitis

See references Immune Enhancement.

Menopause

Menopause before the age of 40 years. Journal de Gynecologie Obstetrique et Biologie de la Reproduction (France), 1997, 26/3 231-237

Endometrial cancer and hormone replacement therapy: Appropriate use of progestins to oppose endogenous and exogenous estrogen. Endocrinology and Metabolism Clinics of North America (USA), 1997, 26/2 (399-412)

Women's hearts are different. Current Problems in Obstetrics, Gynecology and Fertility (USA), 1997,20/3 (72-92)

Estrogen and the prevention and treatment of osteoporosis. Journal of Clinical Rheumatology (USA), 1997, 3/2 SUPPL. (S28-S33)

Neoadjuvant progesterone therapy for primary breast cancer: Rationale for a clinical trial. Clinical Therapeutics (USA), 1997, 19/1 (56-61)

Cardiovascular pathophysiology of ovarian hormones. Schweizerische Rundschau fur Medizin/Praxis (Switzerland), 1997, 86/5 (138-144)

Hemostasis during hormone replacement therapy. Infertility and Reproductive Medicine Clinics of

References

North America (USA), 1997, 8/1 (35-48)

Androgens and the menopause; a study of 40-60-year-old women. Clinical Endocrinology (United Kingdom), 1996, 45/5 (577-587)

Cardiovascular effects of the ovarian hormones. Archives des Maladies du Coeur et des Vaisseaux (France), 1996, 89/SPEC.ISS. 7 (9-16)

The effect of hormones on the lower urinary tract. Archives of STD/HIV Research (USA), 1996, 10/3 (145-150)

Hormone substances and their efficacy in hormonal replacement therapy. Acta Chirurgica Austriaca (Austria), 1996, 28/5 (259-262)

The effects of various hormone replacement therapy regimens on bone mineral density after 2 years of treatment. Marmara Medical Journal (Turkey), 1996, 9/4 (165-168)

A randomized, double-blind, placebo-controlled, crossover study on the effect of oral oestradiol on acute menopausal symptoms. Maturitas (Ireland), 1996, 25/2 (115-123)

The female brain hypoestrogenic continuum from the premenstrual syndrome to menopause: A hypothesis and review of supporting data. Journal of Reproductive Medicine for the Obstetrician and Gynecologist (USA), 1996, 41/9 (633-639)

Treatments for oestoporosis. Revue Francaise de Gynecologie et d'Obstetrique (France), 1996, 91/6 (329-334)

Variations in steroid hormone receptor content throughout age and menopausal periods, and menstrual cycle in breast cancer patients. Neoplasma (Slovak Republic), 1996, 43/3 (163-169)

Hormone therapy and Phytoestrogens. Journal of Clinical Pharmacy and Therapeutics (United Kingdom), 1996,21/2 (101-111)

The menopause and hormone replacement therapy: Lipids, lipoproteins, coagulation and fibrinolytic factors. Maturitas (Ireland), 1996, 23/2 (209-216)

Prevention of cardiovascular disease by hormone replacement therapy in the ostmenopause. Zentralblatt fur Gynakologie (Germany), 1996, 118/4 (188-197)

Menopause and osteoporosis: The role of HRT. Journal of the American Pharmaceutical Association (USA), 1996, 36/4 (234-242)

Characterization of reproductive hormonal dynamics in the perimenopause. Journal of Clinical Endocrinology and Metabolism (USA), 1996, 81/4 (1495-1501)

Clinical evaluation of near-continuous oral micronized progesterone therapy in estrogenized postmenopausal women. Gynecological Endocrinology (United Kingdom), 1996, 10/1 (41-47)

The regulation of adipose tissue distribution in humans. International Journal of Obesity (United Kingdom), 1996, 20/4 (291-302)

Adrenal and gonadal steroid hormone deficiency in the etiopathogenesis of rheumatoid arthritis. Journal of Rheumatology (Canada), 1996, 23/SUPPL. 44 (10-12)

Dietary and behavioral determinants of menopause. Clinical Consultations in Obstetrics and Gynecology (USA), 1996, 8/1(21-26)

References

Alpha-tocopherol and hydroperoxide content in breast adipose tissue from patients with breast tumors. Int J Cancer (UNITED STATES) Jul 17 1996, 67 (2) p170-5

A review of the clinical effects of phytoestrogens. Obstet Gynecol (UNITED STATES) May 1996, 87 (5 Pt 2) p897-904

Value of micronutrient supplements in the prevention or correction of disturbances accompanying the menopause. REV. FR. GYNECOL. OBSTET. (France), 1990, 85/12 (702-705)

Effect of vitamin B-6 on plasma and red blood cell magnesium levels in premenopausal women. ANN. CLIN. LAB. SCI. (USA), 1981, 11/4 333-336

Effect of a natural and artificial menopause on serum, urinary and erythrocyte magnesium. UNITED KINGDOM CLIN. SCI. (ENGLAND), 1980, 58/3 (255-257)

Vitamins as therapy in the 1990s. Journal of the American Board of Family Practice (USA), 1995, 8/3 (206-216)

Functional capacity of the tryptophan niacin pathway in the premenarchial phase and in the menopausal age. EGYPT AMER.J.CLIN.NUTR. (USA), 1975, 28/1 (4-9)

Dehydroepiandrosterone sulphate as a source of steroids in menopause. Acta Ginecologica (Spain), 1995, 52/9 (279-284)

Distribution of glutathione S-transferase isoenzymes in human ovary. J. REPROD. FERTIL. (United Kingdom), 1991, 93/2 (303-311)

Changes in circulating steroids with aging in postmenopausal women. OBSTET. GYNECOL. (USA), 1981, 57/5 (624-628)

Adrenal and gonadal steroid hormone deficiency in the etiopathogenesis of rheumatoid arthritis. Journal of Rheumatology (Canada), 1996, 23/SUPPL. 44 (10-12)

The effects of oral dehydroepiandrosterone on endocrine-metabolic parameters in postmenopausal women. J. CLIN. ENDOCRINOL. METAB. (USA), 1990, 71/3 (696-704)

Catabolic effects and the influence on hormonal variables under treatment with Gynodian-Depot (Reg.trademark) or dehydroepiandrosterone (DHEA) oenanthate. SWEDEN MATURITAS (NETHER-LANDS), 1981, 3/3-4 (225-234)

Nutrition and osteoporosis: An analysis of dietary intake in postmenopausal women. Wiener Klinische Wochenschrift (Austria), 1995, 107/14 (418-422)

Magnesium supplementation and osteoporosis. Nutrition Reviews (USA), 1995, 53/3 (71-74)

Calcium, phosphorus and magnesium intakes correlate with bone mineral content in postmenopausal women. GYNECOL. ENDOCRINOL. (United Kingdom), 1994, 8/1 (55-58)

Incident pain caused by collapsed vertebrae in menopause. The logical background to a personal treatment protocol. ITALY MINERVA ANESTESIOL. (ITALY), 1984, 50/11 (573-576)

Interaction of family history of breast cancer and dietary antioxidants with breast cancer risk (New York, United States). Cancer Causes and Control (United Kingdom), 1995, 6/5 (407-415)

Altered menstrual cycles in rhesus monkeys induced by lead. FUNDAM. APPL. TOXICOL. (USA), 1987, 9/4 (722-729)

Effect of glucocorticoids and calcium intake on bone density and bone, liver and plasma minerals in guinea pigs. J. NUTR. (USA), 1979, 109/7 (1175-1188)

Relationships between usual nutrient intake and bone-mineral content of women 35-65 years of age: Longitudinal and cross-sectional analysis. AM. J. CLIN. NUTR. (USA), 1986, 44/6 (863-876)

Iron deficiency anemia in postmenopausal women. J.AMER.GERIAT.SOC. (USA), 1976, 24/12 (558-559)

Effect of menopause and estrogen substitutional therapy on magnesium metabolsim. DENMARK MINER. ELECTROLYTE METABOL. (SWITZERLAND), 1984, 10/2 (84-87)

Value of micronutrient supplements in the prevention or correction of disturbances accompanying the menopause. REV. FR. GYNECOL. OBSTET. (France), 1990, 85/12 (702-705)

Effect of vitamin B-6 on plasma and red blood cell magnesium levels in premenopausal women. ANN. CLIN. LAB. SCI. (USA), 1981, 11/4 333-336)

Effect of a natural and artificial menopause on serum, urinary and erythrocyte magnesium. UNITED KINGDOM CLIN. SCI. (ENGLAND), 1980, 58/3 (255-257)

Vitamins as therapy in the 1990s. Journal of the American Board of Family Practice (USA), 1995, 8/3 (206-216)

Functional capacity of the tryptophan niacin pathway in the premenarchial phase and in the menopausal age. EGYPT AMER.J.CLIN.NUTR. (USA), 1975, 28/1 (4-9)

Dehydroepiandrosterone sulphate as a source of steroids in menopause. Sulfate de dehidro-epi-androsterona come fuente de esteroides en la menopausia (i). Acta Ginecologica (Spain), 1995, 52/9 (279-284)

Distribution of glutathione S-transferase isoenzymes in human ovary. J. REPROD. FERTIL. (United Kingdom), 1991, 93/2 (303-311)

Changes in circulating steroids with aging in postmenopausal women. OBSTET. GYNECOL. (USA), 1981, 57/5 (624-628)

Adrenal and gonadal steroid hormone deficiency in the etiopathogenesis of rheumatoid arthritis. Journal of Rheumatology (Canada), 1996, 23/SUPPL. 44 (10-12)

The effects of oral dehydroepiandrosterone on endocrine-metabolic parameters in postmenopausal women. J. CLIN. ENDOCRINOL. METAB. (USA), 1990, 71/3 (696- 704)

Catabolic effects and the influence on hormonal variables under treatment with Gynodian-Depot (Reg.trademark) or dehydroepiandrosterone (DHEA) oenanthate. SWEDEN MATURITAS (NETHER-LANDS), 1981, 3/3-4 (225- 234)

Nutrition and osteoporosis: An analysis of dietary intake in postmenopausal women. Wiener Klinische Wochenschrift (Austria), 1995, 107/14 (418-422)

Magnesium supplementation and osteoporosis. Nutrition Reviews (USA), 1995, 53/3 (71-74)

Calcium, phosphorus and magnesium intakes correlate with bone mineral content in postmenopausal women. GYNECOL. ENDOCRINOL. (United Kingdom), 1994, 8/1 (55-58)

Incident pain caused by collapsed vertebrae in menopause. The logical background to a personal treatment protocol. ITALY MINERVA ANESTESIOL. (ITALY), 1984, 50/11 (573-576)

Interaction of family history of breast cancer and dietary antioxidants with breast cancer risk (New York, United States). Cancer Causes and Control (United Kingdom), 1995, 6/5 (407-415)

Altered menstrual cycles in rhesus monkeys induced by lead. FUNDAM. APPL. TOXICOL. (USA), 1987, 9/4 (722-729)

Effect of glucocorticoids and calcium intake on bone density and bone, liver and plasma minerals in guinea pigs. J. NUTR. (USA), 1979, 109/7 (1175-1188)

Relationships between usual nutrient intake and bone-mineral content of women 35-65 years of age: Longitudinal and cross-sectional analysis. AM. J. CLIN. NUTR. (USA), 1986, 44/6 (863-876)

Iron deficiency anemia in postmenopausal women. J.AMER.GERIAT.SOC. (USA), 1976, 24/12 (558-559)

Effect of menopause and estrogen substitutional therapy on magnesium metabolsim. DENMARK MINER. ELECTROLYTE METABOL. (SWITZERLAND), 1984, 10/2 (84-87)

Menstrual Disorders (Premenstrual Syndrome)

Use of nomegestrol acetate in the treatment of menstrual disorders. Our experience of 56 patients. Minerva Ginecologica (Italy), 1997, 49/4 (181-185)

Oral contraception and other factors in relation to hospital referral for menstrual problems without known underlying cause: Findings in a large cohort study. British Journal of Family Planning (United Kingdom), 1997, 22/4 (166-169)

[Risk analysis of menstrual disorders in young women from urban population]. Przegl Epidemiol (POLAND) 1996, 50 (4) p467-74

Severe vaginal bleeding associated with recombinant interferon beta-1B. Ann Pharmacother (UNITED STATES) Jan 1997, 31 (1) p50-2

Prevalence of menstrual dysfunction in Norwegian long-distance runners participating in the Oslo Marathon games. Scand J Med Sci Sports (DENMARK) Jun 1996, 6 (3) p164-71

Effect of vitamin B6 on the side effects of a low-dose combined oral contraceptive. Contraception (UNITED STATES) Apr 1997, 55 (4) p245-8

Effects of a yeast-based dietary supplementation on premenstrual syndrome. A double-blind placebo-controlled study. Gynecologic and Obstetric Investigation (Switzerland), 1997, 43/2 (120-124)

Role of estrogen in postmenopausal depression. Neurology (USA), 1997, 48/5 SUPPL. 7 (S16-S20)

Reduced benzodiazepine sensitivity in patients with premenstrual syndrome: A pilot study. Psychoneuroendocrinology (United Kingdom), 1997, 22/1 (25-38)

Treatment of premenstrual syndrome (PMS) with lisuride maleate. Ginecologia y Obstetricia de Mexico (Mexico), 1996, 64/DEC. (556-560)

Premenstrual syndrome. Trends in Endocrinology and Metabolism (USA), 1996, 7/5 (184-189)

Hormonal approaches to treatment for mood disorders. Infertility and Reproductive Medicine Clinics of North America (USA), 1996, 7/2 (381-395)

Clinical and biochemical effects of nutritional supplementation on the premenstrual syndrome. J. REPROD. MED. (USA), 1987, 32/6 (435-441)

Reduced bone mass in women with premenstrual syndrome. Journal of Women's Health (USA), 1995, 4/2 (161-168)

Calcium-regulating hormones across the menstrual cycle: Evidence of a secondary hyperparathyroidism in women with PMS. Journal of Clinical Endocrinology and Metabolism (USA), 1995, 80/7

Linolenic acid formulations for the treatment of premenstrual syndrome. CURR. OPIN. THER. PAT. (United Kingdom), 1992, 2/12 (2000-2002)

Calcium supplementation in premenstrual syndrome: A randomized crossover trial. J. GEN. INTERN. MED. (USA), 1989, 4/3 (183-189)

Plasma copper, zinc and magnesium levels in patients with premenstrual tension syndrome. ACTA OBSTET. GYNECOL. SCAND. (Denmark), 1994, 73/6 (452-455)

Use of a vitamin-mineral supplement in the management of premenstrual syndrome. BR. J. CLIN. RES. (United Kingdom), 1993, 4/- (219-224)

Oral magnesium successfully relieves premenstrual mood changes. OBSTET. GYNECOL. (USA), 1991, 78/2 (177-181)

Clinical and biochemical effects of nutritional supplementation on the premenstrual syndrome. J. REPROD. MED. (USA), 1987, 32/6 (435-441)

Magnesium and the premenstrual syndrome. ANN. CLIN. BIOCHEM. (UK), 1986, 23/6 (667-670)

The role of essential fatty acids and prostaglandins in the premenstrual syndrome. J. REPROD. MED. (USA), 1983, 28/7 (465-468)

Vitamin B6 in the treatment of the premenstrual syndrome - Review (1). BR. J. OBSTET. GYNAECOL. (United Kingdom), 1991, 98/3 (329-330), BR. J. CLIN. PRACT. (United Kingdom), 1988, 42/11 (448-452)

Clinical and biochemical effects of nutritional supplementation on the premenstrual syndrome.J. REPROD. MED. (USA), 1987, 32/6 (435-441)

Reduced bone mass in women with premenstrual syndrome. Journal of Women's Health (USA), 1995, 4/2 (161-168)

Calcium-regulating hormones across the menstrual cycle: Evidence of a secondary hyperparathyroidism in women with PMS. Journal of Clinical Endocrinology and Metabolism (USA), 1995, 80/7

Linolenic acid formulations for the treatment of premenstrual syndrome. CURR. OPIN. THER. PAT. (United Kingdom), 1992, 2/12 (2000-2002)

Calcium supplementation in premenstrual syndrome: A randomized crossover trial. J. GEN. INTERN. MED. (USA), 1989, 4/3 (183-189)

Plasma copper, zinc and magnesium levels in patients with premenstrual tension syndrome. ACTA OBSTET. GYNECOL. SCAND. (Denmark), 1994, 73/6 (452-455)

Use of a vitamin-mineral supplement in the management of premenstrual syndrome. BR. J. CLIN.

RES. (United Kingdom), 1993, 4/- (219- 224)

Linolenic acid formulations for the treatment of premenstrual syndrome. CURR. OPIN. THER. PAT. (United Kingdom), 1992, 2/12

Oral magnesium successfully relieves premenstrual mood changes. OBSTET. GYNECOL. (USA), 1991, 78/2 (177-181)

Clinical and biochemical effects of nutritional supplementation on the premenstrual syndrome. J. REPROD. MED. (USA), 1987, 32/6 (435-441)

Magnesium and the premenstrual syndrome. ANN. CLIN. BIOCHEM. (UK), 1986, 23/6 (667-670)

The role of essential fatty acids and prostaglandins in the premenstrual syndrome. J. REPROD. MED. (USA), 1983, 28/7 (465-468)

Vitamin B6 in the treatment of the premenstrual syndrome - Review (1). BR. J. OBSTET. GYNAECOL. (United Kingdom), 1991, 98/3 (329-330) BR. J. CLIN. PRACT. (United Kingdom), 1988, 42/11 (448-452)

Migraine

In vivo administration of propranolol decreases exaggerated amounts of serum TNF-alpha in patients with migraine without aura. Possible mechanism of action. Acta Neurol (Napoli); 14(4-6):313-9 1992

Concurrent use of antidepressants and propranolol: case report and theoretical considerations. Biol Psychiatry; 18(2):237-41 1983

Nocturnal melatonin excretion is decreased in patients with migraine without aura attacks associated with menses. Cephalalgia (Norway), 1995, 15/2 (136-139)

Urinary melatonin excretion throughout the ovarian cycle in menstrually related migraine. CEPHA-LALGIA (Norway), 1994

Nocturnal plasma melatonin levels in migraine: A preliminary report. Headache (UNITED STATES) Apr 1989, 29 (4) p242-5

Octopamine and some related noncatecholic amines in invertebrate nervous systems. INT.REV.NEU-ROBIOL. (USA), 1976, Vol.19 (173-224)

Nocturnal melatonin excretion is decreased in patients with migraine without aura attacks associated with menses. Cephalalgia (NORWAY) Apr 1995, 15 (2) p136-9; discussion 79

The co-occurrence of multiple sclerosis and migraine headache: the serotoninergic link. Int J Neurosci (ENGLAND) Jun 1994, 76 (3-4) p249-57

Urinary melatonin excretion throughout the ovarian cycle in menstrually related migraine [see comments] Cephalalgia (NORWAY) Jun 1994, 14 (3) p205-9

The influence of the pineal gland on migraine and cluster headaches and effects of treatment with picoTesla magnetic fields. Int J Neurosci (ENGLAND) Nov-Dec 1992, 67 (1-4) p145-71

Nocturnal plasma melatonin levels in migraine: a preliminary report. Headache (UNITED STATES) Apr 1989, 29 (4) p242-5

Is migraine due to a deficiency of pineal melatonin? Ital J Neurol Sci (ITALY) Jun 1986, 7 (3) p319-23

Melatonin in humans physiological and clinical studies. J Neural Transm Suppl (AUSTRIA) 1978, (13) p289-310

Multiple Sclerosis (MS)

Measurement of low-molecular-weight antioxidants, uric acid, tyrosine and tryptophan in plaques and white matter from patients with multiple sclerosis. Eur Neurol (SWITZERLAND) 1992, 32 (5) p248-52

Dietary polyunsaturated fatty acids and depression: When cholesterol does not satisfy. American Journal of Clinical Nutrition (USA), 1995, 62/1 (1-9)

Health implications of fatty acids. ARZNEIM.-FORSCH. DRUG RES. (Germany), 1994, 44/8 (976-981)

Lipids and neurological diseases. MED. HYPOTHESES (United Kingdom), 1991, 34/3 (272-274)

Plasma lipids and their fatty acid composition in multiple sclerosis. ACTA NEUROL. SCAND. (Denmark), 1988, 78/2 (152-157)

Relevance of essential fatty acids in medicine and nutrition. AKTUEL. ENDOKRINOL. STOFFWECH-SEL (GERMANY, WEST), 1986, 7/1 (18-27)

Essential fatty acids in perspective. HUM. NUTR. CLIN. NUTR. (ENGLAND), 1984, 38/4 (245-260)

Essential fatty acids in the serum and cerebrospinal fluid of multiple sclerosis patients. ACTA NEU-ROL. SCAND. (DENMARK), 1983, 67/3 (151-163)

Polyunsaturated (essential) fatty acids and their importance in pathogenesis, diagnosis and therapy of multiple sclerosis. FORSTSCHR. NEUROL. PSYCHIATR. (GERMANY, WEST), 1982, 50/6 (173-189)

Clinical trials of unsaturated fatty acids in multiple sclerosis. IRCS MED. SCI. (ENGLAND), 1981, 9/12 (1081)

Essential fatty acids in serum and cerebrospinal fluid of patients during multiple sclerosis. NERVE-NARZT (GERMANY, WEST), 1981, 52/2 (100-107)

Abnormality of fatty acid composition of plasma lipid in multiple sclerosis. BRAIN NERVE (TOKYO) (JAPAN), 1979, 31/8 (797-801)

The pineal and regulation of fibrosis: pinealectomy as a model of primary biliary cirrhosis: Roles of melatonin and prostaglandins in fibrosis and regulation of T lymphocytes. MED. HYPOTHESES (ENG-LAND), 1979, 5/4 (403-414)

Multiple sclerosis: The rational basis for treatment with colchicine and evening primrose oil. MED. HYPOTHESES (ENGLAND), 1979, 5/3 (365-378)

Fat deficiency in rats during development of the central nervous system and susceptibility to experi-mental allergic encephalomyelitis. J.NUTR. (USA), 1975, 105/3 (288-300)

Dietary intake of linoleic acid in multiple sclerosis and other diseases. J.NEUROL.NEUROSURG.PSY-CHIAT. (ENGLAND), 1973, 36/4 (668-673)

Fatty acid patterns of serum lipids in multiple sclerosis and other diseases. BIOCHEM.SOC.TRANS. (ENGLAND), 1973, 1/1 (141-143)

Magnesium concentration in brains from multiple sclerosis patients. ACTA NEUROL. SCAND. (Denmark), 1990, 81/3 (197-200)

Zinc, copper and magnesium concentration in serum and CSF of patients with neurological disorders. ACTA NEUROL. SCAND. (Denmark), 1989, 79/5 (373-378)

The susceptibility of the centrocecal scotoma to electrolytes, especially in multiple sclerosis. IDEG-GYOG.SZLE (HUNGARY), 1973, 26/7 (307-312)

Evaluation of a nutrition education programme for people with multiple sclerosis. J. HUM. NUTR. DIET. (United Kingdom), 1993, 6/2 (131-147)

Multiple sclerosis: A diathesis? GAZZ.SANIT. (MILANO) (ITALY), 1973, 22/1 (37-39)

Arachidonic and docosahexanoic acid content of bovine brain myelin: Implications for the pathogenesis of multiple sclerosis. NEUROCHEM. RES. (USA), 1990, 15/1 (7-11)

On the causes of multiple sclerosis. MED. HYPOTHESES (United Kingdom), 1993, 41/2 (93-96)

Multiple sclerosis: vitamin D and calcium as environmental determinants of prevalence (a viewpoint). I.: Sunlight, dietary factors and epidemiology. INT.J.ENVIRON.STUD. (ENGLAND), 1974, 6/1 (19-27)

Biological effects of fish oils in relation to chronic diseases. Lipids (UNITED STATES) Dec 1986, 21 (12) p731-2

Supplementation of polyunsaturated fatty acids in multiple sclerosis. Ital J Neurol Sci (ITALY) Jun 1992, 13 (5) p401-7

Essential fatty acid and lipid profiles in plasma and erythrocytes in patients with multiple sclerosis. Am J Clin Nutr (UNITED STATES) Oct 1989, 50 (4) p801-6

Reduction by linoleic acid of the severity of experimental allergic encephalomyelitis in the guinea pig. J Neurol Sci (NETHERLANDS) Feb 1978, 35 (2-3) p291-308

Red blood cell and adipose tissue fatty acids in mild inactive multiple sclerosis. Acta Neurol Scand (DENMARK) Jul 1990, 82 (1) p43-50

Multiple sclerosis: effect of gamma linolenate administration upon membranes and the need for extended clinical trials of unsaturated fatty acids. Eur Neurol (SWITZERLAND) 1983, 22 (1) p78-83

The nutritional regulation of T lymphocyte function. Med Hypotheses (ENGLAND) Sep 1979, 5 (9) p969-85

Polyunsaturated fatty acids in treatment of acute remitting multiple sclerosis. Br Med J (ENGLAND) Nov 18 1978, 2 (6149) p1390-1

Effect of prolonged ingestion of gamma-linolenate by MS patients. Eur Neurol (SWITZERLAND) 1978, 17 (2) p67-76

Experimental and clinical studies on dysregulation of magnesium metabolism and the aetiopathogenesis of multiple sclerosis. Magnes Res (ENGLAND) Dec 1992, 5 (4) p295-302

Measurement of low-molecular-weight antioxidants, uric acid, tyrosine and tryptophan in plaques and white matter from patients with multiple sclerosis. Eur Neurol (SWITZERLAND) 1992, 32 (5) p248-52

Clinical trials of unsaturated fatty acids in multiple sclerosis. IRCS MED. SCI. (ENGLAND), 1981, 9/12 (1081)

References

Dietary polyunsaturated fatty acids and depression: When cholesterol does not satisfy. American Journal of Clinical Nutrition (USA), 1995, 62/1 (1-9)

Expression and regulation of brain metallothionein. Neurochem Int (ENGLAND) Jul 1995, 27 (1) p1-22

Indirect evidence for nitric oxide involvement in multiple sclerosis by characterization of circulating antibodies directed against conjugated S-nitrosocysteine. J Neuroimmunol (NETHERLANDS) Jul 1995, 60 (1-2) p117-24

Isoprenoid (coQ10) biosynthesis in multiple sclerosis. Acta Neurol Scand (DENMARK) Sep 1985, 72 (3) p328-35

Abnormality of fatty acid composition of plasma lipid in multiple sclerosis. BRAIN NERVE (TOKYO) (JAPAN), 1979, 31/8 (797-801)

The pineal and regulation of fibrosis: pinealectomy as a model of primary biliary cirrhosis: Roles of melatonin and prostaglandins in fibrosis and regulation of T lymphocytes. MED. HYPOTHESES (ENGLAND), 1979, 5/4 (403-414)

Fatty acid patterns of serum lipids in multiple sclerosis and other diseases. BIOCHEM.SOC.TRANS. (ENGLAND), 1973, 1/1 (141-143)

Alternate usages for medications update. Journal of Neurological and Orthopaedic Medicine and Surgery (USA), 1995 16/3 (167-172)

Magnesium concentration in plasma and erythrocytes in MS. Acta Neurologica Scandinavica (Denmark), 1995, 92/1 (109-111)

Comparative findings on serum IMg2+ of normal and diseased human subjects with the NOVA and KONE ISE's for Mg2+. SCAND. J. CLIN. LAB. INVEST. SUPPL. (United Kingdom), 1994, 54/217

Magnesium concentration in brains from multiple sclerosis patients. ACTA NEUROL. SCAND. (Denmark), 1990, 81/3 (197-200)

Zinc, copper and magnesium concentration in serum and CSF of patients with neurological disorders. ACTA NEUROL. SCAND. (Denmark), 1989, 79/5 (373-378)

Multiple sclerosis: Decreased relapse rate through dietary supplementation with calcium, magnesium and vitamin D. MED. HYPOTHESES (UK), 1986, 21/2 (193-200)

Painful tonic seizures in multiple sclerosis. Clinical and electromyographic aspects. MED. CLIN. (BARCELONA) (SPAIN), 1981, 76/10 (454- 456)

On the ion concentration in the cerebrospinal fluid in multiple sclerosis. PSYCHIATR. NEUROL. MED. PSYCHOL. (GERMANY, EAST), 1977, 29/8 (482-489)

Evaluation of a nutrition education programme for people with multiple sclerosis. J. HUM. NUTR. DIET. (United Kingdom), 1993, 6/2 (131-147)

Mineral composition of brains of normal and multiple sclerosis victims. PROC. SOC. EXP. BIOL. MED. (USA), 1980, 165/2 (327- 329)

Multiple sclerosis: A diathesis? GAZZ.SANIT. (MILANO) (ITALY), 1973, 22/1 (37-39)

On the causes of multiple sclerosis. MED. HYPOTHESES (United Kingdom), 1993, 41/2 (93-96)

Dietary polyunsaturated fatty acids and depression: when cholesterol does not satisfy. Am J Clin Nutr (UNITED STATES) Jul 1995, 62 (1) p1-9

Lipids and neurological diseases. Med Hypotheses (ENGLAND) Mar 1991, 34 (3) p272-4

Essential fatty acid and lipid profiles in plasma and erythrocytes in patients with multiple sclerosis. Am J Clin Nutr (UNITED STATES) Oct 1989, 50 (4) p801-6

Plasma lipids and their fatty acid composition in multiple sclerosis. Acta Neurol Scand (DENMARK) Aug 1988, 78 (2) p152-7

The effect of nutritional counselling on diet and plasma EFA status in multiple sclerosis patients over 3 years. Hum Nutr Appl Nutr (ENGLAND) Oct 1987, 41 (5) p297- 310

[Metabolic aspects of multiple sclerosis] Wien Med Wochenschr (AUSTRIA) Jan 31 1985, 135 (1-2) p20-2

Essential fatty acids in the serum and cerebrospinal fluid of multiple sclerosis patients. Acta Neurol Scand (DENMARK) Mar 1983, 67 (3) p151-63

Multiple sclerosis: the rational basis for treatment with colchicine and evening primrose oil. Med Hypotheses (ENGLAND) Mar 1979, 5 (3) p365-78

Multiple sclerosis: some epidemiological clues to etiology. Acta Neurol Latinoam (URUGUAY) 1975, 21 (1-4) p66-85

Red blood cell and adipose tissue fatty acids in mild inactive multiple sclerosis. Acta Neurol Scand (DENMARK) Jul 1990, 82 (1) p43-50

Multiple sclerosis: effect of gamma linolenate administration upon membranes and the need for extended clinical trials of unsaturated fatty acids. Eur Neurol (SWITZERLAND) 1983, 22 (1) p78-83

The nutritional regulation of T lymphocyte function. Med Hypotheses (ENGLAND) Sep 1979, 5 (9) p969-85

Polyunsaturated fatty acids in treatment of acute remitting multiple sclerosis. Br Med J (ENGLAND) Nov 18 1978, 2 (6149) p1390-1

Effect of prolonged ingestion of gamma-linolenate by MS patients. Eur Neurol (SWITZERLAND) 1978, 17 (2) p67-76

Multiple sclerosis patients express increased levels of beta-nerve growth factor in cerebrospinal fluid. Neurosci Lett (NETHERLANDS) Nov 23 1992, 147 (1) p9- 12

Experimental and clinical studies on dysregulation of magnesium metabolism and the aetiopatho-genesis of multiple sclerosis. Magnes Res (ENGLAND) Dec 1992, 5 (4) p295-302

Muscle Building

Ornithine alpha-ketoglutarate in nutritional support. Nutrition (UNITED STATES) Sep-Oct 1991, 7 (5) p313- 22

Anabolic effects of insulin-like growth factor-I (IGF-I) and an IGF-I variant in normal female rats. J Endocrinol (ENGLAND) Jun 1993, 137 (3) p413-21

Arginine needs, physiological state and usual diets. A reevaluation. J Nutr (UNITED STATES) Jan 1986, 116 (1) p36-46

Effects of dietary chromium picolinate supplementation on growth, carcass characteristics, and accretion rates of carcass tissues in growing-finishing swine. J Anim Sci (UNITED STATES) Nov 1995, 73 (11)

Anabolic effects of insulin on bone suggest a role for chromium picolinate in preservation of bone density. Med Hypotheses (ENGLAND) Sep 1995, 45 (3) p241-6

Effect of chromium picolinate on growth, body composition, and tissue accretion in pigs. J Anim Sci (UNITED STATES) Jul 1995, 73 (7) p2033-42

Longevity effect of chromium picolinate—'rejuvenation' of hypothalamic function? Med Hypotheses (ENGLAND) Oct 1994, 43 (4) p253-65

Effects of chromium picolinate on beginning weight training students. Int J Sport Nutr (UNITED STATES) Dec 1992, 2 (4) p343-50

Modulation of immune function and weight loss by L-arginine in obstructive jaundice in the rat. Br J Surg (ENGLAND) Aug 1994, 81 (8) p1199-201

Nutritional ergogenic aids: chromium, exercise, and muscle mass. Int J Sport Nutr (UNITED STATES) Sep 1991, 1 (3) p289-93

Efficacy of chromium supplementation in athletes: emphasis on anabolism. Int J Sport Nutr (UNITED STATES) Jun 1992, 2 (2) p111-22

Dietary supplements: Alternatives to anabolic steroids? PHYSICIAN SPORTSMED. (USA), 1992, 20/3 (189-193+196+198)

Direct anabolic effects of thyroid hormone on isolated mouse heart. AM. J. PHYSIOL. (USA), 1983, 14/3 (C328-C333)

Feeding conjugated linoleic acid to animals partially overcomes catabolic responses due to endotoxin injection. Biochem Biophys Res Commun (UNITED STATES) Feb 15 1994, 198 (3 p1107-12)

Muscular Dystrophy

Two successful double-blind trials with coenzyme Q10 (vitamin Q10) on muscular dystrophies and neurogenic atrophies. Biochim Biophys Acta (NETHERLANDS) May 24 1995

Biochemical rationale and the cardiac response of patients with muscle disease to therapy with coenzyme Q10. Proc Natl Acad Sci U S A (UNITED STATES) Jul 1985

[Efficiency of ubiquinone and p-oxybenzoic acid in prevention of E- hypovitaminosis-induced development of muscular dystrophy] Ukr Biokhim Zh (USSR) Sep-Oct 1981, 53 (5) p73-9

Effect of coenzyme Q on serum levels of creatine phosphokinase in preclinical muscular dystrophy. Proc Natl Acad Sci U S A (UNITED STATES) May 1974

[Some indices of energy metabolism in the tissues of mice with progressive muscular dystrophy under the action of ubiquinone] Vopr Med Khim (USSR) May 1974, 20 (3) p276-84

Free radicals, lipid peroxides and antioxidants in blood of patients ith myotonic dystrophy. J Neurol. 1995 Feb. 242(3). P 119-22

Myasthenia Gravis

Humoral and cellular immunity to intrinsic factor in myasthenia gravis. Scand J Haematol; 23(5):442-448 1979

Dietary precursors and brain neurotransmitter formation. Annu Rev Med (UNITED STATES) 1981, 32 p413-25

[The role of nutrition in the synthesis of neurotransmitters and in cerebral functions: clinical implications] Schweiz Med Wochenschr (SWITZERLAND) Sep 26 1981, 111 (39)

Nails

[Gelatin-cystine, keratogenesis and structure of the hair] Boll Soc Ital Biol Sper (ITALY) Jan 31 1983, 59 (1)

NUTRITION — Miscellanea; HEALTH — Miscellanea. Better Nutrition for Today's Living, Sep94, Vol. 56 Issue 9, p8, 1p, 1c

FOOD — Health aspects. Better Nutrition for Today's Living, Sep94, Vol. 56 Issue 9, p8, 1p, 1c

COSMETICS — Marketing. Environmental Nutrition, Mar96, Vol. 19 Issue 3, p1, 2p

SILICA — Physiological effect. Better Nutrition for Today's Living, Dec95, Vol. 57 Issue 12, p30, 1p, 1c

BIOTIN — Therapeutic use. Prevention, Dec94, Vol. 46 Issue 12, p122, 3p, 2c

Neuropathy

Diabetic polyneuropathy: New therapy plan from alpha lipoic acid. Therapiewoche (Germany), 1995, 45/36 (2118)

Oral alpha lipoic acid preparation proves good bioavailability in diabetic polyneuropathy. Frankfurt am Main Germany Therapiewoche (Germany), 1995, 45/23 (1367- 1370)

Therapy with high dose alpha lipoic acid improves the long-term prognosis in diabetic polyneuropathy. TW NEUROL. PSYCHIATR. (Germany), 1994, 8/12 (699-700)

High dose alpha lipoic acid improves the long-term prognosis in diabetic polyneuropathy. THERAPIEWOCHE (Germany), 1994, 44/38 (2247-2248)

Alpha-lipoic acid: A versatile drug which is proved Alpha lipoic acid. Avoidance and therapy of polyneuropathy in diabetes. Z. ALLGEMEINMED. (Germany), 1993, 69/17 (492-494)

Alternative therapeutic principles in the prevention of microvascular and neuropathic complications. Diabetes Res Clin Pract (IRELAND) Aug 1995, 28 Suppl pS201-7

[Preventive treatment of diabetic microangiopathy: blocking the pathogenic mechanisms] Diabete Metab (FRANCE) 1994, 20 (2 Pt 2) p219-28

[Diabetes mellitus—a free radical-associated disease. Results of adjuvant antioxidant supplementation] Z Gesamte Inn Med (GERMANY) May 1993, 48 (5)

[Treatment of diabetic neuropathy with oral alpha-lipoic acid. MMW Munch Med Wochenschr (GER-

MANY, WEST) May 30 1975

Comparison of the effects of evening primrose oil and triglycerides containing gamma-linolenic acid on nerve conduction and blood flow in diabetic rats. J Pharmacol Exp Ther (UNITED STATES) Apr 1995

The effects of gamma-linolenic acid on breast pain and diabetic neuropathy: possible non-eicosanoid mechanisms. Prostaglandins Leukot Essent Fatty Acids (SCOTLAND) Jan 1993

The use of gamma-linolenic acid in diabetic neuropathy. Agents Actions Suppl (SWITZERLAND) 1992, 37 p120-44

Structural and biochemical effects of essential fatty acid deficiency on peripheral nerve. J Neuropathol Exp Neurol (UNITED STATES) Nov 1980, 39 (6)

Treatment of diabetic neuropathy with gamma-linolenic acid. DIABETES CARE (USA), 1993, 16/1 (8-15)

The effects of gamma-linolenic acid on breast pain and diabetic neuropathy: Possible non-eicosanoid mechanisms. PROSTAGLANDINS LEUKOTRIENES ESSENT. FATTY ACIDS (United Kingdom), 1993, 8/1

The use of gamma-linolenic acid in diabetic neuropathy. AGENTS ACTIONS (Switzerland), 1992, 37/SUPPL. (120-144)

Structural and biochemical effects of essential fatty acid deficiency on peripheral nerve. J. NEUROPATHOL. EXP. NEUROL. (USA), 1980, 39/6 (683-691)

Primary preventive and secondary interventionary effects of acetyl-L- carnitine on diabetic neuropathy in the bio-breeding Worcester rat. J Clin Invest (UNITED STATES) Apr 15 1996, 97 (8) p1900-7

Altered neuroexcitability in experimental diabetic neuropathy: effect of acetyl-L-carnitine. Int J Clin Pharmacol Res (SWITZERLAND) 1992, 12 (5-6)

Acetyl-L-carnitine corrects the altered peripheral nerve function of experimental diabetes. Metabolism: Clinical and Experimental (USA), 1995, 44/5 (677-680)

Diabetic neuropathy in the rat: 1. Alcar augments the reduced levels and axoplasmic transport of substance P Di Giulio A.M.; Lesma E.; Gorio A. RES. (USA), 1995, 40/3

Neural dysfunction and metabolic imbalances in diabetic rats: Prevention by acetyl-L-carnitine. DIABETES (USA), 1994, 43/12 (1469-1477)

Acetyl-L-carnitine prevents substance P loss in the sciatic nerve and lumbar spinal cord of diabetic animals. INT. J. CLIN. PHARMACOL. RES. (Switzerland), 1992, 12/5-6 (243-246)

Altered neuroexcitability in experimental diabetic neuropathy: Effect of acetyl-L-carnitine. INT. J. CLIN. PHARMACOL. RES. (Switzerland), 1992, 12/5-6 (237-241)

Peptide alterations in automatic diabetic neuropathy prevented by acetyl-L-carnitine. CLIN. PHARMACOL. RES. (Switzerland), 1992, 12/5-6 (225-230)

Acetyl-L-carnitine effect on nerve conduction velocity in streptozotocin-diabetic rats. ARZNEIM.-FORSCH. DRUG RES. (Germany), 1993, 43/3 (343-346)

Differential effects of acetyl-L-carnitine, L-carnitine and gangliosides on nerve $Na+,K+$-ATPase impairment in experimental diabetes. DIABETES NUTR. METAB. CLIN. EXP. (Italy), 1992, 5/1 (31-36)

Treatment of symptomatic diabetic peripheral neuropathy with the anti-oxidant alpha-lipoic acid. A 3-week multicentre randomized controlled trial. Diabetologia (Germany), 1995, 38/12 (1425-1433)

Peptide alterations in autonomic diabetic neuropathy prevented by acetyl-L-carnitine. Int J Clin Pharmacol Res (SWITZERLAND) 1992, 12 (5-6)

Primary preventive and secondary interventionary effects of acetyl-L- carnitine on diabetic neuropathy in the bio-breeding Worcester rat. Journal of Clinical Investigation (USA), 1996, 97/8 (1900-1907)

Obesity

Refer to references under Weight Loss.

Organic Brain Syndrome

Refer to references under Alzheimer's Disease.

Osteoporosis

The effectiveness of exercises on treatment of postmenopausal osteoporosis. Fizik Tedavi Rehabilitasyon Dergisi (Turkey), 1997, 21/1 (20-24)

The Bsml vitamin D receptor restriction fragment length polymorphism (bb) influences the effect of calcium intake on bone mineral density. Journal of Bone and Mineral Research (USA), 1997, 12/7 (1049-1057)

The effect of 1,25(OH)2 vitamin D3 on CD4+/CD8+ subsets of T lymphocytes in postmenopausal women. Life Sciences (USA), 1997, 61/2 (147-152)

Acute changes in serum calcium and parathyroid hormone circulating levels induced by the oral intake of five currently available calcium salts in healthy male volunteers. Clinical Rheumatology (Belgium), 1997, 16/3 (249-253)

1-alpha-hydroxyvitamin D3 treatment decreases bone turnover and modulates calcium-regulating hormones in early postmenopausal women. Bone (USA), 1997, 20/6 (557-562)

Nonestrogen management of menopausal symptoms. Endocrinology and Metabolism Clinics of North America (USA), 1997, 26/2 (379-390)

Role of dietary lipid and antioxidants in bone metabolism. Nutrition Research (USA), 1997, 17/7 (1209-1228)

The response to calcitriol therapy in postmenopausal osteoporotic women is a function of initial calcium absorptive status. Calcified Tissue International (USA), 1997, 61/1 (6-9)

Bone mineral density changes during lactation: Maternal, dietary, and biochemical correlates. American Journal of Clinical Nutrition (USA), 1997, 65/6 (1738-1746)

Postprandial parathyroid hormone response to four calcium-rich foodstuffs. American Journal of Clinical Nutrition (USA), 1997, 65/6 (1726-1730)

Complementary medical treatment for Colles' fracture: A comparative, randomized, longitudinal study.

Calcified Tissue International (USA), 1997, 60/6 (567-570)

Treatment of postmenopausal osteoporosis: Spoilt for choice? Part 1 - Foundations for an individually adapted management concept. Munchener Medizinische Wochenschrift (Germany), 1997, 139/20 (33-34+37-38)

Calcium and vitamin D in the prevention and treatment of osteoporosis. Journal of Clinical Rheumatology (USA), 1997, 3/2 SUPPL. (S52-S56)

Calcium intake and fracture risk: Results from the study of osteoporotic fractures. American Journal of Epidemiology (USA), 1997, 145/10 (926-934)

Bone loss and turnover after cardiac transplantation. Journal of Clinical Endocrinology and Metabolism (USA), 1997, 82/5 (1497-1506)

Effect of dietary calcium on urinary oxalate excretion after oxalate loads. American Journal of Clinical Nutrition (USA), 1997, 65/5 (1453-1459)

1alpha-Hydroxyvitamin D2 partially dissociates between preservation of cancellous bone mass and effects on calcium homeostasis in ovariectomized rats. Calcified Tissue International (USA), 1997, 60/5 (449-456)

What's hip in diet and osteoporosis? Scandinavian Journal of Nutrition/Naringsforskning (Sweden), 1997, 41/1 (2-8+12)

Prevention and management of osteoporosis. Current trends and future prospects. Drugs (New Zealand), 1997, 53/5 (727-735)

A high dietary calcium intake is needed for a positive effect on bone density in Swedish postmenopausal women. Osteoporosis International (United Kingdom), 1997, 7/2 (155-161)

Stress injury to bone in the female athlete. Clinics in Sports Medicine (USA), 1997, 16/2 (197-224)

Amelioration of hemiplegia-associated osteopenia more than 4 years after stroke by 1alpha-hydroxyvitamin D3 and calcium supplementation. Stroke (USA), 1997, 28/4 (736-739)

Effects of growth hormone (GH) replacement on bone metabolism and mineral density in adult onset of GH deficiency: Results of a double-blind placebo-controlled study with open follow-up. European Journal of Endocrinology (Norway), 1997, 136/3 (282-289)

Experimental study of glucocorticoid-induced rabbit osteoporosis. Chinese Pharmacological Bulletin (China), 1996, 12/6 (540-542)

Decreased serum IGF-I and dehydroepiandrosterone sulphate may be risk factors for the development of reduced bone mass in postmenopausal women with endogenous subclinical hyperthyroidism. European Journal of Endocrinology (Norway), 1997, 136/3 (277-281)

The usefulness of bone turnover in predicting the response to transdermal estrogen therapy in postmenopausal osteoporosis. Journal of Bone and Mineral Research (USA), 1997, 12/4 (624-631)

Osteoporotic vertebral fractures in postmenopausal women. American Family Physician (USA), 1997, 55/4 (1315-1322)

Proteins and bone health. Pathologie Biologie (France), 1997, 45/1 (57-59)

Osteoporosis: Prevention, diagnosis, and management. American Journal of Medicine (USA), 1997,

102/1 A (35S-39S)

Serum vitamin D metabolites and calcium absorption in normal young and elderly free-living women and in women living in nursing homes. American Journal of Clinical Nutrition (USA), 1997, 65/3 (790-797)

Long-term vegetarian diet and bone mineral density in postmenopausal Taiwanese women. Calcified Tissue International (USA), 1997, 60/3 (245-249)

Effect of 1,25(OH)2 vitamin D3 on circulating insulin-like growth factor-I and beta2 microglobulin in patients with osteoporosis. Calcified Tissue International (USA), 1997, 60/3 (236-239)

Influence of the vitamin D receptor gene alleles on bone mineral density in postmenopausal and osteoporotic women. Journal of Bone and Mineral Research (USA), 1997, 12/2 (241-247)

Connections between phospho-calcium metabolism and bone turnover. Epidemiologic study on osteoporosis (second part). Minerva Medica (Italy), 1996, 87/12 (565-576)

Treatment of post-menopausal osteoporosis with recombinant human growth hormone and salmon calcitonin: A placebo controlled study. Clinical Endocrinology (United Kingdom), 1997, 46/1 (55-61)

Calcium regulation and bone mass loss after total gastrectomy in pigs. Annals of Surgery (USA), 1997, 225/2 (181-192)

Management of osteoporosis in the elderly. Journal of Geriatric Drug Therapy (USA), 1996, 11/1 (5-16)

Osteoporosis and bone mineral metabolism disorders in cirrhotic patients referred for orthotopic liver transplantation. Calcified Tissue International (USA), 1997, 60/2 (148-154)

Effect of hormone replacement therapy on bone mineral content and fractures. Ugeskrift for Laeger (Denmark), 1997, 159/5 (570-576)

Effect of measuring bone mineral density on calcium intake. Japanese Journal of Geriatrics (Japan), 1996, 33/11 (840-846)

Estrogen therapy and osteoporosis: Principles and practice. American Journal of the Medical Sciences (USA), 1997, 313/1 (2-12)

Alternatives to estrogen replacement therapy for preventing osteoporosis. Journal of the American Pharmaceutical Association (USA), 1996,36/12 (707-715)

Osteoporosis: Its pediatric causes and prevention opportunities. Primary Care Update for Ob/Gyns (USA), 1997, 4/1 (15-20)

Estimated dietary calcium intake and food sources for adolescent females: 1980-92. Journal of Adolescent Health (USA), 1997, 20/1 (20-26)

The importance of genetic and nutritional factors in responses to vitamin D and its analogs in osteoporotic patients. Calcified Tissue International (USA), 1997, 60/1 (119-123)

The pathogenesis of age-related osteoporotic fracture: Effects of dietary calcium deprivation. Journal of Clinical Endocrinology and Metabolism (USA), 1997, 82/1 (260-264)

Increased catabolism of 25-hydroxyvitamin D in patients with partial gastrectomy and elevated 1,25-dihydroxyvitamin D levels. Implications for metabolic bone disease. Journal of Clinical Endocrinology and Metabolism (USA), 1997, 82/1 (209-212)

Can the fast bone loss in osteoporotic and osteopenic patients be stopped with active vitamin D metabolites? Calcified Tissue International (USA), 1997, 60/1 (115-118)

Is there a differential response to alfacalcidol and vitamin D in the treatment of osteoporosis? Calcified Tissue International (USA), 1997, 60/1 (111-114)

Rationale for active vitamin D analog therapy in senile osteoporosis. Calcified Tissue International (USA), 1997, 60/1 (100-105)

Efficacy and safety of long-term, open-label treatment of calcitriol in postmenopausal osteoporosis: A retrospective analysis. Current Therapeutic Research - Clinical and Experimental (USA), 1996, 57/11 (857-868)

Osteoporosis prevention and treatment. Pharmacological management and treatment implications. Drugs and Aging (New Zealand), 1996, 9/6 (472-477)

Magnesium deficiency: Possible role in osteoporosis associated with gluten-sensitive enteropathy. Osteoporosis International (United Kingdom), 1996, 6/6 (453-461)

Effects of vitamin B12 on cell proliferation and cellular alkaline phosphatase activity in human bone marrow stromal osteoprogenitor cells and UMR106 osteoblastic cells. Metabolism: Clinical and Experimental (USA), 1996, 45/12 (1443-1446)

Calcium metabolism in the elderly. Giornale di Gerontologia (Italy), 1996, 44/2 (91-96)

Hormones, vitamins, and growth factors in cancer treatment and prevention: A critical appraisal. Cancer (USA), 1996, 78/11 (2264-2280)

Therapy of osteoporosis: Calcium, vitamin D, and exercise. American Journal of the Medical Sciences (USA), 1996, 312/6 (278-286)

Pathophysiology of osteoporosis. American Journal of the Medical Sciences (USA), 1996, 312/6 (251-256)

Involutional osteoporosis in the elderly. Giornale di Gerontologia (Italy), 1996, 44/2 (85-89)

Osteoporosis and hormone replacement therapy. Acta Chirurgica Austriaca (Austria), 1996, 28/5 (263-265)

The effect of season and latitude on in vitro vitamin D formation by sunlight in South Africa. South African Medical Journal (South Africa), 1996, 86/10 (1270-1272)

Risk for osteoporosis in black women. Calcified Tissue International (USA), 1996, 59/6 (415-423)

Age considerations in nutrient needs for bone health: Older adults. Journal of the American College of Nutrition (USA), 1996, 15/6 (575-578)

Osteoporosis in lung transplantation candidates with end-stage pulmonary disease. American Journal of Medicine (USA), 1996, 101/3 (262-269)

Dietary calcium intake and its relation to bone mineral density in patients with inflammatory bowel disease. Journal of Internal Medicine (United Kingdom), 1996, 240/5 (285-292)

Development of clinical practice guidelines for prevention and treatment of osteoporosis. 1 (S30-S33) Calcified Tissue International (USA), 1996, 59/SUPPL.

Harmonization of clinical practice guidelines for the prevention and treatment of osteoporosis and osteopenia in Europe: A difficult challenge. Calcified Tissue International (USA), 1996, 59/SUPPL. 1 (S24-S29)

Clinical practice guidelines for the diagnosis and management of osteoporosis. Canadian Medical Association Journal (Canada), 1996, 155/8 (1113-1129)

Current and potential future drug treatments for osteoporosis. Annals of the Rheumatic Diseases (United Kingdom), 1996, 55/10 (700-714)

Osteoporosis of the lumbar spine. Schweizerische Rundschau fur Medizin/Praxis (Switzerland), 1996, 85/43 (1354-1359)

Common polymorphism of the vitamin D receptor gene is associated with variation of peak bone mass in young Finns. Calcified Tissue International (USA), 1996, 59/4 (231-234)

Diminished effect of etidronate in vitamin D deficient osteopenic postmenopausal women. European Journal of Clinical Pharmacology (Germany), 1996, 51/2 (145-147)

Vitamin D metabolites and analogs in the treatment of osteoporosis. Canadian Medical Association Journal (Canada), 1996, 155/7 (955-961)

Calcium nutrition and osteoporosis. Canadian Medical Association Journal (Canada), 1996, 155/7 (935-939)

Interrelationships of food, nutrition, diet and health: The national association of state universities and land grant colleges white paper. Journal of the American College of Nutrition (USA), 1996, 15/5 (422-433)

Osteoporosis of Crohn's disease: A critical review. Canadian Journal of Gastroenterology (Canada), 1996, 10/5 (317-321)

Effect of Vitamin D receptor gene polymorphism on vitamin D therapy for postmenopausal bone loss. Acta Obstetrica et Gynaecologica Japonica (Japan), 1996, 48/9 (799-805)

The preparation and stability of compound active calcium tablets. Chinese Pharmaceutical Journal (China), 1996, 31/8 (474-477)

Immunosuppression: Tightrope walk between iatrogenic side effects and therapy. Schweizerische Medizinische Wochenschrift (Switzerland), 1996, 126/38 (1603-1609)

Secondary osteoporosis in rheumatic diseases. Ceska Revmatologie (Czech Republic), 1996, 4/2 (51-57)

Does lactose intolerance predispose to low bone density? A population-based study of peri-menopausal Finnish women. Bone (USA), 1996, 19/1 (23-28)

Glucocorticoid-induced osteoporosis. Medecine et Hygiene (Switzerland), 1996, 54/2127 (1490-1495)

Relation of common allelic variation at vitamin D receptor locus to bone mineral density and post-menopausal bone loss: Cross sectional and longitudinal population study. British Medical Journal (United Kingdom), 1996, 313/7057 (586-590)

Nutrition and women's health. Current Problems in Obstetrics, Gynecology and Fertility (USA), 1996, 19/4 (112-166)

Systemic osteoporosis in rheumatoid arthritis. Pathogenetic mechanisms and therapeutic approaches. Zeitschrift fur Rheumatologie (Germany), 1996, 55/3 (149-157)

Current treatment options for osteoporosis. Journal of Rheumatology (Canada), 1996, 23/SUPPL. 45 (11-14)

Treatments for oestoporosis. Revue Francaise de Gynecologie et d'Obstetrique (France), 1996, 91/6 (329-334)

Estrogen replacement may be an alternative to parathyroid surgery for the treatment of osteoporosis in elderly postmenopausal women presenting with primary hyperparathyroidism: A preliminary report. Osteoporosis International (United Kingdom), 1996, 6/4 (329-333)

A comparison of the effects of alfacalcidol treatment and vitamin D2 supplementation on calcium absorption in elderly women with vertebral fractures. Osteoporosis International (United Kingdom), 1996, 6/4 (284-290)

The effect of calcium supplementation and Tanner Stage on bone density, content and area in teenage women. Osteoporosis International (United Kingdom), 1996, 6/4 (276-283)

Corticosteroid induced osteoporosis. Journal of Rheumatology (Canada), 1996, 23/SUPPL. 45 (19-22)

The role of vitamin D in the pathogenesis and treatment of osteoporosis. Journal of Rheumatology (Canada), 1996, 23/SUPPL. 45 (15-18)

Review: Treatment of primary biliary cirrhosis. Journal of Gastroenterology and Hepatology (Australia),1996, 11/7 (605-609)

Osteoporosis. Physical Medicine and Rehabilitation Clinics of North America (USA), 1996, 7/3 (583-599)

Nutritional and biochemical studies on vitamin D and its active derivatives. Yakugaku Zasshi (Japan), 1996, 116/6 (457-472)

Osteoporosis and calcium ingest. Progresos en Obstetricia y Ginecologia (Spain), 1996, 39/4 (289-292)

Lower serum 25-hydroxyvitamin D is associated with increased bone resorption markers and lower bone density at the proximal femur in normal females: A population-based study. Experimental and Clinical Endocrinology and Diabetes (Germany), 1996, 104/3 (289-292)

Hormone therapy and phytoestrogens. Journal of Clinical Pharmacy and Therapeutics (United Kingdom), 1996, 21/2 (101-111)

Recent progress in treatment of osteoporosis. Japanese Journal of Geriatrics (Japan), 1996, 33/4 (240-244)

Vitamin D and calcium in the prevention of corticosteroid induced osteoporosis: A 3 year followup. Journal of Rheumatology (Canada), 1996, 23/6 (995-1000)

Novelties and issues in the drug market 1995. Ricerca e Pratica (Italy), 1996, 12/68 (63-71)

Influence of life style in the MEDOS study. Scandinavian Journal of Rheumatology, Supplement (Norway), 1996, 25/103 (112)

Roles of diet and physical activity in the prevention of osteoporosis. Scandinavian Journal of Rheumatology, Supplement (Norway), 1996, 25/103 (65-74)

The problem: Health impact of osteoporosis. Scandinavian Journal of Rheumatology, Supplement (Norway), 1996, 25/103 (3-5)

Vitamin D in the treatment of osteoporosis revisited. Proceedings of the Society for Experimental Biology and Medicine (USA), 1996, 212/2 (110-115)

Prevention of bone loss in cardiac transplant recipients: A comparison of biphosphonates and vitamin D. Transplantation (USA), 1996, 61/10 (1495-1499)

Prophylaxis of osteoporosis with calcium, estrogens and/or eelcatonin: Comparative longitudinal study of bone mass. Maturitas (Ireland), 1996, 23/3 (327-332)

Open-label, controlled study on the metabolic and absorptiometric effects of calcitriol in involutional osteoporosis. Clinical Drug Investigation (New Zealand), 1996, 11/5 (270-277)

Nutritional prevention of aging osteoporosis. Cahiers de Nutrition et de Dietetique (France), 1996, 31/2 (98-101)

Effects of 2 years' treatment of osteoporosis with 1alpha-hydroxy vitamin D3 on bone mineral density and incidence of fracture: A placebo-controlled, double-blind prospective study. Endocrine Journal (Japan), 1996, 43/2 (211-220)

Osteoporotic fractures: Background and prevention strategies. Maturitas (Ireland), 1996, 23/2 (193-207)

Energy and nutrient intake in patients with CF. Monatsschrift fur Kinderheilkunde (Germany), 1996, 144/4 (396-402)

Current and future nonhormonal approaches to the treatment of osteoporosis. International Journal of Fertility and Menopausal Studies (USA), 1996, 41/2 (148-155)

Dietary protein intake and bone mass in women. Calcified Tissue International (USA), 1996, 58/5 (320-325)

1,25-Dihydroxyvitamin D3 enhances the enzymatic activity and expression of the messenger ribonucleic acid for aromatase cytochrome P450 synergistically with dexamethasone depending on the vitamin D receptor level in cultured human osteoblasts. Endocrinology (USA), 1996, 137/5 (1860-1869)

Effects of hormonal therapies and dietary soy phytoestrogens on vaginal cytology in surgically postmenopausal macaques. Fertility and Sterility (USA), 1996, 65/5 (1031-1035)

Transient osteoporosis of the hip. Case report and review of the literature. Acta Orthopaedica Belgica (Belgium), 1996, 62/1 (56-59)

Osteomalacia and osteoporosis in a woman with ankylosing spondylitis. Journal of Bone and Mineral Research (USA), 1996, 11/5 (697-703)

Evaluation of acceptability, tolerance and observance of a new calcium-vitamine D combination. Rhumatologie (France), 1996, 48/2 (37-42)

Sequential effects of chronic human PTH (1-84) treatment of estrogen-deficiency osteopenia in the rat. Journal of Bone and Mineral Research (USA), 1996, 11/4 (430-439)

References

Effects of vitamin K on bone mass and bone metabolism. Journal of Nutrition (USA), 1996, 126/4 SUPPL. (1187S-1191S)

Calcium and vitamin D nutritional needs of elderly women. Journal of Nutrition (USA), 1996, 126/4 SUPPL. (1165S-1167S)

Vitamin D and bone health. Journal of Nutrition (USA), 1996, 126/4 SUPPL. (1159S-1164S)

Influence of ovariectomy on bone metabolism in very old rats. Calcified Tissue International (USA), 1996, 58/4 (256-262)

Heated oyster shell-seaweed calcium (AAA Ca) on osteoporosis. Calcified Tissue International (USA), 1996, 58/4 (226-230)

Age-related factors in the pathogenesis of senile (type II) femoral neck fractures: An integrated view. American Journal of Orthopedics (USA), 1996, 25/3 (198-204)

Protein consumption and bone fractures in women. American Journal of Epidemiology (USA), 1996, 143/5 (472-479)

The epidemiology of osteoporosis: The oriental perspective in a world context. Clinical Orthopaedics and Related Research (USA), 1996, /323 (65-74)

Comparison of nonrandomized trials with slow-release sodium fluoride with a randomized placebo-controlled trial in postmenopausal osteoporosis. Journal of Bone and Mineral Research (USA), 1996, 11/2 (160-168)

Stimulation of the growth of femoral trabecular bone in ovariectomized rats by the novel parathyroid hormone fragment, hPTH-(1-31)NH2 (Ostabolin). Calcified Tissue International (USA), 1996, 58/2 (81-87)

The lack of influence of long-term potassium citrate and calcium citrate treatment in total body aluminum burden in patients with functioning kidneys. Journal of the American College of Nutrition (USA), 1996, 15/1 (102-106)

Kidney stone clinic: Ten years of experience. Nederlands Tijschrift voor de Klinische Chemie (Netherlands), 1996, 21/1 (8-10)

Calcium deficiency in fluoride-treated osteoporotic patients despite calcium supplementation. Journal of Clinical Endocrinology and Metabolism (USA), 1996, 81/1 (269-275)

Endocrinology. Medecine et Hygiene (Switzerland), 1996, 54/2100 (85-95)

Dietary soybean protein prevents bone loss in an ovariectomized rat model of osteoporosis. Journal of Nutrition (USA), 1996, 126/1 (161-167)

Bone density in children and adolescents with cystic fibrosis. Journal of Pediatrics (USA), 1996, 128/1 (28-34)

Axial bone mass in older women. Annals of Internal Medicine (USA), 1996, 124/2 (187-196)

Bone mineral density in mother-daughter pairs: Relations to lifetime exercise, lifetime milk consumption, and calcium supplements. American Journal of Clinical Nutrition (USA), 1996, 63/1 (72-79)

Is postmenopausal osteoporosis related to pineal gland functions? Int J Neurosci (ENGLAND) Feb 1992, 62 (3-4) p215-25

Glucocorticoid-induced osteoporosis: mechanisms for bone loss; evaluation of strategies for prevention. J Gerontol (UNITED STATES) Sep 1990, 45 (5) pM153-8

Progesterone as a bone-trophic hormone. Endocr Rev (UNITED STATES) May 1990, 11 (2) p386-98

Osteocalcin and its message: relationship to bone histology in magnesium-deprived rats. Am J Physiol (UNITED STATES) Jul 1992, 263 (1 Pt 1) pE107-14

[Influence of active vitamine D3 on bones] Nippon Seikeigeka Gakkai Zasshi (JAPAN) Dec 1979, 53 (12) p1823-37

Relation of magnesium to osteoporosis and calcium urolithiasis. Magnes Trace Elem (SWITZERLAND) 92 1991, 10 (2-4) p281-6

Role of vitamin D, its metabolites, and analogs in the management of osteoporosis. Rheum Dis Clin North Am (UNITED STATES) Aug 1994, 20 (3) p759-75

Anabolic steroids in corticosteroid-induced osteoporosis. Wien Med Wochenschr (AUSTRIA) 1993, 143 (14-15) p395-7

Osteocalcin and its message: relationship to bone histology in magnesium-deprived rats. Am J Physiol (UNITED STATES) Jul 1992, 263 (1 Pt 1) pE107-14

Glucocorticoid-induced osteoporosis: mechanisms for bone loss; evaluation of strategies for prevention. J Gerontol (UNITED STATES) Sep 1990, 45 (5) pM153-8

Nutritional insurance supplementation and corticosteroid toxicity. Med Hypotheses (ENGLAND) Aug 1982, 9 (2) p145-56

Effects of recombinant human growth hormone (GH) on bone and intermediary metabolism in patients receiving chronic glucocorticoid treatment with suppressed endogenous GH response to GH-releasing hormone. J Clin Endocrinol Metab (UNITED STATES) Jan 1995, 80 (1) p122-9

Human marrow stromal osteoblast-like cells do not show reduced responsiveness to in vitro stimulation with growth hormone in patients with postmenopausal osteoporosis. Calcif Tissue Int (UNITED STATES) Jan 1994, 54 (1) p1-6

Growth hormone and bone. Horm Metab Res (GERMANY) Jul 1993, 25 (7) p335-43

Growth hormone and bone. Horm Res (SWITZERLAND) 1991, 36 Suppl 1 p49-55

Aromatase in bone cell: association with osteoporosis in postmenopausal women. J Steroid Biochem Mol Biol (ENGLAND) Jun 1995, 53 (1-6) p165-74

Biological properties and clinical application of propolis. VIII. Experimental observation on the influence of ethanol extract of propolis (EEP) on the regeneration of bone tissue ARZNEIM.-FORSCH. (GERMANY, WEST), 1978, 28/1 (35-37)

Pain

Enhancement of a kappa-opioid receptor agonist-induced analgesia by L-tyrosine and L-tryptophan. Eur J Pharmacol (NETHERLANDS) Jun 13 1994, 258 (3) p173-8

L-Tyrosine-induced antinociception in the mouse: involvement of central delta-opioid receptors and bulbo-spinal noradrenergic system. Eur J Pharmacol (NETHERLANDS) Mar 23 1993, 233 (2-3) p255-

60

L-dopa induces opposing effects on pain in intact rats: (-)-sulpiride, SCH 23390 or alpha-methyl-DL-p-tyrosine methylester hydrochloride reveals profound hyperalgesia in large antinociceptive doses. J Pharmacol Exp Ther (UNITED STATES) Nov 1992, 263 (2) p470-9

Dietary influences on neurotransmission. Adv Pediatr (UNITED STATES) 1986, 33 p23-47

Parathyroid (Hyperparathyroidism)

Different effects of PTH on erythrocyte calcium influx. Italian Journal of Mineral and Electrolyte Metabolism (Italy), 1996, 10/3-4 (149-152)

Hypercalcemia due to constitutive activity of the parathyroid hormone (PTH)/PTH-related peptide receptor: Comparison with primary hyperparathyroidism. Journal of Clinical Endocrinology and Metabolism (USA), 1996, 81/10 (3584-3588)

Osteoclast cytomorphometry in patients with femoral neck fracture. Pathology Research and Practice (Germany), 1996, 192/6 (573-578)

Combined therapy with salmon calcitonin and high doses of active vitamin D3 metabolites in uremic hyperparathyroidism. Polskie Archiwum Medycyny Wewnetrznej (Poland), 1996, 96/1 (23-31)

The PTH-calcium relationship curve in secondary hyperparathyroidism, an index of sensitivity and suppressibility of parathyroid glands. Nephrology Dialysis Transplantation (United Kingdom), 1996, 11/SUPPL. 3 (136-141)

Severe acute pancreatitis as a first symptom of primary hyperparathyroid adenoma: A case report. Journal of Laryngology and Otology (United Kingdom), 1996, 110/6 (602-603)

24,25 dihydroxyvitamin D supplementation corrects hyperparathyroidism and improves skeletal abnormalities in X-linked hypophosphatemic rickets - A clinical research center study. Journal of Clinical Endocrinology and Metabolism (USA), 1996, 81/6 (2381-2388)

1-alpha-hydroxyvitamin D3 treatment decreases bone turnover and modulates calcium-regulating hormones in early postmenopausal women. Bone (USA), 1997, 20/6 (557-562)

Role of parathyroid hormone-related peptide (PTHrP) in hypercalcemia of malignancy and the development of osteolytic metastases. Journal of Clinical Rheumatology (USA), 1997, 3/2 SUPPL. (S109-S113)

Experimental study of glucocorticoid-induced rabbit osteoporosis. Chinese Pharmacological Bulletin (China), 1996, 12/6 (540-542)

Medical parathyroidectomy - The value of vitamin D. Acta Chirurgica Austriaca (Austria), 1996, 28/SUPPL. 124 (8-10)

Oral vitamin D or calcium carbonate in the prevention of renal bone disease? Current Opinion in Nephrology and Hypertension

Estrogen replacement may be an alternative to parathyroid surgery for the treatment of osteoporosis in elderly postmenopausal women presenting with primary hyperparathyroidism: A preliminary report. Osteoporosis International (United Kingdom), 1996, 6/4 (329-333)

References

A comparison of the effects of alfacalcidol treatment and vitamin D2 supplementation on calcium absorption in elderly women with vertebral fractures. Osteoporosis International (United Kingdom), 1996, 6/4 (284-290)

Comparison of effects of calcitriol and calcium carbonate on secretion of interleukin-1beta and tumour necrosis factor-alpha by uraemic peripheral blood mononuclear cells. Nephrology Dialysis Transplantation (United Kingdom), 1996, 11/SUPPL. 3 (15-21)

Hyperparathyroidism. Otolaryngologic Clinics of North America (USA), 1996, 29/4 (663-679)

Intradialytic calcium balances with different calcium dialysate levels. Effects on cardiovascular stability and parathyroid function. Nephron (Switzerland), 1996, 72/4 (530-535)

Influence of ovariectomy on bone metabolism in very old rats. Calcified Tissue International (USA), 1996, 58/4 (256-262)

Biochemical effects of calcium and vitamin D supplementation in elderly, institutionalized, vitamin D-deficient patients. Revue du Rhumatisme (English Edition) (France), 1996, 63/2 (135-140)

Long-term treatment with calcium-alpha-ketoglutarate corrects secondary hyperparathyroidism. Mineral and Electrolyte Metabolism (Switzerland), 1996, 22/1-3 (196-199)

Long-term effect of intravenous calcitriol on the treatment of severe hyperparathyroidism, parathyroid gland mass and bone mineral density in haemodialysis patients. Am J Nephrol (SWITZERLAND) 1997, 17 (2) p118-23

Calcitriol in the management of secondary hyperparathyroidism of renal failure. Pharmacotherapy (UNITED STATES) Jul-Aug 1996, 16 (4) p619-30

Parathyroid hormone increases bone formation and improves mineral balance in vitamin D-deficient female rats. Endocrinology (UNITED STATES) Jun 1997, 138 (6) p2449-57

Effects on bone mineral density of low-dosed oral contraceptives compared to and combined with physical activity. Contraception (UNITED STATES) Feb 1997, 55 (2) p87-90

The importance of genetic and nutritional factors in responses to vitamin D and its analogs in osteoporotic patients. Calcif Tissue Int (UNITED STATES) Jan 1997, 60 (1) p119-23

Effective suppression of parathyroid hormone by 1 alpha-hydroxy-vitamin D2 in hemodialysis patients with moderate to severe secondary hyperparathyroidism. Kidney Int (UNITED STATES) Jan 1997, 51 (1) p317-23

The rise and fall of primary hyperparathyroidism: a population-based study in Rochester, Minnesota, 1965-1992. Ann Intern Med (UNITED STATES) Mar 15 1997, 126 (6) p433-40

Effects of 12 months of growth hormone (GH) treatment on calciotropic hormones, calcium homeostasis, and bone metabolism in adults with acquired GH deficiency: a double blind, randomized, placebo-controlled study. J Clin Endocrinol Metab (UNITED STATES) Sep 1996, 81 (9) p3352-9

Acute biochemical effects of growth hormone treatment compared with conventional treatment in familial hypophosphataemic rickets. Clin Endocrinol (Oxf) (ENGLAND) Jun 1996, 44 (6) p687-96

Calcium, phosphate, vitamin D, and the parathyroid. Pediatric Nephrology (Germany), 1996, 10/3 (364-367)

Vitamin D metabolism in chronic childhood hypoparathyroidism: Evidence for a direct regulatory effect of calcium. J. PEDIATR. (USA), 1990, 116/2 (252-257)

Determinants for serum 1,25-dihydroxycholecalciferol in primary hyperparathyroidism. BONE MINER. (Netherlands), 1989, 5/3 (279-290)

Magnesium hormonal regulation and metabolic interrelations. PRESSE MED. (France), 1988, 17/12 (584-587)

Treatment with active vitamin D (alphacalcidol) in patients with mild primary hyperparathyroidism. ACTA ENDOCRINOL. (Denmark), 1989, 120/2 (250-256)

Intravenous 1,25(OH)2 vitamin D3 therapy in haemodialysis patients: Evaluation of direct and calcium-mediated short-term effects on serum parathyroid hormone concentration.

Calcium, phosphate, vitamin D, and the parathyroid. Pediatric Nephrology (Germany), 1996, 10/3 (364-367)

Vitamin D metabolism in chronic childhood hypoparathyroidism: Evidence for a direct regulatory effect of calcium. J. PEDIATR. (USA), 1990, 116/2 (252-257)

Determinants for serum 1,25-dihydroxycholecalciferol in primary hyperparathyroidism. BONE MINER. (Netherlands), 1989, 5/3 (279-290)

Magnesium hormonal regulation and metabolic interrelations. Regulation hormonale et interrelations metaboliques du magnesium. PRESSE MED. (France), 1988, 17/12 (584-587)

Treatment with active vitamin D (alphacalcidol) in patients with mild primary hyperparathyroidism. ACTA ENDOCRINOL. (Denmark), 1989, 120/2 (250-256)

Intravenous 1,25(OH)2 vitamin D3 therapy in haemodialysis patients: Evaluation of direct and calcium-mediated short-term effects on serum parathyroid hormone concentration. NEPHROL. DIAL. TRANSPLANT. (Germany, Federal Republic of), 1990, 5/6 (457-460)

Parkinson's Disease

Changes in endocrine function after adrenal medullary transplantation to the central nervous system. J. CLIN. ENDOCRINOL. METAB. (USA), 1990, 71/3

Co-dergocrine (Hydergine) regulates striatal and hippocampal acetylcholine release through D2 receptors. NEUROREPORT (United Kingdom), 1994, 5/6 (674-676)

Ergot alkaloids and central monoaminergic receptors. J. PHARMACOL. (FRANCE), 1985, 16/SUPPL. 3 (21-27)

Dementia in the aged. PSYCHIATR. CLIN. NORTH AM. (USA), 1982, 5/1 (67-86)

Alterations of electroencephalographic patterns after intravenous administration of hydergine (dihydroergotoxine). ARG.NEURO-PSIQUIAT. (S.PAULO) (BRAZIL), 1973, 31/2

Phospholipid in Parkinson's disease: Biochemical and clinical data. ITALY PROG. CLIN. BIOL. RES. (USA), 1980, VOL.39 (205-214)

Efficacy and tolerability of amantadine sulfate in the treatment of Parkinson's disease. Nervenheilkunde (Germany), 1995, 14/2 (76-82)

Bromocriptine lessens the incidence of mortality in L-Dopa-treated parkinsonian patients: Prado-study discontinued. EUR. J. CLIN. PHARMACOL. (Germany), 1992, 43/4 (357-363)

Nicotinamidadenindinucleotide (NADH): The new approach in the therapy of Parkinson's disease. ANN. CLIN. LAB. SCI. (USA), 1989, 19/1 (38-43)

Levodopa and dopamine agonists in the treatment of Parkinson's disease: Advantages and disadvantages. EUR. NEUROL. (Switzerland), 1994, 34/SUPPL. 3 (20-28)

Plasma profiles of adrenocorticotropic hormone, cortisol, growth hormone and prolactin in patients with untreated Parkinson's disease. J. NEUROL. (Germany, Federal Republic of), 1991, 238/1

Hypothalamo-pituitary function and dopamine dependence in untreated parkinsonian patients. ACTA NEUROL. SCAND. (Denmark), 1991, 83/3 (145-150)

Effect of dopamine, dimethoxyphenylethylamine, papaverine, and related compounds on mitochondrial respiration and complex I activity. Journal of Neurochemistry (USA), 1996, 66/3 (1174-1181)

Treatment of Parkinson's disease: From theory to practice. USA POSTGRAD. MED. (USA), 1994, 95/5

In vitro oxidation of vitamin E, vitamin C, thiols and cholesterol in rat brain mitochondria incubated with free radicals. USA Neurochemistry International (United Kingdom), 1995, 26/5 (527-535)

Dietary intake and plasma levels of antioxidant vitamins in health and disease: A hospital-based case-control study. India Journal of Nutritional and Environmental Medicine (United Kingdom) 1995, 5/3 (235-242)

Oxidative stress and antioxidant therapy in Parkinson's disease. Progress in Neurobiology (United Kingdom), 1996, 48/1 (1-19)

Clinical pharmacodynamics of acetyl-L-carnitine in patients with Parkinson's disease. Int J Clin Pharmacol Res. 1990. 10(1-2). P 139-43

The significance of eye blink rate in parkinsonism: a hypothesis. Int J Neurosci. 1990 Mar. 51(1-2). P 99-103

Mechanisms of action of ECT in Parkinson's disease: possible role of pineal melatonin. Int J Neurosci. 1990 Jan. 50(1-2). P 83-94

Pineal melatonin functions: possible relevance to Parkinson's disease. Int J Neurosci. 1990 Jan. 50(1-2). P 37-53

Locus coeruleus-pineal melatonin interactions and the pathogenesis of the "on-off" phenomenon associated with mood changes and sensory symptoms in Parkinson's disease. Int J Neurosci. 1989 Nov. 49(1-2). P 95-101

Pineal melatonin and sensory symptoms in Parkinson disease. Ital J Neurol Sci. 1989 Aug. 10(4). P 399-403

[Neuroendocrine and psychopharmacologic aspects of the pineal function. Melatonin and psychiatric disorders]. Acta Psiquiatr Psicol Am Lat. 1989 Jan-Jun. 35(1-2). P 71-9

Impact of deprenyl and tocopherol treatment on Parkinson's disease in DATATOP patients requiring levodopa. Parkinson Study Group. Ann Neurol. 1996 Jan. 39(1). P 37-45

In vivo generation of hydroxyl radicals and MPTP-induced dopaminergic toxicity in the basal ganglia.

References

Ann N Y Acad Sci. 1994 Nov 17. 738P 25-36

Antioxidant mechanism and protection of nigral neurons against MPP+ toxicity by deprenyl (selegiline). Ann N Y Acad Sci. 1994 Nov 17. 738P 214-21

Parkinson's disease: a chronic, low-grade antioxidant deficiency? Med Hypotheses. 1994 Aug. 43(2). P 111-4

Free radicals in brain metabolism and pathology. Br Med Bull. 1993 Jul. 49(3). P 577-87

Free radicals and their scavengers in Parkinson's disease. Eur Neurol. 1993. 33 Suppl 1P 60-8

Phospholipid in Parkinson's disease: Biochemical and clinical data. ITALY PROG. CLIN. BIOL. RES. (USA), 1980, VOL.39 (205-214)

Efficacy and tolerability of amantadine sulfate in the treatment of Parkinson's disease. Nervenheilkunde (Germany), 1995, 14/2 (76-82)

Bromocriptine lessens the incidence of mortality in L-Dopa-treated parkinsonian patients: Prado-study discontinued. EUR. J. CLIN. PHARMACOL. (Germany), 1992, 43/4 (357- 363)

Nicotinamidadenindinucleotide (NADH): The new approach in the therapy of Parkinson's disease. ANN. CLIN. LAB. SCI. (USA), 1989, 19/1 (38-43)

Levodopa and dopamine agonists in the treatment of Parkinson's disease: Advantages and disadvantages. EUR. NEUROL. (Switzerland), 1994, 34/SUPPL. 3 (20- 28)

Plasma profiles of adrenocorticotropic hormone, cortisol, growth hormone and prolactin in patients with untreated Parkinson's disease. J. NEUROL. (Germany, Federal Republic of), 1991, 238/1

Hypothalamo-pituitary function and dopamine dependence in untreated parkinsonian patients. ACTA NEUROL. SCAND. (Denmark), 1991, 83/3 (145-150)

Effect of dopamine, dimethoxyphenylethylamine, papaverine, and related compounds on mitochondrial respiration and complex I activity. Journal of Neurochemistry (USA), 1996, 66/3 (1174- 1181)

Treatment of Parkinson's disease: From theory to practice. USA POSTGRAD. MED. (USA), 1994, 95/5

In vitro oxidation of vitamin E, vitamin C, thiols and cholesterol in rat brain mitochondria incubated with free radicals. USA Neurochemistry International (United Kingdom), 1995, 26/5 (527-535)

Dietary intake and plasma levels of antioxidant vitamins in health and disease: A hospital-based case-control study. India Journal of Nutritional and Environmental Medicine (United Kingdom) 1995, 5/3 (235-242)

Oxidative stress and antioxidant therapy in Parkinson's disease. Progress in Neurobiology (United Kingdom), 1996, 48/1 (1-19)

Co-dergocrine (Hydergine) regulates striatal and hippocampal acetylcholine release through D2 receptors. NEUROREPORT (United Kingdom), 1994, 5/6 (674-676)

Ergot alkaloids and central monoaminergic receptors. J. PHARMACOL. (FRANCE), 1985, 16/SUPPL. 3 (21-27)

Dementia in the aged. PSYCHIATR. CLIN. NORTH AM. (USA), 1982, 5/1 (67-86)

Alterations of electroencephalographic patterns after intravenous administration of hydergine (dihydroergotoxine). ARG.NEURO-PSIQUIAT. (S.PAULO) (BRAZIL), 1973, 31/2

Clinical pharmacodynamics of acetyl-L-carnitine in patients with Parkinson's disease. Int J Clin Pharmacol Res. 1990. 10(1-2). P 139-43

The significance of eye blink rate in parkinsonism: a hypothesis. Int J Neurosci. 1990 Mar. 51(1-2). P 99-103

Mechanisms of action of ECT in Parkinson's disease: possible role of pineal melatonin. Int J Neurosci. 1990 Jan. 50(1-2). P 83-94

Pineal melatonin functions: possible relevance to Parkinson's disease. Int J Neurosci. 1990 Jan. 50(1-2). P 37-53

Locus coeruleus-pineal melatonin interactions and the pathogenesis of the on- off phenomenon associated with mood changes and sensory symptoms in Parkinson's disease. Int J Neurosci. 1989 Nov. 49(1-2). P 95-101

Pineal melatonin and sensory symptoms in Parkinson disease. Ital J Neurol Sci. 1989 Aug. 10(4). P 399-403

[Neuroendocrine and psychopharmacologic aspects of the pineal function. Melatonin and psychiatric disorders] Acta Psiquiatr Psicol Am Lat. 1989 Jan-Jun. 35(1-2). P 71-9

Impact of deprenyl and tocopherol treatment on Parkinson's disease in DATATOP patients requiring levodopa. Parkinson Study Group. Ann Neurol. 1996 Jan. 39(1). P 37-45

In vivo generation of hydroxyl radicals and MPTP-induced dopaminergic toxicity in the basal ganglia. Ann N Y Acad Sci. 1994 Nov 17. 738P 25-36

Antioxidant mechanism and protection of nigral neurons against MPP+ toxicity by deprenyl (selegiline) Ann N Y Acad Sci. 1994 Nov 17. 738P 214-21

Parkinson's disease: a chronic, low-grade antioxidant deficiency? Med Hypotheses. 1994 Aug. 43(2). P 111-4

Free radicals in brain metabolism and pathology. Br Med Bull. 1993 Jul. 49(3). P 577-87

Free radicals and their scavengers in Parkinson's disease. Eur Neurol. 1993. 33 Suppl 1P 60-8

Changes in endocrine function after adrenal medullary transplantation to the central nervous system. J. CLIN. ENDOCRINOL. METAB. (USA), 1990, 71/3

Phospholipid in Parkinson's disease: Biochemical and clinical data. ITALY PROG. CLIN. BIOL. RES. (USA), 1980, VOL.39 (205-214)

Efficacy and tolerability of amantadine sulfate in the treatment of Parkinson's disease. Nervenheilkunde (Germany), 1995, 14/2 (76-82)

Bromocriptine lessens the incidence of mortality in L-Dopa-treated parkinsonian patients: Prado-study discontinued. EUR. J. CLIN. PHARMACOL. (Germany), 1992, 43/4 (357- 363)

Nicotinamidadenindinucleotide (NADH): The new approach in the therapy of Parkinson's disease. ANN. CLIN. LAB. SCI. (USA), 1989, 19/1 (38-43)

Levodopa and dopamine agonists in the treatment of Parkinson's disease: Advantages and disadvantages. EUR. NEUROL. (Switzerland), 1994, 34/SUPPL. 3 (20- 28)

References

Plasma profiles of adrenocorticotropic hormone, cortisol, growth hormone and prolactin in patients with untreated Parkinson's disease. J. NEUROL. (Germany, Federal Republic of), 1991, 238/1

Hypothalamo-pituitary function and dopamine dependence in untreated parkinsonian patients. ACTA NEUROL. SCAND. (Denmark), 1991, 83/3 (145-150)

Effect of dopamine, dimethoxyphenylethylamine, papaverine, and related compounds on mitochondrial respiration and complex I activity. Journal of Neurochemistry (USA), 1996, 66/3 (1174- 1181)

Treatment of Parkinson's disease: From theory to practice. USA POSTGRAD. MED. (USA), 1994, 95/5

In vitro oxidation of vitamin E, vitamin C, thiols and cholesterol in rat brain mitochondria incubated with free radicals. USA Neurochemistry International (United Kingdom), 1995, 26/5 (527-535)

Dietary intake and plasma levels of antioxidant vitamins in health and disease: A hospital-based case-control study. India Journal of Nutritional and Environmental Medicine (United Kingdom) 1995, 5/3 (235-242)

Oxidative stress and antioxidant therapy in Parkinson's disease. Progress in Neurobiology (United Kingdom), 1996, 48/1 (1-19)

Co-dergocrine (Hydergine) regulates striatal and hippocampal acetylcholine release through D2 receptors. NEUROREPORT (United Kingdom), 1994, 5/6 (674-676)

Ergot alkaloids and central monoaminergic receptors. J. PHARMACOL. (FRANCE), 1985, 16/SUPPL. 3 (21-27)

Dementia in the aged. PSYCHIATR. CLIN. NORTH AM. (USA), 1982, 5/1 (67-86)

Alterations of electroencephalographic patterns after intravenous administration of hydergine (dihydroergotoxine). ARG.NEURO-PSIQUIAT. (S.PAULO) (BRAZIL), 1973, 31/2

Clinical pharmacodynamics of acetyl-L-carnitine in patients with Parkinson's disease. Int J Clin Pharmacol Res. 1990. 10(1-2). P 139-43

The significance of eye blink rate in parkinsonism: a hypothesis. Int J Neurosci. 1990 Mar. 51(1-2). P 99-103

Mechanisms of action of ECT in Parkinson's disease: possible role of pineal melatonin. Int J Neurosci. 1990 Jan. 50(1-2). P 83-94

Pineal melatonin functions: possible relevance to Parkinson's disease. Int J Neurosci. 1990 Jan. 50(1-2). P 37-53

Locus coeruleus-pineal melatonin interactions and the pathogenesis of the on- off phenomenon associated with mood changes and sensory symptoms in Parkinson's disease. Int J Neurosci. 1989 Nov. 49(1-2). P 95-101

Pineal melatonin and sensory symptoms in Parkinson disease. Ital J Neurol Sci. 1989 Aug. 10(4). P 399-403

[Neuroendocrine and psychopharmacologic aspects of the pineal function. Melatonin and psychiatric disorders] Acta Psiquiatr Psicol Am Lat. 1989 Jan-Jun. 35(1-2). P 71-9

Impact of deprenyl and tocopherol treatment on Parkinson's disease in DATATOP patients requiring levodopa. Parkinson Study Group. Ann Neurol. 1996 Jan. 39(1). P 37-45

In vivo generation of hydroxyl radicals and MPTP-induced dopaminergic toxicity in the basal ganglia. Ann N Y Acad Sci. 1994 Nov 17. 738P 25-36

Antioxidant mechanism and protection of nigral neurons against MPP+ toxicity by deprenyl (selegiline). Ann N Y Acad Sci. 1994 Nov 17. 738P 214-21

Parkinson's disease: a chronic, low-grade antioxidant deficiency? Med Hypotheses. 1994 Aug. 43(2). P 111-4

Free radicals in brain metabolism and pathology. Br Med Bull. 1993 Jul. 49(3). P 577-87

Free radicals and their scavengers in Parkinson's disease. Eur Neurol. 1993. 33 Suppl 1P 60-8

Phobias

[Beta-blocking drugs and anxiety. A proven therapeutic value] Medications beta-bloquantes et anxiete. Un interet therapeutique certain. Encephale (FRANCE) Sep-Oct 1991, 17 (5) p481-92

Effect of beta-receptor blockade on anxiety with reference to the three-systems model of phobic behavior. Neuropsychobiology (SWITZERLAND) 1985, 13 (4) p187- 93

The treatment of social phobia. Real-life rehearsal with nonprofessional therapists. J Nerv Ment Dis (UNITED STATES) Mar 1981, 169 (3) p180-4

Premenstrual Syndrome

Refer to references under Menstrual Disorders-Premenstrual Syndrome.

Prevention Protocols

Management 1997 of chronic obstructive pulmonary disease. Working Group of the Swiss Society of Pneumology. Schweiz Med Wochenschr (SWITZERLAND) May 3 1997, 127 (18) p766-82

Chemoprevention of colorectal tumors: role of lactulose and of other agents. Scand J Gastroenterol Suppl (NORWAY) 1997, 222 p72-5

Biochemical basis of selenomethionine-mediated inhibition during 2-acetylaminofluorene-induced hepatocarcinogenesis in the rat. Eur J Cancer Prev (ENGLAND) Dec 1996, 5 (6) p455-63

Application of molecular epidemiology to lung cancer chemoprevention. J Cell Biochem Suppl (UNITED STATES) 1996, 25 p63-8

Effects of dietary vitamin C and E supplementation on the copper mediated oxidation of HDL and on HDL mediated cholesterol efflux. Atherosclerosis (IRELAND) Nov 15 1996, 127 (1) p19-26

Antioxidant actions of beta-carotene in liposomal and microsomal membranes: role of carotenoid-membrane incorporation and alpha-tocopherol. Arch Biochem Biophys (UNITED STATES) Feb 15 1997, 338 (2) p244-50

Comparative study of the effect of 21-aminosteroid and alpha-tocopherol on models of acute oxidative renal injury. Free Radic Biol Med (UNITED STATES) 1996, 21 (5) p691-7

Possible prevention of postangioplasty restenosis by ascorbic acid. Am J Cardiol (UNITED STATES) Dec

References

1 1996, 78 (11) p1284-6

Effectiveness of antioxidants (vitamin C and E) with and without sunscreens as topical photoprotectants. Acta Derm Venereol (NORWAY) Jul 1996, 76 (4) p264-8,

Curcumin protects against 4-hydroxy-2-trans-nonenal-induced cataract formation in rat lenses. Am J Clin Nutr (UNITED STATES) Nov 1996, 64 (5) p761-6

Prevention of asthma. Eur Respir J (DENMARK) Jul 1996, 9 (7) p1545-55

Role of oxidant stress in the adult respiratory distress syndrome: evaluation of a novel antioxidant strategy in a porcine model of endotoxin-induced acute lung injury. Shock (UNITED STATES) 1996, 6 Suppl 1 pS23-6

The new paradigm for coronary artery disease: altering risk factors, atherosclerotic plaques, and clinical prognosis. Mayo Clin Proc (UNITED STATES) Oct 1996, 71 (10) p957-65

Synergism between N-acetylcysteine and doxorubicin in the prevention of tumorigenicity and metastasis in murine models. Int J Cancer (UNITED STATES) Sep 17 1996, 67 (6) p842-8

Prevention of dopamine-induced cell death by thiol antioxidants: possible implications for treatment of Parkinson's disease. Exp Neurol (UNITED STATES) Sep 1996, 141 (1) p32-9

Effect of flavonoids on the outcome of myocardial mitochondrial ischemia/reperfusion injury. Res Commun Mol Pathol Pharmacol (UNITED STATES) Jan 1996, 91 (1) p65-75

[The dose-dependent effects of a combination of different classes of antioxidants exemplified by dibunol and beta-carotene]. Izv Akad Nauk Ser Biol (RUSSIA) Mar-Apr 1996, (2) p147-52

Oxidative damage and defense. Am J Clin Nutr (UNITED STATES) Jun 1996, 63 (6) p985S-990S

Dietary fiber and the chemopreventive modelation of colon carcinogenesis. Mutat Res (NETHERLANDS) Feb 19 1996, 350 (1) p185-97

Selenium: a quest for better understanding. Altern Ther Health Med (UNITED STATES) Jul 1996, 2 (4) p59-62, 65-7

[The Mediterranean diet in the prevention of arteriosclerosis]. Recenti Prog Med (ITALY) Apr 1996, 87 (4) p175-81

Change for coronary artery disease. What to tell patients. Postgrad Med (UNITED STATES) Feb 1996, 99 (2) p89-92, 95-6, 102-6

Population nutrient intake approaches dietary recommendations: 1991 to 1995 Framingham Nutrition Studies. J Am Diet Assoc (UNITED STATES) Jul 1997, 97 (7) p742-9

The antioxidant potential of the Mediterranean diet. Eur J Cancer Prev (ENGLAND) Mar 1997, 6 Suppl 1 pS15-9

[Atherogenic factors in the diet of the Costa Rican population, 1991]. Arch Latinoam Nutr (VENEZUELA) Mar 1996, 46 (1) p27-32

Vitamin C intake and cardiovascular disease risk factors in persons with non-insulin-dependent diabetes mellitus. From the Insulin Resistance Atherosclerosis Study and the San Luis Valley Diabetes Study. Prev Med (UNITED STATES) May-Jun 1997, 26 (3) p277-83

The effect of dietary fat, antioxidants, and pro-oxidants on blood lipids, lipoproteins, and atherosclerosis. J Am Diet Assoc (UNITED STATES) Jul 1997, 97 (7 Suppl) pS31-41

Reliability of a food frequency questionnaire to assess dietary antioxidant intake. Ophthalmic Epidemiol (NETHERLANDS) Mar 1997, 4 (1) p33-9

Oxidative stress hypothesis in Alzheimer's disease. Free Radic Biol Med (UNITED STATES) 1997, 23 (1) p134-47

Alcohol, ischemic heart disease, and the French paradox. Clin Cardiol (UNITED STATES) May 1997, 20 (5) p420-4

Dietary antioxidants and Parkinson disease. The Rotterdam Study. Arch Neurol (UNITED STATES) Jun 1997, 54 (6) p762-5

Anti-oxidants and coronary heart disease [letter]. S Afr Med J (SOUTH AFRICA) Jan 1997, 87 (1 Suppl) p103

Randomised trial of alpha-tocopherol and beta-carotene supplements on incidence of major coronary events in men with previous myocardial infraction. Lancet (ENGLAND) Jun 14 1997, 349 (9067) p1715-20

Anti-oxidant therapy for ischaemic heart disease: where do we stand? Lancet (ENGLAND) Jun 14 1997, 349 (9067) p1710-1

Lower ischemic heart disease incidence and mortality among vitamin supplement users. Can J Cardiol (CANADA) Oct 1996, 12 (10) p930-4

Association of serum vitamin levels, LDL susceptibility to oxidation, and autoantibodies against MDA-LDL with carotid atherosclerosis. A case-control study. The ARIC Study Investigators. Atherosclerosis Risk in Communities. Arterioscler Thromb Vasc Biol (UNITED STATES) Jun 1997, 17 (6) p1171-7

Validity of diagnoses of major coronary events in national registers of hospital diagnoses and deaths in Finland. Eur J Epidemiol (NETHERLANDS) Feb 1997, 13 (2) p133-8

Vitamin C and cardiovascular disease: a systematic review. J Cardiovasc Risk (ENGLAND) Dec 1996, 3 (6) p513-21

Biochemical basis of selenomethionine-mediated inhibition during 2-acetylaminofluorene-induced hepatocarcinogenesis in the rat. Eur J Cancer Prev (ENGLAND) Dec 1996, 5 (6) p455-63

Glutathione transferases catalyse the detoxication of oxidized metabolites (o-quinones) of catecholamines and may serve as an antioxidant system preventing degenerative cellular processes. Biochem J (ENGLAND) May 15 1997, 324 (Pt 1) p25-8

Nutrition and newly emerging viral diseases: an overview. J Nutr (UNITED STATES) May 1997, 127 (5 Suppl) p948S-950S

Pathogenesis and treatment of liver fibrosis in alcoholics: 1996 update. Dig Dis (SWITZERLAND) Jan-Apr 1997, 15 (1-2) p42-66

Adenocarcinomas of the esophagus and gastric cardia: the role of diet. Nutr Cancer (UNITED STATES) 1997, 27 (3) p298-309

Vitamin C, neutrophil function, and upper respiratory tract infection risk in distance runners: the missing link. Exerc Immunol Rev (UNITED STATES) 1997, 3 p32-5

Equine degenerative myeloencephalopathy. Vet Clin North Am Equine Pract (UNITED STATES) Apr 1997, 13 (1) p43-52

Intake of fatty acids and risk of coronary heart disease in a cohort of Finnish men. The Alpha-Tocopherol, Beta-Carotene Cancer Prevention Study. Am J Epidemiol (UNITED STATES) May 15 1997, 145 (10) p876-87

Functional effects of food components and the gastrointestinal system: chicory fructooligosaccharides. Nutr Rev (UNITED STATES) Nov 1996, 54 (11 Pt 2) pS38-42

[Coronary heart disease--a free radical associated disease? What is the value of antioxidant substances?]. Med Monatsschr Pharm (GERMANY) Mar 1997, 20 (3) p66-70

Antioxidant flavonols and ischemic heart disease in a Welsh population of men: the Caerphilly Study. Am J Clin Nutr (UNITED STATES) May 1997, 65 (5) p1489-94

[Vitamin E as a possible aid in the control of disease problems on pig farms: a field test]. Tijdschr Diergeneeskd (NETHERLANDS) Apr 1 1997, 122 (7) p190-2

Antioxidants and dementia. Lancet (ENGLAND) Apr 26 1997, 349 (9060) p1189-90

[Is supplemental vitamin E for prevention of coronary heart disease ov value?]. Internist (Berl) (GERMANY) Feb 1997, 38 (2) p168-76; discussion 176

The 'diet heart' hypothesis in secondary prevention of coronary heart disease. Eur Heart J (ENGLAND) Jan 1997, 18 (1) p13-8

Tea and health: a historical perspective. Cancer Lett (IRELAND) Mar 19 1997, 114 (1-2) p315-7

[Prevalence and risk factors in the population of Graz (Austrian Stroke Prevention Study)]. Wien Med Wochenschr (AUSTRIA) 1997, 147 (2) p36-40

Beta-2-agonists have antioxidant function in vitro. 2. The effect of beta-2-agonists on oxidant-mediated cytotoxicity and on superoxide anion generated by human polymorphonuclear leukocytes. Respiration (SWITZERLAND) 1997, 64 (1) p23-8

Antioxidant vitamins and cardiovascular disease: current perspectives and future directions [editorial]. Eur Heart J (ENGLAND) Feb 1997, 18 (2) p177-9

Protective effects of silymarin against photocarcinogenesis in a mouse skin model. J Natl Cancer Inst (UNITED STATES) Apr 16 1997, 89 (8) p556-66

Which changes in diet prevent coronary heart disease? A review of clinical trials of dietary fats and antioxidants. Acta Cardiol (BELGIUM) 1996, 51 (6) p467-90

Antioxidants in the prevention of atherosclerosis. Curr Opin Lipidol (UNITED STATES) Dec 1996, 7 (6) p374-80

[Cardio-protective effect of red wine as reflected in the literature]. Orv Hetil (HUNGARY) Mar 16 1997, 138 (11) p673-8

Tea and heart disease [letter]. Lancet (ENGLAND) Mar 8 1997, 349 (9053) p735

Application of molecular epidemiology to lung cancer chemoprevention. J Cell Biochem Suppl (UNITED STATES) 1996, 25 p63-8

Cancer risk factors for selecting cohorts for large-scale chemoprevention trials. J Cell Biochem Suppl

(UNITED STATES) 1996, 25 p29-36

Protection against induction of mouse skin papillomas with low and high risk of conversion to malignancy by green tea polyphenols. Carcinogenesis (ENGLAND) Mar 1997, 18 (3) p497-502

Effects of dietary vitamin C and E supplementation on the copper mediated oxidation of HDL and on HDL mediated cholesterol efflux. Atherosclerosis (IRELAND) Nov 15 1996, 127 (1) p19-26

Efficacy of a dentifrice and oral rinse containing sanguinaria extract in conjunction with initial periodontal therapy. Aust Dent J (AUSTRALIA) Feb 1997, 42 (1) p47-51

The impact of zinc supplementation on Schistosoma mansoni reinfection rate and intensities: a randomized, controlled trial among rural Zimbabwean schoolchildren. Eur J Clin Nutr (ENGLAND) Jan 1997, 51 (1) p33-7

Methylenetetrahydrofolate reductase polymorphism, dietary interactions, and risk of colorectal cancer. Cancer Res (UNITED STATES) Mar 15 1997, 57 (6) p1098-102

Nutrition in women. Assessment and counseling. Prim Care (UNITED STATES) Mar 1997, 24 (1) p37-51

Hypertension and borderline isolated systolic hypertension increase risks of cardiovascular disease and mortality in male physicians. Circulation (UNITED STATES) Mar 4 1997, 95 (5) p1132-7

Bronchial reactivity and dietary antioxidants. Thorax (ENGLAND) Feb 1997, 52 (2) p166-70

Effects of bisaramil on coronary-occlusion-reperfusion injury and free-radical-induced reactions. Pharmacol Res (ENGLAND) Jun 1996, 33 (6) p327-36

Whole-grain consumption and chronic disease: protective mechanisms. Nutr Cancer (UNITED STATES) 1997, 27 (1) p14-21

Dietary manipulation of plasma carotenoid concentrations of squirrel monkeys (Saimiri sciureus). J Nutr (UNITED STATES) Jan 1997, 127 (1) p122-9

Mechanisms of spontaneous human cancers. Environ Health Perspect (UNITED STATES) May 1996, 104 Suppl 3 p633-7

Molecular epidemiology in environmental carcinogenesis. Environ Health Perspect (UNITED STATES) May 1996, 104 Suppl 3 p441-3

Vitamin C intake and susceptibility to the common cold. Br J Nutr (ENGLAND) Jan 1997, 77 (1) p59-72

Antioxidant actions of beta-carotene in liposomal and microsomal membranes: role of carotenoid-membrane incorporation and alpha-tocopherol. Arch Biochem Biophys (UNITED STATES) Feb 15 1997, 338 (2) p244-50

[Alcohol and free radicals: from basic research to clinical prospects]. Ann Gastroenterol Hepatol (Paris) (FRANCE) May-Jun 1996, 32 (3) p128-33; discussion 133-4

Melatonin reduces mortality from Aleutian disease in mink (Mustela vison). J Pineal Res (DENMARK) Nov 1996, 21 (4) p214-7

Exercise causes blood glutathione oxidation in chronic obstructive pulmonary disease: prevention by O2 therapy. J Appl Physiol (UNITED STATES) Nov 1996, 81 (5) p2198-202

Comparative study of the effect of 21-aminosteroid and alpha-tocopherol on models of acute oxidative renal injury. Free Radic Biol Med (UNITED STATES) 1996, 21 (5) p691-7

Prospective study of moderate alcohol consumption and risk of peripheral arterial disease in US male physicians. Circulation (UNITED STATES) Feb 4 1997, 95 (3) p577-80

Oxidized low-density lipoprotein and atherosclerosis. Int J Clin Lab Res (GERMANY) 1996, 26 (3) p178-84

Serum levels of antioxidant vitamins in relation to coronary artery disease: a case control study of Koreans. Biomed Environ Sci (UNITED STATES) Sep 1996, 9 (2-3) p229-35

Antioxidants in food and chronic degenerative diseases. Biomed Environ Sci (UNITED STATES) Sep 1996, 9 (2-3) p117-23

Randomized trials of dietary antioxidants in cardiovascular disease prevention and treatment. J Cardiovasc Risk (ENGLAND) Aug 1996, 3 (4) p368-71

Basic research in antioxidant inhibition of steps in atherogenesis. J Cardiovasc Risk (ENGLAND) Aug 1996, 3 (4) p352-7

General background on diet and cancer. ECP (UK) Headquarters, Lady Sobell GI Unit, Wexham Park Hospital 1996, 5 (5) p 413-4

Oxidative susceptibility of low-density lipoproteins--influence of regular alcohol use. Alcohol Clin Exp Res (UNITED STATES) Sep 1996, 20 (6) p980-4

Molecular epidemiology and retinoid chemoprevention of head and neck cancer. J Natl Cancer Inst (UNITED STATES) Feb 5 1997, 89 (3) p199-211

Do hydroxy-carotenoids prevent coronary heart disease? A comparison between Belfast and Toulouse. Int J Vitam Nutr Res (SWITZERLAND) 1996, 66 (2) p113-8

Role of dietary phyto oestrogens in the protection against cancer and heart disease. Biochem Soc Trans (ENGLAND) Aug 1996, 24 (3) p795-800

Role of dietary flavonoids in protection against cancer and coronary heart disease. Biochem Soc Trans (ENGLAND) Aug 1996, 24 (3) p785-9

Can carotenoids reduce oxidation-induced cataract? Biochem Soc Trans (ENGLAND) Aug 1996, 24 (3) p385S

Rationale and design of a large study to evaluate the renal and cardiovascular effects of an ACE inhibitor and vitamin E in high-risk patients with diabetes. The MICRO-HOPE Study. Microalbuminuria, cardiovascular, and renal outcomes. Heart Outcomes Prevention Evaluation. Diabetes Care (UNITED STATES) Nov 1996, 19 (11) p1225-8

Vitamin E ameliorates renal injury in an experimental model of immunoglobulin A nephropathy. Pediatr Res (UNITED STATES) Oct 1996, 40 (4) p620-6

Demonstration of organotropic effects of chemopreventive agents in multiorgan carcinogenesis models. IARC Sci Publ (FRANCE) 1996, (139) p143-50

The Leon Golberg Memorial Lecture. Antioxidants and disease prevention. Food Chem Toxicol (ENGLAND) Oct 1996, 34 (10) p1013-20

Effect of nicotine on antioxidant defence mechanisms in rats fed a high-fat diet. Pharmacology (SWITZERLAND) Mar 1996, 52 (3) p153-8

New carotenoid values for foods improve relationship of food frequency questionnaire intake estimates to plasma values. Cancer Epidemiol Biomarkers Prev (UNITED STATES) Nov 1996, 5 (11) p907-12

Wheat kernel ingestion protects from progression of muscle weakness in mdx mice, an animal model of Duchenne muscular dystrophy. Pediatr Res (UNITED STATES) Sep 1996, 40 (3) p444-9

Effects of the 21-amino steroid tirilazad mesylate (U-74006F) on brain damdema after perinatal hypoxia-ischemia in the rat. Pediatr Res (UNITED STATES) Sep 1996, 40 (3) p399-403

What dose of vitamin E is required to reduce susceptibility of LDL to oxidation? Aust N Z J Med (AUSTRALIA) Aug 1996, 26 (4) p496-503

Preliminary studies on the isolation and characterization of predominant prostatic proteins. Department of Veterans Affairs Medical Center, Bay Pines Flo) Dec 1996, 2 9 (6) p381-5

Cardioprotective effects of individual conjugated equine estrogens through their possible modulation of insulin resistance and oxidation of low-density lipoprotein. Fertil Steril (UNITED STATES) Jan 1997, 67 (1) p57-62

Antioxidants in cardiovascular disease: randomized trials. Nutrition (UNITED STATES) Sep 1996, 12 (9) p583-8

Possible prevention of postangioplasty restenosis by ascorbic acid. Am J Cardiol (UNITED STATES) Dec 1 1996, 78 (11) p1284-6

Does coronary artery screening by electron beam computed tomography motivate potentially beneficial lifestyle behaviors? [see comments]. Am J Cardiol (UNITED STATES) Dec 1 1996, 78 (11) p1220-3, Comment in Am J Cardiol 1996 Dec 1;78(11):1265-6

Inhibition of steroid-induced cataract in rat eyes by administration of vitamin-E ophthalmic solution. Ophthalmic Res (SWITZERLAND) 1996, 28 Suppl 2 p64-71

Anticataract action of vitamin E: its estimation using an in vitro steroid cataract model. Ophthalmic Res (SWITZERLAND) 1996, 28 Suppl 2 p16-25

[Effect of antioxidants on the relative risk of coronary heart disease]. Harefuah (ISRAEL) Nov 15 1996, 131 (10) p408-12

randomized trial of antioxidants in the primary prevention of Alzheimer disease warranted? Alzheimer Dis Assoc Disord (UNITED STATES) Fall 1996, 10 Suppl 1 p45-9

Effectiveness of antioxidants (vitamin C and E) with and without sunscreens as topical photoprotectants. Acta Derm Venereol (NORWAY) Jul 1996, 76 (4) p264-8

Human nutrition and its discontents: a personal view. Perspect Biol Med (UNITED STATES) Autumn 1996, 40 (1) p1-6

Inhibitory effect of a traditional Chinese medicine, Juzen-taiho-to, on progressive growth of weakly malignant clone cells derived from murine fibrosarcoma. Jpn J Cancer Res (JAPAN) Oct 1996, 87 (10) p1039-44

Diet and the prevention and treatment of breast cancer. Altern Ther Health Med (UNITED STATES) Nov 1996, 2 (6) p32-8

Beyond cholesterol reduction in coronary heart disease: is vitamin E the answer? Heart (ENGLAND) Oct 1996, 76 (4) p293-4

Influence of heat shock protein 70 and metallothionein induction by zinc-bis-(DL-hydrogenaspartate) on the release of inflammatory mediators in a porcine model of recurrent endotoxemia. Biochem Pharmacol (ENGLAND) Oct 25 1996, 52 (8) p1201-10

Intake of dietary fiber and risk of coronary heart disease in a cohort of Finnish men. The Alpha-Tocopherol, Beta-Carotene Cancer Prevention Study. Circulation (UNITED STATES) Dec 1 1996, 94 (11) p2720-7

The hypocholesterolemic and antiatherogenic effects of topically applied phosphatidylcholine in rabbits with heritable hypercholesterolemia. Artery (UNITED STATES) 1996, 22 (1) p1-23

Curcumin protects against 4-hydroxy-2-trans-nonenal-induced cataract formation in rat lenses. Am J Clin Nutr (UNITED STATES) Nov 1996, 64 (5) p761-6

Delayed tumor onset in transgenic mice fed an amino acid-based diet supplemented with red wine solids. Am J Clin Nutr (UNITED STATES) Nov 1996, 64 (5) p748-56

Study design and baseline characteristics of the study to evaluate carotid ultrasound changes in patients treated with ramipril and vitamin E: SECURE. Am J Cardiol (UNITED STATES) Oct 15 1996, 78 (8) p914-9

Ascorbic acid and atherosclerotic cardiovascular disease. Subcell Biochem (ENGLAND) 1996, 25 p331-67

Increased pancreatic metallothionein and glutathione levels: protecting against cerulein- and tauro-cholate-induced acute pancreatitis in rats. Pancreas (UNITED STATES) Aug 1996, 13 (2) p173-83

Inhibition of LDL oxidation by cocoa [letter]. Lancet (ENGLAND) Nov 30 1996, 348 (9040) p1514

Alpha-Tocopherol and beta-carotene supplements and lung cancer incidence in the alpha-tocopherol, beta-carotene cancer prevention study: effects of base-line characteristics and study compliance [see comments]. J Natl Cancer Inst (UNITED STATES) Nov 6 1996, 88 (21) p1560-70

Risk factors for lung cancer and for intervention effects in CARET, the Beta-Carotene and Retinol Efficacy Trial [see comments]. J Natl Cancer Inst (UNITED STATES) Nov 6 1996, 88 (21) p1550-9

Inhibition of phagocyte-endothelium interactions by oxidized fatty acids: a natural anti-inflammatory mechanism? J Lab Clin Med (UNITED STATES) Jul 1996, 128 (1) p27-38

Effect of a mediterranean type of diet on the rate of cardiovascular complications in patients with coronary artery disease. Insights into the cardioprotective effect of certain nutriments [see comments]. J Am Coll Cardiol (UNITED STATES) Nov 1 1996, 28 (5) p1103-8

Lipid peroxidation and antioxidant vitamins C and E in hypertensive patients. Ir J Med Sci (IRELAND) Jul-Sep 1996, 165 (3) p210-2

[Alcohol, lipid metabolism and coronary heart disease]. Herz (GERMANY) Aug 1996, 21 (4) p217-26

Prevention of asthma. Eur Respir J (DENMARK) Jul 1996, 9 (7) p1545-55

Epidemiological evidence for beta-carotene in prevention of cancer and cardiovascular disease. Eur J Clin Nutr (ENGLAND) Jul 1996, 50 Suppl 3 pS57-61

Selenium as a risk factor for cardiovascular diseases. J Cardiovasc Risk (ENGLAND) Feb 1996, 3 (1) p42-7

Role of oxidant stress in the adult respiratory distress syndrome: evaluation of a novel antioxidant strategy in a porcine model of endotoxin-induced acute lung injury. Shock (UNITED STATES) 1996, 6 Suppl 1 pS23-6

Zinc administration prevents wasting in stressed mice. Arch Med Res (MEXICO) Autumn 1996, 27 (3) p319-25

Vitamin E in humans: demand and delivery. Annu Rev Nutr (UNITED STATES) 1996, 16 p321-47

The resistance of low density lipoprotein to oxidation promoted by copper and its use as an index of antioxidant therapy. Atherosclerosis (IRELAND) Jan 26 1996, 119 (2) p169-79

[Selenium, glutathione peroxidase, peroxides and platelet functions]. Ann Biol Clin (Paris) (FRANCE) 1996, 54 (5) p181-7

Is there a fountain of youth? A review of current life extension strategies. Pharmacotherapy (UNITED STATES) Mar-Apr 1996, 16 (2) p183-200

Pathogenic mechanisms in familial amyotrophic lateral sclerosis due to mutation of Cu, Zn superoxide dismutase. Pathol Biol (Paris) (FRANCE) Jan 1996, 44 (1) p51-6

Update on dietary antioxidants and cancer. Pathol Biol (Paris) (FRANCE) Jan 1996, 44 (1) p42-5

Antioxidants in cardiovascular disease: randomized trials. Nutr Rev (UNITED STATES) Jun 1996, 54 (6) p175-7

Advances in diagnosis and treatment of cancer and cardiovascular disease as well as increased understanding of the mechanisms of the diseases have provided and will certainly continue to provide enormous benefit to affected individuals. At the same time, interventions that may prevent common cancers or atherosclerosis from developing in healthy people could, at least in theory, afford even greater benefits to society as a whole. (6 The new paradigm for coronary artery disease: altering risk factors, atherosclerotic plaques, and clinical prognosis. Mayo Clin Proc (UNITED STATES) Oct 1996, 71 (10) p957-65

Deliberations and evaluations of the approaches, endpoints and paradigms for selenium and iodine dietary recommendations. J Nutr (UNITED STATES) Sep 1996, 126 (9 Suppl) p2427S-2434S

Antioxidants in health and disease [see comments]. J Am Optom Assoc (UNITED STATES) Jan 1996, 67 (1) p50-7

Multicenter ophthalmic and nutritional age-related macular degeneration study--part 2: antioxidant intervention and conclusions. J Am Optom Assoc (UNITED STATES) Jan 1996, 67 (1) p30-49

Multicenter ophthalmic and nutritional age-related macular degeneration study--part 1: design, subjects and procedures. J Am Optom Assoc (UNITED STATES) Jan 1996, 67 (1) p12-29

Vegetables, fruit, and cancer prevention: a review. J Am Diet Assoc (UNITED STATES) Oct 1996, 96 (10) p1027-39

Synergism between N-acetylcysteine and doxorubicin in the prevention of tumorigenicity and metastasis in murine models. Int J Cancer (UNITED STATES) Sep 17 1996, 67 (6) p842-8

Chemoprevention of stomach cancer. IARC Sci Publ (FRANCE) 1996, (136) p35-9

Prevention of dopamine-induced cell death by thiol antioxidants: possible implications for treatment of Parkinson's disease. Exp Neurol (UNITED STATES) Sep 1996, 141 (1) p32-9

Effect of flavonoids on the outcome of myocardial mitochondrial ischemia/reperfusion injury. Res Commun Mol Pathol Pharmacol (UNITED STATES) Jan 1996, 91 (1) p65-75

The Inuit diet. Fatty acids and antioxidants, their role in ischemic heart disease, and exposure to organochlorines and heavy metals. An internatedersen. Arctic Med Res (FINLAND) 1996, 55 Suppl 1 p20-4

All vitamins, cancer, and cardiovascular disease [letter]. N Engl J Med (UNITED STATES) Oct 3 1996, 335 (14) p1066-7

Antioxidant vitamins, cancer, and cardiovascular disease [letter]. N Engl J Med (UNITED STATES) Oct 3 1996, 335 (14) p1065-6

[The dose-dependent effects of a combination of different classes of antioxidants exemplified by dibunol and beta-carotene]. Izv Akad Nauk Ser Biol (RUSSIA) Mar-Apr 1996, (2) p147-52

Nutritional support to prevent and treat multiple organ failure. World J Surg (UNITED STATES) May 1996, 20 (4) p474-81

Oxidative damage and defense. Am J Clin Nutr (UNITED STATES) Jun 1996, 63 (6) p985S-990S

Do antioxidant micronutrients protect against the development and progression of knee osteoarthritis? Arthritis Rheum (UNITED STATES) Apr 1996, 39 (4) p648-56

Beta-carotene, carotenoids, and disease prevention in humans. FASEB J (UNITED STATES) May 1996, 10 (7) p690-701

Vegetable, fruit, and cereal fiber intake and risk of coronary heart disease among men [see comments]. JAMA (UNITED STATES) Feb 14 1996, 275 (6) p447-51

Dietary non-tocopherol antioxidants present in extra virgin olive oil increase the resistance of low density lipoproteins to oxidation in rabbits. Atherosclerosis (IRELAND) Feb 1996, 120 (1-2) p15-23

Antioxidants, Helicobacter pylori and stomach cancer in Venezuela. Eur J Cancer Prev (ENGLAND) Feb 1996, 5 (1) p57-62

Dietary fiber and the chemopreventive modelation of colon carcinogenesis. Mutat Res (NETHERLANDS) Feb 19 1996, 350 (1) p185-97

Antioxidant vitamins, cancer, and cardiovascular disease [editorial; comment]. N Engl J Med (UNITED STATES) May 2 1996, 334 (18) p1189-90, 10/L/184

Effects of a combination of beta carotene and vitamin A on lung cancer and cardiovascular disease [see comments]. N Engl J Med (UNITED STATES) May 2 1996, 334 (18) p1150-5

Lack of effect of long-term supplementation with beta carotene on the incidence of malignant neoplasms and cardiovascular disease [see comments]. N Engl J Med (UNITED STATES) May 2 1996, 334 (18) p1145-9

Ascorbic acid protects against male infertility in a teleost fish. Experientia (SWITZERLAND) Feb 15 1996, 52 (2) p97-100

Clinical evaluation of in-feed zinc bacitracin for the control of porcine intestinal adenomatosis in growing/fattening pigs. Vet Rec (ENGLAND) May 18 1996, 138 (20) p489-92

The effect of modest vitamin E supplementation on lipid peroxidation products and other cardiovascular risk factors in diabetic patients. Lipids (UNITED STATES) Mar 1996, 31 Suppl pS87-90

The role of oxidized lipoproteins in atherogenesis. Free Radic Biol Med (UNITED STATES) 1996, 20 (5) p707-27

Inhibition of naphthalene cataract in rats by aldose reductase inhibitors. Curr Eye Res (ENGLAND) Apr 1996, 15 (4) p423-32

Selenium: a quest for better understanding. Altern Ther Health Med (UNITED STATES) Jul 1996, 2 (4) p59-62, 65-7

Primary and secondary prevention of myocardial infarction. Clin Exp Hypertens (UNITED STATES) Apr-May 1996, 18 (3-4) p547-58

Tuberculosis in Siberia: 2. Diagnosis, chemoprophylaxis and treatment. Tuber Lung Dis (SCOTLAND) Aug 1996, 77

Antioxidants, oxidants and free radical stress in cardiovascular disease. J Assoc Physicians India (INDIA) Jan 1996, 44 (1) p43-8

Lipid peroxidation: a review of causes, consequences, measurement and dietary influences. Int J Food Sci Nutr (ENGLAND) May 1996, 47 (3) p233-61

Female lung cancer. Annu Rev Public Health (UNITED STATES) 1996, 17 p97-114

The role of metals in ischemia/reperfusion injury of the liver. Semin Liver Dis (UNITED STATES) Feb 1996, 16 (1) p31-8

[Bronchopulmonary dysplasia]. Rev Mal Respir (FRANCE) Jul 1996, 13 (3) p243-9

[LDL oxidation in homozygous familial hypercholesterolemia: effects of selective LDL-apheresis treatment]. Cardiologia (ITALY) May 1996, 41 (5) p435-9

Dietary antioxidants in disease prevention. Nat Prod Rep (ENGLAND) Aug 1996, 13 (4) p265-73

Oxidative stress as a mechanism of cardiac failure in chronic volume overload in canine model. J Mol Cell Cardiol (ENGLAND) Feb 1996, 28 (2) p375-85

Vascular incorporation of alpha-tocopherol prevents endothelial dysfunction due to oxidized LDL by inhibiting protein kinase C stimulation. J Clin Invest (UNITED STATES) Jul 15 1996, 98 (2) p386-94

[The significance of ixidized low density lipoprotein in atherosclerosis]. Ugeskr Laeger (DENMARK) May 6 1996, 158 (19) p2706-10

Nutrition and immunity with emphasis on infection and autoimmune disease. Nutr Health (ENGLAND) 1996, 10 (4) p285-312

In vivo antioxidant treatment suppresses nuclear factor-kappa B activation and neutrophilic lung inflammation. J Immunol (UNITED STATES) Aug 15 1996, 157 (4) p1630-7

Effect of radiation on red cell membrane and intracellular oxidative defense systems. Free Radic Res (SWITZERLAND) Mar 1996, 24 (3) p199-204

Oxidatively modified LDL and atherosclerosis: an evolving plausible scenario. Crit Rev Food Sci Nutr

(UNITED STATES) Apr 1996, 36 (4) p341-55

The effects of alpha tocopherol supplementation on monocyte function. Decreased lipid oxidation, interleukin 1 beta secretion, and monocyte adhesion to endothelium. J Clin Invest (UNITED STATES) Aug 1 1996, 98 (3) p756-63

Metallopanstimulin as a novel tumor marker in sera of patients with various types of common cancers: implications for prevention and therapy. Anticancer Res (GREECE) Jul-Aug 1996, 16 (4B) p2177-85

Antioxidants and age-related eye disease. Current and future perspectives. Ann Epidemiol (UNITED STATES) Jan 1996, 6 (1) p60-6

Hyperlipidemia. When does treatment make a difference? Postgrad Med (UNITED STATES) Jul 1996, 100 (1) p138-49

[Free radicals in the central nervous system]. Cesk Fysiol (CZECH REPUBLIC) Mar 1996, 45 (1) p4-12

[Can vitamin E prevent development of coronary heart disease?]. Tidsskr Nor Laegeforen (NORWAY) Mar 30 1996, 116 (9) p1109-13

Protection by multiple antioxidants against lipid peroxidation in rat liver homogenate. Lipids (UNITED STATES) Jan 1996, 31 (1) p47-50

Effect of selenium on 1,2-dimethylhydrazine-induced intestinal cancer in rats. Dis Colon Rectum (UNITED STATES) Jun 1996, 39 (6) p628-31

[The Mediterranean diet in the prevention of arteriosclerosis]. Recenti Prog Med (ITALY) Apr 1996, 87 (4) p175-81

Serum high density lipoprotein cholesterol, alcohol, and coronary mortality in male smokers [see comments]. BMJ (ENGLAND) May 11 1996, 312 (7040) p1200-3

Lifestyle change for coronary artery disease. What to tell patients. Postgrad Med (UNITED STATES) Feb 1996, 99 (2) p89-92, 95-6, 102-6

Inhibition of Ca2+-pump ATPase and the Na+/K+-pump ATPase by iron-generated free radicals. Protection by 6,7-dimethyl-2,4-DI-1-pyrrolidinyl-7H-pyrrolo[2,3-d] pyrimidine sulfate (U-89843D), a potent, novel, antioxidant/free radical scavenger. Biochem Pharmacol (ENGLAND) Feb 23 1996, 51 (4) p471-6

Long-term oral vitamin E supplementation in cystic fibrosis patients: RRR-alpha-tocopherol compared with all-rac-alpha-tocopheryl acetate preparations. Am J Clin Nutr (UNITED STATES) May 1996, 63 (5) p722-8

The HOPE (Heart Outcomes Prevention Evaluation) Study: the design of a large, simple randomized trial of an angiotensin-converting enzyme inhibitor (ramipril) and vitamin E in patients at high risk of cardiovascular events. The HOPE study investigators. Can J Cardiol (CANADA) Feb 1996, 12 (2) p127-37

Dietary antioxidant vitamins and death from coronary heart disease in postmenopausal women [see comments]. N Engl J Med (UNITED STATES) May 2 1996, 334 (18) p1156-62

Mortality associated with low plasma concentration of beta carotene and the effect of oral supplementation. JAMA (UNITED STATES) Mar 6 1996, 275 (9) p699-703

Effect of vitamin E and beta carotene on the incidence of angina pectoris. A randomized, double-blind, controlled trial. JAMA (UNITED STATES) Mar 6 1996, 275 (9) p693-8

[Overview--suppression effect of essential trace elements on arteriosclerotic development and it's mechanism]. Nippon Rinsho (JAPAN) Jan 1996, 54 (1) p59-66

Prevention of doxorubicin induced cardiotoxicity by catechin. Cancer Lett (IRELAND) Jan 19 1996, 99 (1) p1-6

Relative resistance of the hamster to aortic atherosclerosis in spite of prolonged vitamin E deficiency and dietary hypercholesterolemia. Putative effect of increased HDL? Biochim Biophys Acta (NETHERLANDS) Jan 19 1996, 1299 (2) p216-22

Gastroprotective activity of melatonin and its precursor, L-tryptophan, against stress-induced and ischaemia-induced lesions is mediated by scavenge of oxygen radicals. Scand J Gastroenterol (NORWAY) May 1997, 32 (5) p433-8

Comparison between dietary soybean protein and casein of the inhibiting effect on atherogenesis in the thoracic aorta of hypercholesterolemic (ExHC) rats treated with experimental hypervitarnin D. Biosci Biotechnol Biochem (JAPAN) Mar 1997, 61 (3) p514-9

Melatonin: media hype or therapeutic breakthrough? Nurse Pract (UNITED STATES) Feb 1997, 22 (2) p66-7, 71-2, 77

[Guidelines of drug therapies for Parkinson's disease]. Nippon Rinsho (JAPAN) Jan 1997, 55 (1) p52-7

Myocardium-protective effects of Ginkgo biloba extract (EGb 761) in old rats against acute isobaric hypoxia. An electron microscopic morphometric study. II. Protection of microvascular endothelium. Exp Toxicol Pathol (GERMANY) Jan 1996, 48 (1) p81-6

Myocardium-protective effects of Ginkgo biloba extract (EGb 761) in old rats against acute isobaric hypoxia. An electron microscopic morphometric study. I. Protection of cardiomyocytes. Exp Toxicol Pathol (GERMANY) Jan 1996, 48 (1) p33-9

The effect of coenzyme Q10 on infarct size in a rabbit model of ischemia/reperfusion. Cardiovasc Res (NETHERLANDS) Nov 1996, 32 (5) p861-8

Prevention of cytokine-induced hypotension in cancer patients by the pineal hormone melatonin. Support Care Cancer (GERMANY) Jul 1996, 4 (4) p313-6

Protection by coenzyme Q10 of tissue reperfusion injury during abdominal aortic cross-clamping. J Cardiovasc Surg (Torino) (ITALY) Jun 1996, 37 (3) p229-35

A review of the clinical effects of phytoestrogens. Obstet Gynecol (UNITED STATES) May 1996, 87 (5 Pt 2) p897-904

Protection by multiple antioxidants against lipid peroxidation in rat liver homogenate. Lipids (UNITED STATES) Jan 1996, 31 (1) p47-50

The making of a user friendly MAOI diet. J Clin Psychiatry (UNITED STATES) Mar 1996, 57 (3) p99-104

Neuroprotective strategy for Alzheimer disease: intranasal administration of a fatty neuropeptide. Proc Natl Acad Sci U S A (UNITED STATES) Jan 9 1996, 93 (1) p427-32

Effects of green tea catechins (Polyphenon 100) on cerulein-induced acute pancreatitis in rats. Pancreas (UNITED STATES) Apr 1997, 14 (3) p276-9

Characterization of early pulmonary hyperproliferation and tumor progression and their inhibition by black tea in a 4-(methylnitrosamino)-1-(3-pyridyl)-1-butanone-induced lung tumorigenesis model with

References

A/J mice. Cancer Res (UNITED STATES) May 15 1997, 57 (10) p1889-94

Tea and health: a historical perspective. Cancer Lett (IRELAND) Mar 19 1997, 114 (1-2) p315-7

[Cardio-protective effect of red wine as reflected in the literature]. Orv Hetil (HUNGARY) Mar 16 1997, 138 (11) p673-8

Delayed tumor onset in transgenic mice fed an amino acid-based diet supplemented with red wine solids. Am J Clin Nutr (UNITED STATES) Nov 1996, 64 (5) p748-56

[Alcohol, lipid metabolism and coronary heart disease]. Herz (GERMANY) Aug 1996, 21 (4) p217-26

Oxidative damage and defense. Am J Clin Nutr (UNITED STATES) Jun 1996, 63 (6) p985S-990S

Dietary non-tocopherol antioxidants present in extra virgin olive oil increase the resistance of low density lipoproteins to oxidation in rabbits. Atherosclerosis (IRELAND) Feb 1996, 120 (1-2) p15-23

Chemopreventive effects of green and black tea on pulmonary and hepatic carcinogenesis. Fundam Appl Toxicol (UNITED STATES) Feb 1996, 29 (2) p244-50Increased brain damage after stroke or excitotoxic seizures in melatonin-deficient rats. FASEB Journal (USA), 1996, 10/13 (1546-1551)

Oxidative damage caused by free radicals produced during catecholamine autoxidation: Protective effects of O-methylation and melatonin. Free Radical Biology and Medicine (USA), 1996, 21/2 (241-249)

Oxidative processes and antioxidative defense mechanisms in the aging brain. FASEB Journal (USA), 1995, 9/7 (526-533)

Melatonin, hydroxyl radical-mediated oxidative damage, and aging: A hypothesis. J. PINEAL RES. (Denmark), 1993, 14/4 (151-168)

Neuroimmunotherapy of human cancer with interleukin-2 and the neurohormone melatonin: Its efficacy in preventing hypotension. ANTICANCER RES. (Greece), 1990, 10/6 (1759-1761)

Loss of delta-6-desaturase activity as a key factor in aging. MED. HYPOTHESES (ENGLAND), 1981, 7/9 (1211-1220)

Betaine:homocysteine methyltransferase - A new assay for the liver enzyme and its absence from human skin fibroblasts and peripheral blood lymphocytes. CLIN. CHIM. ACTA (Netherlands), 1991, 204/1-3 (239-250)

Dimethylglycine and chemically related amines tested for mutagenicity under potential nitrosation conditions. MUTAT. RES. (Netherlands), 1989, 222/4 (343-350)

Homocystinuria due to cystathionine beta-synthase deficiency - The effects of betaine treatment in pyridoxine-responsive patients. METAB. CLIN. EXP. (USA), 1985, 34/12 (1115-1121)

Prevention of strychnine-induced seizures and death by the N-methylated glycine derivatives betaine, dimethylglycine and sarcosine. PHARMACOL. BIOCHEM. BEHAV. (USA), 1985, 22/4 (641-643)

Serenoa repens (Permixon (R)). A review of its pharmacology and therapeutic efficacy in benign prostatic hyperplasia. Drugs and Aging (New Zealand), 1996, 9/5 (379-395)

The extract of serenoa repens in the treatment of benign prostatic hyperplasia: A multicenter open study. CURR. THER. RES. CLIN. EXP. (USA), 1994, 55/7 (776-785)

Influence of dietary components on occurrence of and mortality due to neoplasms in male F344 rats. Aging - Clinical and Experimental Research (Italy), 1996, 8/4 (254-262)

Soy isoflavonoids and cancer prevention: Underlying biochemical and pharmacological issues. Advances in Experimental Medicine and Biology (USA), 1996, 401/-(87-100)

A review of the clinical effects of phytoestrogens. Obstetrics and Gynecology (USA), 1996, 87/5 II SUPPL. (897-904)

Perspectives on soy protein as a nonpharmacological approach for lowering cholesterol. Journal of Nutrition (USA), 1995, 125/3 SUPPL. (675S-678S)

Overview: Dietary approaches for reducing cardiovascular disease risks. Journal of Nutrition (USA), 1995, 125/3 SUPPL. (656S-665S)

Protective effects of soy protein on the peroxidizability of lipoproteins in cerebrovascular diseases. Journal of Nutrition (USA), 1995, 125/3 SUPPL. (639S-646S)

Modern applications for an ancient bean: Soybeans and the prevention and treatment of chronic disease. Journal of Nutrition (USA), 1995, 125/3 SUPPL. (567S-569S)

Green tea consumption and serum lipid profiles: A cross-sectional study in Northern Kyushu, Japan. PREV. MED. (USA), 1992, 21/4 (526-531)

Use of soya-beans for the dietary prevention and management of malnutrition in Nigeria. ACTA PAEDIATR. SCAND. SUPPL. (Sweden), 1991, 80/374 (175-182)

Increasing use of soyfoods and their potential role in cancer prevention. J. AM. DIET. ASSOC. (USA), 1991, 91/7 (836-840)

Diet and serum lipids in vegan vegetarians: A model for risk reduction. J. AM. DIET. ASSOC. (USA), 1991, 91/4 (447-453)

Nutritional contributors to cardiovascular disease in the elderly. J. AM. GERIATR. SOC. (USA), 1986, 34/1 (27-36)

Human and laboratory studies on the causes and prevention of gastrointestinal cancer. SCAND. J. GASTROENTEROL. SUPPL. (NORWAY), 1984, 19/104 (15-26)

Preventive nutrition: Disease-specific dietary interventions for older adults. GERIATRICS (USA), 1992, 47/11 (39-49)

Significance of active and passive prevention of cancer, arteriosclerosis and senility. MINERVA MED. (ITALY), 1982, 73/41 (2867-2872)

Increased brain damage after stroke or excitotoxic seizures in melatonin-deficient rats. FASEB Journal (USA), 1996, 10/13 (1546-1551)

Oxidative processes and antioxidative defense mechanisms in the aging brain. FASEB Journal (USA), 1995, 9/7 (526-533)

Partial restoration of choline acetyltransferase activities in aging and AF64A-lesioned rat brains by vitamin E. NEUROCHEM. INT. (United Kingdom), 1993, 22/5 (487-491)

Do antioxidant micronutrients protect against the development and progression of knee osteoarthritis?. Arthritis and Rheumatism (USA), 1996, 39/4 (648-656)

Dietary flavonoids, antioxidant vitamins, and incidence of stroke: The Zutphen study. Archives of Internal Medicine (USA), 1996, 156/6 (637-642)

Free radicals, oxidative stress, oxidized low density lipoprotein (LDL), and the heart: Antioxidants and other strategies to limit cardiovascular damage. Connecticut Medicine (USA), 1995, 59/10 (579-588)

Causes and prevention of premature aging. GERIATRIKA (Spain), 1994, 10/7 (19-24)

Antioxidant vitamins and disease - Risks of a suboptimal supply. THER. UMSCH. (Switzerland), 1994, 51/7 (467-474)

Tracking the daily supplement. TODAY'S LIFE SCI. (Australia), 1994, 6/3 (24-31)

Preventive nutrition: Disease-specific dietary interventions for Older adults. GERIATRICS (USA), 1992, 47/11 (39-49)

Experimental approaches to nutrition and cancer: Fats, calories, vitamins and minerals. MED. ONCOL. TUMOR PHARMACOTHER. (United Kingdom), 1990, 7/2-3 (183-192)

Vitamin D requirements for the elderly. CLIN. NUTR. (USA), 1986, 5/3 (121-129)

Vitamin D deficiency and hip fractures. TIJDSCHR. GERONTOL. GERIATR. (NT), 1985, 16/6 (239-245)

The physiologic and pharmacologic factors protecting the lens transparency and the update approach to the prevention of experimental cataracts: A review. METAB. PEDIATR. SYST. OPHTHALMOL. (USA), 1983, 7/2 (115-124)

Prostate Cancer (Early Stage)

Effects of protein kinase and phosphatase inhibitors on the growth of human prostatic cancer cells. Medical Science Research (United Kingdom), 1997, 25/5 (353-354)

Phyto-oestrogens and Western diseases. Annals of Medicine (United Kingdom), 1997, 29/2 (95-120)

Genistein inhibits proliferation and in vitro invasive potential of human prostatic cancer cell lines. Anticancer Research (Greece), 1997, 17/2 A (1199-1204)

Soy and rye diets inhibit the development of Dunning R3327 prostatic adenocarcinoma in rats. Cancer Letters (Ireland), 1997, 114/1-2 (313-314)

Measurement and metabolism of isoflavonoids and lignans in the human male. Cancer Letters (Ireland), 1997, 114/1-2 (145-151):

Inhibition of N-methyl-N-nitrosourea-induced mammary tumors in rats by the soybean isoflavones. Anticancer Research (Greece), 1996, 16/6 A (3293-3298)

Genistein-induced apoptosis of prostate cancer cells is preceded by a specific decrease in focal adhesion kinase activity. Molecular Pharmacology (USA), 1997, 51/2 (193-200)

Genistein-stimulated adherence of prostate cancer cells is associated with the binding of focal adhesion kinase to beta-1-integrin. Clinical and Experimental Metastasis (United Kingdom), 1996, 14/4 (389-398)

Quantification of genistein and genistin in soybeans and soybean products. Food and Chemical Toxicology (United Kingdom), 1996, 34/5 (457-461)

Molecular effects of genistein on estrogen receptor mediated pathways. Carcinogenesis (United Kingdom), 1996, 17/2 (271-275)

References

Effects of soya consumption for one month on steroid hormones in premenopausal women: Implications for breast cancer risk reduction. Cancer Epidemiology Biomarkers and Prevention (USA), 1996, 5/1 (63-70)

Early di. An update. Medecine Biologie Environnement (Italy), 1996, 24/2 (139-152)

Prostate-specific antigen as a screening test for prostate cancer: The United States experience. Urologic Clinics of North America (USA), 1997, 24/2 (299-306)

Prostate cancer screening: The controversy. Revue Medicale Libanaise (Lebanon), 1996, 8/3 (152-154)

Clinical utility of measurements of free and total prostate-specific. Prostate (USA), 1996, 29/SUPPL. 7 (64-69)

Detection of human papillomavirus DNA and p53 gene mutations in human prostate cancer. Prostate (USA), 1996, 28/5 (318-324)

Effects of potent vitamin D3 analogs on clonal proliferation of human prostate cancer cell lines. Prostate (USA), 1997, 31/2 (77-83)

1,25-Dihydroxyvitamin D3 and 9-cis-retinoic acid act synergistically to inhibit the growthcause accumulation of cells in G1. Endocrinology (USA), 1997, 138/4 (1491-1497)

Vitamin D receptor content and transcriptional activity do not fully predict antiproliferative effects of vitamin D in human prostate cancer cell lines. Molecular and Cellular Endocrinology (Ireland), 1997, 126/1 (83-90)

A preliminary report on the use of transfer factor for treating stage D3 hormone-unr metastatic prostate cancer. Biotherapy (Netherlands), 1996, 9/1-3 (123-132)

The role of vitamin D in normal prostate growth and differentiation. Cell Growth and Differentiation (USA), 1996, 7/11 (1563-1570)

Effects of 1,25 dihydroxyvitamin D3 and its analogues on induction of apoptosis in breast cancer cells. Journal of Steroid Biochemistry and Molecular Biology (United Kingdom), 1996, 58/4 (395-401)

Vitamin D receptor expression is required for growth modulation by 1alpha,25-dihydroxyvitamin D3 in the human prostatic carcinoma cell line ALVA-31. Journal of Steroid Biochemistry and Molecular Biology (United Kingdom), 1996, 58/3 (277-288)

Induction of transforming growth factor-beta autocrine activity by all-trans-retinoic acid and 1alpha,25-dihydroxyvitamin D3 in NRP-152 rat prostatic epithelial cells. Journal of Cellular Physiology (USA), 1996, 166/1 (231-239)

Biologically active acylglycerides from the berries of saw-palmetto (Serenoa repens). Journal of Natural Products (USA), 1997, 60/4 (417-418)

Effects of the lipidosterolic extract of Serenoa repens (Permixon (R)) on human prostatic cell lines. Prostate (USA), 1996, 29/4 (219-230)

Comparison of in vitro effects of the pure antiandrogens OH-flutamide, casodex, and nilutamide on androgen-sensitive parameters. Urology (USA), 1997, 49/4 (580-589)

Casodex (R) (Bicalutamide): Overview of a new antiandrogen developed for the treatment of prostate cancer. European Urology (Switzerland), 1997, 31/SUPPL. 2 (30-39)

References

Recommended dose of flutamide with LH-RH agonist therapy in patients with advanced prostate cancer. International Journal of Urology (Japan), 1996, 3/6 (468-471)

Bicalutamide (Casodex). Expert Opinion on Investigational Drugs (United Kingdom), 1996, 5/12 (1707-1722)

U.S. Drug and biologic approvals in 1994-1995. Drug Development Research (USA), 1996, 37/4 (197-207)

Cryosurgery of prostate cancer. Use of adjuvant hormonal therapy and temperature monitoring—A one year follow-up. Anticancer Research (Greece), 1997, 17/3 A (1511-1515)

The potential role of lycopene for human health. Journal of the American College of Nutrition (USA), 1997, 16/2 (109-126)

Lycopene: A biologically important carotenoid for humans? Archives of Biochemistry and Biophysics (USA), 1996, 336/1 (1-9)

cis-trans lycopene isomers, carotenoids, and retinol in the human prostate. Cancer Epidemiology Biomarkers and Prevention (USA), 1996, 5/10 (823-833)

How is individual risk for prostate cancer assessed? Hematology/Oncology Clinics of North America (USA), 1996, 10/3 (537-548)

A tomato a day for preventing prostate cancer? Diet may be key. Geriatrics (USA), 1996, 51/2 (21)

Intake of carotenoids and retinol in relation to risk of prostate cancer. Journal of the National Cancer Institute (USA), 1995, 87/23 (1767-1776)

Whatever happened to beta carotene? Journal of the National Cancer Institute (USA), 1995, 87/23 (1739-1741)

Vegetable and fruit consumption in relation to prostate cancer risk in Hawaii: A reevaluation of the effect of dietary beta-carotene. AM. J. EPIDEMIOL. (USA), 1991, 133/3 (215-219)

Serologic precursors of cancer. Retinol, carotenoids, and tocopherol and risk of prostate cancer. J. NATL. CANCER INST. (USA), 1990, 82/11 (941-946)

Carcinogenicity of oral cadmium in the male Wistar (WF/NCr) rat: Effect of chronic dietary zinc deficiency. FUNDAM. APPL. TOXICOL. (USA), 1992, 19/4 (512-520)

Nutrition and prostate cancer: A case-control study. PROSTATE (USA), 1985, 6/1 (7-17)

Zinc, vitamin A and prostatic cancer. BR. J. UROL. (ENGLAND), 1983, 55/5 (525-528)

Influence of isoflavones in soy protein isolates on development of induced prostate-related cancers in L-W rats. Nutrition and Cancer (USA), 1997, 28/1 (41-45)

Peptide growth factors: Clinical and therapeutic strategies. Minerva Urologica e Nefrologica (Italy), 1997, 49/2 (63-72)

Cancer risk factors for selecting cohorts for large-scale chemoprevention trials. Journal of Cellular Biochemistry (USA), 1996, 63/SUPPL. 25 (29-36)

Inhibition of liposomal lipid peroxidation by isoflavonoid type phyto-oestrogens from soybeans of different countries of origin. Biochemical Society Transactions (United Kingdom), 1996, 24/3 (392S)

Phytoestrogens: Epidemiology and a possible role in cancer protection. Environmental Health Perspectives (USA), 1995, 103/SUPPL. 7 (103-112)

Differential sensitivity of human prostatic cancer cell lines to the effects of protein kinase and phosphatase inhibitors. Cancer Letters (Ireland), 1995, 98/1 (103-110):

Genetic damage and the inhibition of 7,12-dimethylbenz(a)anthracene-induc ed genetic damage by the phytoestrogens, genistein and daidzein, in female ICR mice. Cancer Letters (Ireland), 1995, 95/1-2 (125-133)

Rationale for the use of genistein-containing soy matrices in chemoprevention trials for breast and prostate cancer. Journal of Cellular Biochemistry (USA), 1995, 58/SUPPL. 22 (181-187)

A simplified method to quantify isoflavones in commercial soybean diets and human urine after legume consumption. Cancer Epidemiology Biomarkers and Prevention (USA), 1995, 4/5 (497-503)

Rapid HPLC analysis of dietary phytoestrogens from legumes and from human urine. PROC. SOC. EXP. BIOL. MED. (USA), 1995, 208/1 (18-26)

Soy intake and cancer risk: A review of the in vitro and in vivo data. NUTR. CANCER (USA), 1994, 21/2 (113-131)

Plasma concentrations of phyto-oestrogens in Japanese men. LANCET (United Kingdom), 1993, 342/8881 (1209-1210)

Genistein is an effective stimulator of sex hormone-binding globulin production in hepatocarcinoma human liver cancer cells and suppresses proliferation of these cells in culture. STEROIDS (USA), 1993, 58/7 (301-304)

Genistein and biochanin A inhibit the growth of human prostate cancer cells but not epidermal growth factor receptor tyrosine autophosphorylation. PROSTATE (USA), 1993, 22/4 (335-345)

Surrogate endpoint biomarkers for phase II cancer chemoprevention trials. J. CELL. BIOCHEM. (USA), 1994, 56/SUPPL. 19 (1-9)

The 16-ene vitamin D analogs. Current Pharmaceutical Design (Netherlands), 1997, 3/1 (99-123)

Signal transduction inhibitors as modifiers of radiation therapy in human prostate carcinoma xenografts. Radiation Oncology Investigations (USA), 1996, 4/5 (221-230)

Calcium regulation of androgen receptor expression in the human prostate cancer cell line LNCaP. Endocrinology (USA), 1995, 136/5 (2172-2178)

The role of calcium, pH, and cell proliferation in the programmed (apoptotic) death of androgen-independent prostatic cancer cells induced by thapsigarin. CANCER RES. (USA), 1994, 54/23 (6167-6175)

Programmed cell death as a new target for prostatic cancer therapy. CANCER SURV. (USA), 1991, 11/- (265-277):

Hyperparathyroidism in metastases of prostatic carcinoma: A biochemical, hormonal and histomorphometric study. EUR. UROL. (Switzerland), 1990, 17/1 (35-39)

In vitro studies of human prostatic epithelial cells: Attempts to identify distinguishing features of malignant cells. GROWTH FACTORS (United Kingdom), 1989, 1/3 (237-250)

Hypocalcemia associated with estrogen therapy for metastatic adenocarcinoma of the prostate. J.

UROL. (USA), 1988, 140/5 PART I (1025-1027)

Hypercalcemia in carcinoma of the prostate: Case report and review of the literature. J. UROL. (BALTIMORE) (USA), 1987, 137/2 (309-311)

Calcium excretion in metastatic prostatic carcinoma. BR. J. UROL. (ENGLAND), 1984, 56/6 (687-689)

Osteomalacia associated with prostatic cancer and osteoblastic metastases. UROLOGY (USA), 1983, 21/1 (65-67)

Carcinoma of the prostate: The treatment of bone metastases by radiophosphorus. CLIN. RADIOL. (SCOTLAND), 1981, 32/6 (695-697)

Management of cancer of the prostate. BRIT.J.HOSP.MED. (ENGLAND), 1974, 11/3 (357-372)

Intracavitary irradiation of prostate carcinomas. REV. MED. SUISSE ROMANDE (SWITZERLAND), 1980, 100/9

Epidemiology of prostatic cancer: A case-control study. PROSTATE (USA), 1990, 17/3 (189-206)

Demonstration of specifically sensitized lymphocytes in patients treated with an aqueous mistletoe extract (Viscum album L.). KLIN. WOCHENSCHR. (Germany), 1991, 69/9 (397-403)

An urodynamic study of patients with benign prostatic hypertrophy treated conservatively with phytotherapy or testosterone. WIEN. KLIN. WOCHENSCHR. (AUSTRIA), 1979, 91/18 (622-627)

Rationale for the use of genistein-containing soy matrices in chemoprevention trials for breast and prostate cancer. Journal of Cellular Biochemistry (USA), 1995, 58/SUPPL. 22

Phytoestrogens are partial estrogen agonists in the adult male mouse. Environmental Health Perspectives (USA), 1995, 103/SUPPL. 7

Soy intake and cancer risk: A review of the in vitro and in vivo data. NUTR. CANCER (USA), 1994, 21/2 (113-131)

Plasma concentrations of phyto-oestrogens in Japanese men. LANCET (United Kingdom), 1993, 342/8881 (1209-1210)

Urinary excretion of lignans and isoflavonoid phytoestrogens in Japanese men and women consuming a traditional Japanese diet. AM. J. CLIN. NUTR. (USA), 1991, 54/6

How is individual risk for prostate cancer assessed? Hematology/Oncology Clinics of North America (USA), 1996, 10/3

Control of LNCaP proliferation and differentiation: Actions and interactions of androgens, 1alpha,25-dihydroxycholecalciferol, all-trans retinoid acid, 9-cis retinoic acid, and phenylacetate. Prostate (USA), 1996, 28/3 (182-194)

1,25-Dihydroxy-16-ene-23-yne-vitamin D3 and prostate cancer cell proliferation in vivo. Urology (USA), 1995, 46/3 (365-369)

Recent advances in hormonal therapy for cancer. Current Opinion in Oncology (USA), 1995, 7/6

Endocrine control of prostate cancer. Cancer Surveys (USA), 1995, 23/- (43-62)

Vitamin D and prostate cancer. Advances in Experimental Medicine, 1995, 375/-

Actions of vitamin D3 analogs on human prostate cancer cell lines: Comparison with 1,25-dihydroxyvitamin D3. ENDOCRINOLOGY (USA), 1995, 136/1 (20-26)

Vitamin D and cancer. REV. FR. ENDOCRINOL. CLIN. NUTR. METAB. (France), 1994, 35/4-5

Human prostate cancer cells: Inhibition of proliferation by vitamin D analogs. ANTICANCER RES. (Greece), 1994, 14/3 A (1077-1081)

Vitamin D and prostate cancer: 1,25 Dihydroxyvitamin D3 receptors and actions in human prostate cancer cell lines. ENDOCRINOLOGY (USA), 1993, 132/5 (1952-1960)

Is vitamin D deficiency a risk factor for prostate cancer? (hypothesis). ANTICANCER RES. (Greece), 1990, 10/5 A (1307-1312)

The in vitro response of four antisteroid receptor agents on the hormone-responsive prostate cancer cell line LNCaP. Oncology Reports (Greece), 1995, 2/2 (295-298)

Combination treatment in M1 prostate cancer. CANCER (USA), 1993, 72/12 SUPPL. (3880-3885)

Antiandrogenic drugs. CANCER (USA), 1993, 71/3 SUPPL. (1046-1049)

The effects of flutamide on total DHT and nuclear DHT levels in the human prostate. PROSTATE (USA), 1981, 2/3 (309-314)

Endocrine profiles during administration of the new non-steroidal anti-androgen Casodex in prostate cancer. CLIN. ENDOCRINOL. (United Kingdom), 1994, 41/4 (525-530)

Antiandrogenic drugs. CANCER (USA), 1993, 71/3 SUPPL. (1046-1049)

Prostate Cancer (Metastasized/Late Stage)

Refer to references under Cancer Treatment.

Prostate Enlargement
(Benign Prostatic Hypertrophy)

NOTE: PERMIXON and SERENOA REPENS are synonyms for SAW PALMETTO EXTRACT.

Comparison of androgen-independent growth and androgen-dependent growth in BPH and cancer tissue from the same radical prostatectomies in sponge-gel matrix histoculture. Prostate (UNITED STATES) Jun 1 1997, 31 (4) p250-4

Alpha-1 adrenoceptor subtypes (high, low) in human benign prostatic hypertrophy tissue according to the affinities for prazosin. Prostate (UNITED STATES) Jun 1 1997, 31 (4) p216-22

[Urethral opening pressure: its clinical significance in prostatic obstruction]. Nippon Hinyokika Gakkai Zasshi (JAPAN) Apr 1997, 88 (4) p496-502

Free and total serum PSA values in patients with prostatic intraepithelial neoplasia (PIN), prostate cancer and BPH. Is F/T PSA a potential probe for dormant and manifest cancer? Anticancer Res (GREECE) May-Jun 1997, 17 (3A) p1531-4

Optimising the medical management of benign prostatic hyperplasia. Br J Clin Pract (ENGLAND) Mar 1997, 51 (2) p116-8

[Inferior vena cava obstruction syndrome caused by urinary retention]. Arch Esp Urol (SPAIN) Jan-Feb 1997, 50 (1) p61-2

[Diagnostic efficacy of free SPA/total PSA ratio in the diagnosis of prostatic carcinoma]. Arch Ital Urol Androl (ITALY) Feb 1997, 69 Suppl 1 p93-5

[Laser-assisted endoscopic resection: a new surgical technique for the treatment of benign prostatic hypertrophy. Preliminary results of a study involving 100 patients]. Arch Ital Urol Androl (ITALY) Feb 1997, 69 (1) p15-21

Blood haemoglobin and the long-term incidence of acute myocardial infarction after transurethral resection of the prostate. Eur Urol (SWITZERLAND) 1997, 31 (2) p199-203

Insulin-like growth factor-binding protein-2 in patients with prostate carcinoma and benign prostatic hyperplasia. Clin Endocrinol (Oxf) (ENGLAND) Feb 1997, 46 (2) p145-54

[Ureteral jet in patients with benign prostatic hypertrophy: prognostic evaluation during single and combined therapy]. Arch Ital Urol Androl (ITALY) Dec 1996, 68 (5 Suppl) p175-8

[Laser treatment of benign prostatic hypertrophy: the correlation of histologic results to nuclear magnetic resonance imaging]. Ann Urol (Paris) (FRANCE) 1997, 31 (1) p19-26

[Laser-tissue interactions in urology]. Ann Urol (Paris) (FRANCE) 1997, 31 (1) p11-8

Effect of Serenoa repens extract (Permixon) on estradiol/testosterone-induced experimental prostate enlargement in the rat. Pharmacol Res (ENGLAND) Sep-Oct 1996, 34 (3-4) p171-9

Immunohistochemical analysis of beta-tubulin isotypes in human prostate carcinoma and benign prostatic hypertrophy. Prostate (UNITED STATES) Mar 1 1997, 30 (4) p263-8

[LH-RH agonists as therapeutic alternative in patients with benign prostatic hyperplasia (BPH) and surgical contraindication. Long term follow up]. Arch Esp Urol (SPAIN) Nov 1996, 49 (9) p923-7

c-erbB-2 oncoprotein: a potential biomarker of advanced prostate cancer. Prostate (UNITED STATES) Feb 15 1997, 30 (3) p195-201

Role of m1 receptor-G protein coupling in cell proliferation in the prostate. Life Sci (ENGLAND) 1997, 60 (13-14) p963-8

Transurethral prostatectomy--new trends. Geriatr Nurs (UNITED STATES) Mar-Apr 1997, 18 (2) p78-80

[Sabal serrulata extract in the management of symptoms of prostatic hypertrophy]. Orv Hetil (HUNGARY) Feb 16 1997, 138 (7) p419-21

[Comparative effects of transurethral incision (TUIP) and the combination of TUIP and LHRH agonists in the treatment of benign prostatic hypertrophy]. J Urol (Paris) (FRANCE) 1996, 102 (3) p111-6

Immunochemical detection of 5 alpha-reductase in human serum. Steroids (UNITED STATES) Nov 1996, 61 (11) p651-6

Nd:YAG laser transurethral evaporation of the prostate (TUEP) for urinary retention. Lasers Surg Med (UNITED STATES) 1996, 19 (4) p480-6

Possible mechanisms of action of transurethral needle ablation of the prostate on benign prostatic hyperplasia symptoms: a neurohistochemical study. J Urol (UNITED STATES) Mar 1997, 157 (3) p894-

9

Histopathologic evaluation of the canine prostate following electrovaporization. J Urol (UNITED STATES) Mar 1997, 157 (3) p1144-8

Transurethral vaporization of the prostate: a promising new technique. Br J Urol (ENGLAND) Feb 1997, 79 (2) p186-9

Early experience with high-intensity focused ultrasound for the treatment of benign prostatic hypertrophy. Br J Urol (ENGLAND) Feb 1997, 79 (2) p172-6

Detection of bladder tumor by urine cytology in cases of prostatic hypertrophy. Diagn Cytopathol (UNITED STATES) Dec 1996, 15 (5) p409-11

Quantification and distribution of alpha 1-adrenoceptor subtype mRNAs in human prostate: comparison of benign hypertrophied tissue and non-hypertrophied tissue. Br J Pharmacol (ENGLAND) Nov 1996, 119 (5) p797-803

Prostate-specific antigen and age. Is there a correlation? And why does it seem to vary? Eur Urol (SWITZERLAND) 1996, 30 (3) p296-300

Colocalization of immunoglobulin binding factor and prostate specific antigen in human prostate gland. Arch Androl (UNITED STATES) Nov-Dec 1996, 37 (3) p149-54

A study of the efficacy and safety of transurethral needle ablation (TUNA) treatment for benign prostatic hyperplasia. Neurourol Urodyn (UNITED STATES) 1996, 15 (6) p619-28

[Diagnostic values and limitations of conventional urodynamic studies (uroflowmetry.residual urine measurement.cystometry) in benign prostatic hypertrophy]. Nippon Hinyokika Gakkai Zasshi (JAPAN) Dec 1996, 87 (12) p1321-3

Alpha 1a-adrenoceptor polymorphism: pharmacological characterization and association with benign prostatic hypertrophy. Br J Pharmacol (ENGLAND) Jul 1996, 118 (6) p1403-8

[Double-blind evaluation of mepartricin 150.000 U (40 mg) compared with placebo in benign prostatic hypertrophy]. Minerva Urol Nefrol (ITALY) Dec 1996, 48 (4) p207-11

[Alternative treatment of benign prostatic hypertrophy]. Minerva Urol Nefrol (ITALY) Dec 1996, 48 (4) p177-82

Transition zone ratio and prostate-specific antigen density: the index of response of benign prostatic hypertrophy to an alpha blocker. Int J Urol (JAPAN) Sep 1996, 3 (5) p361-6

A case of prostate cancer diagnosed one and half year after retropubic prostatectomy for benign prostatic hypertrophy]. Hinyokika Kiyo (JAPAN) Nov 1996, 42 (11) p907-9

The use of alpha-adrenoceptor antagonists in the pharmacological management of benign prostatic hypertrophy: an overview. Pharmacol Res (ENGLAND) Mar 1996, 33 (3) p145-60

Clinical application of basic arginine amidase in human male urine. Biol Pharm Bull (JAPAN) Aug 1996, 19 (8) p1083-5

Free to total prostate-specific antigen (PSA) ratio is superior to total-PSA in differentiating benign prostate hypertrophy from prostate cancer. Prostate Suppl (UNITED STATES) 1996, 7 p30-4

Clinical study on estramustine binding protein (EMBP) in human prostate. Prostate (UNITED STATES)

Sep 1996, 29 (3) p169-76

Three-year followup of patients treated with lower energy microwave thermotherapy. J Urol (UNITED STATES) Dec 1996, 156 (6) p1959-63

Detection of Chlamydia trachomatis in the prostate by in-situhybridization and by transmission electron microscopy. Int J Androl (ENGLAND) Apr 1996, 19 (2) p109-12

Breast and prostate cancer in the relatives of men with prostate cancer. Br J Urol (ENGLAND) Oct 1996, 78 (4) p552-6

Effect of finasteride on free and total serum prostate-specific antigen in men with benign prostatic hyperplasia. Br J Urol (ENGLAND) Sep 1996, 78 (3) p405-8

The safety of finasteride used in benign prostatic hypertrophy: a non-interventional observational cohort study in 14,772 patients. Br J Urol (ENGLAND) Sep 1996, 78 (3) p379-84

[Transurethral thermotherapy with microwaves in patients with benign prostatic hypertrophy and urinary retention: comparative study between high energy (25) and standard energy (2.0)]. Arch Esp Urol (SPAIN) May 1996, 49 (4) p337-46

Detection of alpha 1-adrenoceptor subtypes in human hypertrophied prostate by insituhybridization. Histochem J (ENGLAND) Apr 1996, 28 (4) p283-8

Safety profile of 3 months' therapy with alfuzosin in 13,389 patients suffering from benign prostatic hypertrophy. Eur Urol (SWITZERLAND) 1996, 29 (1) p29-35

Estramustine-binding protein in carcinoma and benign hyperplasia of the human prostate. Eur Urol (SWITZERLAND) 1996, 29 (1) p106-10

Surface-epitope masking and expression cloning identifies the human prostate carcinoma tumor antigen gene PCTA-1 a member of the galectin gene family. Proc Natl Acad Sci U S A (UNITED STATES) Jul 9 1996, 93 (14) p7252-7

[The significance of free-type PSA and complex-type PSA in patients with prostatic carcinoma--the characteristics of ACS-PSA method compared with that of Delfia- and Eiken-PSA method]. Rinsho Byori (JAPAN) Apr 1996, 44 (4) p345-50

The Oxford Laser Prostate Trial: a double-blind randomized controlled trial of contact vaporization of the prostate against transurethral resection; preliminary results. Br J Urol (ENGLAND) Mar 1996, 77 (3) p382-5

A case-control study of cancer of the prostate in Somerset and east Devon. Br J Cancer (ENGLAND) Aug 1996, 74 (4) p661-6

Usefulness of PSA density and PSA excess in the differential diagnosis between prostate cancer and benign prostatic hypertrophy. Int J Biol Markers (ITALY) Jan-Mar 1996, 11 (1) p12-7

[Detection of prostate cancer in urological practice: clinical establishment of serum PSA reference values by age]. Nippon Hinyokika Gakkai Zasshi (JAPAN) Mar 1996, 87 (3) p702-9

Free-to-total prostate specific antigen ratio as a single test for detection of significant stage T1c prostate cancer. J Urol (UNITED STATES) Sep 1996, 156 (3) p1042-7; discussion 1047-9

[Transurethral thermotherapy with microwaves in symptomatic prostatic benign hypertrophy: comparison between the high-energy (2.5) protocol and the standard protocol (2.0)]. Arch Esp Urol (SPAIN)

Mar 1996, 49 (2) p99-109

Two-dimensional outcome analysis as a guide for quality assurance of prostatectomy. Int J Qual Health Care (ENGLAND) Feb 1996, 8 (1) p67-73

Alpha blockers: a reassessment of their role in therapy. Am Fam Physician (UNITED STATES) Jul 1996, 54 (1) p263-6

Effect of prostatic growth factor, basic fibroblast growth factor, epidermal growth factor, and steroids on the proliferation of human fetal prostatic fibroblasts. Prostate (UNITED STATES) Jun 1996, 28 (6) p352-8

The impact of prostate-specific antigen density in predicting prostate cancer when serum prostate-specific antigen levels are less than 10 ng/ml. Eur Urol (SWITZERLAND) 1996, 29 (2) p189-92

Usefulness of prostate-specific antigen density as a diagnostic test of prostate cancer. Tumour Biol (SWITZERLAND) 1996, 17 (1) p20-6

The extract of serenoa repens in the treatment of benign prostatic hyperplasia: A multicenter open study. CURR. THER. RES. CLIN. EXP. (USA), 1994, 55/7 (776- 785)

Prostaserene (R). Treatment for BPH. DRUGS FUTURE (Spain), 1994, 19/5 (452-453)

The effect of Permixon on androgen receptors. ACTA OBSTET. GYNECOL. SCAND. (Sweden), 1988, 65/6

Pharmacological combinations in the treatment of benign prostatic hypertrophy. J. UROL. (France), 1993, 99/6 (316-320)

Inhibition of androgen metabolism and binding by a liposterolic extract of 'Serenoa repens B' in human foreskin fibroblasts. J. STEROID BIOCHEM. (ENGLAND), 1984, 20/1 (515-519)

Testosterone metabolism in primary cultures of human prostate epithelial cells and fibroblasts. J Steroid Biochem Mol Biol (ENGLAND) Dec 1995, 55 (3-4) p375-83

The effect of Permixon on androgen receptors. Acta Obstet Gynecol Scand (SWEDEN) 1988, 67 (5) p397-9

Binding of Permixon, a new treatment for prostatic benign hyperplasia, to the cytosolic androgen receptor in the rat prostate. J Steroid Biochem (ENGLAND) Jan 1984, 20 (1) p521-3

Inhibition of androgen metabolism and binding by a liposterolic extract of Serenoa repens B in human foreskin fibroblasts. J Steroid Biochem (ENGLAND) Jan 1984, 20 (1) p515-9

Testosterone metabolism in primary cultures of human prostate epithelial cells and fibroblasts. Journal of Steroid Biochemistry and Molecular Biology (United Kingdom), 1995, 55/3-4 (375-383)

Human prostatic steroid 5alpha-reductase isoforms - A comparative study of selective inhibitors. Journal of Steroid Biochemistry and Molecular Biology (United Kingdom) 1995, 54/5-6 (273-279)

The lipidosterolic extract from Serenoa repens interferes with prolactin receptor signal. Journal of Biomedical Science (Switzerland), 1995, 2/4 (357-365)

Lack of effects of a lyposterolic extract of Serenoa repens on plasma levels of testosterone, follicle-stimulating hormone, and luteinizing hormone. CLIN. THER. (USA), 1988, 10/5 (585-588)

Serenoa repens capsules: A bioequivalence study. ACTA TOXICOL. THER. (Italy), 1994, 15/1 (21-39)

Rectal bioavailability and pharmacokinetics in healthy volunteers of serenoa repens new formulation. ARCH. MED. INTERNA (Italy), 1994, 46/2 (77-86)

Clinical controlled trial on therapeutical bioequivalence and tolerability of Serenoa repens oral capsules 160 mg or rectal capsules 640 mg. ARCH. MED. INTERNA (Italy), 1994, 46/2 (61-75)

Evidence that serenoa repens extract displays an antiestrogenic activity in prostatic tissue of benign prostatic hypertrophy patients. EUR. UROL. (Switzerland), 1992, 21/4 (309-314)

Liposterolic extract of Serenoa Repens in management of benign prostatic hypertrophy. UROLOGIA (Italy), 1988, 55/5 (547-552)

Lack of effects of a lyposterolic extract of Serenoa repens on plasma levels of testosterone, follicle-stimulating hormone, and luteinizing hormone. CLIN. THER. (USA), 1988, 10/5 (585-588)

Binding of permixon, a new treatment for prostatic benign hyperplasia, to the cytosolic androgen receptor in the rat prostate. J. STEROID BIOCHEM. (ENGLAND), 1984, 20/1 (521-523)

Effect of Pygeum africanum extract on A23187-stimulated production of lipoxygenase metabolites from human polymorphonuclear cells. J Lipid Mediat Cell Signal. 1994 May. 9(3). P 285-90.

Combined extracts of Urtica dioica and Pygeum africanum in the treatment of benign prostatic hyperplasia: double-blind comparison of two doses. Clin Ther. 1993 Nov-Dec. 15(6). P 1011-20

[Urological and sexual evaluation of treatment of benign prostatic disease using Pygeum africanum at high doses]. Arch Ital Urol Nefrol Androl. 1991 Sep. 63(3). P 341-5

[Efficacy of Pygeum africanum extract in the medical therapy of urination disorders due to benign prostatic hyperplasia: evaluation of objective and subjective parameters. A placebo-controlled double-blind multicenter study] Wien Klin Wochenschr. 1990 Nov 23. 102(22). P 667-73

Pulmonary Insufficiencies

Refer to references under Emphysema and Chronic Obstructive Pulmonary Disease.

Retinopathy

A deficiency of vitamin B6 is a plausible molecular basis of the retinopathy of patients with diabetes mellitus. Biochem Biophys Res Commun. 1991 Aug 30. 179(1). P 615-9

Pharmacological prevention of diabetic microangiopathy, MECANISMES PATHOGENIQUES, DIABETE METABOL. (France), 1994, 20/2 BIS (219-228)

Clinical study of vitamin influence in diabetes mellitus. Journal of the Medical Society of Toho University (Japan), 1996, 42/6

Erythrocyte and plasma antioxidant activity in type I diabetes mellitus. Presse Medicale (France), 1996, 25/5 (188-192)

Lipid peroxidation in insulin-dependent diabetic patients with early retina degenerative lesions: Effects of an oral zinc supplementation. European Journal of Clinical Nutrition (United Kingdom), 1995, 49/4 (282-288)

Angioid streaks associated with abetalipoproteinemia. OPHTHALMIC GENET. (Netherlands), 1994, 15/3-4 (151- 159)

Comparison of gamma-glutamyl transpeptidase in retina and cerebral cortex, and effects of antioxidant therapy. CURR. EYE RES. (United Kingdom), 1994, 13/12 (891- 896)

Status of antioxidants in patients with diabetes mellitus with and without late complications. AKTUEL. ERNAHR.MED. KLIN. PRAX. (Germany), 1994, 19/3 (155-159)

Vitamins for seeing. COMPR. THER. (USA), 1990, 16/4 (62)

The regional distribution of vitamins E and C in mature and premature human retinas. INVEST. OPHTHALMOL. VISUAL SCI. (USA), 1988, 29/1 (22-26)

Oral vitamin E supplements can prevent the retinopathy of abetalipoproteinaemia. BR. J. OPHTHALMOL. (UK), 1986, 70/3 (166-173)

The role of taurine in developing rat retina. Ophtalmologie (France), 1995, 9/3 (283-286)

Taurine: Review and therapeutic applications (Part I). J. FARM. CLIN. (Spain), 1990, 7/7 (580-600)

Supplemental taurine in diabetic rats: Effects on plasma glucose and triglycerides. BIOCHEM. MED. METAB. BIOL. (USA), 1990, 43/1 (1-9+8)

Taurine deficiency retinopathy in the cat. J. SMALL ANIM. PRACT. (ENGLAND), 1980, 21/10 (521-534)

[Clinical experimentation with pyridoxylate in treatment of various chorioretinal degenerative disorders (50 cases)]. Bull Soc Ophtalmol Fr. 1969 Dec. 69(12). P 1145-50

Rationales for micronutrient supplementation in diabetes. Med Hypotheses. 1984 Feb. 13(2). P 139-51

Magnesium and potassium in diabetes and carbohydrate metabolism. Review of the present status and recent results. Magnesium. 1984. 3(4-6). P 315-23

Seasonal Affective Disorder (SAD)

L-tryptophan augmentation of light therapy in patients with seasonal affective disorder. Can J Psychiatry (CANADA) Apr 1997, 42 (3) p303-6

Prediction of acute and late responses to light therapy from vocal (pitch) and self-rated activation in seasonal affective disorder. J Affect Disord (NETHERLANDS) Feb 1997, 42 (2-3) p117-26

A controlled trial of light therapy for the treatment of pediatric seasonal affective disorder. J Am Acad Child Adolesc Psychiatry (UNITED STATES) Jun 1997, 36 (6) p816-21

Effects of tryptophan depletion on drug-free patients with seasonal affective disorder during a stable response to bright light therapy. Arch Gen Psychiatry (UNITED STATES) Feb 1997, 54 (2) p133-8

Sunny hospital rooms expedite recovery from severe and refractory depressions. J Affect Disord (NETHERLANDS) Sep 9 1996, 40 (1-2) p49-51

The importance of full summer remission as a criterion for the diagnosis of seasonal affective disorder. Psychopathology (SWITZERLAND) 1996, 29 (4) p230-5

Light therapy in bulimia nervosa: a double-blind, placebo-controlled study. Psychiatry Res (IRELAND) Feb 28 1996, 60 (1) p1-9

Predictors of response and nonresponse to light treatment for winter depression. Am J Psychiatry (UNITED STATES) Nov 1996, 153 (11) p1423-9

'Natural' light treatment of seasonal affective disorder. J Affect Disord (NETHERLANDS) Apr 12 1996, 37 (2-3) p109-20

[Phototherapy in psychiatry: clinical update and review of indications]. Encephale (FRANCE) Mar-Apr 1996, 22 (2) p143-8

Seasonal affective disorder and season-dependent abnormalities of melatonin suppression by light. Lancet (1990 Sep 22) 336(8717):703-6. (For additional references on treating seasonal affective disorder, refer to Depression, above.)

Skin Aging

Skin photosensitizing agents and the role of reactive oxygen species in photoaging. J. PHOTOCHEM. PHOTOBIOL. B BIOL. (Switzerland), 1992, 14/1-2 (105-124)

An in vitro model to test relative antioxidant potential: Ultraviolet- induced lipid peroxidation in liposomes. ARCH. BIOCHEM. BIOPHYS. (USA), 1990, 283/2 (234-240)

Diminished stimulation of hyaluronic acid synthesis by PDGF, IGF-I or serum in the senescence phase of skin fibroblasts in vitro. Z. GERONTOL. (Germany), 1994, 27/3 (177-181)

Ultrastructural study of hyaluronic acid before and after the use of a pulsed electromagnetic field, electrorydesis, in the treatment of wrinkles. INT. J. DERMATOL. (Canada), 1994, 33/9 (661-663)

Hyaluronic acid in cutaneous intrinsic aging. INT. J. DERMATOL. (Canada), 1994, 33/2 (119-122)

Stimulation of cell proliferation by hyaluronidase during in vitro aging of human skin fibroblasts. EXP. GERONTOL. (USA), 1993, 28/1 (59-68)

Topical retinoic acid treatment of photoaged skin: Its effects on hyaluronan distribution in epidermis and on hyaluronan and retinoic acid in suction blister fluid. ACTA DERM.-VENEREOL. (Norway), 1992, 72/6 (423-427)

Werner's syndrome: Biochemical and cytogenetic studies. ARCH. DERMATOL. (USA), 1985, 121/5 (636-641)

Urinary acidic glycosaminoglycans in Werner's syndrome. EXPERIENTIA (SWITZERLAND), 1982, 38/3 (313-314)

Non-enzymatic degradation of acid-soluble calf skin collagen by superoxide ion: Protective effect of flavonoids. BIOCHEM. PHARMACOL. (ENGLAND), 1983, 32/1 (53-58)

In vitro cytotoxic effects of enzymatically induced oxygen radicals in human fibroblasts: Experimental procedures and protection by radical scavengers. TOXICOL. VITRO (United Kingdom), 1989, 3/2 (103-109)

Antiviral activity of plant components. 1st Communication: flavonoids. ANTIVIRALE WIRKUNG VON PFLANZENINHALTSSTOFFEN. 1. MITTEILUNG: FLAVONOIDE. ARZNEIM.-FORSCH. (GERMANY,

WEST), 1978, 28/3 (347-350)

Therapy of radiation damage in mice with O (L hydroxyethyl) rutoside. STRAHLENTHERAPIE (GERMANY, WEST), 1973, 145/6 (731-734)

Anti-ageing active principals by the oral route. Myth or reality? NOUV. DERMATOL. (France), 1994, 13/6 (423-425)

Topical 8% glycolic acid and 8% L-lactic acid creams for the treatment of photodamaged skin: A double-blind vehicle-controlled clinical trial. Archives of Dermatology (USA), 1996, 132/6 (631-636)

Alpha hydroxy acids in the cosmetic treatment of photo-induced skin ageing. Journal of Applied Cosmetology (Italy), 1996, 14/1 (1-8)

Effects of alpha-hydroxy acids on photoaged skin: A pilot clinical, histologic, and ultrastructural study. Journal of the American Academy of Dermatology (USA), 1996, 34/2 I (187- 195)

Topical gelatin-glycine and alpha-hydroxy acids for photoaged skin. J. APPL. COSMETOL. (Italy), 1994, 12/1 (1-10)

Antioxidants, fat and skin cancer. Skin Cancer (Portugal), 1995, 10/2 (97-101)

An in vitro model to test relative antioxidant potential: Ultraviolet- induced lipid peroxidation in liposomes. ARCH. BIOCHEM. BIOPHYS. (USA), 1990, 283/2 (234-240)

Photoprotective effect of superoxide scavenging antioxidants against ultraviolet radiation-induced chronic skin damage in the hairless mouse. Photodermatology Photoimmunology Photomedicine (Denmark), 1990, 7/2 (56-62)

Impairment of enzymic and nonenzymic antioxidants in skin by UVB irradiation. J. INVEST. DERMATOL. (USA), 1989, 93/6 (769-773)

Low levels of essential fatty acids are related to impaired delayed skin hypersensitivity in malnourished chronically ill elderly people. EUR. J. CLIN. INVEST. (United Kingdom), 1994, 24/9 (615-620)

Two concentrations of topical tretinoin (retinoic acid) cause similar improvement of photoaging but different degrees of irritation: A double- blind, vehicle-controlled comparison of 0.1% and 0.025% tretinoin creams. Archives of Dermatology (USA), 1995, 131/9 (1037-1044)

Topical tretinoin (retinoic acid) treatment for liver spots associated with photodamage. NEW ENGL. J. MED. (USA), 1992, 326/6 (368-374)

The effects of an abrasive agent on normal skin and on photoaged skin in comparison with topical tretinoin. BR. J. DERMATOL. (United Kingdom), 1990, 123/4 (457-466)

Aging and the skin. POSTGRAD. MED. (USA), 1989, 86/1 (131-144)

Topical tretinoind and photoaged skin. CUTIS (USA), 1989, 43/5 (476-482)

Stress

Refer to references under Anxiety.

Stroke (Hemorrhagic)

Putaminal and thalamic hemorrhage in ethnic chinese living in Hong Kong. Surg Neurol (UNITED STATES) Nov 1996, 46 (5) p441-5

Diet and heart disease. The role of fat, alcohol, and antioxidants. Cardiol Clin (UNITED STATES) Feb 1996, 14 (1) p69-83,.777

[Effect of piracetam on inorganic phosphates and phospholipids in the blood of patients with cerebral infarction in the earliest period of the disease]. Neurol Neurochir Pol (POLAND) Nov-Dec 1991, 25 (6)

Effect of piracetam on recovery and rehabilitation after stroke: A double- blind, placebo-controlled study. CLIN. NEUROPHARMACOL. (USA, 1994, 17/4 (320-331)

Ergoloids (Hydergine) and ischaemic strokes; Efficacy and mechanism of action. Journal of International Medical Research (United Kingdom), 1995, 23/3 (154-160)

Satellite symposium 'Piracetam and acute stroke : Pass' within the framework of the 3rd International Conference on stroke, 18-21 October 1995 in Prague satelliten-symposium 'Piracetam and acute stroke: Pass' im rahmen der 3. International Conference on stroke, 18.-21. Oktober 1995, Prag. Nervenheilkunde (Germany, 1996, 15/1

The nootropic agent piracetam in the treatment of acute stroke.NOOTROPIKA. PIRACETAM BEIM AKUTEN SCHLAGANFALL. TW Neurologie Psychiatrie (Germany, 1996, 10/1-2 (81)

Cerebroprotective effect of piracetam: The acute and chronic administrations of piracetam during short-term and long-term transient ischaemia. Turkish Journal of Medical Sciences (Turkey), 1995, 24/SUPPL.(39)

Stroke (Thrombotic)

Diminished production of malondialdehyde after carotid artery surgery as a result of vitamin administration. Medical Science Research (United Kingdom), 1996, 24/11 (777-780)

Spermine partially normalizes in vivo antioxidant defense potential in certain brain regions in transiently hypoperfused rat brain. Neurochemical Research (USA), 1996, 21/12 (1497-1503)

Positron-labeled antioxidant 6-deoxy-6-(18F)fluoro-L-ascorbic acid: Increased uptake in transient global ischemic rat brain. Nuclear Medicine and Biology (USA), 1996, 23/4 (479-486)

Stroke is an emergency. Disease-a-Month (USA), 1996, 42/4 (202-264)

Antithrombotic agents in cerebral ischemia. American Journal of Cardiology (USA), 1995, 75/6 (34B-38B)

Platelet activity and stroke severity. J. NEUROL. SCI. (Netherlands), 1992, 108/1 (1-6)

The use of antithrombotic drugs in artery disease. CLIN. HAEMATOL. (UK), 1986, 15/2 (509-559)

Medical management in the endovascular treatment of carotid-cavernous aneurysms. Journal of Neurosurgery (USA), 1996, 84/5 (755-761)

Mechanism of hydrogen peroxide and hydroxyl free radical-induced intracellular acidification in cultured rat cardiac myoblasts. Circulation Research (USA), 1996, 78/4 (564-572)

Thrombolysis of the cervical internal carotid artery before balloon angioplasty and stent placement: Report of two cases. Neurosurgery (USA), 1996, 38/3 (620-624)

Aspirin at any dose above 30 mg offers only modest protection after cerebral ischaemia. Journal of Neurology Neurosurgery and Psychiatry (United Kingdom), 1996, 6 0/2 (197-199)

Mild hyperhomocysteinemia and hemostatic factors in patients witharterial vascular diseases. Thromb Haemost (GERMANY) Mar 1997, 77 (3) p466-71

Vitamin E plus aspirin compared with aspirin alone in patients with transient ischemic attacks. American Journal of Clinical Nutrition (USA), 1995, 62/6 SUPPL.

Poor plasma status of carotene and vitamin C is associated with higher mortality from ischemic heart disease and stroke: Basel Prospective Study. CLIN. INVEST. (Germany), 1993, 71/1 (3-6)

The treatment of acute cerebral ischemia. Ginkgo: Free radical scavenger and PAF antagonist. THERAPIEWOCHE (Germany), 1994, 44/24 (1394-1396) CODEN: THEWA

Efficiency of ginkgo biloba extract (EGb 761) in antioxidant protection against myocardial ischemia and reperfusion injury. Biochemistry and Molecular Biology International (Australia), 1995, 35/1 (125-134)

Magnesium content of erythrocytes in patients with vasospastic angina. CARDIOVASC. DRUGS THER. (USA), 1991, 5/4 (677-680)

Neuroprotective properties of Ginkgo biloba - Constituents. Z. PHYTOTHER. (Germany), 1994, 15/2 (92-96)

Variant angina due to deficiency of intracellular magnesium. CLIN. CARDIOL. (USA), 1990, 13/9 (663-665)

Magnesium and sudden death. S. AFR. MED. J. (SOUTH AFRICA), 1983, 64/18 (697-698)

Magnesium deficiency produces spasms of coronary arteries: Relationship to etiology of sudden death ischemic heart disease. SCIENCE (USA), 1980, 208/4440 (198-200)

Effect of vitamin E on hydrogen peroxide production by human vascular endothelial cells after hypoxia/reoxygenation. Free Radical Biology and Medicine (USA), 1996, 20/1 (99-105)

On the mechanism of the anticlotting action of vitamin E quinone. Proceedings of the National Academy of Sciences of the United States of America (USA), 1995, 92/18 (8171-8175)

Vitamin E may enhance the benefits of aspirin in preventing stroke. American Family Physician (USA), 1995, 51/8 (1977

Antioxidant vitamins and disease - Risks of a suboptimal supply. THER. UMSCH. (Switzerland), 1994, 51/7 (467-474)

Vitamin E consumption and the risk of coronary disease in women. NEW ENGL. J. MED. (USA), 1993, 328/20 (1444-1449)

Increased risk of cardiovascular disease at suboptimal plasma concentrations of essential antioxidants: An epidemiological update with special attention to carotene and vitamin C. AM. J. CLIN. NUTR. (USA), 1993, 57/5 SUPPL. (787S-797S)

Lipid peroxide, phospholipids, glutathione levels and superoxide dismutase activity in rat brain after ischaemia: Effect of ginkgo biloba extract. Pharmacological Research (United Kingdom), 1995, 32/5 (273-278)

Protection of hypoxia-induced ATP decrease in endothelial cells by ginkgo biloba extract and bilobalide. Biochemical Pharmacology (United Kingdom), 1995, 50/7 (991-999)

Lipid peroxidation in experimental spinal cord injury. Comparison of treatment with Ginkgo biloba, TRH and methylprednisolone. Research in Experimental Medicine (Germany), 1995, 195/2 (117-123)

Effects of natural antioxidant Ginkgo biloba extract (EGb 761) on myocardial ischemia-reperfusion injury. FREE RADIC. BIOL. MED. (USA), 1994, 16/6 (789-794)

Experimental model of cerebral ischemia. Preventive activity of Ginkgo biloba extract.Rapin J.R.; Le Poncin-Lafitte M. SEM. HOP. (FRANCE), 1979, 55/43-44 (2047-2050)

On brain protection of co-dergocrine mesylate (Hydergine (R)) against hypoxic hypoxidosis of different severity: Double-blind placebo-controlled quantitative EEG and psychometric studies. INT. J. CLIN. PHARMACOL. THER. TOXICOL. (Germany, Federal Republic of), 1990, 28/12 (510-524)

Pharmacodynamics of the cerebral circulation. Effects of ten drugs on cerebral blood flow and metabolism in cerebrovascular insufficiency. PATH.BIOL. (PARIS) (FRANCE), 1974, 22/9 (815-825)

Effects of ionic and nonionic contrast media on clot structure, platelet function and thrombolysis mediated by tissue plasminogen activator in plasma clots. Haemostasis (Switzerland), 1995, 25/4 (172-181)

Thrombolytic therapy: Recent advances. Treatment of myocardial infarction. APPL. CARDIOPULM. PATHOPHYSIOL. (Netherlands), 1991/92, 4/3 (193-204)

Selective decrease in lysis of old thrombi after rapid administration of tissue-type plasminogen activator. J. AM. COLL. CARDIOL. (USA), 1989, 14/5 (1359-1364)

Antioxidant Curcuma extracts decrease the blood lipid peroxide levels of human subjects. Age (USA), 1995, 18/4 (167-169)

Inhibition of tumor necrosis factor by curcumin, a phytochemical. Biochemical Pharmacology (United Kingdom), 1995, 49/11 (1551-1556)

Inhibitory effect of curcumin, an anti-inflammatory agent, on vascular smooth muscle cell proliferation. EUR. J. PHARMACOL. (Netherlands), 1992, 221/2-3 (381-384)

Change of fatty acid composition, platelet aggregability and RBC function in elderly subjects with administration of low dose fish oil concentrate and comparison with those in younger subjects. JPN. J. GERIATR. (Japan), 1994, 31/8 (596-603)

Premature Carotid Atherosclerosis: Does It Occur in Both Familial Hypercholesterolemia and Homocystinuria? Ultrasound Assessment of Arterial Intima-Media Thickness and Blood Flow Velocity. Stroke, May 1994;25(5):943-950.

Fibrinogen, Arterial Risk Factor in Clinical Practice.Clinical Hemorrheology, 1994;14(6):739-767

Fibrinogen and Cardiovascular Disorders. Quarterly Journal of Medicine, 1995;88:155-165.

Can Lowering Homocysteine Levels Reduce Cardiovascular Risk? The New England Journal of Medicine, February 2, 1995;332(5):328-329.

Fibrinogen, Arterial Risk Factor in Clinical Practice.Potron,G., et al. Clinical Hemorrheology, 1994;14(6):739-767

The Lipoprotein(a). Significance and Relation to Atherosclerosis.Heller, F.R., et al. ACTA Clinica Belgica, 1991;46(6):371-383.

Surgical Precautions

Refer to references under Anesthesia and Surgical Precautions.

Thyroid Deficiency

Protein tyrosine phosphorylation influences adhesive junction assembly and follicular organization of cultured thyroid epithelial cells Endocrinology (USA), 1997, 138/6 (2315-2324)

An extract of soy flour influences serum cholesterol and thyroid hormones in rats and hamsters. Journal of Nutrition (USA), 1996, 126/12 (3046-3053)

Identification of hormonogenic tyrosines in fragment 1218-1591 of bovine thyroglobulin by mass spectrometry. Hormonogenic acceptor Tyr-1291 and donor Tyr-1375. Journal of Biological Chemistry (USA), 1997, 272/1 (639-646)

Selectivity in tyrosyl iodination sites in human thyroglobulin. Archives of Biochemistry and Biophysics (USA), 1996, 334/2 (284-294)

Soy protein concentrate and isolated soy protein similarly lower blood serum cholesterol but differently affect thyroid hormones in hamsters. Journal of Nutrition (USA), 1996, 126/8 (2007-2011)

Involvement of tyrosine phosphorylation in the regulation of 5'- deiodinases in FRTL-5 rat thyroid cells and rat astrocytes. Endocrinology (USA), 1996, 137/4 (1313-1318)

Characterization of a melanosomal transport system in murine melanocytes mediating entry of the melanogenic substrate tyrosine. Journal of Biological Chemistry (USA), 1996, 271/8 (4002-4008)

Influence of the thyroid hormone status on tyrosine hydroxylase in central and peripheral catecholaminergic structures. Neurochemistry International (United Kingdom), 1996, 28/3 (277-281)

Soy protein, thyroid regulation and cholesterol metabolism. Journal of Nutrition (USA), 1995, 125/3 SUPPL. (619S-623S)

Comparative pharmacology of the thyroid hormones. ANN. THORAC. SURG. (USA), 1993, 56/1 SUPPL. (S2-S8)

Primary hypothyroidism in an adult patient with protein-calorie malnutrition: A study of its mechanism and the effect of amino acid deficiency. METAB. CLIN. EXP. (USA), 1988, 37/1 (9-14)

Preferential formation of triiodothyronine residues in newly synthesized (14C)tyrosine-labeled thyroglobulin molecules in follicles reconstructed in a suspension culture of hog thyroid cells. MOL. CELL. ENDOCRINOL. (Ireland), 1988, 59/1-2 (117-124)

Importance of the content and localization of tyrosine residues for thyroxine formation within the N-terminal part of human thyroglobulin den. European Journal of Endocrinology (Norway), 1995, 132/5 (611-617)

Melatonin and the endocrine role of the pineal organ. ARGENTINA CURR.TOPICS EXP.ENDOCRIN. (USA), 1974, Vol. 2 (107-128)

Brief report: Circadian melatonin, thyroid-stimulating hormone, prolactin, and cortisol levels in serum of young adults with autism. Israel Journal of Autism and Developmental Disorders (USA), 1995, 25/6 (641-654)

Effects of melatonin and thyroxine replacement on thyrotropin, luteinizing hormone, and prolactin in male hypothyroid hamsters. ENDOCRINOLOGY (USA), 1985, 117/6 (2402-2407)

Influence of phytogenic substances with thyreostatic effects in combination with iodine on the thyroid hormones and somatomedin level in pigs. EXP. CLIN. ENDOCRINOL. (GERMANY, EAST), 1985, 85/2 (183-190)

Soy protein, thyroid regulation and cholesterol metabolism. Journal of Nutrition (USA), 1995, 125/3 SUPPL. (619S-623S)

Comparative pharmacology of the thyroid hormones. ANN. THORAC. SURG. (USA), 1993, 56/1 SUPPL. (S2-S8)

Primary hypothyroidism in an adult patient with protein-calorie malnutrition: A study of its mechanism and the effect of amino acid deficiency. METAB. CLIN. EXP. (USA), 1988, 37/1 (9-14)

Preferential formation of triiodothyronine residues in newly synthesized (14C)tyrosine-labeled thyroglobulin molecules in follicles reconstructed in a suspension culture of hog thyroid cells. MOL. CELL. ENDOCRINOL. (Ireland), 1988, 59/1-2 (117- 124)

Importance of the content and localization of tyrosine residues for thyroxine formation within the N-terminal part of human thyroglobulin den. European Journal of Endocrinology (Norway), 1995, 132/5 (611-617)

Melatonin and the endocrine role of the pineal organ. ARGENTINA CURR.TOPICS EXP.ENDOCRIN. (USA), 1974, Vol. 2 (107-128)

Brief report: Circadian melatonin, thyroid-stimulating hormone, prolactin, and cortisol levels in serum of young adults with autism. Israel Journal of Autism and Developmental Disorders (USA), 1995, 25/6 (641-654)

Effects of melatonin and thyroxine replacement on thyrotropin, luteinizing hormone, and prolactin in male hypothyroid hamsters. ENDOCRINOLOGY (USA), 1985, 117/6 (2402-2407)

Influence of phytogenic substances with thyreostatic effects in combination with iodine on the thyroid hormones and somatomedin level in pigs. EXP. CLIN. ENDOCRINOL. (GERMANY, EAST), 1985, 85/2 (183-190)

Importance of the content and localization of tyrosine residues for thyroxine formation within the N-terminal part of human thyroglobulin. European Journal of Endocrinology (Norway), 1995, 132/5 (611-617)

Preferential formation of triiodothyronine residues in newly synthesized (14C)tyrosine-labeled thyroglobulin molecules in follicles reconstructed in a suspension culture of hog thyroid cells. MOL. CELL. ENDOCRINOL. (Ireland), 1988, 59/1-2 (117- 124)

Primary hypothyroidism in an adult patient with protein-calorie malnutrition: A study of its mechanism and the effect of amino acid deficiency. METAB. CLIN. EXP. (USA), 1988, 37/1 (9-14)

Comparative pharmacology of the thyroid hormones. ANN. THORAC. SURG. (USA), 1993, 56/1 SUPPL. (S2-S8)

Tinnitus

Attenuation of salicylate-induced tinnitus by Ginkgo biloba extract in rats. Audiology and Neuro-Otology (Germany), 1997, 2/4 (197-212)

[Hydergine in pathology of the inner ear]. An Otorrinolaringol Ibero Am (1990) 17(1):85-98 (Published in Spanish)

Tinnitus rehabilitation in sensorineural hearing loss. Based on 400 patients. Otorinolaringologia (Italy), 1994, 44/5 (227-229)

The value of rheological, vasoactive and metabolically active substances in the initial treatment of acute acoustic trauma. HNO (GERMANY, WEST), 1986, 34/10 (424-428)

Trental and Cavinton in the therapy of cochleovestibular disorders. CESK. OTOLARYNGOL. (CZECHOSLOVAKIA), 1984, 33/4 (264-267)

Prospects of using Cavinton in Meniere's disease. VESTN. OTORINOLARINGOL. (USSR), 1980, 42/3 (18-22)

Results of combined low-power laser therapy and extracts of Ginkgo biloba in cases of sensorineural hearing loss and tinnitus. In: Adv Otorhinolaryngol (1995) 49:101-4

[Hydergine in pathology of the inner ear] Hydergina en patologia del oido interno. An Otorrinolaringol Ibero Am (1990) 17(1):85-98 (Published in Spanish)

Tinnitus rehabilitation in sensorineural hearing loss. Based on 400 patients. Otorinolaringologia (Italy), 1994, 44/5 (227-229)

The value of rheological, vasoactive and metabolically active substances in the initial treatment of acute acoustic trauma. HNO (GERMANY, WEST), 1986, 34/10 (424-428)

Trental and Cavinton in the therapy of cochleovestibular disorders. CESK. OTOLARYNGOL. (CZECHOSLOVAKIA), 1984, 33/4 (264-267)

Prospects of using Cavinton in Meniere's disease. VESTN. OTORINOLARINGOL. (USSR), 1980, 42/3 (18-22)

Results of combined low-power laser therapy and extracts of Ginkgo biloba in cases of sensorineural hearing loss and tinnitus. In: Adv Otorhinolaryngol (1995) 49:101-4

Trauma

Effect of dietary vitamin C on compression injury of the spinal cord in a rat mutant unable to synthe-size ascorbic acid and its correlation with that of vitamin E. Japan Spinal Cord (United Kingdom), 1996, 34/4 (234- 238)

Effect of allopurinol, sulphasalazine, and vitamin C on aspirin induced gastroduodenal injury in human volunteers. United Kingdom Gut (United Kingdom), 1996, 38/4 (518-524

Hemodynamic effects of delayed initiation of antioxidant therapy (beginning two hours after burn) in extensive third-degree burns. Journal of Burn Care and Rehabilitation (USA), 1995, 16/6 (610-615)

Dietary intake and plasma levels of antioxidant vitamins in health and disease: A hospital-based case-control study. Journal of Nutritional and Environmental Medicine (United Kingdom), 1995, 5/3

Vitamin C and pressure sores.Journal of Dermatological Treatment (United Kingdom), 1995, 6/3

Supplementation with vitamins C and E suppresses leukocyte oxygen free radical production in patients with myocardial infarction. European Heart Journal (United Kingdom), 1995, 16/8 (1044-1049)

Antioxidant therapy using high dose vitamin C: Reduction of postburn resuscitation fluid volume requirements. World Journal of Surgery (USA), 1995, 19/2 (287-291)

Vitamin C reduces ischemia-reperfusion injury in a rat epigastric island skin flap model. ANN. PLAST. SURG. (USA), 1994, 33/6 (620-623)

An experimental study on the protection against reperfusion myocardial ischemia by using large doses of vitamin C. CHIN. J. CARDIOL. (China), 1994, 22/1 (52-54+80)

Vitamins as radioprotectors in vivo. I. Protection by vitamin C against internal radionuclides in mouse testes: Implications to the mechanism of damage caused by the auger effect. USA RADIAT. RES. (USA), 1994, 137/3 (394-399)

Experimental studies on the treatment of frostbite in rats. INDIAN J. MED. RES. SECT. B BIOMED. RES. OTHER THAN INFECT. DIS. (India), 1993, 98/AUG. (178-184)

The effects of high-dose vitamin C therapy on postburn lipid peroxidation. USA J. BURN CARE REHA-BIL. (USA), 1993, 14/6 (624- 629)

Effect of antioxidant vitamin supplementation on muscle function after eccentric exercise. EUR. J. APPL. PHYSIOL. OCCUP. PHYSIOL. (Germany), 1993, 67/5 (426-430)

Vitamin C as a radioprotector against iodine-131 in vivo. J. NUCL. MED. (USA), 1993, 34/4 (637-640)

Effects of high-dose vitamin C administration on postburn microvascular fluid and protein flux. REHA-BIL. (USA), 1992, 13/5 (560-566)

Modification of the daily photoreceptor membrane shedding response in vitro by antioxidants. INVEST. OPHTHALMOL. VISUAL SCI. (USA), 1992, 33/10 (3005-3008)

Ascorbate treatment prevents accumulation of phagosomes in RPE in light damage. INVEST. OPH-THALMOL. VISUAL SCI. (USA), 1992, 33/10 (2814-2821)

Topical vitamin C protects porcine skin from ultraviolet radiation-induced damage. BR. J. DERMA-TOL. (United Kingdom), 1992, 127/3 (247- 253)

The synergism of gamma-interferon and tumor necrosis factor in whole body hyperthermia with vita-min C to control toxicity. MED. HYPOTHESES (United Kingdom), 1992, 38/3 (257- 258)

Tirilazad mesylate protects vitamins C and E in brain ischemia- reperfusion injury. J. NEUROCHEM. (USA), 1992, 58/6 (2263-2268)

Vitamin C supplementation in the patient with burns and renal failure. J. BURN CARE REHABIL. (USA), 1992, 13/3 (378-380)

High-dose vitamin C therapy for extensive deep dermal burns. USA BURNS (United Kingdom), 1992, 18/2 (127-131)

Metabolic and immune effects of enteral ascorbic acid after burn trauma. BURNS (United Kingdom), 1992, 18/2 (92-97)

Reduced fluid volume requirement for resuscitation of third-degree burns with high-dose vitamin C. J. BURN CARE REHABIL. (USA), 1991, 12/6 (525-532)

Biochemical basis of ozone toxicity. FREE RADIC. BIOL. MED. (USA), 1990, 9/3 (245-265)

Decreases in tissue levels of ubiquinol-9 and -10, ascorbate and alpha-tocopherol following spinal cord impact trauma in rats. USA NEUROSCI. LETT. (Netherlands), 1990, 108/1-2 (201-206)

Nutritional considerations for the burned patient. SURG. CLIN. NORTH AM. (USA), 1987, 67/1 (109-131)

Nutritional considerations for the burned patient. SURG. CLIN. NORTH AM. (USA), 1987, 67/2 (109-131)

Ascorbic acid metabolism in trauma. INDIAN J. MED. RES. (INDIA), 1982, 75/5 (748-751)

Multiple pathologic fractures in osteogenesis imperfecta. ORTHOPADE (GERMANY, WEST), 1982, 11/3 (101-108)

Effect of zinc supplementation in fracture healing. INDIAN J. ORTHOP. (INDIA), 1980, 14/1 (62-71)

Treatment results of spinal cord injuries in the Swiss paraplegic centre of Basle. PARAPLEGIA (EDINB.) (SCOTLAND), 1976, 14/1 (58-65)

Effect of piracetam on electroshock induced amnesia and decrease in brain acetylcholine in rats. INDIAN J. EXP. BIOL. (India), 1993, 31/10 (822-824)

Use of piracetam in treatment of head injuries. Observations in 903 cases. CLIN. TER. (ITALY), 1985, 114/6 (481-487)

Urinary Tract Infections

Effect of cranberry juice on urinary pH in older adults. Home Healthc Nurse (UNITED STATES) Mar 1997, 15 (3) p198-202

Cranberry juice and its impact on peri-stomal skin conditions for urostomy patients. Ostomy Wound Manage (UNITED STATES) Nov-Dec 1994, 40 (9) p60-2, 64, 66-8

Infection control. The therapeutic uses of cranberry juice. Nurs Stand (ENGLAND) May 17-23 1995, 9 (34) p33-5

Urinary problems after formation of a Mitrofanoff stoma. Prof Nurse (ENGLAND) Jan 1995, 10 (4) p221-4

New support for a folk remedy: cranberry juice reduces bacteriuria and pyuria in elderly women. Nutr Rev (UNITED STATES) May 1994, 52 (5) p168-70

An examination of the anti-adherence activity of cranberry juice on urinary and nonurinary bacterial isolates. Microbios (ENGLAND) 1988, 55 (224-225) p173-81

Inhibitory activity of cranberry juice on adherence of type 1 and type P fimbriated Escherichia coli to eucaryotic cells. Antimicrob Agents Chemother (UNITED STATES) Jan 1989, 33 (1) p92-8

Inhibition of bacterial adherence by cranberry juice: potential use for the treatment of urinary tract infections. J Urol (UNITED STATES) May 1984, 131 (5) p1013-6

Knight-Ridder Info. Effect of cranberry juice on urinary pH. Nurs Res (UNITED STATES) Sep-Oct 1979, 28 (5) p287-90

First-time urinary tract infection and sexual behavior. Epidemiology (UNITED STATES) Mar 1995, 6 (2) p162-8

Anti-Escherichia coli adhesin activity of cranberry and blueberry juices [letter] N Engl J Med (1991 May 30) 324(22):1599

Effect of cranberry juice on urinary pH. Nurs Res (1979 Sep-Oct) 28(5):287-90

Inhibition of bacterial adherence by cranberry juice: potential use for the treatment of urinary tract infections. J Urol (1984 May) 131(5):1013-6

Anti-Escherichia coli adhesin activity of cranberry and blueberry juices [letter]. N Engl J Med (1991 May 30) 324(22):1599

Effect of cranberry juice on urinary pH. Nurs Res (1979 Sep-Oct) 28(5):287-90

Inhibitory activity of cranberry juice on adherence of type 1 and type P fimbriated Escherichia coli to eucaryotic cells. Antimicrob Agents Chemother (1989 Jan) 33(1):92-8

An examination of the anti-adherence activity of cranberry juice on urinary and nonurinary bacterial isolates. Microbios (1988) 55(224-225):173-81

Valvular Insufficiency/Heart Valve Defects

[Doppler echocardiography of heart valve defects in the dog]. Tierarztl Prax (GERMANY) Apr 1996, 24 (2) p177-89

Also, refer to references under Congestive Heart Failure/Cardiomyopathy

Vertigo

Piracetam in patients with chronic vertigo. Results of a double-blind,placebo-controlled study. Clinical Drug Investigation (New Zealand), 1996, 11/5 (251-260)

Nootropics: Efficacy and tolerability of products from three active substance classes. Journal of Drug Development and Clinical Practice (United Kingdom), 1996, 8/2 (77-94)

The effect of ginkgo biloba glycoside on the blood viscosity and erythrocyte deformability. Clinical Hemorheology (USA), 1996, 16/3 (271-276)

[Clinical trial of the use of the combination of piracetam and dihydroergocristine in vertigo from different causes]. An Otorrinolaringol Ibero Am (SPAIN) 1989, 16 (3)

Treatment of vertigo syndrome with Nootropil]. Otolaryngol Pol (POLAND) 1988, 42 (5) p312-7

The use of piracetam in vertigo. S Afr Med J (SOUTH AFRICA) Nov 23 1985, 68 (11) p806-8

The efficacy of piracetam in vertigo. A double-blind study in patients with vertigo of central origin. Arzneimittelforschung (GERMANY, WEST) 1980, 30 (11)

Piracetam in the treatment of post-concussional syndrome. A double-blind study. Eur Neurol (SWITZERLAND) 1978, 17 (1) p50-5

[Evaluation of the therapeutic effectiveness of a piracetam plus dihydroergocristine combination in the treatment of vertigo]. Acta Otorrinolaringol Esp (SPAIN) Jul-Aug 1988, 39 (4)

[Hydergine in pathology of the inner ear]. An Otorrinolaringol Ibero Am (1990) 17(1):85-98

[The elimination of chemotherapy side effects in pulmonary tuberculosis patients]. Vrach Delo (USSR) Apr 1990, (4) p71-3

The treatment of minocycline-induced brainstem vertigo by the combined administration of piracetam and ergotoxin. Acta Otolaryngol Suppl (Stockh) (SWEDEN) 1989, 468

[Clinical trial of the use of the combination of piracetam and dihydroergocristine in vertigo from different causes] An Otorrinolaringol Ibero Am (SPAIN) 1989, 16 (3)

Treatment of vertigo syndrome with Nootropil] Otolaryngol Pol (POLAND) 1988, 42 (5) p312-7

The use of piracetam in vertigo. S Afr Med J (SOUTH AFRICA) Nov 23 1985, 68 (11) p806-8

The efficacy of piracetam in vertigo. A double-blind study in patients with vertigo of central origin. Arzneimittelforschung (GERMANY, WEST) 1980, 30 (11)

Piracetam in the treatment of post-concussional syndrome. A double-blind study. Eur Neurol (SWITZERLAND) 1978, 17 (1) p50-5

[Evaluation of the therapeutic effectiveness of a piracetam plus dihydroergocristine combination in the treatment of vertigo] Acta Otorrinolaringol Esp (SPAIN) Jul-Aug 1988, 39 (4)

[Hydergine in pathology of the inner ear] An Otorrinolaringol Ibero Am (1990) 17(1):85-98

[The elimination of chemotherapy side effects in pulmonary tuberculosis patients] Vrach Delo (USSR) Apr 1990, (4) p71-3

The treatment of minocycline-induced brainstem vertigo by the combined administration of piracetam and ergotoxin. Acta Otolaryngol Suppl (Stockh) (SWEDEN) 1989, 468

Weight Loss

Magnesium and carbohydrate metabolism. THERAPIE (France), 1994, 49/1 (1-7)

Disorders of magnesium metabolism. Endocrinology and Metabolism Clinics of North America (USA), 1995, 24/3

Magnesium deficiency produces insulin resistance and increased thromboxane synthesis. HYPERTENSION (USA), 1993, 21/6 II (1024-1029)

Magnesium and glucose homeostasis. DIABETOLOGIA (Germany, Federal Republic of), 1990, 33/9 (511-514)

Effect of thyroxine supplementation on the response to perfluoro-n-decanoic acid (PFDA) in rats. J. TOXICOL. ENVIRON. HEALTH (USA), 1988, 24/4 (491- 498)

References

The role of thyroid hormones and insulin in the regulation of energy metabolism. AM. J. CLIN. NUTR. (USA), 1983, 38/6 (1006-1017)

The effect of triiodothyronine on weight loss and nitrogen balance of obese patients on a very low calorie liquid formula diet. INT. J. OBESITY (ENGLAND), 1981, 5/3 (279-282)

The effect of a low-calorie diet alone and in combination with triiodothyronine therapy on weight loss and hypophyseal thyroid function in obesity. INT. J. OBESITY (ENGLAND), 1983, 7/2 (123-131)

The effect of triiodothyronine on weight loss, nitrogen balance and muscle protein catabolism in obese patients on a very low calorie diet. NUTR. REP. INT. (USA), 1981, 24/1 (145-151)

Effect of triiodothyronine on some metabolic responses of obese patients. AMER.J.CLIN.NUTR. (USA), 1973, 26/7 (715-721)

The variability of weight reduction during fasting: Predictive value of thyroid hormone measurements. INT. J. OBESITY (ENGLAND), 1982, 6/1 (101-111)

The effects of triiodothyronine on energy expenditure, nitrogen balance and rates of weight and fat loss in obese patients during prolonged caloric restriction. INT. J. OBESITY (EN), 1985, 9/6 (433-442)

Desiccated thyroid in a nutritional supplement. J. FAM. PRACT. (USA), 1994, 38/3 (287-288)

Factors determining energy expenditure during very-low-calorie diets. AM. J. CLIN. NUTR. (USA), 1992, 56/1 SUPPL. (224S-229S)

Resting metabolic rate, body composition and thyroid hormones. Short term effects of very low calorie diet. HORM. METAB. RES. (Germany, Federal Republic of), 1990, 22/12 (632- 635)

Decrease in resting metabolic rate during rapid weight loss is reversed by low dose thyroid hormone treatment. METAB. CLIN. EXP. (USA), 1986, 35/4 (289-291)

Relationship between the changes in serum thyroid hormone levels and protein status during prolonged protein supplemented caloric deprivation. CLIN. ENDOCRINOL. (OXFORD) (ENGLAND), 1985, 22/1 (1-15)

Thyroid hormone changes in obese subjects during fasting and a very-low-calorie diet. INT. J. OBESITY (ENGLAND), 1981, 5/3 (305-311)

The role of Tsub 3 and its receptor in efficient metabolisers receiving very-low-calorie diets. INT. J. OBESITY (ENGLAND), 1981, 5/3 (283-286)

Effects of total fasting in obese women. III. Response of serum thyroid hormones to thyroxine and triiodothyronine administration. ENDOKRINOLOGIE (GERMANY, EAST), 1979, 73/2 (221-226)

Thyroidal hormone metabolism in obesity during semi-starvation. CLIN. ENDOCRINOL. (OXFORD) (ENGLAND), 1978, 9/3 (227-231)

Clinical characteristics of hyperthyroidism. A study of 100 patients. REV.CUBA.MED. (CUBA), 1973, 12/1 (39-52)

The effect of triiodothyronine (Tsub 3) on protein turnover and metabolic rate. INT. J. OBESITY (ENGLAND), 1985, 9/6 (459-463)

Soy protein, thyroid regulation and cholesterol metabolism. Journal of Nutrition (USA), 1995, 125/3 SUPPL.

Overview of proposed mechanisms for the hypocholesterolemic effect of soy. Journal of Nutrition (USA), 1995, 125/3 SUPPL.

Endocrinological response to soy protein and fiber in mildly hypercholesterolemic men. NUTR. RES. (USA), 1993, 13/8 (873-884)

Response of hormones modulating plasma cholesterol to dietary casein or soy protein in minipigs. J. NUTR. (USA), 1990, 120/11 (1387-1392)

Dietary protein effects on cholesterol and lipoprotein concentrations: A review. J. AM. COLL. NUTR. (USA), 1986, 5/6 (533-549)

Comparison of dietary casein or soy protein effects on plasma lipids and hormone concentrations in the gerbil (Meriones unguiculatus). J. NUTR. (USA), 1986, 116/7 (1165-1171)

Hypolipidemic effect of casein vs. soy protein in the hyperlipidemic hypothyroid chick model. NUTR. REP. INT. (USA), 1980, 21/4 (497-503)

Characterization of the insulin resistance of glucose utilization in adipocytes from patients with hyper- and hypothyroidism. Acta Endocrinol (Copenh) (DENMARK) Oct 1988

Thyroid hormone action on intermediary metabolism. Part I: respiration, thermogenesis and carbohydrate metabolism. Klin Wochenschr (GERMANY, WEST) Jan 2 1984

Relative roles of the thyroid hormones and noradrenaline on the thermogenic activity of brown adipose tissue in the rat. J Endocrinol (ENGLAND) Jun 1995, 145

Age-related differences in body weight loss in response to altered thyroidal status. Exp Gerontol (ENGLAND) 1990, 25 (1)

Long-term weight regulation in treated hyperthyroid and hypothyroid subjects. Am J Med (UNITED STATES) Jun 1984, 76 (6)

Chromium improves insulin response to glucose in rats. Metabolism (UNITED STATES) Oct 1995, 44 (10)

Enhancing central and peripheral insulin activity as a strategy for the treatment of endogenous depression—an adjuvant role for chromium picolinate? Med Hypotheses (ENGLAND) Oct 1994, 43 (4)

Homologous physiological effects of phenformin and chromium picolinate. Med Hypotheses (ENGLAND) Oct 1993, 41 (4)

Chromium in human nutrition: a review. J Nutr (UNITED STATES) Apr 1993, 123 (4)

Use of the artificial beta cell (ABC) in the assessment of peripheral insulin sensitivity: effect of chromium supplementation in diabetic patients. Gen Pharmacol (ENGLAND) 1984, 15 (6)

Wound Healing
(Surgical Wounds, Trauma, Burns)

Nutritional intake and status of clients in the home with open surgical wounds. J Community Health Nurs (UNITED STATES) 1990, 7 (2)

High-dose vitamin C therapy for extensive deep dermal burns. Burns (ENGLAND) Apr 1992, 18 (2)

Yeast Infections

Refer to references under Candida Infection.

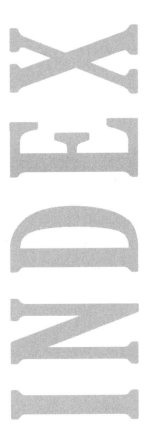

Notes

Notes

Notes